PATHOLOGY
Quick Review and MCQs
SECOND EDITION

Based on
Textbook of Pathology
5th Edition

Harsh Mohan MD, MNAMS, FICPath, FUICC
Professor & Head
Department of Pathology
Government Medical College
Sector-32 A, Chandigarh-160030
INDIA
&
Editor-in-Chief
The Indian Journal of Pathology & Microbiology
E-mail: drharshmohan@ya

JAYPEE BROTHERS
MEDICAL PUBLISHERS (P) LTD
New Delhi

Tunbridge Wells
UK

First published in the UK by

Anshan Ltd
in 2005
6 Newlands Road
Tunbridge Wells
Kent TN4 9AT, UK

Tel/Fax: +44 (0)1892 557767
E-mail: info@anshan.co.uk
www.anshan.co.uk

ISBN 1 904798 209

British Library Cataloguing in Publication Data
A catalogue record for this book is available from the British Library

Printed in India by Gopsons Papers Ltd., A-14, Sector 60, Noida

> He whose deeds are virtuous,
> is rewarded with purity and knowledge.
> The actions done with passion cause misery,
> while he whose deeds are dark is cursed with ignorance.
>
> (The Bhagavadgita, Chapter XIV: Verse 16)

To my daughters:
Sugandha and Tanya
for their understanding and patience.

To all my students
who help me keep the joy of learning fresh and exciting.

Preface

It is with feelings of fulfillment as I write the preface of the Second Edition of *Pathology Quick Review with MCQs* simultaneous to the release of the *Fifth Edition* of its parent book, *Textbook of Pathology*. In fact, the satisfied users of its maiden edition for over last four years, by their patronage, have encouraged me and the publishers to make it a convention of keeping this baby-book in the lap of its mother-book in the same package.

The small book is the abridged version of fifth revised edition of my textbook and has been aimed to serve the following twin purposes:

■ For young students of Pathology, after they have undertaken an in-depth study earlier, as an aid to revise the subject quickly when they are short of time.

■ For senior students and interns preparing for their postgraduate and other entrance examinations who are confronted with revision of all medical subjects besides pathology in a limited time, this book is expected to act the main source material for quick revision of essential pathology for them.

Pathology Quick Review book has the same 29 chapters (1-10 General Pathology, 11-29 Systemic Pathology) and an Appendix containing important Normal Values as in the main textbook and has cross-references of page numbers of the 5th edition of my textbook so that an avid and inquisitive reader interested in simultaneous in-depth study of the topic or for clarification of a doubt, may refer to it conveniently. In the revised edition, many new tables listing important conditions, classifications and contrasting features of closely simulating conditions which have been added in the main book have been included in the baby book as well. Self Assessment by MCQs given at the end of every chapter, which keeps this book apart from other similar books, has also many newer questions, increasing their number from 500 to about 600 in the revised edition. All this along with increased knowledge condensed from the added material in the main textbook has lamentably resulted in slight increase in the volume of this book. However, only a few select graphic representations have been retained to restrict the girth of this book. It is hoped that the book with enhanced and updated contents continues to be user-friendly in learning the essential aspects of pathology, while at the same time, maintaining the ease with which it can be conveniently carried by the users in the pocket of their white aprons.

Preparation of this little book necessitated selection from vast body of information contained in the revised edition of my textbook and therefore, required application of my discretion, combined with suggestions from colleagues and users of earlier edition. In particular, valuable and selfless assistance rendered by my diligent colleague, Dr. Amanjit, MD, DNB, Senior Lecturer in the department, is gratefully acknowledged.

I must thank profusely the entire staff of M/s Jaypee Brothers Medical Publishers (P) Ltd. for their ever smiling support and cooperation and adjusting to my inconsistencies and vagaries. It is owing to their tireless and continuous hard work which has made it possible for me to come out with the revised edition of this book in such a short time when we had barely finished with the Herculean task of the fifth revised edition of the textbook.

Finally, although sincere effort has been made to be as accurate as possible, element of human error is still likely; I shall humbly welcome all suggestions directed at further improvements of its contents.

Government Medical College   **Harsh Mohan**
Sector-32 A   MD, MNAMS, FICPath, FUICC
Chandigarh-160030   Professor & Head
INDIA   Department of Pathology

E-mail: drharshmohan@yahoo.com

Contents

Abbreviations Used

Throughout the book following abbreviations have been used:

G/A for Gross Appearance.

M/E for Microscopic Examination.

EM for Electron Microscopy.

IF for Immunofluorescence Microscopy.

1

Introduction to Pathology

INTRODUCTION (p. 3)

The word 'Pathology' is derived from two Greek words—*pathos* meaning suffering, and *logos* meaning study. Pathology is, thus, scientific study of structure and function of the body in disease; it deals with causes, effects, mechanisms and nature of disease.

Since pathology is the study of disease, then what is *disease*? In simple language, disease is opposite of health i.e. what is not healthy is disease. *Health* is a condition when the individual is in complete accord with the surroundings, while *disease* is loss of ease to the body (dis-ease).

■ *Lesions* are the characteristic changes in tissues and cells produced by disease in an individual or experimental animal.

■ *Pathologic changes* or *morphology* consist of examination of diseased tissues by gross appearance (G/A) and microscopic examination (M/E).

■ The causal factors responsible for the lesions are included in *etiology* of disease ('why' of disease).

■ The mechanism by which the lesions are produced is termed *pathogenesis* of disease ('how' of disease).

■ The functional implications of the lesion felt by the patient are *symptoms* and those discovered by the clinician are the *physical signs*.

EVOLUTION OF PATHOLOGY (p. 4)

FROM RELIGIOUS BELIEFS TO RATIONAL APPROACH (ANTIQUITY TO AD 1500) (p. 4)

The earliest concepts of disease were the religious beliefs that affliction or disease was the outcome of 'curse' or 'evil eye of spirits.'

The real practice of medicine began with *Hippocrates* (460–377 BC), the great Greek clinical genius of all times and regarded as 'the father of medicine'. He first stressed study of patient's symptoms and described methods of diagnosis.

Hippocrates introduced ethical concepts in the practice of medicine and is revered by the medical profession by taking *'Hippocratic Oath'* at the time of entry into practice of medicine.

Cornelius Celsus (53 BC-7 AD) first described four cardinal signs of inflammation—rubor (redness), tumour (swelling), calor (heat), and dolor (pain).

The hypothesis of disequilibrium of elements constituting the body *(Dhatus)* similar to Hippocratic doctrine finds mention in ancient Indian medicine books—*Charaka Samhita*, and *Sushruta Samhita*, compiled about AD 200.

Cladius Galen (130–200 AD) in Rome postulated humoral theory, later called Galenic theory, suggesting that the illness resulted from imbalance between *four humours* (or body fluids): blood, lymph, black bile (believed to be from the spleen), and biliary secretion from the liver.

ERA OF GROSS PATHOLOGY (AD 1500 TO 1800) (p. 5)

Dissection of human body was started by *vesalius* (1514-1564). *von Leeuwenhoek* (1632–1723), draper by profession, during his spare time invented the first ever microscope by grinding the lenses himself.

The credit for beginning of the study of morbid anatomy (pathologic anatomy), however, goes to Italian anatomist-pathologist, *Giovanni B. Morgagni*

1

(1682–1771). With Morgagni, pathology made its beginning on the autopsy table and the concept of clinicopathologic correlation (CPC) had been introduced, establishing a coherent sequence of cause, lesions, symptoms, and outcome of disease.

Sir Percival Pott (1714–1788), famous surgeon in England, identified the first ever occupational cancer in the chimney sweeps in 1775 and discovered chimney soot as the first carcinogenic agent.

John Hunter (1728–1793) together with his elder brother *William Hunter* (1718–1788) developed the first museum of comparative anatomy and pathology in the world which later became the Hunterian Museum in England.

R.T.H. Laennec (1781–1826), described several lung diseases (tubercles, caseous lesions, miliary lesions, pleural effusion, bronchiectasis), chronic sclerotic liver disease (later called Laennec's cirrhosis) and invented stethoscope.

Carl F. von Rokitansky (1804–1878), performed nearly 30,000 autopsies and described acute yellow atrophy of the liver, wrote an outstanding monograph on diseases of arteries and congenital heart defects.

Richard Bright (1789–1858) described non-suppurative nephritis, later termed glomerulonephritis or Bright's disease.

Thomas Addison (1793–1860) gave an account of chronic adrenocortical insufficiency termed Addison's disease.

Thomas Hodgkin (1798–1866), observed the complex of chronic enlargement of lymph nodes, often with enlargement of the liver and spleen, later called Hodgkin's disease.

ERA OF TECHNOLOGY DEVELOPMENT AND CELLULAR PATHOLOGY (AD 1800 TO 1950s) *(p. 7)*

The discovery of existence of disease-causing micro-organisms was made by French chemist *Louis Pasteur* (1822–1895). Subsequently, *G.H.A. Hansen* (1841–1912) identified Hansen's bacillus as causative agent for leprosy (Hansen's disease) in 1873.

Christian Gram (1853–1938), Danish physician, developed bacteriologic staining by crystal violet.

D.L. Romanowsky (1861–1921), Russian physician, developed stain for peripheral blood film using eosin and methylene blue derivatives.

Robert Koch (1843–1910), discovered tubercle bacilli in 1882 and cholera vibrio organism in 1883.

May-Grunwald in 1902 and *Giemsa* in 1914 developed blood stains.

Sir William Leishman (1865–1926) described Leishman's stain for blood films in 1914 and observed Leishman-Donovan bodies (LD bodies) in leishmaniasis.

Robert Feulgen (1884–1955) described Feulgen reaction for DNA staining.

Rudolf Virchow (1821–1905) in Germany is credited with the beginning of histopathology as a method of investigation by examination of diseased tissues at cellular level. Virchow is aptly known as the 'father of cellular pathology'.

Until the end of the 19th century, the study of morbid anatomy had remained largely autopsy-based and thus had remained a retrospective science. Soon, knowledge and skill gained by giving accurate diagnosis on postmortem findings was applied to surgical biopsy and thus emerged the discipline of surgical pathology.

The concept of frozen section examination was introduced by Virchow's student, *Julius Cohnheim* (1839–1884).

Karl Landsteiner (1863–1943) described the existence of human blood groups in 1901 and was awarded Nobel Prize in 1930.

Ruska and *Lorries* in 1933 developed electron microscope which aided the pathologist to view ultrastructure of cell and its organelles.

The development of exfoliative cytology for early detection of cervical cancer began with *George N. Papanicolaou* in 1930s and is known as 'father of exfoliative cytology'.

MODERN PATHOLOGY (1950s TO DAWN OF 21ST CENTURY) *(p. 8)*

In recent times, there have been major advances in molecular biology in the field of diagnosis and treatment of genetic disorders, immunology and in cancer.

The structure of DNA of the cell was described by *Watson* and *Crick* in 1953.

Identification of chromosomes and their correct number in humans (46) was done by *Tijo* and *Levan* in 1956.

Identification of Philadelphia chromosome t(9;22) in chronic myeloid leukaemia by *Nowell* and *Hagerford* in 1960 was the first chromosomal abnormality in any cancer.

In situ Hybridization was introduced in 1969 in which a labeled probe is employed to detect and localize specific RNA or DNA sequences.

Recombinant DNA technique was developed in 1972 using restriction enzymes to cut and paste bits of DNA.

In 1983, Kary Mullis introduced *polymerase chain reaction* (PCR).

The flexibility and dynamism of DNA was invented by *Barbara McClintock*.

In 1997, *Ian Wilmut*, successfully used a technique of somatic cell nuclear transfer to create the clone of a sheep; the cloned sheep was named Dolly. This has set in the era of *mammalian cloning*.

In June 2000, discovery of chemicals of the approximately 80,000 genes that make up the human body, their structure and position on chromosomes (i.e. *mapping of the human genome*) has been successfully carried out.

Recent report in April 2004 suggests that Prof Wilmut's group, which first cloned the sheep Dolly, has applied to the regulatory authorities for *therapeutic cloning of human embryos* and is being introduced soon for use in treating human diseases. Due to availability of *human stem cell research* in which embryonic stem cells obtained from *in vitro* fertilisation will be used for cell therapy, it seems that time is not far when organs for transplant may be 'harvested' from the embryo.

Modern day human molecular biology is closely linked to information technology; the best recent example is the availability of molecular profiling by *cDNA microarrays* in which by a small silicon chip, expression of thousands of genes can be simultaneously measured.

Chapter One

SUBDIVISIONS OF PATHOLOGY *(p. 9)*

Human pathology is the largest branch of pathology. It is conventionally divided into *General Pathology* dealing with general principles of disease, and *Systemic Pathology* that includes study of diseases pertaining to the specific organs and body systems.

Histopathology, used synonymously with anatomic pathology, pathologic anatomy, or morbid anatomy, is the classic method of study and still the most useful one which has stood the test of time. It includes 3 main subdivisions:

1. *Surgical pathology* deals with the study of tissues removed from the living body.

2. *Forensic pathology and autopsy work* includes the study of organs and tissues removed at postmortem.

3. *Cytopathology*, includes study of cells shed off from the lesions (exfoliative cytology) and fine-needle aspiration cytology (FNAC) of superficial and deep-seated lesions for diagnosis.

Haematology deals with the diseases of blood.

The detection and diagnosis of abnormalities at the level of DNA of the cell is included in *molecular pathology*.

■ SELF ASSESSMENT

1. **The concept of clinicopathologic correlation (CPC) by study of morbid anatomy was introduced by:**
   A. Hippocrates
   B. Virchow
   C. John Hunter
   D. Morgagni

2. **The first ever museum of pathologic anatomy was developed by:**
   A. John Hunter
   B. Rokitansky
   C. Rudolf Virchow
   D. Morgagni

3. **ABO human blood group system was first described by:**
   A. Edward Jenner
   B. Karl Landsteiner
   C. Hippocrates
   D. Laennec

4. **Frozen section was first introduced by:**
   A. Cohnheim
   B. Ackerman
   C. Virchow
   D. Feulgen

5. **Electron microscope was first developed by:**
   A. Barbara McClintock
   B. Watson and Crick
   C. Tijo and Levan
   D. Ruska and Lorries

6. **Structure of DNA of the cell was described by:**
   A. Watson and Crick
   B. Tijo and Levan
   C. Ruska and Lorries
   D. Barbara McClintock

7. **Flexibilty and dynamism of DNA was invented by:**
   A. Watson and Crick
   B. Tijo and Levan
   C. Ruska and Lorries
   D. Barbara McClintock

8. **Father of cellular pathology is:**
   A. Carl Rokitansky
   B. Rudolf Virchow
   C. G. Morgagni
   D. FT Schwann

9. **Humans genome consists of following number of genes:**
   A. 60,000
   B. 80,000
   C. 100,000
   D. Innumerable

10. **Stem cell research consists of:**
    A. Human cells grown *in vitro*
    B. Plant cells grown *in vitro*
    C. Cadaver cells grown *in vitro*
    D. Synonymous with PCR

KEY

1 = D	2 = A	3 = B	4 = A
5 = D	6 = A	7 = D	8 = B
9 = B	10 = A		

2

Techniques for the Study of Pathology

AUTOPSY PATHOLOGY *(p. 13)*

Professor William Boyd in his unimitable style wrote 'Pathology had its beginning on the autopsy table'. The significance of study of autopsy in pathology is summed up in Latin inscription in an autopsy room reproduced in English as "The place where death delights to serve the living'.

There are two methods for carrying out autopsy:
1. Block extraction of abdominal and thoracic organs.
2. *In situ* organ-by-organ dissection.

In conditions where multiple organs are expected to be involved, complete autopsy should be performed. But if a particular organ-specific disease is suspected, a mini-autopsy or limited autopsy may be sufficient.

The study of autopsy throws new light on the knowledge and skills of both physician as well as pathologist. The main **purposes** of autopsy are as under:

1. *Quality assurance of patientcare.*
2. *Education of the entire team* involved in patientcare.

Declining autopsy rate throughout world in the recent times is owing to:

1. Higher diagnostic confidence made possible by advances in imaging techniques e.g. CT, MRI etc.
2. Physician's fear of legal liability on being wrong.

SURGICAL PATHOLOGY *(p. 14)*

Surgical pathology is the classic and time-tested method of tissue diagnosis made on gross and microscopic study of tissues. With technology development and advances made in the dye industry in the initial years of this century, the speciality of diagnostic surgical pathology by biopsy developed. Surgical pathology services in any large hospital depend largely on inputs from surgeons and physicians familiar with the scope and limitations inherent in the speciality.

SURGICAL PATHOLOGY PROTOCOL *(p. 14)*

1. REQUEST FORM. It must contain the entire relevant information about the case and the disease (history, physical and operative findings, results of other relevant biochemical/haematological/radiological investigations, and clinical and differential diagnosis).

2. TISSUE ACCESSION. Tissue received in the surgical pathology laboratory must have proper identification of the specimen matching with that on the accompanied request form. For routine tissue processing by paraffin-embedding technique, the tissue must be either in appropriate fixative solution (most commonly 10% formol-saline or 10% buffered formalin) or received fresh-unfixed. For frozen section, the tissue is always transported fresh-unfixed. Microwave fixation may also be used in the laboratory for rapid fixation of routine surgical specimens.

3. GROSS ROOM. Proper gross dissection, description and selection of tissue sample is a crucial part of the pathologic examination of tissue submitted.

Calcified tissues and bone are subjected to decalcification to remove the mineral and soften the tissue by treatment with decalcifying agents such as acids and chelating agents (most often aqueous nitric acid).

It is mandatory that all the gross-room personnel follow strict precautions in handling the tissues infected with tuberculosis, hepatitis, HIV and other viruses.

4. HISTOPATHOLOGY LABORATORY. Majority of histopathology departments use automated tissue processors having 12 separate stages completing the cycle in about 18 hours by overnight schedule:

■ 10% formalin for fixation;

■ ascending grades of alcohol (70%, 95% through 100%) for dehydration for about 5 hours in 6-7 jars,

■ xylene/toluene/chloroform for clearing for 3 hours in two jars; and

■ paraffin impregnation for 6 hours in two thermostat-fitted waxbaths.

Embedding of tissue is done in molten wax, blocks of which are prepared using L (Leuckhart's) mould. The blocks are then trimmed followed by sectioning by microtomy, most often by rotary microtome, employing fixed knife or disposable blades.

Cryostat or frozen section eliminates all the steps of tissue processing and paraffin-embedding. Instead the tissue is frozen to ice at about –25°C which acts as embedding medium and then sectioned. It is a quick diagnostic procedure for tissues before proceeding to a major radical surgery. This is also used for demonstration of some special substances in the cells and tissues e.g. fat, enzymes.

Paraffin-embedded sections are routinely stained with haematoxylin and eosin (H & E). Frozen section is stained with rapid H & E or toluidine blue routinely. Special stains are employed for either of the two methods according to need. The sections are mounted and submitted for microscopic study.

5. SURGICAL PATHOLOGY REPORT. The ideal report must contain:

i) Precise gross description, ii) brief microscopic findings, and iii) morphologic diagnosis which must include the organ for indexing purposes using SNOMED (*Scientific Nomenclature in Medicine*) codes.

6. QUALITY CONTROL. An internal quality control by mutual discussion in controversial cases and self-check on the quality of sections are important for accuracy and efficacy of the procedure.

7. HISTOPATHOLOGIST AND THE LAW. Problem of allegations of negligence and malpractice in laboratory medicine too have come to the forefront now just as with other clinical disciplines.

SPECIAL STAINS (p. 16)

In certain 'special' circumstances when the pathologist wants to demonstrate certain specific substances/constituents of the cells/tissues to confirm etiologic, histogenic or pathogenetic components, special stains are employed.

ENZYME HISTOCHEMISTRY (p. 16)

Enzyme histochemical techniques for tissue section require special preparations of fresh tissues and can not be applied to paraffin-embedded sections or formalin-fixed tissues since enzymes are damaged rapidly.

BASIC MICROSCOPY (p. 16)

The usual type of microscope used in clinical laboratories is called *light microscope*, which may have some variations.

Simple microscope. This is a simple hand magnifying lens. The magnification power of hand lens is from 2x to 200x.

Compound microscope. This has a battery of lenses which are fitted in a complex instrument. One type of lens remains near the object (objective lens) and another type of lens near the observer's eye (eye piece lens). The eye piece and objective lenses have different magnification.

Dark ground illumination (DGI). This method is used for examination of unstained living micro-organisms e.g. *Treponema pallidum.*

Polarising microscope. This method is used for demonstration of birefringence e.g. amyloid, foreign body, hair etc. The light is made plane polarised.

IMMUNOFLUORESCENCE *(p. 18)*

Immunofluorescence technique is employed to localise antigenic molecules on the cells by microscopic examination. This is done by using specific antibody against the antigenic molecule forming antigen-antibody complex at the specific antigenic site which is made visible by employing a fluorochrome which has the property to absorb radiation in the form of ultraviolet light so as to be within the visible spectrum of light in microscopic examination.

FLUORESCENCE MICROSCOPE. Fluorescence microscopy is based on the principle that the exciting radiation from ultraviolet light of shorter wavelength (360 nm) or blue light (wavelength 400 nm) causes fluorescence of certain substances and thereafter re-emits light of a longer wavelength.

Source of light. Mercury vapour and xenon gas lamps are used as source of light for fluorescence microscopy. A variety of filters are used between the source of light and objective.

Dark-ground condenser is used in fluorescence microscope so that no direct light falls into the objective and instead gives dark contrast background to the fluorescence.

TECHNIQUES. There are two types of fluorescence techniques both of which are performed on cryostat sections of fresh unfixed tissue:

■ In *direct technique,* first introduced by Coons (1941) who did the original work on immunofluorescence, antibody against antigen is directly conjugated with the fluorochrome and then examined under fluorescence microscope.

■ In *indirect technique,* also called sandwich technique, there is interaction between tissue antigen and specific antibody, followed by a step of washing and then addition of fluorochrome for completion of reaction. Indirect immuno-fluorescence technique is applied to detect autoantibodies in patient's serum.

APPLICATIONS. Immunofluorescence methods are applied for the following purposes:

1. *Detection of autoantibodies in the serum.*
2. *In renal diseases* for detection of deposits of immunoglobulins, complement and fibrin in various types of glomerular diseases.
3. *In skin diseases* to detect deposits of immunoglobulin.
4. For study of *mononuclear cell surface markers.*
5. For specific diagnosis of *infective disorders.*

IMMUNOHISTOCHEMISTRY *(p. 20)*

Immunohistochemistry is the application of immunologic techniques to the cellular pathology. The technique is used to detect the status and localisation of particular antigen in the cells by use of specific antibodies which then helps in determining cell lineage specifically, or is used to confirm a specific infection.

Applications of Immunohistochemistry *(p. 21)*

1. *Tumours of uncertain histogenesis.* Immunohistochemical stains for *intermediate filaments* (keratin, vimentin, desmin, neurofilaments and glial

Chapter Two

fibillary acidic proteins) expressed by the tumour cells are of immense value besides others listed in Table 2.1

2. Prognostic markers in cancer
3. Prediction of response to therapy
4. Infections.

TABLE 2.1: Common Immunohistochemical Stains for Tumours of Uncertain Origin.

	TUMOUR	IMMUNOSTAIN
1.	**Epithelial tumours (Carcinomas)**	i) Pankeratin
		ii) Epithelial membrane antigen (EMA)
		iii) Carcinoembryonic antigen (CEA)
		iv) Neuron-specific enolase (NSE)
2.	**Mesenchymal tumours (Sarcomas)**	i) Vimentin (general mesenchymal)
		ii) Desmin (for general myogenic)
		iii) Muscle specific actin (for general myogenic)
		iv) Myoglobin (for skeletal myogenic)
		v) α-1-anti-chymotrypsin (for malignant fibrous histiocytoma)
		vi) Factor VIII (for vascular tumours)
3.	**Special groups**	
	a) Melanoma	i) Vimentin
		ii) S-100
		iii) HMB-45 (most specific)
	b) Lymphoma	i) Leucocyte common antigen (LCA/CD45)
		ii) Pan-B
		iii) Pan-T
		iv) RS cell marker (for Hodgkin's)
	c) Neural and neuroendocrine tumours	i) Neurofilaments (NF)
		ii) NSE
		iii) GFAP (for glial tumours)
		iv) Chromogranin (for neuroendocrine)
		v) Synaptophysin

ELECTRON MICROSCOPY *(p. 21)*

Electron microscope (EM) first developed in 1930s in Germany has undergone modifications so as to add extensive new knowledge to our understanding the structure and function of normal and diseased cells at the level of cell organelles:

1. In renal pathology in conjunction with light microscopy and immunofluorescence, 2. ultrastructure of tumours of uncertain histogenesis, 3. subcellular study of macrophages in storage diseases, and 4. for research purposes.

There are two main types of EM:

1. Transmission electron microscope (TEM). The magnification obtained by TEM is 2,000 to 10,000 times.

2. Scanning electron microscope (SEM). SEM scans the cell surface architecture and provides three-dimensional image. For example, for viewing the podocytes in renal glomerulus.

Some of the relevant salient technical considerations pertaining to EM are:

1. Whenever it is planned to undertake EM examination of tissue, small thin piece of tissue not more than 1 mm thick should be fixed in 2-4% buffered glutaraldehyde. **2.** Tissue is plastic-embedded with resin on grid. **3.** First, semithin sections are cut at a thickness of 1 μm and stained with methylene blue or toluidine blue. **4.** For ultrastructural examination, ultrathin sections are cut by use of diamond knife.

CYTOGENETICS *(p. 22)*

Human somatic cells are diploid and contain 46 chromosomes: 22 pairs of autosomes and one pair of sex chromosomes (XX in the case of female and XY in the males). Gametes (sperm and ova) contain 23 chromosomes and are called *haploid cells*. All ova contain 23X while sperms contain 23X or 23Y chromosomes. Thus the sex of the offspring is determined by paternal chromosomal contribution i.e. if the ovum is fertilised by X-bearing sperm, female zygote results, while an ovum fertilised by Y-bearing sperm forms male zygote.

Karyotype is defined as the sequence of chromosomal alignment on the basis of size, centromeric location and banding pattern. Determination of karyotype of an individual is an important tool in cytogenetic analysis. Broad outlines of karyotyping are as under:

1. Cell selection. Cells capable of growth and division are selected for cytogenetic analysis. These include: cells from amniotic fluid, chorionic villus sampling (CVS), peripheral blood lymphocytes, bone marrow, lymph node, solid tumours etc.

2. Cell culture. The sample so obtained is cultured in mitogen media. A *mitogen* is a substance which induces mitosis in the cells e.g. PPD, phytohaemagglutinin (PHA), pokeweed mitogen (PWM) etc. The dividing cells are then arrested in metaphase.

3. Staining/banding. When stained, the chromosomes have the property of forming alternating dark and light bands. For this purpose, the fixed metaphase preparation is stained by one of the following banding techniques:
a) *Giemsa banding* or *G-banding*, b) *quinacrine banding* or *Q-banding*, c) *constitutive banding* or *C-banding*, and d) *reverse staining Giemsa banding* or *R-banding*.

4. Microscopic analysis. Chromosomes are then photographed by examining the preparation under the microscope. From the photograph, chromosomes are cut and then arranged according to their size, centromeric location and banding patterns.

Applications *(p. 23)*

Karyotyping is employed for:
i) Chromosomal numerical abnormalities, ii) chromosome structural abnormalities, and iii) cancer.

MOLECULAR PATHOLOGY *(p. 23)*

These techniques detect abnormalities at the level of DNA or RNA of the cell.

1. *IN SITU* HYBRIDISATION. *In situ* hybridisation (ISH) is a molecular hybridisation technique which allows localisation of nucleic acid sequence directly in *the intact cell* (i.e. *in situ*) without DNA extraction. Its applications are:
i) In *viral infections* e.g. HPV, EBV, HIV, CMV, HCV etc.
ii) In *human tumours* for detection of gene expression and oncogenes.
iii) In *chromosomal disorders*, particularly by use of fluorescent *in situ* hybridisation (FISH).

2. FILTER HYBRIDISATION. In this method, target DNA or RNA is extracted from the tissue, and analysed by
i) Slot and dot blots, ii) southern blot, iii) northern blot, and iv) Western blot.

Chapter Two

These techniques have widespread applications in diagnostic pathology e.g.: i) In neoplasia, ii) in infectious diseases, iii) in inherited genetic diseases, and iv) In identity determination.

3. POLYMERASE CHAIN REACTION. The technique is based on the *principle* that a single strand of DNA has limitless capacity to duplicate itself to form millions of copies. In PCR, a single strand of DNA generates another by DNA polymerase using a short complementary DNA fragment; this is done using a *primer* which acts as an initiating template.

A *cycle of PCR* consists of three steps:

i) *Heat denaturation* of DNA (at 94°C for 60-90 seconds).

ii) *Annealing* of the primers to their complementary sequences (at 55°C for 30-120 seconds).

iii) *Extension* of the annealed primers with DNA polymerase (at 72°C for 60-180 seconds).

Repeated cycling can be done in automated thermal cycler and yields large accumulation of the target sequence.

PCR analysis has the same applications as for filter hybridisation techniques and has many advantages over them in being more rapid, can be automated by thermal cyclers and a need for low level of starting DNA/RNA. However, PCR suffers from the risk of contamination.

FLOW CYTOMETRY *(p. 24)*

Flow cytometry is a more recent tool in the study of properties of cells suspended in a single moving stream.

Flow cytometer has a laser-light source for fluorescence, cell transportation system in a single stream, monochromatic filters, lenses, mirrors and a computer for data analysis. Flow cytometer acts like a cell sorter to physically sort out cells from liquid suspension flowing in a single-file.

Currently, flow cytometric analysis finds uses in clinical practice in: 1. Immunophenotyping, 2. diagnosis and prognostication of immunodeficiency, 3. to diagnose the cause of allograft rejection in renal transplantation, 4. diagnosis of autoantibodies, 5. measurement of nucleic acid content, and 6. DNA ploidy studies.

OTHER METHODS FOR CELL PROLIFERATION ANALYSIS *(p. 24)*

Besides flow cytometry, the degree of proliferation of cells in tumours can be determined by various other methods. These include the following: 1. Mitotic count, 2. radioautography, 3. microspectrophotometric analysis, 4. Immunohistochemistry. Ki-67, Ki-S1, and cyclins, and 5. nucleolar organiser region (NOR).

COMPUTERS IN PATHOLOGY LABORATORY *(p. 25)*

It is, imperative that a modern pathology laboratory has laboratory information system (LIS) which should be ideally connected to hospital information system (HIS).

LIS includes: computer system, speech recognition system and image analysis system.

There are two main purposes of having computers in the laboratory:
- for the *billing* of patients' investigations; and
- for *reporting* of results of tests in numeric, narrative and graphic format.

Application of computers in the pathology laboratory has several advantages as under:
1. The laboratory as well as the hospital staff have access to information pertaining to the patient which helps in *improving patientcare*.

2. The *turn-around time* of any test is shortened.
3. It *improves productivity* of laboratory staff at all levels.
4. *Coding and indexing* of results and data of different tests is possible.
5. For *research purposes* and getting accreditation so as to get grants.

SPEECH RECOGNITION SYSTEM. Computer systems are now available which can recognise and transform spoken words of gross and microscopic description of reports through dictaphone into text.

IMAGE ANALYSERS. Image analyser is a form of computer that can capture image formed by microscopic viewing of slide and transform it into digital image which can be used for

1. Morphometric studies of cells.
2. Quantitative nuclear DNA ploidy measurement.
3. Evaluation of immunohistochemical staining quantitatively.
4. Storage and retrieval of laboratory data.

The concept of *'tele-pathology'* instantaneously moves information on pathology work and also pass relevant literature on-line from one place to another far off place through internet information superhighway.

cDNA MICROARRAYS ANALYSIS. This is the latest application of silicon chip technology for simultaneous analysis of large volume of data pertaining to human genes for molecular profiling of tumours.

■ SELF ASSESSMENT

1. **Frozen section is employed for the following purposes** *except:*
   A. Fat demonstration
   B. Amyloid
   C. Rapid diagnosis
   D. Enzymes

2. **For frozen section, the tissue should be sent to the laboratory as under:**
   A. In 10% formalin
   B. In Carnoy's fixative
   C. In saline
   D. Fresh unfixed

3. **Decalcification of calcified tissue and bone is done by the following methods** *except:*
   A. Aqueous nitric acid
   B. Chelating agents
   C. Glacial acetic acid
   D. Microwave

4. **Fluorescent microscopy is employed for the following purposes** *except:*
   A. Glomerular diseases
   B. Tumour of uncertain origin
   C. Bullous dermatosis
   D. Serum autoantibodies

5. **Usual chromogens used in immunohistochemical staining techniques impart the following colour to indicate positivity:**
   A. Pink
   B. Blue
   C Brown
   D. Red

6. **Immunohistochemistry is employed for the following purpose:**
   A. To distinguish neoplastic from non-neoplastic lesion
   B. To distinguish benign and malignant lesion
   C. To localise the cell of origin of tumour
   D. To detect autoantibodies in the serum

7. **Tissues for electron microscopy are fixed in:**
   A. Carnoy's fixative
   B. 10% buffered formalin
   C. Saline
   D. 4% glutaraldehyde

8. **For karyotyping, the dividing cells are arrested by addition of colchicine in the following mitotic phase:**
   A. Prophase
   B. Metaphase
   C. Anaphase
   D. Telophase

9. **For counting of CD4 + T cells in AIDS, the following technique is often employed:**
   A. *In situ* hybridisation
   B. Polymerase chain reaction
   C. Flow cytometry
   D. Electron microscopy

10. **DNA extraction is a pre-requisite for the following molecular techniques *except:***
    A. PCR technique
    B. *In situ* hybridisation
    C. Western blot technique
    D. Southern blot technique

KEY

1 = B	2 = D	3 = C	4 = B
5 = C	6 = C	7 = D	8 = B
9 = C	10 = B		

3

Cell Injury and Cellular Adaptations

Cell injury is defined as a variety of stresses a cell encounters as a result of changes in its internal and external environment. All cells of the body have inbuilt mechanism to deal with changes in environment to an extent. The cellular response to stress varies and depends upon:

i) the type of cell and tissue involved; and

ii) on extent and type of cell injury.

Cellular responses to injury may be as shown in Fig. 3.1 below.

Fig. 3.1: Cellular responses to cell injury.

THE NORMAL CELL *(p. 26)*

I. CELL MEMBRANE *(p. 26)*

Electron microscopy has shown that cell membrane or plasma membrane has a trilaminar structure having a total thickness of about 7.5 nm and is known as *unit membrane*. Biochemically, the cell membrane is composed of complex mixture of phospholipids, glycolipids, cholesterol, proteins and carbohydrates. Proteins and glycoproteins of the cell membrane may act as antigens (e.g. blood group antigens), or may form receptors (e.g. for viruses, bacterial products, hormones, immunoglobulins and many enzymes). Bundle of micro-filaments along with cytoplasm and protein of cell membrane may form projections on the surface of the cell called *microvilli*.

II. NUCLEUS *(p. 27)*

The outer layer of the nuclear membrane is studded with ribosomes and is continuous with endoplasmic reticulum.

The main substance of the nucleus is comprised by the *nuclear chromatin* which is in the form of shorter pieces of thread-like structures called *chromosomes* of which there are 23 pairs (46 chromosomes) together measuring about a metre in length in a human diploid cell. Of these, there are 22 pairs (44 chromosomes) of *autosomes* and one pair of *sex chromosomes*, either XX (female) or XY (male). Each chromosome is composed of two chromatids connected at the centromere to form 'X' configuration having variation in location of the centromere. Depending upon the length of chromosomes and centromeric location, 46 chromosomes are categorised into 7 groups from A to G according to *Denver classification* (adopted at a meeting in Denver, USA).

Chromosomes are composed of 3 components: deoxyribonucleic acid (DNA) comprising about 20%, ribonucleic acid (RNA) about 10%, and the remaining 70% consists of nuclear proteins that include a number of basic proteins (histones), neutral proteins, and acid proteins. DNA of the cell is largely contained in the nucleus. The only other place in the cell that contains small amount of DNA is mitochondria. During cell division, one half of DNA molecule acts as a template for the manufacture of the other half by the enzyme, DNA polymerase, so that the genetic characteristics are transmitted to the next progeny of cells *(replication)*.

The **DNA molecule** as proposed by Watson and Crick in 1953 consists of two complementary polypeptide chains forming a double helical strand which is wound spirally around an axis composed of pentose sugar-phosphoric acid chains. The molecule is spirally twisted in a ladder-like pattern the steps of which are composed of *4 nucleotide bases: two purines* (adenine and guanine i.e. A and G) and *two pyrimidines* (cytosine and thymine i.e. C and T); however, A pairs specifically with T while G pairs with C. The sequence of these nucleotide base pairs in the chain, of which there are thousands, determines the information contained in the DNA molecule or constitutes the genetic code.

In the interphase nucleus (i.e. between mitosis), part of the chromatin that remains relatively inert metabolically and appears deeply basophilic due to condensation of chromosomes is called *heterochromatin,* while the part of chromatin that is lightly stained or vesicular due to dispersed chromatin is called *euchromatin.*

The nucleus may contain one or more nucleoli which are the site of synthesis of ribosomal RNA.

III. CYTOSOL AND ORGANELLES *(p. 29)*

The cytosol or the cytoplasm is the gel-like ground substance in which the organelles of the cells are suspended.

1. CYTOSKELETON. Microfilaments, intermediate filaments, and microtubules are responsible for maintaining cellular form and movement and are collectively referred to as cytoskeleton.

i)   Microfilaments are long filamentous structures having a diameter of 6-8 nm. They are composed of contractile proteins, actin and myosin.

ii)   Intermediate filaments are filamentous structures, 10 nm in diameter, and are cytoplasmic constituent of a number of cell types. They are composed of proteins. There are 5 principal types of intermediate filaments:

a)   Cytokeratin (found in epithelial cells).

b)   *Desmin* (found in skeletal, smooth and cardiac muscle).

c)   *Vimentin* (found in cells of mesenchymal origin).

d)   Glial fibrillary acidic protein (present in astrocytes and ependymal cells).

e)   *Neurofilaments* (seen in neurons of central and peripheral nervous system).

iii)   Microtubules are long hollow tubular structures about 25 nm in diameter. They are composed of protein, tubulin. *Cilia* and *flagella* which project from the surface of cell are composed of microtubules enclosed by plasma membrane and are active in locomotion of the cells.

2. MITOCHONDRIA. Mitochondria are oval structures and are more numerous in metabolically active cells. They are enveloped by two layers of membrane—the outer smooth and the inner folded into incomplete septa or sheaf-like ridges called *cristae.* The matrix of the mitochondria contains enzymes required in the Krebs' cycle by which the products of carbohydrate, fat and protein metabolism are oxidised to produce energy which is stored in the form of ATP in the lollipop-like globular structures.

3. RIBOSOMES. Ribosomes are spherical particles which contain 80-85% of the cell's RNA. They may be present in the cytosol as 'free' unattached form, or in 'bound' form when they are attached to membrane of endoplasmic reticulum. Ribosomes are the protein-synthesising units.

4. ENDOPLASMIC RETICULUM. Morphologically, there are 2 forms of endoplasmic reticulum: rough or granular, and smooth or agranular.

i) *Rough endoplasmic reticulum (RER)* is so-called because its outer surface is rough or granular due to attached ribosomes on it. RER is especially well developed in cells active in protein synthesis e.g. Russell bodies of plasma cells, Nissl granules of nerve cells.

ii) *Smooth endoplasmic reticulum (SER)* is devoid of ribosomes on its surface. SER and RER are generally continuous with each other. SER contains many enzymes which metabolise drugs, steroids, cholesterol, and carbohydrates and partake in muscle contraction.

5. GOLGI APPARATUS OR COMPLEX. The Golgi apparatus or complex is generally located close to the nucleus. The Golgi apparatus is particularly well developed in exocrine glandular cells. Its main functions are synthesis of carbohydrates and complex proteins and packaging of proteins synthesised in the RER into vesicles.

6. LYSOSOMES. Lysosomes are rounded to oval membrane-bound organelles containing powerful lysosomal digestive (hydrolytic) enzymes.

i) *Primary lysosomes or storage vacuoles* are formed from the various hydrolytic enzymes synthesised by the RER and packaged in the Golgi apparatus.

ii) *Secondary lysosomes or autophagic vacuoles* are formed by fusion of primary lysosomes with the parts of damaged or worn-out cell components.

iii) *Residual bodies* are indigestible materials in the lysosomes e.g. lipofuscin.

IV. INTERCELLULAR JUNCTIONS (p. 30)

Plasma membranes of epithelial and endothelial cells, though closely apposed, are separated from each other by 20 nm wide space. These cells communicate across this space through intercellular junctions or junctional complexes visible under electron microscope and are of 4 types:

1. Occluding junctions (Zonula occludens), 2. adhering junctions (Zonula adherens), 3. desmosomes (Macula densa), and 4. gap junctions (Nexus).

MOLECULAR INTERACTIONS BETWEEN CELLS (p. 31)

All cells in the body, including those in circulation, constantly exchange information with each other. This process is accomplished in the cells by chemical agents, also called as molecular agents or factors.

1. CELL ADHESION MOLECULES (CAMs). These are chemicals which mediate the interaction between cells (cell-cell interaction) as well as between cells and extracellular matrix (cell-ECM interaction).The *ECM* is the ground substance or matrix of connective tissue which provides environment to the cells.

There are 5 groups of CAMs:

i) Integrins: They have a role in cell-ECM interactions and in leucocyte-endothelial cell interaction.

ii) Cadherins: These are calcium-dependent adhesion molecules which bind adjacent cells together and prevent invasion of ECM by cancer cells. Various types of cadherins include: E-cadherin (epithelial cell), N-cadherin (nerve cell), M-cadherin (muscle cell), P-cadherin (placenta).

iii) Selectins: Their major role is in movement of leucocytes and platelets and develop contact with endothelial cells. Selectins are of 3 types: *P-selectin* (from platelets, also called CD62), *E-selectin* (from endothelial cells, also named ECAM), and *L-selectin* (from leucocytes, also called LCAM).

ChapterThree

iv) Immunoglobulin superfamily: These partake in cell-to-cell contact through various other CAMs and cytokines. They have a major role in recognition and binding of immunocompetent cells. This group includes ICAM-1,2 (intercellular adhesion molecule, also called CD54), VCAM (vascular cell adhesion molecule, also named CD106), NCAM (neural cell adhesion molecule).

v) CD44: The last group of adhesion molecules is a break away from immunoglobulin superfamily. It is involved in leucocyte-leucocyte-endothelial interactions as well as in cell-ECM interactions.

2. CYTOKINES. These are soluble proteins secreted by haemopoietic and non-haemopoietic cells in response to various stimuli. Their main role is in activation of immune system. Presently, about 50 cytokines have been identified which are grouped in 6 categories: i) interferons (IFN), ii) interleukins (IL), iii) tumour necrosis factor (TNF, cachectin), iv) transforming growth factor (TGF), v) colony stimulating factor (CSF), and vi) the growth factors e.g. platelet-derived growth factor (PDGF), epidermal growth factor (EGF), fibroblast growth factor (FGF), endothelial-derived growth factor (EDGF).

3. CELL MEMBRANE RECEPTORS. Cell receptors are molecules consisting of proteins, glycoproteins or lipoproteins and may be located on the outer cell membrane, inside the cell, or may be trans-membranous. These receptor molecules are synthesised by the cell itself depending upon their requirement, and thus there may be upregulation or downregulation of number of receptors. There are 3 main types of receptors:

i) Enzyme-linked receptors: These receptors are involved in control of cell growth e.g. tyrosine kinase associated receptors take part in activation of synthesis and secretion of various hormones.

ii) Ion channels: The activated receptor for ion exchange such as for sodium, potassium and calcium and certain peptide hormones determines inward or outward movement of these molecules.

iii) G-protein receptors: These are trans-membranous receptors and activate phosphorylating enzymes for metabolic and synthetic functions of cells. The activation of adenosine monophosphate-phosphatase cycle (c-AMP) by the G-proteins (guanosine nucleotide binding regulatory proteins) is the most important signal system, also known as 'second messenger' activation.

CELL CYCLE *(p. 32)*

Multiplication of the somatic (mitosis) and germ (meiosis) cells is the most complex of all cell functions. Mitosis is controlled by genes which encode for release of specific proteins molecules that promote or inhibit the process of mitosis at different steps. Mitosis promoting protein molecules are *cyclins A, B and E*. These cyclins activate *cyclin-dependent kinases (CDKs)* which act in conjunction with cyclins. After the mitosis is complete, cyclins and CDKs are degraded and the residues of used molecules are taken up by cytoplasmic caretaker proteins, *ubiquitin,* to the peroxisome for further degradation.

Period between the mitosis is called *interphase.* The *cell cycle* is the phase between two consecutive divisions. There are 4 sequential phases in the cell cycle: G_1 (gap 1) phase, S (synthesis) phase, G_2 (gap 2) phase, and M (mitotic) phase.

G_1 **(Pre-mitotic gap) phase** is the stage when messenger RNAs for the proteins and the proteins themselves required for DNA synthesis (e.g. DNA polymerase) are synthesised. The process is under control of cyclin E and CDKs.

S phase involves replication of nuclear DNA. Cyclin A and CDKs control it.

G_2 (Pre-mitotic gap) phase is the short gap phase in which correctness of DNA synthesised is assessed. This stage is promoted by cyclin B and CDKs.

M phase is the stage in which process of mitosis to form two daughter cells is completed. This occurs in 4 sequential stages: *prophase, metaphase, anaphase*, and *telophase* (i.e. PMAT).

G_0 phase. The daughter cells may continue to remain in the cell cycle and divide further, or may go out of the cell cycle into resting phase, called G_0 phase.

ETIOLOGY OF CELL INJURY *(p. 33)*

The causes of cell injury, reversible or irreversible, may be broadly classified into two large groups:
A. Genetic causes
B. Acquired causes

Based on underlying agent, the acquired causes of cell injury can be further categorised as under:

1. HYPOXIA AND ISCHAEMIA. Hypoxia is the most common cause of cell injury.
■ The most common mechanism of hypoxic cell injury is by reduced supply of blood to cells i.e. ischaemia.
■ However, oxygen deprivation of tissues may result from other causes as well e.g. in anaemia, carbon monoxide poisoning, cardiorespiratory insufficiency, and increased demand of tissues.

2. PHYSICAL AGENTS. Physical agents in causation of disease are: mechanical trauma (e.g. road accidents); thermal trauma (e.g. by heat and cold); electricity; radiation (e.g. ultraviolet and ionising); and rapid changes in atmospheric pressure.

3. CHEMICALS AND DRUGS. An ever increasing list of chemical agents and drugs may cause cell injury. Important examples include: chemical poisons such as cyanide, arsenic, mercury; strong acids and alkalis; environmental pollutants; insecticides and pesticides; oxygen at high concentrations; hypertonic glucose and salt; social agents such as alcohol and narcotic drugs; and therapeutic administration of drugs.

4. MICROBIAL AGENTS. Injuries by microbes include infections caused by bacteria, rickettsiae, viruses, fungi, protozoa, metazoa, and other parasites.

5. IMMUNOLOGIC AGENTS. Immunity is a 'double-edged sword'—it protects the host against various injurious agents but it may also turn lethal and cause cell injury e.g. hypersensitivity reactions; anaphylactic reactions; and autoimmune diseases.

6. NUTRITIONAL DERANGEMENTS. A deficiency or an excess of nutrients may result in nutritional imbalances.

7. PSYCHOLOGIC FACTORS. There are no specific biochemical or morphologic changes in common acquired mental diseases due to mental stress, strain, anxiety, overwork and frustration e.g. depression, schizophrenia. However, problems of drug addiction, alcoholism, and smoking result in various organic diseases such as liver damage, chronic bronchitis, lung cancer, peptic ulcer, hypertension, ischaemic heart disease etc.

PATHOGENESIS OF CELL INJURY *(p. 34)*

The following principles apply in pathogenesis of most forms of cell injury by various agents:

ChapterThree

1.   Type, duration and severity of injurious agent: small dose of chemical toxin or short duration of ischaemia cause reversible cell injury while large dose of the same chemical agent or persistent ischaemia cause cell death.

2.   Type, status and adaptability of target cell: e.g. skeletal muscle can withstand hypoxic injury for long time while cardiac muscle suffers irreversible cell injury after 30-60 minutes of persistent ischaemia.

3.   Underlying intracellular phenomena: Two essential biochemical phenomena underlie all forms of cell injury to distinguish between reversible and irreversible cell injury:
i)   Inability to reverse mitochondrial dysfunction by reperfusion or reoxygenation.
ii)   Disturbance in membrane function in general, and in plasma membrane in particular.

4.   Morphologic consequences: The ultrastructural changes become apparent earlier than the light microscopic alterations.

Pathogenesis of Ischaemic and Hypoxic Injury *(p. 35)*

Ischaemia and hypoxia are common causes of cell injury.

REVERSIBLE CELL INJURY. If the ischaemia or hypoxia is of short duration, the effects are reversible on rapid restoration of circulation e.g. in coronary artery occlusion, myocardial contractility, metabolism and ultrastructure are reversed if the circulation is quickly restored. The sequential changes in reversible cell injury are as under (Fig. 3.2):

Fig. 3.2: Sequence of events in the pathogenesis of reversible cell injury caused by hypoxia/ischaemia.

1.   Decreased generation of cellular ATP. ATP in human cell is derived from 2 sources—*firstly,* by aerobic respiration or oxidative phosphorylation (which requires oxygen) in the mitochondria, and *secondly,* by anaerobic glycolytic pathway. Ischaemia and hypoxia both limit the supply of oxygen to the cells, thus causing decreased ATP generation from ADP. But in *ischaemia,* aerobic respiration as well as glucose availability are both compromised resulting in more severe effects of cell injury. On the other hand, in *hypoxia* anaerobic glycolytic energy production continues and thus cell injury is less severe. Secondly, highly specialised cells such as myocardium, proximal tubular cells of the kidney, and neurons of the CNS are dependent on aerobic respiration for ATP generation and thus these tissues suffer from ill-effects of ischaemia more severely and rapidly.

2. Reduced intracellular pH. Due to low oxygen supply to the cell, aerobic respiration by mitochondria fails first. This is followed by switch to anaerobic glycolytic pathway for the energy (i.e. ATP) requirement. This results in rapid depletion of glycogen and accumulation of lactic acid lowering the intracellular pH. Early fall in intracellular pH (i.e. intracellular acidosis) results in clumping of nuclear chromatin.

3. Damage to plasma membrane sodium pump. Normally, the energy (ATP)-dependent sodium pump ($Na^+ - K^+$ ATPase) operating at the plasma membrane allows active transport of sodium out of the cell and diffusion of potassium into the cell. Lowered ATP in the cell and consequent increased ATPase activity interfere with this membrane-regulated process. This results in intracellular accumulation of sodium and diffusion of potassium out of cell. The accumulation of sodium in the cell leads to increase in intracellular water to maintain iso-osmotic conditions (hydropic swelling).

4. Reduced protein synthesis. As a result of continued hypoxia, ribosomes are detached from granular endoplasmic reticulum and polysomes are degraded to monosomes, thus causing reduced protein synthesis.

5. Functional consequences. Reversible cell injury may result in functional disturbances e.g. myocardial contractility ceases within 60 seconds of coronary occlusion but can be reversed if circulation is restored.

6. Ultrastructural changes. Reversible injury to the cell causes the following ultrastructural changes:

i) *Endoplasmic reticulum:* Distension of cisternae by fluid and detachment of membrane-bound polyribosomes from the surface of RER.

ii) *Mitochondria:* Mitochondrial swelling and phospholipid-rich amorphous densities.

iii) *Plasma membrane:* Loss of microvilli and focal projections of the cytoplasm ('blebs').

iv) *Myelin figures:* These are structures lying in the cytoplasm or present outside the cell. They are derived from membranes (plasma or organellar) enclosing water and dissociated lipoproteins between the lamellae of injured membranes.

v) *Nucleolus:* There is segregation of granular and fibrillar components of nucleolus and reduced synthesis of ribosomal RNA.

IRREVERSIBLE CELL INJURY. Persistence of ischaemia or hypoxia results in irreversible changes in structure and function of the cell (cell death).

1. Mitochondrial dysfunction. As a result of continued hypoxia, a large cytosolic influx of Ca^{++} ions occurs, especially after reperfusion of irreversibly injured cell, which is taken up by mitochondria and is the cause of mitochondrial dysfunction. Morphologically, mitochondrial changes seen are vacuoles in the mitochondria and deposits of amorphous calcium salts in the mitochondrial matrix.

2. Membrane damage. Defect in membrane function in general, and plasma membrane in particular, is the most important event in irreversible cell injury in ischaemia. The mechanisms underlying membrane damage are as under (Fig. 3.3): i) Accelerated degradation of membrane phospholipid, ii) cytoskeletal damage, iii) toxic oxygen radicals, iv) break down products of lipid, and v) reperfusion damage.

3. Hydrolytic enzymes. Damage to lysosomal membranes is followed by liberation of *hydrolytic enzymes* (RNAase, DNAase, proteases, glycosidases, phosphatases, and cathepsin) which on activation cause enzymatic digestion of cellular components and induce the nuclear changes (pyknosis, karyolysis and karyorrhexis) and hence cell death. The dead cell is eventually replaced

Fig. 3.3: Possible sequence of events in the pathogenesis of irreversible cell injury with ischaemia.

by masses of phospholipids called *myelin figures* which are either phagocytosed by macrophages or there may be formation of calcium soaps.

4. Serum estimation of liberated intracellular enzymes. Liberated enzymes just mentioned leak across the abnormally permeable cell membrane into the serum, the estimation of which may be used as clinical parameters of cell death. For example, in myocardial infarction, estimation of elevated serum glutamic oxaloacetic transaminase (SGOT), lactic dehydrogenase (LDH), isoenzyme of creatine kinase (CK-MB), and more recently cardiac troponins (cTn) are useful guides for death of heart muscle.

Ischaemia-Reperfusion Injury *(p. 37)*

Depending upon the duration of ischaemia/hypoxia, restoration of blood flow may result in the following 3 different consequences:

1. *When the period of ischaemia is of short duration,* reperfusion with resupply of oxygen restores the structural and functional state of the injured cell i.e. reversible cell injury.

2. *When ischaemia is for longer duration,* then rather than restoration of structure and function of the cell, reperfusion paradoxically deteriorates the already injured cell. This is termed ischaemia-reperfusion injury. The main proposed mechanism in ischaemia-reperfusion injury is that upon reoxygenation there is increased generation of oxygen free radicals or activated oxygen species (superoxide, H_2O_2, hydroxyl radicals) from incoming inflammatory cells. Alternatively, during reperfusion activated oxygen species may be generated by adhesion and activation of circulating neutrophils. Besides, ischaemia also damages the cellular antioxidant defense mechanism favouring further accumulation of oxygen free radicals.

3. *Longer period of ischaemia* may also produce irreversible cell injury *during ischaemia itself* without any role of reperfusion.

Free Radical-Mediated Cell Injury *(p. 38)*

Although oxygen is the lifeline of all cells and tissues, its molecular forms as oxygen free radicals (or reactive oxygen intermediates) can be most devastating for the cells. Free radical-mediated cell injury plays an important role in the following situations: i) In ischaemic reperfusion injury, ii) in ionising radiation by causing radiolysis of water, iii) in chemical toxicity, iv) hyperoxia (toxicity due to oxygen therapy), v) cellular aging, vi) killing of exogenous biologic agents, vii) inflammatory damage, viii) destruction of tumour cells, ix) chemical carcinogenesis, and x) atherosclerosis.

Generation of oxygen free radicals begins within mitochondrial inner membrane when cytochrome oxidase catalyses the four electron reduction of oxygen (O_2) to water (H_2O). Intermediate between reaction of O_2 to H_2O, three partially reduced species of oxygen are generated depending upon the number of electrons transferred. These are:

■ Superoxide oxygen (O'_2): one electron
■ Hydrogen peroxide (H_2O_2): two electrons
■ Hydroxyl radical (OH^-): three electrons.

The three partially reduced intermediate species between O_2 to H_2O are derived from enzymatic and non-enzymatic reaction as shown in Fig. 3.4:

The hydroxyl radical is the most reactive species. It may produce membrane damage by lipid peroxidation, protein oxidation, DNA damage and cytoskeletal damage.

ANTI-OXIDANTS. These are endogenous or exogenous substances which inactivate the free radicals e.g.

■ Vitamins E, A and C (ascorbic acid)
■ Sulfhydryl-containing compounds e.g. cysteine and glutathione.
■ Serum proteins e.g. ceruloplasmin and transferrin.

Free radicals are formed in physiologic as well as pathologic processes. However, oxygen radicals are basically unstable and are destroyed

Fig. 3.4: Mechanisms of generation of free radicals by free radicals. (SOD = *superoxide dismutase;* GSH = *glutathione peroxidase*).

ChapterThree

spontaneously. The net effect of free radical injury in physiologic and disease states, therefore, depends upon the rate of free radical formation and rate of their elimination.

Pathogenesis of Chemical Injury *(p. 40)*

Chemicals induce cell injury by one of the following two mechanisms:

DIRECT CYTOTOXIC EFFECTS. The direct cytotoxic damage is usually greatest to cells which are involved in the metabolism of such chemicals e.g. in mercuric chloride poisoning, the greatest damage occurs to cells of the alimentary tract and kidney. Cyanide kills the cell by poisoning mitochondrial cytochrome oxidase thus blocking oxidative phosphorylation.

CONVERSION TO REACTIVE TOXIC METABOLITES. The target cells in this group of chemicals may not be the same cell that metabolised the toxin. Example of cell injury by conversion of reactive metabolites is toxic liver necrosis caused by carbon tetrachloride (CCl_4), acetaminophen (commonly used analgesic and antipyretic) and bromobenzene.

Pathogenesis of Physical Injury *(p. 40)*

Radiation injury to human by accidental or therapeutic exposure is of importance in treatment of persons with malignant tumours as well as may have carcinogenic influences. Killing of cells by *ionising radiation* is the result of direct formation of hydroxyl radicals from radiolysis of water. These hydroxyl radicals damage the cell membrane as well as may interact with DNA of the target cell.

MORPHOLOGY OF CELL INJURY *(p. 41)*

Depending upon the severity of cell injury, degree of damage and residual effects on cells and tissue are variable.

MORPHOLOGY OF REVERSIBLE CELL INJURY *(p. 41)*

Cellular Swelling *(p. 41)*

This is the commonest and earliest form of cell injury from almost all causes. The common causes of cellular swelling include: bacterial toxins, chemicals, poisons, burns, high fever, intravenous administration of hypertonic glucose or saline etc. Cloudy swelling results from impaired regulation of cellular volume, especially for sodium.

G/A The affected organ such as kidney, liver or heart muscle is enlarged due to swelling. The cut surface bulges outwards and is slightly opaque.

M/E 1. The cells are swollen and the microvasculature compressed.
2. Small clear vacuoles are seen in the cells and hence the term vacuolar degeneration. These vacuoles represent distended cisternae of the endoplasmic reticulum.

Hyaline Change *(p. 42)*

Hyaline is a descriptive histologic term for glassy, homogeneous, eosinophilic appearance of material in haematoxylin and eosin-stained sections and does not refer to any specific substance. Hyaline change is associated with heterogeneous pathologic conditions and may be intracellular or extracellular.

INTRACELLULAR HYALINE. Intracellular hyaline is mainly seen in epithelial cells e.g.

1. *Hyaline droplets* in the proximal tubular epithelial cells in cases of excessive reabsorption of plasma proteins.

2. *Hyaline degeneration* of voluntary muscle, also called Zenker's degeneration, occurs in rectus abdominalis muscle in typhoid fever. The muscle loses its fibrillar staining and becomes glassy and hyaline.

3. *Mallory's hyaline* represents aggregates of intermediate filaments in the hepatocytes in alcoholic liver cell injury.

4. Nuclear or cytoplasmic *hyaline inclusions* seen in some viral infections.

5. *Russell's bodies* representing excessive immunoglobulins in the rough endoplasmic reticulum of the plasma cells.

EXTRACELLULAR HYALINE. Extracellular hyaline is seen in connective tissues e.g.

1. Hyaline degeneration in *leiomyomas* of the uterus.

2. Hyalinised *old scar* of fibrocollagenous tissues.

3. *Hyaline arteriolosclerosis* is renal vessels in hypertension and diabetes mellitus.

4. Hyalinised glomeruli in *chronic glomerulonephritis*.

5. *Corpora amylacea* seen in the prostate in the elderly, in the brain and in the spinal cord in old age, and in old infarcts of the lung.

Mucoid Change *(p. 42)*

Mucus secreted by mucous glands is a combination of proteins complexed with mucopolysaccharides. *Mucin*, a glycoprotein, is its chief constituent. Mucin is normally produced by epithelial cells of mucous membranes and mucous glands, as well as by some connective tissues like in the umbilical cord. Epithelial mucin stains positively with periodic acid-Schiff (PAS), while connective tissue mucin is PAS negative but is stained positively with colloidal iron. Both are, however, stained by alcian blue.

EPITHELIAL MUCIN e.g

1. Catarrhal inflammation of mucous membrane (e.g. of respiratory tract, alimentary tract, uterus).

2. Obstruction of duct leading to mucocele in the oral cavity and gall bladder.

3. Cystic fibrosis of the pancreas.

4. Mucin-secreting tumours (e.g. of ovary, stomach, large bowel etc).

CONNECTIVE TISSUE MUCIN e.g.

1. Mucoid or myxoid degeneration in some tumours e.g. myxomas, neurofibromas soft tissue sarcomas etc.

2. Dissecting aneurysm of aorta due to Erdheim's medial degeneration and Marfan's syndrome.

3. Myxomatous change in the dermis in myxoedema.

4. Myxoid change in the synovium in ganglion on the wrist.

INTRACELLULAR ACCUMULATIONS *(p. 43)*

Intracellular accumulation of substances in abnormal amounts can occur within the cytoplasm (especially lysosomes) or nucleus of the cell.

Such abnormal intracellular accumulations can be divided into 3 groups:

i) *Accumulation of constituents of normal cell metabolism produced in excess* e.g. accumulations of lipids (fatty change, cholesterol deposits), proteins and carbohydrates. In addition, deposits of amyloid and urate are discussed later.

ii) *Accumulation of abnormal substances* produced as a result of abnormal metabolism due to lack of some enzymes e.g. storage diseases or inborn errors of metabolism.

iii) *Accumulation of pigments* e.g. endogenous pigments under special circumstances, and exogenous pigments due to lack of enzymatic mechanisms to degrade the substances or transport them to other sites.

FATTY CHANGE (STEATOSIS) *(p. 44)*

Fatty change, steatosis or fatty metamorphosis is the intracellular accumulation of neutral fat within parenchymal cells. It is especially common in the liver but may occur in other non-fatty tissues like the heart, skeletal muscle, kidneys (lipoid nephrosis or minimum change disease) and other organs.

Fatty Liver *(p. 44)*

Liver is the commonest site for accumulation of fat because it plays central role in fat metabolism. Depending upon the cause and amount of accumulation, fatty change may be mild and reversible, or severe producing irreversible cell injury and cell death.

ETIOLOGY. The common causes of fatty liver include the following:
i) Excess alcohol consumption (most common); ii) starvation; iii) malnutrition; iv) obesity; v) diabetes mellitus; vi) chronic illnesses (e.g. tuberculosis); vii) late pregnancy; viii) hypoxia (e.g. anaemia, cardiac failure); ix) hepatotoxins (e.g. carbon tetrachloride, chloroform, ether, aflatoxins and other poisons); x) certain drugs (e.g. administration of oestrogen, steroids, tetracycline etc); and xi) Reye's syndrome.

PATHOGENESIS. Lipids as free acids enter the liver cell from either of the following 2 sources:
■ *From diet* as chylomicrons (containing triglycerides and phospholipids) and as free fatty acids; and
■ *From adipose tissue* as free fatty acids.

Normally, a small part of fatty acids is synthesised from acetate in the liver cells. Most of fatty acid is esterified to triglycerides by the action of α-glycerophosphate and only a small part is changed into cholesterol, phospholipids and ketone bodies. Intracellular triglycerides require 'lipid acceptor protein' to form lipoprotein, the form in which lipids are normally excreted from the liver cells.

In fatty liver, intracellular accumulation of triglycerides can occur due to defect at one or more of the following *6 steps* in the normal fat metabolism as shown in Fig. 3.5.

In most cases of fatty liver, one of the above mechanisms is operating. But in the case of liver cell injury by chronic alcoholism, many factors are implicated which includes: increased lipolysis; increased free fatty acid synthesis; decreased triglyceride utilisation; decreased fatty acid oxidation to ketone bodies; and block in lipoprotein excretion.

An alcoholic who has not developed progressive fibrosis in the form of cirrhosis, the enlarged fatty liver may return to normal if the person becomes teetotaller.

G/A The fatty liver is enlarged with a tense, glistening capsule and rounded margins. The cut surface bulges slightly and is pale-yellow to yellow and is greasy to touch.

M/E There are numerous lipid vacuoles in the cytoplasm of hepatocytes.
i) The vacuoles are initially small and are present around the nucleus *(microvesicular)*.
ii) But with progression of the process, the vacuoles become larger pushing the nucleus to the periphery of the cells *(macrovesicular)*.
iii) At times, the hepatocytes laden with large lipid vacuoles may rupture and lipid vacuoles coalesce to form fatty cysts.
iv) Infrequently, *lipogranulomas* may appear consisting of collections of lymphocytes, macrophages, and some multinucleated giant cells.
v) Fat in the tissue can be demonstrated by frozen section followed by *fat stains* such as Sudan dyes (Sudan III, IV, Sudan black), oil red O and osmic acid.

Fig. 3.5: Lipid metabolism in the pathogenesis of fatty liver. Defects in any of the six numbered steps can produce fatty liver by different etiologic agents.

Stromal Fatty Infiltration (p. 45)

Stromal fatty infiltration is the deposition of mature adipose cells in the stromal connective tissue in contrast to intracellular deposition of fat in the parenchymal cells in fatty change. The condition occurs most often in patients with obesity. The two commonly affected organs are the heart and the pancreas.

INTRACELLULAR ACCUMULATION OF PROTEINS (p. 45)

Pathologic accumulation of proteins in the cytoplasm of cells may occur in the following conditions.

1. In *proteinuria*, there is excessive renal tubular reabsorption of proteins by the proximal tubular epithelial cells which show pink hyaline droplets in their cytoplasm.
2. The cytoplasm of actively functioning plasma cells shows pink hyaline inclusions called *Russell's bodies* representing synthesised immunoglobulins.
3. In *antitrypsin deficiency*, the cytoplasm of hepatocytes shows eosinophilic globular deposits of a mutant protein.
4. *Mallory's body* or alcoholic hyaline in the hepatocytes is intracellular accumulation of intermediate filaments of cytokeratin.

INTRACELLULAR ACCUMULATION OF GLYCOGEN (p. 46)

1. In *diabetes mellitus*, there is intracellular accumulation of glycogen in different tissues because normal cellular uptake of glucose is impaired.

Deposits of glycogen produce clear vacuoles in the cytoplasm of the affected cells. Best's carmine and periodic acid-Schiff (PAS) staining may be employed to confirm the presence of glycogen in the cells.

2. In *glycogen storage diseases or glycogenosis*, there is defective metabolism of glycogen due to genetic disorders.

PIGMENTS *(p. 46)*

There are 2 broad categories of pigments: endogenous and exogenous.

A. ENDOGENOUS PIGMENTS *(p. 46)*

Melanin *(p. 46)*

Melanin is the brown-black, non-haemoglobin-derived pigment normally present in the hair, skin, choroid of the eye, meninges and adrenal medulla. It is synthesised in the melanocytes and dendritic cells, both of which are present in the basal cells of the epidermis and is stored in the form of cytoplasmic granules in the phagocytic cells called the melanophores, present in the underlying dermis. Melanocytes possess the enzyme tyrosinase necessary for synthesis of melanin from tyrosine.

Various disorders of melanin pigmentation cause generalised and localised hyperpigmentation and hypopigmentation:

i) Generalised hyperpigmentation: e.g. In Addison's disease, Chloasma and chronic arsenical poisoning.

ii) Focal hyperpigmentation: e.g. Cäfe-au-lait spots, Peutz-Jeghers syndrome, melanosis coli, melanotic tumours, lentigo and dermatopathic lymphadenitis.

iii) Generalised hypopigmentation: Albinism is an extreme degree of generalised hypopigmentation in which tyrosinase activity of the melanocytes is genetically defective and no melanin is formed. Albinos have blond hair, poor vision and severe photophobia. They are highly sensitive to sunlight. Chronic sun exposure may lead to precancerous lesions and squamous and basal cell cancers of the skin in such individuals.

iv) Localised hypopigmentation: e.g. leucoderma, vitiligo and acquired focal hypopigmentation from various causes such as leprosy, healing of wounds, DLE, radiation dermatitis etc.

Ochronosis *(p. 47)*

Ochronosis is an autosomal recessive disorder in which there is deficiency of an oxidase enzyme required for break down of homogentisic acid which then accumulates in the tissues and is excreted in the urine. Most commonly affected tissues are the cartilages, capsules of joints, ligaments and tendons. In almost all the cases, alkaptonuria is present in which homogentisic acid is excreted by the kidneys.

Haemoprotein-derived Pigments *(p. 47)*

Haemoproteins are the most important endogenous pigments derived from haemoglobin, cytochromes and their break down products.

1. HAEMOSIDERIN. Iron is stored in the tissues in 2 forms:

■ *Ferritin,* which is iron complexed to apoferritin and can be identified by electron microscopy.

■ *Haemosiderin,* which is formed by aggregates of ferritin and is identifiable by light microscopy as golden-yellow to brown, granular pigment, especially within the mononuclear phagocytes of the bone marrow, spleen and liver where break down of senescent red cells takes place. Haemosiderin is ferric iron that can be demonstrated by Prussian blue reaction.

Excessive storage of haemosiderin occurs in situations when there is increased break down of red cells, or systemic overload of iron due to primary (idiopathic, hereditary) haemochromatosis, and secondary (acquired) causes such as in thalassaemia, sideroblastic anaemia, alcoholic cirrhosis, multiple blood transfusions etc.

The effects of haemosiderin excess are as shown in Fig. 3.6.

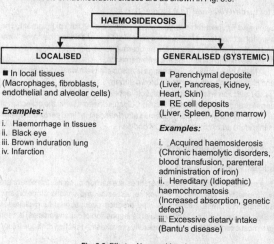

Fig. 3.6: Effects of haemosiderosis.

2. ACID HAEMATIN (HAEMOZOIN). Acid haematin or haemozoin is a haemoprotein-derived brown-black pigment containing haem iron in ferric form in acidic medium. But it differs from haemosiderin because it can not be stained by Prussian blue (Perl's) reaction, probably because of formation of complex with a protein so that it is unable to react in the stain. Haematin pigment is seen most commonly in chronic malaria and in mismatched blood transfusions.

3. BILIRUBIN. Bilirubin is the normal non-iron containing pigment present in the bile. Normal level of bilirubin in blood is less than 1 mg/dl. Excess of bilirubin causes an important clinical condition called jaundice. Briefly, jaundice appears in one of the following 3 ways:

a) *Prehepatic or haemolytic,* when there is excessive destruction of red cells.

b) *Posthepatic or obstructive,* which results from obstruction to the outflow of conjugated bilirubin.

c) *Hepatocellular* that results from failure of hepatocytes to conjugate bilirubin and inability of bilirubin to pass from the liver to intestine.

In infants, rise in unconjugated bilirubin may produce toxic brain injury called *kernicterus.*

4. PORPHYRINS. Porphyrins are tetrapyrrols.

Porphyria results from genetic deficiency of one of the enzymes required for the synthesis of haem so that there is excessive production of porphyrins. Porphyrias are broadly of 2 types:

(a) Erythropoietic porphyrias. These have defective synthesis of haem in the erythrocytes. These may be further of 2 subtypes: congenital type, and erythropoietic protoporphyria.

(b) Hepatic porphyrias. These are more common and have a defect in synthesis of haem in the liver. Its further subtypes include acute intermittent porphyria, variegate porphyria hereditary coproporphyria and porphyria cutanea tarda.

Lipofuscin (Wear and Tear Pigment) *(p. 49)*

Lipofuscin or lipochrome is yellowish-brown intracellular lipid pigment. The pigment is often found in atrophied cells of old age and hence the name 'wear and tear pigment'. It is seen in the myocardial fibres, hepatocytes, Leydig cells of the testes and in neurons in senile dementia.

In the heart muscle, the change is associated with wasting of the muscle and is commonly referred to as 'brown atrophy'.

By electron microscopy, lipofuscin appears as intralysosomal electron-dense granules in perinuclear location. Lipofuscin represents the collection of indigestible material in the lysosomes after intracellular lipid peroxidation and is therefore an example of residual bodies.

B. EXOGENOUS PIGMENTS *(p. 49)*

Inhaled Pigments *(p. 49)*

The most commonly inhaled substances are carbon or coal dust; others are silica or stone dust, iron or iron oxide, asbestos and various other organic substances. These substances may produce occupational lung diseases called pneumoconiosis. *Anthracosis* (i.e. deposition of cabon particles) is seen in almost every adult lung and generally provokes no reaction of tissue injury.

Ingested Pigments *(p. 49)*

Chronic ingestion of certain metals may produce pigmentation e.g. argyria, chronic lead poisoning, melanosis coli and carotenaemia.

Injected Pigments (Tattooing) *(p. 49)*

Pigments like India ink, cinnabar and carbon are introduced into the dermis in the process of tattooing where the pigment is taken up by macrophages and lies permanently in the connective tissue.

MORPHOLOGY OF IRREVERSIBLE
CELL INJURY (CELL DEATH) *(p. 50)*

Cell death is a state of irreversible injury. It may occur in the living body as a local or focal change (i.e. autolysis, necrosis and apoptosis) and the changes that follow it (i.e. gangrene and pathologic calcification), or result in end of the life (somatic death).

AUTOLYSIS *(p. 50)*

Autolysis *('self-digestion')* is disintegration of the cell by its own hydrolytic enzymes liberated from lysosomes. Autolysis can occur in the living body when it is surrounded by inflammatory reaction *(vital reaction)*, or may occur as postmortem change in which there is complete absence of surrounding inflammatory response. Autolysis is *rapid* in some tissues rich in hydrolytic enzymes such as in the pancreas, and gastric mucosa; *intermediate* in tissues like the heart, liver and kidney; and *slow* in fibrous tissue.

NECROSIS *(p. 50)*

Necrosis is defined as focal death along with degradation of tissue by hydrolytic enzymes liberated by cells. It is invariably accompanied by inflammatory reaction.

Necrosis can be caused by various agents such as hypoxia, chemical and physical agents, microbial agents and immunological injury. Two essential changes bring about irreversible cell injury in necrosis—cell digestion by lytic enzymes and denaturation of proteins. These processes are morphologically identified by characteristic cytoplasmic and nuclear changes in necrotic cell. The cytoplasm appears homogeneous and intensely eosinophilic. Occasionally, it may show vacuolation or dystrophic calcification. The nuclear changes include condensation of nuclear chromatin *(pyknosis)* which may either undergo dissolution *(karyolysis)* or fragmentation into many granular clumps *(karyorrhexis)*.

Types of Necrosis *(p. 50)*

Morphologically, 5 distinct types of necrosis are identified.

1. COAGULATIVE NECROSIS. This is the most common type of necrosis caused by irreversible focal injury, mostly from sudden cessation of blood flow (ischaemia), and less often from bacterial and chemical agents. The organs commonly affected are the heart, kidney, and spleen.

G/A Foci of coagulative necrosis in the early stage are pale, firm, and slightly swollen. With progression, they become more yellowish, softer, and shrunken.

M/E The hallmark of coagulative necrosis is the conversion of normal cells into their 'tombstones' i.e. outlines of the cells are retained so that the cell type can still be recognised but their cytoplasmic and nuclear details are lost. The necrosed cells are swollen and appear more eosinophilic than the normal, along with nuclear changes described above. Eventually, the necrosed focus is infiltrated by inflammatory cells and the dead cells are phagocytosed leaving granular debris and fragments of cells.

2. LIQUEFACTION (COLLIQUATIVE) NECROSIS. Liquefaction or colliquative necrosis occurs commonly due to ischaemic injury and bacterial or fungal infections. It occurs due to degradation of tissue by the action of powerful hydrolytic enzymes e.g. infarct brain and abscess cavity.

G/A The affected area is soft with liquefied centre containing necrotic debris. Later, a cyst wall is formed.

M/E The cystic space contains necrotic cell debris and macrophages filled with phagocytosed material. The cyst wall is formed by proliferating capillaries, inflammatory cells, and gliosis (proliferating glial cells) in the case of brain and proliferating fibroblasts in the case of abscess cavity.

3. CASEOUS NECROSIS. Caseous necrosis is found in the centre of foci of tuberculous infections. It combines features of both coagulative and liquefactive necrosis.

G/A Foci of caseous necrosis, as the name implies, resemble dry cheese and are soft, granular and yellowish.

M/E The necrosed foci are structureless, eosinophilic, and contain granular debris. The surrounding tissue shows characteristic granulomatous inflammatory reaction consisting of epithelioid cells with interspersed giant cells of Langhans' or foreign body type and peripheral mantle of lymphocytes.

4. FAT NECROSIS. Fat necrosis is a special form of cell death occurring at two anatomically different locations but morphologically similar lesions. These are: following *acute pancreatic necrosis,* and *traumatic fat necrosis* commonly in breasts.

ChapterThree

G/A Fat necrosis appears as yellowish-white and firm deposits.

M/E The necrosed fat cells have cloudy appearance and are surrounded by an inflammatory reaction.

5. FIBRINOID NECROSIS. Fibrinoid necrosis or fibrinoid degeneration is characterised by deposition of fibrin-like material which has the staining properties of fibrin. It is encountered in various examples of immunologic tissue injury (e.g. in immune complex vasculitis, autoimmune diseases, Arthus reaction etc), arterioles in hypertension, peptic ulcer etc.

M/E Fibrinoid necrosis is identified by brightly eosinophilic, hyaline-like deposition in the vessel wall or on the luminal surface of a peptic ulcer.

APOPTOSIS (p. 52)

Apoptosis is a form of 'coordinated and internally programmed cell death' which is of significance in a variety of physiologic and pathologic conditions.

The characteristic morphologic changes in apoptosis as seen in histo-logic and electron microscopic examination are as under:

1. Involvement of *single cells or small clusters of cells* in the background of viable cells.
2. *Shrinkage of cell* with dense cytoplasm and almost-normal organelles.
3. Convolutions of the cell membrane with formation of membrane-bound near-spherical bodies called *apoptotic bodies* containing compacted organelles.
4. *Chromatin condensation* around the periphery of nucleus.
5. Characteristically, there is *no acute inflammatory reaction*.
6. *Phagocytosis* of apoptotic bodies by macrophages takes place at varying speed.

Biochemical Changes

1. Proteolysis of cytoskeletal proteins.
2. Protein-protein cross linking.
3. Fragmentation of nuclear chromatin by activation of nuclease.
4. Appearance of phosphatidylserine on the outer surface of cell membrane.
5. In some forms of apoptosis, appearance of an adhesive glycoprotein thrombospondin on the outer surface of apoptotic bodies.
6. Appearance of phosphatidylserine and thrombospondin on the outer surface of apoptotic cell facilitates early recognition by macrophages for phagocytosis prior to appearance of inflammatory cells.

Identifying Apoptotic Cells.

1. Staining of chromatin condensation (by haematoxylin, Feulgen, or acridine orange).
2. Flow cytometry to visualise rapid cell shrinkage.
3. DNA changes detected by *in situ* techniques or by gel electrophoresis.
4. Annexin V as marker for apoptotic cell membrane having phosphatidylserine on the cell exterior.

MOLECULAR MECHANISMS OF APOPTOSIS. These are shown in Fig. 3.7.

1. Initiators of apoptosis. Stimuli for signalling programmed cell death act either at the cell membrane or intracellularly.

i) Absence of stimuli required for normal cell survival (e.g. absence of certain hormones, growth factors, cytokines).
ii) Activators of programmed cell death (e.g. receptors for TNF).
iii) Intracellular stimuli include heat, radiation, hypoxia etc.

2. Regulators of apoptosis. These include the following:

i) *BCL-2.* BCL-2 protein is a human counterpart of *CED-9* (cell death) gene found in programmed cell death of nematode worm *C. elegans*. BCL-2 is

Fig. 3.7: Mechanism of apoptosis.

located in the outer mitochondrial membrane and may regulate the apoptotic process by binding to some other related proteins e.g to *BAX* and *BAD* for promoting apoptosis, and *BCL-XL* for inhibiting apoptosis. Another important *BCL-2* binding protein in the cytosol is the pro-apoptotic *protease activating factor (apaf-1)*.

ii) *Other apoptotic regulator proteins* are *TP53 (p53)* protein, *caspases, BAX* and certain viruses (adenovirus, papillomavirus, hepatitis B virus).

3. Programmed cell death. The final outcome of apoptotic regulators in the programmed cell death involves the following pathways: i) FAS receptor activation, ii) ceramide generation, and iii) DNA damage.

4. Phagocytosis. The dead apoptotic cells and their fragments possess cell surface receptors which facilitate their identification by adjacent phagocytes. The phagocytosis is unaccompanied by any other inflammatory cells.

Apoptosis in Biologic Processes

Physiologic Processes:

1. In sculpting of tissues during *development of embryo.*
2. Physiologic involution of cells in *hormone-dependent tissues* e.g. endometrial shedding, regression of lactating breast after withdrawal of breast feeding.
3. *Replacement proliferation* such as in intestinal epithelium.
4. *Involution of the thymus* in early age.

Pathologic Processes:

1. Cell death in tumours exposed to *chemotherapeutic agents.*
2. *Cell death by cytotoxic T cells* in immune mechanisms such as in graft-versus-host disease and rejection reactions.

3. *Cell death in viral infections* e.g. formation of Councilman bodies in viral hepatitis.

4. *Pathologic atrophy* of organs and tissues on withdrawal of stimuli e.g. prostatic atrophy after orchiectomy.

5. Progressive *depletion of CD4+T cells* in the pathogenesis of AIDS.

6. Cell death in response to *injurious agents* involved in causation of necrosis e.g. radiation, hypoxia and mild thermal injury.

7. In *degenerative diseases of CNS* e.g. in Alzheimer's disease, Parkinson's disease, and chronic infective dementias.

The contrasting features of apoptosis and necrosis are summarised in Table 3.1.

TABLE 3.1: Contrasting Features of Apoptosis and Necrosis.

	FEATURE	APOPTOSIS	NECROSIS
1.	**Definition**	Programmed and coordinated cell death	Cell death along with degradation of tissue by hydrolytic enzymes
2.	**Causative agents**	Physiologic and pathologic processes	Hypoxia, toxins
3.	**Morphology**	i) No Inflammatory reaction	i) Inflammatory reaction always present
		ii) Death of single cells	ii) Death of many adjacent cells
		iii) Cell shrinkage	iii) Cell swelling initially
		iv) Cytoplasmic blebs on membrane	iv) Membrane disruption
		v) Apoptotic bodies	v) Damaged organelles
		vi) Chromatin condensation	vi) Nuclear disruption
		vii) Phagocytosis of apoptotic bodies by macrophages	vii) Phagocytosis of cell debris by macrophages
4.	**Molecular changes**	i) Lysosomes and other organelles intact	i) Lysosomal breakdown with liberation of hydrolytic enzymes
		ii) Genetic activation by proto-oncogenes and oncosuppressor genes, and cytotoxic T cell-mediated target cell killing	ii) Cell death by ATP depletion, membrane damage, free radical injury

GANGRENE *(p. 54)*

Gangrene is a form of necrosis of tissue with superadded putrefaction. The type of necrosis is usually coagulative due to ischaemia. There are 3 main forms of gangrene:

Dry Gangrene *(p. 54)*

This form of gangrene begins in the distal part of a limb due to ischaemia. The typical example is the dry gangrene in the toes and feet of an old patient due to arteriosclerosis. Other causes of dry gangrene foot include thromboangiitis obliterans (Buerger's disease), Raynaud's disease, trauma, ergot poisoning.

G/A The affected part is dry, shrunken and dark black, resembling the foot of a mummy.

M/E There is necrosis with smudging of the tissue. The line of separation consists of inflammatory granulation tissue.

Wet Gangrene *(p. 55)*

This occurs in naturally moist tissues and organs such as the mouth, bowel, lung, cervix, vulva etc. Diabetic foot is another example of wet gangrene due to high sugar content in the necrosed tissue which favours growth of bacteria. *Bed sores* occurring in a bed-ridden patient due to pressure on sites like the sacrum, buttocks and heels are the other important clinical conditions included in wet gangrene. Wet gangrene usually develops rapidly due to blockage of venous and less commonly arterial blood flow from thrombosis or embolism.

G/A The affected part is soft, swollen, putrid, rotten and dark. The classic example is gangrene of bowel, commonly due to strangulated hernia, volvulus or intussusception.

M/E There is coagulative necrosis with stuffing of affected part with blood. There is ulceration of the mucosa and intense inflammatory infiltration. Lumen of the bowel contains mucus and blood. The line of demarcation between gangrenous segment and viable bowel is generally not clear-cut.

Contrasting features of two main forms of gangrene are summarised in Table 3.2.

TABLE 3.2: Contrasting Features of Dry and Wet Gangrene.

	FEATURE	DRY GANGRENE	WET GANGRENE
1.	*Site*	Commonly limbs	More common in bowel
2.	*Mechanisms*	Arterial occlusion	More commonly venous obstruction, less often arterial occlusion
3.	*Macroscopy*	Organ dry, shrunken and black	Part moist, soft, swollen, rotten and dark
4.	*Putrefaction*	Limited due to very little blood supply	Marked due to stuffing of organ with blood
5.	*Line of demarcation*	Present at the junction between healthy and gangrenous part	No clear line of demarcation
6.	*Bacteria*	Bacteria fail to survive	Numerous present
7.	*Prognosis*	Generally better due to little septicaemia	Generally poor due to profound toxaemia

Gas Gangrene *(p. 56)*

Gas gangrene is a special form of wet gangrene caused by gas-forming clostridia (gram-positive anaerobic bacteria) which gain entry into the tissues through open contaminated wounds, especially in the muscles, or as a complication of operation on colon which normally contains clostridia.

G/A The affected area is swollen, oedematous, painful and crepitant due to accumulation of gas bubbles within the tissues. Subsequently, the affected tissue becomes dark black and foul smelling.

M/E The muscle fibres undergo coagulative necrosis with liquefaction. Large number of gram-positive bacilli can be identified.

PATHOLOGIC CALCIFICATION *(p. 56)*

Deposition of calcium salts in tissues other than osteoid or enamel is called pathologic or heterotopic calcification. Two distinct types of pathologic calcification are recognised:

Chapter Three

■ *Dystrophic calcification*, which is characterised by deposition of calcium salts in dead or degenerated tissues with normal calcium metabolism and normal serum calcium levels.

■ *Metastatic calcification*, on the other hand, occurs in apparently normal tissues and is associated with deranged calcium metabolism and hypercalcaemia.

M/E In routine H and E stained sections, calcium salts appear as deeply basophilic, irregular and granular clumps. Calcium deposits can be confirmed by special stains like silver impregnation method of *von-Kossa* producing black colour, and *alizarin red S* that produces red staining.

Etiopathogenesis *(p. 56)*

DYSTROPHIC CALCIFICATION. It may occur due to 2 types of causes:

Calcification in dead tissue: e.g. 1. *Caseous necrosis* in tuberculosis is the most common site for dystrophic calcification, 2. *liquefaction necrosis* in chronic abscesses, 3. *fat necrosis* following acute pancreatitis or traumatic fat necrosis in the breast, 4. *infarcts,* 5. *thrombi,* especially in the veins, may produce phleboliths, 6. *haematomas* in the vicinity of bones, 7. *dead parasites* like in hydatid cyst, Schistosoma eggs, and cysticercosis, 8. calcification in *breast cancer* detected by mammography, and 9. *congenital toxoplasmosis* involving the central nervous system.

Calcification in degenerated tissues: e.g.
1. *Dense old scars.*
2. *Atheromas* in the aorta and coronaries.
3. *Mönckeberg's sclerosis* shows calcification in the tunica media of muscular arteries in elderly people.
4. *Stroma of tumours* such as uterine fibroids, breast cancer, thyroid adenoma, goitre etc show calcification. Some tumours show characteristic spherules of calcification called *psammoma bodies* or *calcospherites* such as in meningioma, papillary serous cystadenocarcinoma of the ovary and papillary carcinoma of the thyroid.
5. *Cysts* which have been present for a long time e.g. epidermal and pilar cysts.
6. *Calcinosis cutis* in which there are irregular nodular deposits of calcium salts in the skin and subcutaneous tissue.
7. *Senile degenerative changes* in costal cartilages, tracheal or bronchial cartilages, and pineal gland in the brain etc.

The **pathogenesis** of dystrophic calcification has been likened to the formation of normal hydroxyapatite in the bone involving 2 phases:

■ *Initiation* is the phase in which calcium and phosphates begin to accumulate intracellularly in the mitochondria, or extracellularly in membrane-bound vesicles.

■ *Propagation* is the phase in which minerals deposited in the initiation phase are propagated to form mineral crystals.

METASTATIC CALCIFICATION. Since metastatic calcification occurs in normal tissues due to hypercalcaemia, its causes would include one of the following two conditions:

Excessive mobilisation of calcium from the bone: e.g.
1. *Hyperparathyroidism*
2. *Bony destructive lesions* such as multiple myeloma, metastatic carcinoma.
3. *Prolonged immobilisation* of a patient.

Excessive absorption of calcium from the gut: e.g.
1. *Hypervitaminosis D* results in increased calcium absorption.

2. *Milk-alkali syndrome*
3. *Hypercalcaemia of infancy*

Metastatic calcification affects the following organs more commonly:

■ *Kidneys*, especially at the basement membrane of tubular epithelium and in the tubular lumina causing nephrocalcinosis.

■ *Lungs*, especially in the alveolar walls.

■ *Stomach*, on the acid-secreting fundal glands.

■ *Blood vessels*, especially on the internal elastic lamina.

■ *Cornea* is another site affected by metastatic calcification.

The **pathogenesis** of metastatic calcification at the above mentioned sites is based on the hypothesis that these sites have relatively high (alkaline) pH which favours the precipitation of calcium.

The distinguishing features between the two types of pathologic calcification are summarised in Table 3.3.

TABLE 3.3: Differences between Dystrophic and Metastatic Calcification.

	FEATURE	DYSTROPHIC CALCIFICATION	METASTATIC CALCIFICATION
1.	*Definition*	Deposits of calcium salts in dead and degenerated tissues	Deposits of calcium salts in normal tissues
2.	*Calcium metabolism*	Normal	Deranged
3.	*Serum calcium level*	Normal	Hypercalcaemia
4.	*Causes*	Necrosis (caseous, liquefactive, fat), infarcts, thrombi, haematomas, dead parasites, old scars, atheromas, Mönckeberg's sclerosis, certain tumours, cysts, calcinosis cutis	Hyperparathyroidism (due to adenoma, hyperplasia, CRF), bony destructive lesions (e.g. myeloma, metastatic carcinoma), prolonged immobilisation, hypervitaminosis D, milk-alkali syndrome, hypercalcaemia of infancy
5.	*Pathogenesis*	Akin to formation of normal hydroxyapatite involving phases of initiation and propagation	Favoured by relatively high pH (alkaline) at certain sites e.g. in lungs, stomach, blood vessels and cornea

ChapterThree

CELLULAR ADAPTATIONS *(p. 58)*

For the sake of survival on exposure to stress, the cells make adjustments with the changes in their environment (i.e. adapt) to the physiologic needs *(physiologic adaptation)* and to non-lethal pathologic injury *(pathologic adaptation)*. Broadly speaking, such physiologic and pathologic adaptations occur by:

■ Decreasing or increasing their size i.e. *atrophy* and *hypertrophy* respectively, or by increasing their number i.e. *hyperplasia.*

■ By changing the pathway of phenotypic differentiation of cells i.e. *metaplasia* and *dysplasia.*

In general, the adaptive responses are reversible on withdrawal of stimulus. However, if the irritant stimulus persists for long time, the cell may not be able to survive and may either die or progress further.

ATROPHY *(p. 59)*

Reduction of the number and size of parenchymal cells of an organ or its parts which was once normal is called atrophy

A. Physiologic atrophy. Atrophy is a normal process of aging in some tissues which could be due to loss of endocrine stimulation or arteriosclerosis. For example: i) Atrophy of lymphoid tissue in lymph nodes, appendix and thymus, ii) atrophy of gonads after menopause, and iii) atrophy of brain.

B. Pathologic atrophy e.g.

1. *Starvation atrophy.*

2. *Ischaemic atrophy* e.g. i) Small atrophic kidney in atherosclerosis of renal artery, and ii) atrophy of brain in cerebral atherosclerosis.

3. *Disuse atrophy* e.g. i) wasting of muscles of limb immobilised in cast, and ii) atrophy of the pancreas in obstruction of pancreatic duct.

4. *Neuropathic atrophy* e.g. i) poliomyelitis, ii) motor neuron disease, and iii) nerve section.

5. *Endocrine atrophy* e.g. i) hypopituitarism may lead to atrophy of thyroid, adrenal and gonads, and ii) hypothyroidism may cause atrophy of the skin and its adnexal structures.

6. *Pressure atrophy* e.g. i) erosion of spine by tumour in nerve root, ii) erosion of skull by meningioma arising from pia-arachnoid, and iii) erosion of sternum by aneurysm of arch of aorta.

7. *Idiopathic atrophy* e.g. i) myopathies, and ii) testicular atrophy.

G/A The organ is small, often shrunken.

M/E The cells become smaller in size but are not dead cells. Shrinkage in cell size is due to reduction in cell organelles, chiefly mitochondria, myofilaments and endoplasmic reticulum.

HYPERTROPHY *(p. 59)*

Hypertrophy is an increase in the size of parenchymal cells resulting in enlargement of the organ or tissue, without any change in the number of cells.

A. Physiologic hypertrophy. Enlarged size of the uterus in pregnancy is an excellent example of physiologic hypertrophy as well as hyperplasia.

B. Pathologic hypertrophy. e.g.

1. *Hypertrophy of cardiac muscle* in: i) systemic hypertension, ii) aortic valve disease (stenosis and insufficiency), and iii) mitral insufficiency.

2. *Hypertrophy of smooth muscle* e.g. i) cardiac achalasia (in oesophagus), ii) pyloric stenosis (in stomach), iii) intestinal strictures, and iv) muscular arteries in hypertension.

3. *Hypertrophy of skeletal muscle* in athletes and manual labourers.

4. *Compensatory hypertrophy* e.g.
i) Following nephrectomy on one side in a young patient, there is compensatory hypertrophy as well as hyperplasia of the nephrons of the other kidney.
ii) Adrenal hyperplasia following removal of one adrenal gland.

G/A The affected organ is enlarged and heavy. For example a hypertrophied heart of a patient with systemic hypertension may weigh 700-800 g as compared to average normal adult weight of 350 g.

M/E There is enlargement of muscle fibres as well as of nuclei.

HYPERPLASIA *(p. 60)*

Hyperplasia is an increase in the number of parenchymal cells resulting in enlargement of the organ or tissue. Quite often, both hyperplasia and hypertrophy occur together. Hyperplasia occurs due to increased recruitment of cells from G_0 (resting) phase of the cell cycle to undergo mitosis, when stimulated. Hyperplasia persists so long as stimulus is present.

A. Physiologic hyperplasia. e.g.

1. *Hormonal hyperplasia* i.e. hyperplasia occurring under the influence of hormonal stimulation e.g.

i) Hyperplasia of female breast at puberty, during pregnancy and lactation.

ii) Hyperplasia of pregnant uterus.

iii) Proliferative activity of normal endometrium after a normal menstrual cycle.

iv) Prostatic hyperplasia in old age.

2. *Compensatory hyperplasia* i.e. hyperplasia occurring following removal of part of an organ or a contralateral organ in paired organ e.g.

i) Regeneration of the liver following partial hepatectomy

ii) Regeneration of epidermis after skin abrasion

iii) Following nephrectomy on one side.

B. Pathologic hyperplasia e.g.

i) Endometrial hyperplasia following oestrogen excess.

ii) In wound healing, there is formation of granulation tissue due to proliferation of fibroblasts and endothelial cells.

iii) Formation of skin warts from hyperplasia of epidermis due to human papilloma virus.

iv) Pseudocarcinomatous hyperplasia of the skin.

v) Intraductal epithelial hyperplasia in the breast in fibrocystic breast disease.

G/A There is enlargement of the affected organ or tissue.

M/E There is increase in the number of cells which is due to increased rate of DNA synthesis and hence increased mitoses of the cells.

METAPLASIA *(p. 61)*

Metaplasia is defined as a reversible change of one type of epithelial or mesenchymal adult cells to another type of adult epithelial or mesenchymal cells, usually in response to abnormal stimuli, and often *reverts back to normal on removal of stimulus.*

Metaplasia is broadly divided into 2 types:

A. EPITHELIAL METAPLASIA. This is the more common type. The metaplastic change may be patchy or diffuse and usually results in replacement by stronger but less well-specialised epithelium. Some common types of epithelial metaplasia are as under:

1. Squamous metaplasia. For example:

i) In *bronchus* (normally lined by pseudostratified columnar ciliated epithelium) in chronic smokers.

ii) In *uterine endocervix* (normally lined by simple columnar epithelium) in prolapse of the uterus and in old age.

iii) In *gallbladder* (normally lined by simple columnar epithelium) in chronic cholecystitis with cholelithiasis.

iv) In *prostate* (ducts normally lined by simple columnar epithelium) in chronic prostatitis and oestrogen therapy.

v) In *renal pelvis* and *urinary bladder* (normally lined by transitional epithelium) in chronic infection and stones.

vi) In *vitamin A deficiency*, apart from xerophthalmia, there is squamous metaplasia in the nose, bronchi, urinary tract, lacrimal and salivary glands.

2. Columnar metaplasia. For example:

i) Intestinal metaplasia in healed chronic gastric ulcer.

ChapterThree

ii) Conversion of pseudostratified columnar epithelium in chronic bronchitis and bronchiectasis to columnar type.

iii) In cervical erosion (congenital and adult type), there is variable area of endocervical glandular mucosa everted into the vagina.

B. MESENCHYMAL METAPLASIA. Less often, there is transformation of one adult type of mesenchymal tissue to another.

1. Osseous metaplasia. Osseous metaplasia is formation of bone in fibrous tissue, cartilage and myxoid tissue e.g.

i)   In arterial wall in old age (Mönckeberg's medial calcific sclerosis)

ii) In soft tissues in myositis ossificans

iii) In cartilage of larynx and bronchi in elderly people

iv) In scar of chronic inflammation of prolonged duration

v) In the fibrous stroma of tumour.

2. Cartilaginous metaplasia. In healing of fractures, cartilaginous metaplasia may occur where there is undue mobility.

DYSPLASIA *(p. 62)*

Dysplasia means 'disordered cellular development', often accompanied with metaplasia and hyperplasia; it is therefore also referred to as *atypical hyperplasia*. Dysplasia occurs most often in epithelial cells. Epithelial dysplasia is characterised by cellular proliferation and cytologic changes:

1.   Increased number of layers of epithelial cells

2.   Disorderly arrangement of cells from basal layer to the surface layer

3.   Loss of basal polarity i.e. nuclei lying away from basement membrane

4.   Cellular and nuclear pleomorphism

5.   Increased nucleocytoplasmic ratio

6.   Nuclear hyperchromatism

7.   Increased mitotic activity.

The two most common examples of dysplastic changes are the *uterine cervix* and *respiratory tract*.

Dysplastic changes often occur due to chronic irritation or prolonged inflammation. On removal of the inciting stimulus, the changes may disappear. In a proportion of cases, however, dysplasia progresses into carcinoma *in situ* (cancer confined to layers superficial to basement membrane) or invasive cancer.

The differences between dysplasia and metaplasia are contrasted in Table 3.4.

CELLULAR AGING *(p. 62)*

Old age is a concept of longevity in human beings. The consequences of aging appear after reproductive age. The average age of death of primitive man was barely 20-25 years compared to life-expectancy now which is approaching 80 years, survival being longer in women than men (3:2).

In general, the life expectancy of an individual depends upon the following factors:

1.   *Intrinsic genetic process* i.e the genes controlling response to endogenous and exogenous factors initiating apoptosis in senility

2.   *Environmental factors* e.g. consumption and inhalation of harmful substances, diet, role of antioxidants etc.

3.   *Lifestyle of the individual* such as diseases due to alcoholism (e.g.cirrhosis, hepatocellular carcinoma), smoking (e.g. bronchogenic carcinoma and other respiratory diseases), drug addiction.

4.   *Age-related diseases* e.g. atherosclerosis and ischaemic heart disease, diabetes mellitus, hypertension, osteoporosis, Alzheimer's disease, Parkinson's disease etc.

TABLE 3.4: Differences between Metaplasia and Dysplasia.

	FEATURE	METAPLASIA	DYSPLASIA
i)	**Definition**	Change of one type of epithelial or mesenchymal cell to another type of adult epithelial or mesenchymal cell	Disordered cellular development, may be accompanied with hyperplasia or metaplasia
ii)	**Types**	Epithelial (squamous, columnar) and mesenchymal (osseous, cartilaginous)	Epithelial only
iii)	**Tissues affected**	Most commonly affects bronchial mucosa, uterine endocervix; others mesenchymal tissues (cartilage, arteries)	Uterine cervix, bronchial mucosa
iv)	**Cellular changes**	Mature cellular development	Disordered cellular development (pleomorphism, nuclear hyperchromasia, mitosis, loss of polarity)
v)	**Natural history**	Reversible on withdrawal of stimulus	May regress on removal of inciting stimulus, or may progress to higher grades of dysplasia or carcinoma *in situ*

CELLULAR BASIS (p. 63)

With age, structural and functional changes occur in different organs and systems of the human body. Although no definitive biologic basis of aging is established, most acceptable theory is the functional decline of non-dividing cells such as neurons and myocytes.

1. Experimental cellular senescence. By *in vitro* studies of tissue culture, it has been observed that cultured human fibroblasts replicate for upto 50 population doublings and then the culture dies out. It means that *in vitro* there is reduced functional capacity to proliferate with age. Studies have shown that there is either loss of chromosome 1 or deletion of its long arm (1q). Alternatively with every cell division there is progressive shortening of *telomere* present at the tips of chromosomes which in normal cell is repaired by the presence of RNA enzyme, *telomerase*.

2. Genetic control in invertebrates. Clock *(clk)* genes responsible for controlling the rate and time of aging have been identified in lower invertebrates e.g. *clk-1* gene mutation in the metazoa, *Caenorhabditis elegans*, results in prolonging the lifespan of the worm and slowing of some metabolic functions.

3. Diseases of accelerated aging. Aging is under genetic control in human beings supported by the observation of high concordance in lifespan of identical twins. A heritable condition associated with signs of accelerated aging process is termed *progeria* and is characterised by baldness, cataracts, and coronary artery disease. Another example is Werner syndrome, a rare autosomal recessive disease, characterised by similar features of premature aging, atherosclerosis and risk for development of various cancers.

4. Oxidative stress hypothesis. In normal cells, very small amount (3%) of total oxygen consumption by the cell is converted into reactive oxygen species. The rate of generation of reactive oxygen species is directly correlated with metabolic rate of the organisms. With aging, there is low metabolic rate with generation of toxic oxygen radicals which fail to get eliminated causing their accumulation and cell damage.

ORGAN CHANGES IN AGING *(p. 63)*

1. *Cardiovascular system:* Atherosclerosis, arteriosclerosis with calcification, Mönckeberg's medial calcification, brown atrophy of heart, loss of elastic tissue from aorta and major arterial trunks causing their dilatation.

2. *Nervous system:* Atrophy of gyri and sulci, Alzheimer's disease, Parkinson's disease.

3. *Musculoskeletal system:* Degenerative bone diseases, frequent fractures due to loss of bone density, age related muscular degeneration.

4. *Eyes:* Deterioration of vision due to cataract and vascular changes in retina.

5. *Hearing:* Disability in hearing due to senility is related to otosclerosis.

6. *Immune system:* reduced IgG response to antigens, frequent and severe infections.

7. *Skin:* Laxity of skin due to loss of elastic tissue.

8. *Cancers:* 80% of cancers occur in the age range of 50 and 80 years.

■ SELF ASSESSMENT

1. **Besides nucleus, the only other place in the cell having DNA is:**
   - A. Ribosome
   - B. Golgi apparatus
   - C. Mitochondria
   - D. Endoplasmic reticulum
2. **The DNA molecule is a double helical strand having the following nucleotide bases:**
   - A. Cytosine, thymine, alanine, guanine
   - B. Adenine, guanine, valine, thymine
   - C. Cytosine, lysine, adenine, guanine
   - D. Adenine, guanine, cytosine, thymine
3. **Actin and myosin proteins are found in:**
   - A. Microtubules
   - B. Microfilaments
   - C. Intermediate filaments
   - D. Ribosomes
4. **For cell injury by ischaemia and hypoxia, the following is correct statement:**
   - A. Ischaemia and hypoxia both cause cell injury at the same rate
   - B. Ischaemia tends to injure tissues faster than hypoxia
   - C. Hypoxia tends to injure tissues faster than ischaemia
   - D. Glycolytic energy production continues in ischaemia but not in hypoxia
5. **In ischaemia-reperfusion cell injury, there are:**
   - A. Increased Ca^{++}ions in the extracellular fluid
   - B. Increased Ca^{++}ions in the cytosol
   - C. Ca^{++}ions are equal in the cytosol and in extracellular fluid
   - D. Ca^{++}ion equilibrium is unaffected
6. **The major mechanism of damage to plasma membrane in ischaemia is:**
   - A. Reduced intracellular pH
   - B. Increased intracellular accumulation of sodium
   - C. Increased Ca^{++} ions in the cytosol
   - D. Reduced aerobic respiration
7. **Out of various free radical species, the following radical is most reactive:**
   - A. Superoxide ($O_2^{\cdot}$)
   - B. Hydrogen peroxide (H_2O_2)
   - C. Hydroxyl (OH^-)
   - D. Nitric oxide (NO)

8. In fatty liver due to chronic alcoholism, the following mechanisms are involved *except:*
   A. Increased free fatty acid synthesis
   B. Decreased triglyceride utilization
   C. Increased α-glycerophosphate
   D. Block in lipoprotein excretion

9. The following pigments are stainable by Prussian blue reaction *except:*
   A. Haemosiderin   B. Ferritin
   C. Haematin   D. Haemochromatosis

10. Enzymatic digestion is the predominant event in the following type of necrosis:
    A. Coagulative necrosis   B. Liquefactive necrosis
    C. Caseous necrosis   D. Fat necrosis

11. Mechanism of mammalian apoptosis involves the most important role of the following protein:
    A. Receptor for TNF   B. *BCL-2*
    C. *TP53*   D. *CED-9*

12. Apoptosis has the following features *except:*
    A. There is cell shrinkage in apoptosis
    B. There are no acute inflammatory cells surrounding apoptosis
    C. There may be single cell loss or affect clusters of cells
    D. Apoptosis is seen in pathologic processes only

13. Diabetic foot is an example of:
    A. Dry gangrene   B. Wet gangrene
    C. Gas gangrene   D. Necrotising inflammation

14. Idiopathic calcinosis cutis is an example of:
    A. Necrotising inflammation   B. Dystrophic calcification
    C. Metastatic calcification   D. Calcified thrombi in veins

15. In atrophy, the cells are:
    A. Dead cells   B. Shrunken cells
    C. Irreversibly injured cells   D. Reversibly injured cells

16. For metaplasia the following holds true:
    A. It is a disordered growth
    B. It affects only epithelial tissues
    C. It is a reversible change
    D. It is an irreversible and progressive change

17. In cell cycle, signal transduction system is activated by:
    A. G protein receptors   B. Selectins
    C. Cadherins   D. Integrins

18. Immune system in the body is activated by:
    A. Cell adhesion molecules   B. Cyptokines
    C. G-protein receptors   D. Ion channels

Chapter Three

KEY

1 = C	2 = D	3 = B	4 = B
5 = B	6 = C	7 = C	8 = C
9 = C	10 = B	11 = B	12 = D
13 = B	14 = B	15 = B	16 = C
17 = A	18 = B		

4

Immunopathology Including Amyloidosis

Immunity and immunopathology are proverbial two edges of 'double-edged sword'.

■ An **antigen (Ag)** is defined as a substance, usually protein in nature, which when introduced into the tissues stimulates antibody production.

■ **Hapten** is a non-protein substance which has no antigenic properties, but on combining with a protein can form a new antigen capable of forming antibodies.

■ An **antibody (Ab)** is a protein substance produced as a result of antigenic stimulation. Circulating antibodies are immunoglobulins (Igs) of which there are 5 classes: IgG, IgA, IgM, IgE and IgD.

■ Alternatively, an antigen may induce **specifically sensitised cells** having the capacity to recognise, react and neutralise the injurious agent or organisms.

■ The antigen may combine with antibody to form **antigen-antibody complex**.

COMPONENTS OF IMMUNE SYSTEM (p. 64)

Broadly speaking, immunity or body defense mechanism is divided into 2 types:

I.   Nonspecific or innate immunity is considered as the first line of defense without antigenic specificity. Its major components are:

a) *Humoral:* comprised by complement.

b) *Cellular:* consists of neutrophils, macrophages, and natural killer (NK) cells.

II.   Specific or adaptive immunity is characterised by antigenic specificity. Its main components are:

a) *Humoral:* consisting of antibodies formed by B cells.

b) *Cellular:* mediated by T cells.

Lymphocytes (p. 65)

Morphologically, lymphocytes appear as a homogeneous group but functionally two major lymphocyte populations are identified—T and B lymphocytes (Table 4.1).

Hybridoma Monoclonal Antibodies (p. 65)

Hybridoma technique is the *in vitro* method of obtaining monoclonal antibodies against any antigen by mixing (hybridising) B cells of required clone of antibodies with myeloma cells as source for continued secretion of immunoglobulin to immortalise the cell lineage. Antibodies labelled specifically to kappa (κ) and lambda (λ) light chains, both of which are normally present on B cells, can be used to determine whether the lesion is:

■ *polyclonal*, if arising from stimulation of several clones containing κ as well as λ light chains e.g. in non-neoplastic or reactive proliferations; or

■ *monoclonal*, if arising from stimulation of only one clone and thus one light chain type only e.g. in malignant tumours.

Effector Lymphocyte Subpopulations (p. 66)

Different subpopulations of sensitised lymphocytes (T_{DTH}, CD4+ T cells, or helper T cells; T_{CTL}, CD8+ T cells, or cytotoxic lymphocytes) and unsensitised

TABLE 4.1: Differences between T and B Lymphocytes.

	FEATURE	T CELLS	B CELLS
1.	**Origin**	Bone marrow → Thymus	Bone marrow → Bursa (in fowl); mucosa-associated lymphoid tissue (MALT)
2.	**Life span**	Small T cells: months to years	Small B cells: less than 1 month
		T cell blasts: several days	B cell blasts : several days
3.	**Location**		
	(i) *Lymph nodes*	Perifollicular (paracortical)	Germinal centres, medullary cords
	(ii) *Spleen*	Periarteriolar	Germinal centres, red pulp
	(iii) *Peyer's patches*	Perifollicular	Central follicles
4.	**Presence in**		
	(i) *Blood*	80%	20%
	(ii) *Bone marrow*	Rarely present	Numerous
	(iii) *Lymph nodes*	85%	15%
	(iv) *Spleen*	65%	35%
	(v) *Thymus*	90%	10%
5.	**Surface markers**		
	(i) *Ag receptors*	Present	Absent
	(ii) *Surface Ig*	Absent	Present
	(iii) *Fc receptor*	Absent	Present
	(iv) *Complement receptor*	Absent	Present
	(v) *Rosettes*	E-rosettes (sheep erythrocytes)	EAC-rosettes (mouse erythrocytes)
	(vi) *CD markers*	TH CD4, 3, 7, 2 TS CD8, 3, 7, 2	CD19, 21, 23
6.	**Functions**	(i) CMI via cytotoxic T cells positive for CD3 and CD4	(i) Role in humoral immunity by synthesis of specific antibodies (Igs)
		(ii) Delayed hypersensitivity via CD4+ T cells	(ii) Precursors of plasma cells
		(iii) Immunoregulation of other T cells, B cells and stem cells via T helper (CD4+) or T suppressor (CD8+) cells	

cells (NK or natural killer cells) can mediate the specific immune responses (Table 4.2).

Macrophage *(p. 66)*

The macrophage subpopulations like the dendritic cells found in the lymphoid tissue and Langerhans' cells seen in the epidermis, are characterised by the presence of dendritic cytoplasmic processes and are active in the immune system.

i) They *recognise the antigen* for presenting to immunocompetent T or B cells.

ii) The *phagocytic function* of macrophage is performed due to location of surface receptor for Fc fragment of IgG and C_3 complement.

iii) Macrophages produce *interleukin*-1 which has a role in differentiation stage of T and B lymphocytes.

TABLE 4.2: Effector Lymphocyte Subpopulations.

SUBPOPULATION	FUNCTIONS
1. T_{DTH} *(CD4+, helper T) cells*	60% peripheral T cells
	Release lymphokines
	Activate macrophages
	Mediate delayed hypersensitivity reactions
2. T_{CTL} *(CD8+, cytotoxic suppressor T) cells*	30% peripheral T cells
	Specific cell-mediated cytotoxicity
3. *NK (CD11, 45, 46, 57) cells*	React without previous sensitisation
	React and lyse the target cells e.g. tumour cells, virus-infected cells and some normal cells
4. *K (Fc Ig receptor) cells*	Antibody-dependent cell-mediated cytotoxicity e.g. autoimmune thyroiditis
5. *TIL (activated NK) cells*	Lysis of cells more effective than NK cells

CD= Cluster of differentiation; CTL= cytotoxic T lymphocytes; NK= natural killer; K= killer; TIL= tumour infiltrating lymphocytes; Fc Ig= crystalisable fragment of immunoglobulin.

iv) Macrophages are capable of *lysing tumour cells* by secretion of toxic metabolites.

v) They act as powerful effector cells in some forms of *cell-mediated immunity* e.g. in delayed hypersensitivity reactions.

vi) They act as *mediators of inflammation* in release of prostaglandins, activation of coagulation factors and in secretion of acute phase reactant proteins by the liver.

HUMAN LEUCOCYTE ANTIGEN (HLA) SYSTEM *(p. 66)*

HLA stands for Human Leucocyte Antigens because these antigens were first discovered on leucocytes. The major importance of human histocompatibility antigens of HLA system lies in matching donor and recipient for organ transplant.

Out of the various genes for histocompatibility antigens, most of the transplantation antigens are located on a portion of *chromosome 6* of all nucleated cells of the body and platelets. This is called *major histocompatibility complex (MHC)* or *HLA complex*. These genes occupy four regions or loci—A, B, C and D, on the short (p) arm of chromosome 6 and exhibit marked variation in allelic genes at each locus.

■ **Class I MHC antigens** have loci as HLA-A, HLA-B and HLA-C. CD8 lymphocytes carry receptors for class I MHC and are used to identify the cells having them.

■ **Class II MHC antigens** have single locus as HLA-D. These antigens have further 3 loci, DR, DQ and DP. Class II MHC is identified by B cells and CD4 or T helper cells.

■ **Class III MHC antigens** are some components of the complement system (C2 and C4) coded on HLA complex but are not associated with HLA expression and are not used in antigen identification.

ROLE OF HLA COMPLEX. The HLA complex is significant in a number of ways:

1. Organ transplantation. Historically, the major importance of HLA system is in matching donor and recipient for tissue transplantation.

2. Regulation of the immune system. Class I and II histocompatibility antigens play a role in regulating both cellular and humoral immunity.

3. Association of diseases with HLA. An increasing number of diseases has been found to have association with some specific histocompatibility antigens. These disorders include: *inflammatory, autoimmune disorders* and *inherited disorders of metabolism.*

DISEASES OF IMMUNITY *(p. 68)*

The word *immunity* is synonymous with *resistance* meaning protection from particular diseases or injuries, whereas the term *hypersensitivity* is interchangeable with *allergy* meaning a state of exaggerated or altered immune response to a given agent. The diseases of the immune system are broadly classified into the following 4 groups:

I. Immunodeficiency disorders comprised by a list of *primary and secondary immunodeficiency diseases* including the dreaded *acquired immunodeficiency syndrome (AIDS).*

II. Hypersensitivity reactions

III. Autoimmune diseases

IV. Possible immune disorders classical example of this group being amyloidosis.

ACQUIRED IMMUNODEFICIENCY SYNDROME (AIDS) *(p. 68)*

EPIDEMIOLOGY. Although AIDS was first described in the US, the disease has now attained pandemic proportions involving all continents. Presently, developing countries comprise majority of cases and Africa alone constitutes 50% of all positive cases globally. According to a rough estimate, 1 in every 100 sexually active adults worldwide is infected with HIV. Half of all serologically positive cases are in women while children comprise 5% of all cases.

ETIOLOGIC AGENT. AIDS is caused by a retrovirus called human immuno-deficiency virus (HIV) which is a type of human T cell leukaemia-lymphoma virus (HTLV).

HIV resembles other HTLVs in shape and size and both have *tropism for CD4 molecules* present on subpopulation of T cells which are the particular targets of attack by HIV. However, *HIV differs from HTLV in being cytolytic for T cells causing immunodeficiency (cytopathic virus) while HTLV may transform the target cells into T cell leukaemia (transforming virus).* Two forms of HIV have been described, HIV1 being the etiologic agent for AIDS in the US and Central Africa, while HIV2 causes a similar disease in West Africa and parts of India.

Three important genes coding for the respective components of virion are: *gag* for core proteins, *pol* for reverse transcriptase, and *env* for the envelope proteins. These genes and viral components act as markers for the laboratory diagnosis of HIV infection. Besides, there is *tat* gene (transacti-vator) for viral functions such as amplification of viral genes, viral budding and replication.

ROUTES OF TRANSMISSION. Transmission of HIV infection occurs by one of following three routes:

1. Sexual contact. Sexual contact in the main mode of spread and constitutes 75% of all cases of HIV transmission. Most cases of AIDS in the industrialised world like in the US occur in *homosexual* or *bisexual males* while *heterosexual promiscuity* seems to be the dominant mode of HIV infection in Africa and Asia.

2. Parenteral transmission. This mode of transmission is the next largest group (25%) and occurs in 3 groups of high risk populations: *intravenous drug abusers, haemophiliacs* and *recipients of blood and blood products.*

3.   **Perinatal transmission.** HIV infection occurs from infected mother to the newborn during pregnancy *transplacentally*, or in immediate post-partum period *through contamination* with maternal blood, infected amniotic fluid or breast milk.

Besides blood, *HIV has been isolated from a number of body fluids and tissues* such as: semen, vaginal secretions, cervical secretions, breast milk, CSF, synovial, pleural, peritoneal, pericardial and amniotic fluid.

In order to allay the fear in the public regarding spread of HIV infection, *AIDS cannot be transmitted by* casual non-sexual contact like shaking hands, hugging, sharing household facilities like beds, toilets, utensils etc.

HIV contaminated waste products can be *sterilised and disinfected by* most of the chemical germicides used in laboratories at a much lower concentration. These are: sodium hypochlorite (liquid chlorine bleach), formaldehyde (5%), ethanol (70%), glutaraldehyde (2%), β-propionolactone. HIV is also heat-sensitive and can be inactivated at 56°C for 30 min.

PATHOGENESIS. The pathogenesis of HIV infection is largely related to the *depletion of CD4+ T cells (helper T cells) resulting in profound immuno-suppression.*

1.   **Selective tropism and internalisation.** HIV on entering the body via any route described above has *selective tropism for CD4+ cells* and certain population of monocytes and macrophages.

2.   **Uncoating and proviral DNA integration.** The virus is then uncoated and its genomic RNA is transcribed to proviral DNA by enzyme reverse transcriptase. The proviral DNA so formed may initially remain *unintegrated* in the affected cell and later gets *integrated* into the T cell genome.

3.   **Budding and syncytia formation.** On activation, the infected CD4+ T cells bear budding viral particles due to multiplication which further attract more number of CD4+ T cells resulting in syncytia formation.

4.   **Cytopathic effects.** In an inactive T cell, the infection may remain in *latent phase* for a long time, accounting for the long incubation period. An antigenically-activated and infected T cell develops into *cytopathic phase.* The cytopathic effects on T cells are two fold: *firstly*, there is quantitative depletion of CD4+ T cells due to direct cytolysis; and *secondly*, there is qualitative defect in the form of inability of these T cells to respond to antigens.

5.   **Effects on monocytes and macrophages.** Besides the cytopathic effects on CD4+ T cells, CD4 molecule-bearing subpopulations of monocytes and macrophages (e.g. dendritic cells, microglial cells) are also attacked by HIV but without causing cytopathic effects on these cells.

6.   **HIV infection of nervous system.** Out of non-lymphoid organ involvement, HIV infection of nervous system is the most serious and can occur as a result of the following:

i)   Infection carried to the microglia of the nervous system by *HIV infected CD4+ monocyte-macrophage subpopulation or endothelial cells.*

ii)   *Direct infection* of astrocytes and oligodendrocytes.

iii) Neurons are not invaded by HIV but are affected due to gp120 and by release of *cytokines* by macrophages.

75-90% of AIDS patients may demonstrate some form of neurological involvement at autopsy.

7.   **B cell dysfunctions.** Besides affecting CD4+ cells, gpl20 of HIV envelope also produces derangements of B cell functions resulting in decreased immunoglobulin production, hypergammaglobulinaemia, polyclonal activation, circulating immune complexes.

NATURAL HISTORY. As per the WHO, AIDS is defined as the existence of at least two major signs associated with at least one minor sign, in the absence of known secondary causes of immunosuppression.

- *Major signs* include:
i) weight loss of > 10% of body weight;
ii) chronic diarrhoea of > 1 month's duration; and
iii) prolonged fever (intermittent or continuous) for > 1 month.

- *Minor signs* are:
i) recurrent oropharyngeal candidiasis;
ii) persistent generalised lymphadenopathy;
iii) persistent cough for > one month;
iv) generalised pruritic dermatitis;
v) recurrent herpes zoster; and
vi) progressive disseminated herpes simplex infection.

The following 3 phases are recognised (Table 4.3):

TABLE 4.3: Natural History of HIV Infection.

PHASE	EARLY, ACUTE	MIDDLE, CHRONIC	FINAL, CRISIS
Period after infection	3-6 weeks	10 to 12 years	Any period up to death
CDC category	Group I: Acute HIV syndrome	Group II: Asymptomatic infection Group III: PGL	Group IV: 5 Subgroups: A: Constitutional symptoms B: Neurologic disease C: Secondary infection D: Secondary neoplasms E: Other conditions
Plasma viraemia	High	Moderate	High
CD4 counts	Suddenly reduced	Moderate loss	Severely reduced (< 200/μl)

(CDC = Centres for Disease Control, Atlanta, USA; PGL = Persistent generalised lymphadenopathy).

1. Acute HIV syndrome (3-12 weeks).

2. Middle chronic phase (10-12 years).

3. Final crisis phase. This phase is characterised by profound immuno-suppression and onset of full-blown AIDS and has the following features:

i) Marked increase in *viraemia*.

ii) The time period between HIV infection developing into chronic phase followed by full-blown AIDS may last *7-10 years and culminates in death.*

iii) *CD 4+ T cells* are markedly reduced (below 200 per μl).

iv) *Clinically*, the features of the final phase are categorised into following 5 subgroups (CDC group IV):

Subgroup A: *Constitutional disease* characterised by fever of more than one month duration, weight loss of more than 10% of body weight, and chronic diarrhoea lasting more than one month.

Subgroup B: *Neurologic disease* present in majority of cases and include viral meningoencephalitis, aseptic meningitis, peripheral neuropathy, AIDS-dementia complex.

Subgroup C: *Secondary opportunistic infections* such as fungal, viral, bacterial and parasitic.

Subgroup D: *Secondary neoplasms* such as Kaposi's sarcoma (Chapter 8), Non-Hodgkin's lymphoma (Burkitt's, immunoblastic), Hodgkin's lymphoma, primary CNS lymphoma.

Subgroup E: This recent subgroup includes < 200 CD 4+ T lymphocytes/μl, pulmonary tuberculosis and recurrent pneumonia.

The average survival after the onset of full-blown AIDS is 18-24 months.

PATHOLOGIC CHANGES. The morphological changes in AIDS are non-specific and variable depending upon the stage of the disease:

1. *Lymphoid tissues* (lymph nodes, spleen, thymus and bone marrow) show predominant changes *viz.:*
- *In early stage*, there is B cell hyperplasia.
- *The full-blown AIDS* is characterised by universal lymphoid cell depletion.

2. Widespread opportunistic infections.

3. AIDS-associated cancers e.g. HPV-associated cancers such as carcinoma of uterine cervix, vagina, anus.

4. Neurological manifestations includes AIDS-associated dementia.

5. AIDS associated nephropathy characterised by focal segmental glomerulosclerosis.

Laboratory Diagnosis of AIDS

1. *Specific tests:*

i) Serologic tests by ELISA, Western blot and immunofluorescence test

ii) Antigen detection tests using envelope and core proteins of HIV by recombinant DNA techniques

iii) Virus isolation and culture in neoplastic T cell line

iv) Polymerase chain reaction (PCR).

2. *Indirect tests:*

i) CD4 and CD8 cell counts; reversal of CD4 to CD8 cell ratio

ii) Lymphopenia

iii) Lymph node biopsy

iv) Platelet count revealing thrombocytopenia

v) Increased β-2 microglobulin levels.

HYPERSENSITIVITY REACTIONS (IMMUNOLOGIC TISSUE INJURY) *(p. 74)*

A state of balance in the immune responses (humoral or cell-mediated) is essential for protection against endogenous and exogenous antigens. *Hypersensitivity is defined as a state of exaggerated immune response to an antigen.* The lesions of hypersensitivity (immunologic tissue injury) are produced due to interaction between antigen and product of the immune response.

Depending upon the *rapidity* and *duration* of the immune response, two distinct forms of hypersensitivity reactions are recognised:

1. Immediate type in which on administration of antigen, the reaction occurs immediately (within seconds to minutes). Immune response in this type is mediated largely by *humoral antibodies*. Immediate type of hypersensitivity is further of 3 types—*type I, II and III.*

2. Delayed type in which the reaction is slower in onset and develops within 24-48 hours and the effect is prolonged. It is mainly mediated by *cellular response. Type IV reaction* is the delayed hypersensitivity reaction.

The mechanisms and examples of immunologic tissue injury by the 4 types of hypersensitivity reactions are summarised in Table 4.4.

AUTOIMMUNE DISEASES *(p. 76)*

Autoimmunity is a state in which the body's immune system fails to distinguish between 'self' and 'non-self' and reacts by formation of autoantibodies against one's own tissue antigens. In other words, there is loss of tolerance to one's own tissues; *autoimmunity is the opposite of immune tolerance.*

Immune tolerance is a normal phenomenon present since foetal life and is defined as the ability of an individual to recognise self tissue and antigens.

TABLE 4.4: Mechanisms of Immunologic Tissue Injury.

TYPE	MECHANISM	EXAMPLES
Type I **(Anaphylactic, atopic)**	Humoral Abs of IgE type → basophils/mast cells sensitised → release of anaphylactic mediators	i. Systemic anaphylaxis (administration of antisera and drugs, stings) ii. Local anaphylaxis (hay fever, bronchial asthma, food allergy, cutaneous, angioedema)
Type II **(Cytotoxic)**	i. Cytotoxic auto- and iso- antibodies to blood cells	i. Autoimmune haemolytic anaemia, transfusion reactions, erythroblastosis foetalis, ITP, leucopenia, drug-induced
	ii. Cytotoxic Abs to tissue components	ii. Myasthenia gravis, male sterility
	iii. Ab-dependent cell-mediated cytotoxicity (ADCC)	iii. Tumour cells, parasites
Type III **(Immune-complex)**	i. Local (Arthus reaction) Ag-Ab complexes	i. Injection of ATS, farmer's lung
	ii. Systemic (circulating) Ag-Ab complexes or serum sickness	ii. Glomerulonephritis, collagen diseases, Goodpasture's syndrome, arthritis, uveitis, skin diseases
Type IV **(Cell-mediated)**	i. Classical delayed hypersensitivity mediated by CD4 + T cells	i. Tuberculin reaction, tuberculosis, tuberculoid leprosy, typhoid, contact dermatitis
	ii. T cell mediated cytotoxicity by CD8+ T cells	ii. Virus-infected cells, tumour cells, transplant rejection

PATHOGENESIS OF AUTOIMMUNITY *(p. 77)*

The mechanisms by which the immune tolerance of the body is broken causes autoimmunity. These mechanisms may be immunological, genetic, and microbial, all of which may be interacting.

1. **Immunological factors:**
i) Polyclonal activation of B cells.
ii) Generation of self-reacting B cell clones.
iii) Decreased T suppressor and increased T helper cell activity.
iv) Fluctuation of anti-idiotype network control.
v) Sequestered antigen released from tissues.

2. **Genetic factors:**
i) Increased expression of *Class II HLA antigens* on tissues involved in autoimmunity.
ii) Increased *familial incidence* of some of the autoimmune disorders.

3. **Microbial factors.** Infection with microorganisms, particularly viruses (e.g. EBV infection), and less often bacteria (e.g. streptococci, *Klebsiella*) and mycoplasma, has been implicated.

TYPES AND EXAMPLES OF AUTOIMMUNE DISEASES *(p. 77)*

1. **Organ specific diseases.** In these, the autoantibodies formed react specifically against an organ or target tissue component and cause its chronic inflammatory destruction.

2. Non-organ specific diseases. These are diseases in which a number of autoantibodies are formed which react with antigens in many tissues and thus cause systemic lesions. The examples of this group are various systemic collagen diseases.

Systemic Lupus Erythematosus (SLE) *(p. 77)*

Two forms of lupus erythematosus are described:

1. Systemic or disseminated form is characterised by acute and chronic inflammatory lesions widely scattered in the body and there is presence of various nuclear and cytoplasmic autoantibodies in the plasma.

2. Discoid form is characterised by chronic and localised skin lesions involving the bridge of nose and adjacent cheeks without any systemic manifestations. Rarely, discoid form may develop into disseminated form.

ETIOLOGY. The exact etiology of SLE is not known. However, autoantibodies against nuclear and cytoplasmic components of the cells are demonstrable in plasma by immunofluorescence tests in almost all cases of SLE.

i) Antinuclear antibodies (ANA) are the antibodies against common nuclear antigen that includes DNA as well as RNA.

ii) Antibodies to double-stranded (anti-dsDNA) or single-stranded DNA (anti-ssDNA) is the most specific, present in half the cases of SLE.

iii) Anti-Smith antigen antibodies (anti-SmAg), in which antibodies appear against Smith antigen which is part of ribonucleoproteins.

iv) Anti-ribonucleoproteins (anti-RNP) are not specific for SLE but are seen more often in Sjögren's syndrome.

v) Anti-histone antibodies, seen particularly in cases of drug-induced SLE.

vi) Anti-nucleolar antibodies to nucleolar antigens.

vii) Antiphospholipid antibodies or lupus anticoagulant are quite specific for SLE and are responsible for thrombotic complications in cases of SLE.

The source of these autoantibodies as well as hypergammaglobulinaemia in SLE is the **polyclonal activation of B cells** brought about by:

1. *immunologic factors.*
2. *genetic factors.*
3. *other factors* such as certain drugs e.g. penicillamine D; certain viral infections e.g. EBV infection; and certain hormones e.g. oestrogen.

Two types of immunologic tissue injury can occur in SLE:

1. *Type II hypersensitivity* is characterised by formation of autoantibodies against blood cells (red blood cells, platelets, leucocytes) and results in haematologic derangement in SLE.

2. *Type III hypersensitivity* is characterised by antigen-antibody complex (commonly DNA-anti-DNA antibody; sometimes Ig-anti-Ig antibody complex) which is deposited at sites such as renal glomeruli, walls of small blood vessels etc.

LE CELL PHENOMENON. The test is based on the principle that ANAs cannot penetrate the intact cells and thus cell nuclei should be exposed to bind them with the ANAs. The binding of exposed nucleus with ANAs results in homogeneous mass of nuclear chromatin material which is called *LE body or haematoxylin body.*

■ If this mass is engulfed by a neutrophil, displacing the nucleus of neutrophil to the rim of the cell, it is called *LE cell.*

■ If the mass, more often an intact lymphocyte, is phagocytosed by a monocyte, it is called *Tart cell.*

LE cell test is positive in 70% cases of SLE while newer and more sensitive immunofluorescence tests for autoantibodies are positive in almost 100% cases of SLE.

The manifestations of SLE are widespread in different visceral organs as well as show erythematous cutaneous eruptions. The principal lesions are renal, vascular, cutaneous and cardiac; other organs and tissues involved are serosal linings (pleuritis, pericarditis); joints (synovitis); spleen (vasculitis); liver (portal triaditis); lungs (interstitial pneumonitis, fibrosing alveolitis), CNS (vasculitis) and in blood (autoimmune haemolytic anaemia, thrombocytopaenia) (Table 4.5).

M/E The characteristic lesion in SLE is *fibrinoid necrosis* which may be seen in the connective tissue, beneath the endothelium in small blood vessels, under the mesothelial lining of pleura and pericardium, under the endothelium in endocardium, or under the synovial lining cells of joints.

TABLE 4.5: Morphology of Major Lesions in SLE.

ORGANS (MAIN LESION)	MORPHOLOGIC FEATURES
1. **Renal lesions** (Lupus nephritis)	EM-shows large deposits in mesangium, subepithelial or subendothelial. IM-shows granular deposits of immune complex (IgG and C3) on capillaries, mesangium and tubular basement membranes. Six patterns: i. Minimal disease: LM shows no change. ii. Mesangial GN: LM shows increase in matrix; mesangial hypercellularity. iii. Focal proliferative GN: LM shows focal (parts of 50% glomeruli) endothelial and mesangial cell proliferation; infiltration with neutrophils. iv. Diffuse proliferative GN: LM shows all glomeruli affected; proliferation of endothelial, mesangial and epithelial cells; epithelial crescents. v. Membranous lupus GN: LM shows diffuse basement membrane thickening; features of nephrotic syndrome. vi. Sclerosing nephropathy: LM shows hyalinisation of whole of glomeruli.
2. **Small blood vessels** (Acute necrotising vasculitis)	Affects all tissues; commonly skin and muscles involved; LM shows fibrinoid deposits in the vessel wall; perivascular infiltrate of mononuclear cells.
3. **Cutaneous lesions** (Erythematous eruptions)	Butterfly area on nose and cheek; LM shows liquefactive degeneration of basal layer of epidermis; oedema at dermoepidermal junction; acute necrotising vasculitis in dermis; IM shows immune complex deposits (IgG and C3) at dermo-epidermal junction.
4. **Cardiac lesions** (Libman-Sacks endocarditis)	Vegetations on mitral and tricuspid valves, may extend to mural endocardium, chordae tendineae; LM of vegetations shows fibrinoid material, necrotic debris, inflammatory cells, haematoxylin bodies may be present; connective tissue of endocardium and myocardium may show focal inflammation and necrotising vasculitis.

(EM = electron microscopy, LM = light microscopy; IM = immunofluorescence microscopy; GN = glomerulonephritis).

Scleroderma (Progressive Systemic Sclerosis) *(p. 79)*

Two main types are recognised:

1. *Diffuse scleroderma* in which the skin shows widespread involvement and may progress to involve visceral structures.

2. *CREST syndrome* of progressive systemic sclerosis characterised by Calcinosis (C), Raynaud's phenomenon (R), Esophageal hypomotility (E), Sclerodactyly (S) and Telangiectasia (T).

Chapter Four

Immunologic mechanisms have been implicated in the pathogenesis of lesions in systemic sclerosis which finally cause activation of fibroblasts in the following ways:

1. *Elaboration of cytokines* such as by fibroblast growth factor and chemotactic factors by activated T cells and macrophages.

2. *Endothelial cell injury* due to cytotoxic damage to endothelium from autoantibodies or antigen-antibody complexes.

Disseminated visceral involvement as well as cutaneous lesions are seen in systemic sclerosis.

1. **Skin changes.** Skin is involved diffusely, beginning distally from fingers and extending proximally to arms, shoulders, neck and face. In advanced stage, the fingers become claw-like and face mask-like.

M/E

- *Early stage* shows oedema and degeneration of collagen.
- *Late stage* reveals thin and flat epidermis.

2. **Kidney changes.** The lesions are prominent in the walls of interlobular arteries which develop changes resembling malignant hypertension.

3. **Smooth muscle of GIT.** Muscularis of the alimentary tract, particularly oesophagus, is progressively atrophied and replaced by fibrous tissue.

Polymyositis-Dermatomyositis *(p. 81)*

This disease is a combination of symmetric muscle weakness and skin rash. The affected muscles are infiltrated by sensitised T lymphocytes of both T helper and T suppressor type which are considered to bring about inflammatory destruction of muscle. The skeletal muscles usually affected are of pelvis, shoulders, neck, chest and diaphragm.

M/E Vacuolisation and fragmentation of muscle fibres and numerous inflammatory cells are present.

Sjögren's Syndrome *(p. 81)*

Sjögren's syndrome is characterised by the *triad* of dry eyes *(keratoconjunctivitis sicca)*, dry mouth *(xerostomia)*, and *rheumatoid arthritis*. The combination of the former two symptoms is called *sicca syndrome*.

Antinuclear antibodies are found in about 90% of cases; test for rheumatoid factor is positive in 25% of cases. The lesions in lacrimal and salivary glands are mediated by T lymphocytes, B cells and plasma cells.

In early stage, the lacrimal and salivary glands show periductal infiltration by lymphocytes and plasma cells, which at times may form lymphoid follicles (pseudolymphoma). *In late stage*, glandular parenchyma is replaced by fat and fibrous tissue.

Reiter's Syndrome *(p. 81)*

This syndrome is characterised by *triad of arthritis, conjunctivitis* and *urethritis*.

TRANSPLANT REJECTION *(p. 81)*

1. *Autografts* are grafts in which the donor and recipient is the same individual.

2. *Isografts* are grafts between the donor and recipient of the same genotype.

3. *Allografts* are those in which the donor is of the same species but of a different genotype.

4. *Xenografts* are those in which the donor is of a different species from that of the recipient.

All types of grafts have been performed in human beings but xenografts have been found to be rejected invariably due to genetic disparity. Presently, surgical skills exist for skin grafts and for organ transplants such as kidney, heart, lungs, liver, pancreas, cornea and bone marrow.

Besides the rejection reaction, a peculiar problem occurring especially in bone marrow transplantation is graft-versus-host reaction (GVH). In humans, GVH reaction results when immunocompetent cells are transplanted to an immunodeficient recipient e.g. when severe combined immunodeficiency is treated by bone marrow transplantation. The clinical features of GVH reaction include: fever, weight loss, anaemia, dermatitis, diarrhoea, intestinal malabsorption, pneumonia and hepatosplenomegaly.

The development of immunosuppressive drugs has made the survival of allografts in recipients possible. Rejection of allografts involves both cell-mediated and humoral immunity.

Types of Rejection Reactions *(p. 82)*

Based on the underlying mechanism and time period, rejection reactions are classified into 3 types:

1. HYPERACUTE REJECTION. Hyperacute rejection appears within minutes to hours of placing the transplant and destroys it. It is mediated by preformed humoral antibody against donor-antigen.

G/A Hyperacute rejection is recognised by the surgeon soon after the vascular anastomosis of the graft is performed to the recipient's vessels. The organ becomes swollen, oedematous, haemorrhagic, purple and cyanotic rather than gaining pink colour.

M/E The characteristics of Arthus reaction are present. There are numerous neutrophils around dilated and obstructed capillaries which are blocked by fibrin and platelet thrombi.

2. ACUTE REJECTION. This usually becomes evident within a few days to a few months of transplantation. Acute graft rejection may be mediated by cellular or humoral mechanisms.

Acute cellular rejection is more common and is characterised by extensive infiltration in the interstitium of the transplant by lymphocytes (mainly T cells), a few plasma cells, monocytes and a few polymorphs. There is damage to the blood vessels and there are foci of necrosis in the transplanted tissue.

3. CHRONIC REJECTION. Chronic rejection may follow repeated attacks of acute rejection or may develop slowly over a period of months to a year or so.

AMYLOIDOSIS *(p. 83)*

Amyloidosis is the term used for a group of diseases characterised by extracellular deposition of fibrillar proteinaceous substance called amyloid having common morphological appearance, staining properties and physical structure but with variable protein (or biochemical) composition.

By *light microscopy* with H&E staining, amyloid appears as extracellular, homogeneous, structureless and eosinophilic hyaline material, which is *positive with Congo red* staining and shows apple-green birefringence on *polarising microscopy*.

PHYSICAL AND CHEMICAL NATURE OF AMYLOID *(p. 83)*

It emerges that on the basis of morphology and physical characteristics all forms of amyloid are similar in appearance, but they are chemically hetero-geneous. Based on these analysis, amyloid is composed of 2 main types of complex proteins:

I. Fibril Proteins *(p. 83)*

By electron microscopy, it became apparent that major component of all forms of amyloid (about 95%) consists of meshwork of fibril proteins. The *fibrils* are delicate, randomly dispersed, non-branching, each measuring 7.5-10 nm in diameter and having indefinite length. Each fibril is further composed of double helix of two pleated sheets in the form of *twin filaments* separated by a clear space. By X-ray crystallography and infra-red spectroscopy, the fibrils are shown to have *cross-β-pleated* sheet configuration which produces 1000 A° periodicity that gives the characteristic staining properties of amyloid with Congo red and birefringence under polarising microscopy. Based on these features amyloid is also referred to as *β-fibrillosis*.

Chemically two major forms of amyloid fibril proteins were first identified in 1970s while currently 20 biochemically different proteins are known to form amyloid fibrils.

AL PROTEIN. AL amyloid fibril protein is derived from immunoglobulin light chain, which in most cases includes amino-terminal segment of the immunoglobulin light chain and part of C region. AL fibril protein is more frequently derived from the lambda (λ) light chain than kappa (κ), the former being twice more common. However, in any given case, there is amino acid sequence homology. AL type of fibril protein is produced by immunoglobulin-secreting cells and is therefore seen in association with plasma cell dyscrasias and is seen in primary systemic amyloidosis.

AA PROTEIN. AA fibril protein is composed of protein with molecular weight of 8.5-kD which is derived from larger precursor protein in the serum called SAA (serum amyloid-associated protein) with a molecular weight of 12.5-kD. Unlike AL amyloid, the deposits of AA amyloid do not have sequence homology. In the plasma, SAA circulates in association with HDL_3 (high-density lipoprotein). SAA is an acute phase reactant protein synthesised in the liver, its level being high in chronic inflammatory and traumatic conditions. SAA fibril protein is found in secondary amyloidosis which includes the largest group of diseases associated with amyloidosis.

OTHER PROTEINS. Apart from the two major forms of amyloid fibril proteins, a few other forms of proteins are found in different clinical states:

1. **Transthyretin (TTR)** is a serum protein synthesised in the liver and *transports thyroxine* and *retinol* normally (trans-thy-retin). Single amino acid substitution mutations in the structure of TTR results in variant form of protein which is responsible for amyloidosis i.e. ATTR. About 60 such mutations have been described. ATTR is the most common form of heredofamilial amyloidosis e.g. in familial amyloid polyneuropathies.

2. **Aβ₂-microglobulin (Aβ₂M)** is amyloid seen in cases of long-term haemodialysis (8-10 years). As the name suggests, $β_2M$ is a small protein which is a normal component of major histocompatibility complex (MHC) and has β -pleated sheet structure. Although the deposit due to $Aβ_2M$ may be systemic in distribution, it has predilection for bones and joints.

3. **β-amyloid protein (Aβ)** is distinct from $Aβ_2M$ and is seen in cerebral plaques as well as cerebral blood vessels in Alzheimer's disease.

4. **Immunoglobulin heavy chain amyloid (AH)** derived from truncated heavy chain of immunoglobulin is an uncommon form of systemic amyloidosis.

5. **Amyloid from hormone precursor proteins** such as pro-calcitonin, islet amyloid polypeptide, pro-insulin, prolactin, atrial notriuretic factor, and lactoferrin has also been reported in amyloid.

6. **Amyloid of prion protein (APrP)** is derived from precursor prion protein which is a plasma membrane glycoprotein. Prion proteins are proteinaceous infectious particles lacking in RNA or DNA.

7. **Miscellaneous heredofamilial forms of amyloid** These include amyloid derived from: apolipoprotein I (AApoAI), gelsolin (Agel), lysozyme (ALys), fibrinogen α-chain (AFib), and cystatin C (ACys) etc.

II. Non-fibrillar Components (p. 85)

Non-fibrillar components comprise about 5% of the amyloid material. These include the following:

1. *Amyloid P (AP)-component* synthesised in the liver and is present in all types of amyloid. It is derived from circulating serum amyloid P-component, a glycoprotein resembling the normal serum α_1-glycoprotein and is PAS-positive. It is structurally related to C-reactive protein, an acute phase reactant, but is not similar to it. By electron microscopy, it has a pentagonal profile (P-component).

2. *Apolipoprotein-E (apoE):* It is a regulator of lipoprotein metabolism and is found in all types of amyloid.

3. *Sulfated glycosaminoglycans(GAGs):* These are constituents of matrix proteins; particulary associated is heparan sulfate in all types of tissue amyloid.

4. *α-1 anti-chymotrypsin:* It is only seen in cases of AA deposits but negative in primary amyloidosis.

5. *Protein X:* This protein has been shown to be present in cases of prionoses.

PATHOGENESIS OF AMYLOIDOSIS (p. 85)

Deposition of AL Amyloid (p. 85)

1. The stimulus for production of AL amyloid is some disorder of *immunoglobulin synthesis* e.g. multiple myeloma, B cell lymphoma, other plasma cell dyscrasias.

2. Excessive immunoglobulin production is in the form of *monoclonal gammopathy* i.e. there is production of either intact immunoglobulin, or λ light chain, or κ light chain, or rarely heavy chains.

3. *Partial degradation* in the form of limited proteolysis of larger protein molecules occurs in macrophages which are anatomically closely associated with AL amyloid.

4. *Non-fibrillar components* like AP and GAGs play some role in folding and aggregation of fibril proteins.

Deposition of AA Amyloid (p. 85)

1. AA amyloid is directly related to *SAA levels.* SAA is a high density lipoprotein the levels of which are elevated in long-standing tissue destruction accompanied by chronic inflammation.

2. SAA is synthesised by the liver in response to *cytokines,* notably interleukin 1 and 6, from activated macrophages.

3. As in AL amyloid, *partial degradation* in the form of limited proteolysis takes place in reticuloendothelial cells.

4. In AA amyloid, a significant role is played by another glycoprotein, *amyloid enhancing factor (AEF).*

5. As in AL amyloid, there is a role of *AP component* and *glycosaminoglycans* in the fibril protein aggregation and to protect it from disaggregation again.

CLASSIFICATION OF AMYLOIDOSIS (p. 86)

With availability of biochemical composition of various forms of amyloid, a biochemical-based *clinicopathologic classification* is widely acceptable (Table 4.6). According to this classification, amyloidosis can be divided into 2 major categories, each found in distinct clinical settings:

A. SYSTEMIC AMYLOIDOSIS (p. 87)

1. Primary Systemic (AL) Amyloidosis (p. 87)

Primary amyloidosis consisting of AL fibril proteins is systemic or generalised in distribution. About 30% cases of AL amyloid have some form of plasma cell

Chapter Four

TABLE 4.6: Classification of Amyloidosis.

CATEGORY	ASSOCIATED DISEASE	BIOCHEM.TYPE	ORGANS COMMONLY INVOLVED
A. SYSTEMIC (GENERALISED) AMYLOIDOSIS			
1. *Primary*	Plasma cell dyscrasias	AL type	Heart, bowel, skin, nerves, kidney
2. *Secondary (Reactive)*	Chronic inflammation, cancers	AA type	Liver, spleen, kidneys, adrenals
3. *Haemodialysis associated*	Chronic renal failure	$A\beta_2M$	Synovium, joints, tendon sheaths
4. *Heredofamilial*			
i. *Hereditary polyneuropathies*	—	ATTR	Peripheral and autonomic nerves, heart
ii. *Familial Mediterranean fever*	—	AA type	Liver, spleen, kidneys, adrenals
iii. *Rare hereditary forms*	—	AApoAI, AGel, ALys, AFib, ACys	Systemic amyloidosis
B. LOCALISED AMYLOIDOSIS			
1. *Senile cardiac*	Senility	ATTR	Heart
2. *Senile cerebral*	Alzheimer's, transmissible encephalopathy	$A\beta$, APrP	Cerebral vessels, plaques, neurofibrillary tangles
3. *Endocrine*	Medullary carcinoma	Procalcitonin	Thyroid
	Diabetes type II	Proinsulin	Islets of Langerhans
4. *Tumour-forming*	Lungs, larynx, skin, urinary bladder, tongue, eye	AL	Respective anatomic location

AL= Amyloid light chain; AA= Amyloid-associated protein; $A\beta_2M$= Amyloid β_2-microglobulin; ATTR= Amyloid transthyretin; APrP= Amyloid of prion proteins, $A\beta$= β-amyloid protein).

dyscrasias, most commonly multiple myeloma (in about 10% cases), and less often other monoclonal gammopathies such as Waldenström's macroglobulinaemia, heavy chain disease, solitary plasmacytoma and nodular malignant lymphoma (B cell lymphoma). The neoplastic plasma cells usually are a single clone and, therefore, produce the same type of immunoglobulin light chain or part of light chain. Almost all cases of multiple myeloma have either λ or κ light chains (Bence Jones proteins) in the serum and are excreted in the urine. However, in contrast to normal or myeloma light chains, AL is twice more frequently derived from λ light chains. The remaining 70% cases of AL amyloid do not have evident B-cell proliferative disorder or any other associated diseases and are thus cases of true 'primary' (idiopathic) amyloidosis.

AL amyloid is most prevalent type of systemic amyloidosis in the USA. Primary amyloidosis is often severe in the heart, kidney, bowel, skin, peripheral nerves, respiratory tract, skeletal muscle, and other organs.

Treatment of AL amyloid is targetted at reducing the underlying clonal expansion of plasma cells.

2. Secondary/ Reactive (AA) Systemic Amyloidosis (p. 88)

The second form of systemic or generalised amyloidosis is reactive or inflammatory or secondary in which the fibril proteins contain AA amyloid. Secondary or reactive amyloidosis occurs typically as a complication of chronic infectious (e.g. tuberculosis, bronchiectasis, chronic osteomyelitis, chronic pyelonephritis, leprosy, chronic skin infections), non-infectious chronic inflammatory conditions associated with tissue destruction (e.g. autoimmune disorders such as rheumatoid arthritis, inflammatory bowel disease), some tumours (e.g. renal cell carcinoma, Hodgkin's disease) and in familial Mediterranean fever, an inherited disorder (discussed below).

Secondary amyloidosis is typically distributed in solid abdominal viscera like the kidney, liver, spleen and adrenals. Secondary reactive amyloidosis is seen less frequently in developed countries due to containment of infections before they become chronic but this is the most common type of amyloidosis worldwide, particularly in underdeveloped and developing countries of the world.

The contrasting features of the two main forms of systemic amyloidosis are given in Table 4.7.

3. Haemodialysis-Associated (Aβ₂M) Amyloidosis (p. 88)

Patients on long-term dialysis for more than 10 years for chronic renal failure may develop systemic amyloidosis derived from β_2-microglobulin which is normal component of MHC. The amyloid deposits are preferentially found in the vessel walls at the synovium, joints, tendon sheaths and subchondral bones.

4. Heredofamilial Amyloidosis (p. 88)

i)   Hereditary polyneuropathic (ATTR) amyloidosis. This is an autosomal dominant disorder in which amyloid is deposited in the peripheral and autonomic nerves resulting in muscular weakness, pain and paraesthesia, or may have cardiomyopathy. This type of amyloid is derived from transthyretin (ATTR) with single amino acid substitution in the structure of TTR.

ii)   Familial Mediterranean fever (AA). This is an autosomal recessive disease and is seen in people of Mediterranean region. The condition is characterised by periodic attacks of fever and polyserositis. Amyloidosis occurring in these cases is AA type, suggesting relationship to secondary amyloidosis due to chronic inflammation.

iii) Rare hereditary forms. Heredofamilial mutations of several normal proteins have been reported.

TABLE 4.7: Contrasting Features of Primary and Secondary Amyloidosis.

	FEATURE	PRIMARY AMYLOID	SECONDARY AMYLOID
1.	**Biochemical composition**	AL (Light chain proteins); lambda chains more common than kappa; sequence homology of chains	AA (Amyloid associated proteins); derived from larger precursor protein SAA; No sequence homology of polypeptide chain
2.	**Associated diseases**	Plasma cell dyscrasias e.g. multiple myeloma, B cell lymphomas, others	Chronic inflammation e.g. infections (TB, leprosy, osteomyelitis, brochiectasis), autoimmune diseases (rheumatoid arthritis, IBD), cancers (RCC, Hodgkin's disease), FMF
3.	**Pathogenesis**	Stimulus → Monoclonal B cell proliferation → Excess of Igs and light chains → Partial degradation → Insoluble AL fibril	Stimulus → Chronic inflammation → Activation of macrophages → Cytokines (IL1,6) → Partial degradation → AEF → Insoluble AA fibril
4.	**Incidence**	Most common in US and other developed countries	Most common worldwide (particularly third world countries)
5.	**Organ distribution**	Kidney, heart, bowel, nerves	Kidney, liver, spleen, adrenals
6.	**Stains to distinguish**	Congophilia persists after permanganate treatment of section; specific immuno-stains anti-λ, anti-κ	Congophilia disappears after permanganate treatment of section; specific immunostain anti-AA

B. LOCALISED AMYLOIDOSIS *(p. 89)*

1. Senile cardiac amyloidosis (ATTR). It is seen in 50% of people above the age of 70 years. The deposits are seen in the heart and aorta. The type of amyloid in these cases is ATTR but without any change in the protein structure of TTR.

2. Senile cerebral amyloidosis (Aβ, APrP). It is heterogeneous group of amyloid deposition of varying etiologies that includes sporadic, familial, hereditary and infectious. Some of the important diseases associated with cerebral amyloidosis and the corresponding amyloid proteins are:Alzheimer's disease (Aβ), Down's syndrome (Aβ) and transmissible spongiform encephalopathies (APrP).

In Alzheimer's disease, deposit of amyloid is seen as Congophilic angiopathy (amyloid material in the walls of cerebral blood vessels), neurofibrillary tangles and in senile plaques.

3. Endocrine amyloidosis (Hormone precursors). Some endocrine tumours are associated with microscopic deposits of amyloid e.g. in medullary carcinoma of the thyroid (procalcitonin), islet cell tumour of the pancreas (islet amyloid polypeptide), type 2 diabetes mellitus and insulinoma (pro-insulin), pituitary amyloid (prolactin).

4. Localised tumour forming amyloid (AL). Sometimes, isolated tumour like formation of amyloid deposits are seen e.g. in lungs, larynx, skin, urinary bladder, tongue, eye, isolated atrial amyloid. In most of these cases, the amyloid type is AL.

STAINING CHARACTERISTICS OF AMYLOID *(p. 89)*

1. STAIN ON GROSS. The oldest method since the time of Virchow for demonstrating amyloid on cut surface of a gross specimen, or on the frozen/

paraffin section is iodine stain. Lugol's iodine imparts *purple* colour to the amyloid-containing area which on addition of dilute sulfuric acid turns blue. This starch-like property of amyloid is due to AP component, a glycoprotein, present in all forms of amyloid.

2. H & E. Amyloid by light microscopy with haematoxylin and eosin staining appears as extracellular, homogeneous, structureless and eosinophilic hyaline material, especially in relation to blood vessels.

3. METACHROMATIC STAINS (ROSANILINE DYES). Amyloid has the property of metachromasia i.e. the dye reacts with amyloid and undergoes a colour change. Metachromatic stains employed are rosaniline dyes such as methyl violet and crystal violet which impart *rose-pink* colouration to amyloid deposits.

4. CONGO RED AND POLARISED LIGHT. All types of amyloid have affinity for Congo red stain; therefore this method is used for confirmation of amyloid of all types. The stain may be used on both gross specimens and microscopic sections; amyloid of all types stains *red colour*. If the stained section is viewed in polarised light, the amyloid characteristically shows *apple-green birefringence* due to cross-β-pleated sheet configuration of amyloid fibrils.

5. FLUORESCENT STAINS. Fluorescent stain thioflavin-T binds to amyloid and fluoresce *yellow* under ultraviolet light i.e. amyloid emits secondary fluorescence. Thioflavin-S is less specific.

6. IMMUNOHISTOCHEMISTRY. More recently, type of amyloid can be classified by immunohistochemical stains. Various antibody stains against the specific antigenic protein types of amyloid are commercially available. However, more useful ones are *anti-AP* for confirmation of presence of amyloid of all types, and *anti-AA*, and *anti-lambda (λ)* and *anti-kappa (κ)* antibody stains for fibril protein of specific types.

DIAGNOSIS OF AMYLOIDOSIS *(p. 90)*

1. BIOPSY EXAMINATION. Histologic examination of biopsy material is the commonest and confirmatory method for diagnosis in a suspected case of amyloidosis. Biopsy of an obviously *affected organ* is likely to offer the best results e.g. *kidney biopsy* in a case on dialysis, sural nerve biopsy in familial polyneuropathy. In systemic amyloidosis, renal biopsy provides the best detection rate, but *rectal biopsy* also has a good pick up rate. However, *gingiva* and *skin biopsy* have poor result. More recently, fine needle aspiration of abdominal *subcutaneous fat* followed by Congo red staining and polarising microscopic examination for confirmation has become an acceptable simple and useful technique with excellent result.

2. IN VIVO CONGO RED TEST. A known quantity of Congo red dye may be injected intravenously in living patient. If amyloidosis is present, the dye gets bound to amyloid deposits and its levels in blood rapidly decline.

PATHOLOGIC CHANGES IN AMYLOIDOSIS OF ORGANS *(p. 90)*

Amyloidosis of Kidneys *(p. 90)*

Amyloidosis of the kidney accounts for about 20% of deaths from amyloidosis. Even small quantities of amyloid deposits in the glomeruli can cause proteinuria and nephrotic syndrome.

G/A The kidneys may be normal-sized, enlarged or terminally contracted due to ischaemic effect of narrowing of vascular lumina. Cut surface is pale, waxy and translucent.

M/E

■ *In the glomeruli*, the deposits initially appear on the basement membrane of the glomerular capillaries, but later extend to produce luminal narrowing and distortion of the glomerular capillary tuft.

■ *In the tubules,* the amyloid deposits likewise begin close to the tubular epithelial basement membrane.

■ The *vascular involvement* affects chiefly the walls of small arterioles and venules, producing narrowing of their lumina and consequent ischaemic effects.

Amyloidosis of Spleen *(p. 92)*

1. **'SAGO SPLEEN'.** The splenomegaly is not marked and cut surface shows characteristic translucent pale and waxy nodules resembling sago grains and hence the name.

M/E The amyloid deposits begin in the walls of the arterioles of the white pulp and may subsequently replace the follicles.

2. **'LARDACEOUS SPLEEN'.** There is generally moderate to marked spleno-megaly (weight up to 1 kg). Cut surface of the spleen shows map-like areas of amyloid.

M/E The deposits involve the walls of splenic sinuses and the small arteries and in the connective tissue of the red pulp.

Amyloidosis of Liver *(p. 91)*

G/A The liver is often enlarged, pale, waxy and firm.

M/E
■ The amyloid initially appears in the space of Disse.
■ Later, as it increases, it compresses the cords of hepatocytes. However, hepatic function remains normal even at an advanced stage of the disease.

Amyloidosis of Heart *(p. 91)*

Heart is involved in systemic amyloidosis quite commonly, more so in the primary than in secondary systemic amyloidosis.

Amyloidosis of Alimentary Tract *(p. 92)*

Involvement of the gastrointestinal tract by amyloidosis may occur at any level from the oral cavity to the anus. Rectal and gingival biopsies are the common sites for diagnosis of systemic amyloidosis. The deposits are initially located around the small blood vessels but later may involve adjacent layers of the bowel wall. Tongue may be the site for tumour-forming amyloid, producing macroglossia.

■ SELF ASSESSMENT

1. **Transplantation antigens are located on portion of:**
   A. Chromosome 1   B. Chromosome 6
   C. Chromosome 9   D. Chromosome 22
2. **Class I HLA antigens are located on:**
   A. All nucleated cells of the body   B. B and T lymphocytes
   C. Macrophages   D. Complement system
3. **HIV contaminated waste products can be decontaminated by the following agents *except*:**
   A. Sodium hypochlorite   B. Methanol
   C. Formaldehyde   D. Glutaraldehyde
4. **CD4 bearing subpopulation of macrophages are attacked by HIV and cause the following *except*:**
   A. Cytopathic effects
   B. Act as reservoir of HIV infection

    C. Act as source of infection in nervous system

    D. Defects in CD4+ T lymphocytes

5. **In autoimmune haemolytic anaemia, the following type of immunologic tissue injury is involved:**
    A. Type I (anaphylactic)   B. Type II (cytotoxic)
    C. Type III (immune complex)   D. Type IV (cell mediated)

6. **Out of various antinuclear antibodies, pathognomonic of SLE is:**
    A. Antibody to single-stranded DNA
    B. Antibody to double-stranded DNA
    C. Antibody to histones
    D. Antibody to nucleolar antigen

7. **In cases of renal failure on long-term haemodialysis, there is development of following type of amyloid:**
    A. Amyloid light chain (AL)
    B. Amyloid-associated protein (AA)
    C. Amyloid β_2 microglobulin ($A\beta_2m$)
    D. β amyloid protein ($A\beta$)

8. **The most common form of amyloid in third world countries is:**
    A. Primary   B. Secondary
    C. Hereditary   D. Localised

9. **Cardiac amyloidosis often produces:**
    A. Dilated cardiomyopathy   B. Constrictive cardiomyopathy
    C. Restrictive cardiomyopathy   D. Ischaemic cardiomyopathy

10. **In senile cardiac amyloidosis, the biochemical form of amyloid is:**
    A. AL   B. AA
    C. ATTR   D. $A\beta_2M$

11. **In Alzheimer's disease, cerebral plaques consist of:**
    A. ATTR protein   B. $A\beta_2M$ protein
    C. $A\beta$ protein   D. Prion protein

12. **Amyloid enhancing factor (AEF) plays a significant role in:**
    A. Primary amyloid
    B. Secondary amyloid
    C. Senile cerebral amyloid
    D. Haemodialysis-associated amyloid

KEY

1 = B	2 = A	3 = B	4 = A	5 = B
6 = B	7 = C	8 = B	9 = C	10 = C
11 = C	12 = B			

Chapter Four

5

Haemodynamic Disorders

INTERNAL ENVIRONMENT (p. 93)

The mechanism by which the constancy of the internal environment is maintained and ensured is called the *homeostasis*. For this purpose, living membranes with varying permeabilities such as vascular endothelium and the cell wall play important role in exchange of fluids, electrolytes, nutrients and metabolites across the compartments of body fluids.

The normal composition of internal environment is as under:

1. WATER. Water is the principal and essential constituent of the body. The total body water in a normal adult male comprises 50-70% (average 60%) of the body weight and about 10% less in a normal adult female (average 50%). The total body water (assuming average of 60%) is distributed into 2 main compartments of body fluids separated from each other by membranes freely permeable to water.

i) Intracellular fluid compartment. This comprises about 33% of the body weight.

ii) Extracellular fluid compartment. This constitutes the remaining 27% of body weight containing water. Included in this are the following 4 subdivisions of extracellular fluid (ECF):

a) Interstitial fluid including lymph fluid constitutes the major proportion of ECF (12% of body weight).

b) Intravascular fluid or blood plasma comprises about 5% of the body weight. Thus plasma content is about 3 litres of fluid out of 5 litres of total blood volume.

c) Mesenchymal tissues such as dense connective tissue, cartilage and bone contain body water that comprises about 9% of the body weight.

d) Transcellular fluid constitutes 1% of body weight. This is the fluid contained in the secretions of secretory cells of the body.

2. ELECTROLYTES. *In the intracellular fluid,* the main cations are potassium and magnesium and the main anions are phosphates and proteins. It has low concentration of sodium and chloride.

In the extracellular fluid, the predominant cation is sodium and the principal anions are chloride and bicarbonate. Besides these, a small proportion of non-diffusible proteins and some diffusible nutrients and metabolites such as glucose and urea are present in the ECF.

The essential difference between the two main subdivisions of ECF is the higher protein content in the plasma than in the interstitial fluid which plays an important role in maintaining fluid balance.

ACID-BASE BALANCE (p. 95)

The pH of the blood is kept constant at 7.4 ± 0.05 in health by the following factors:

1. BUFFER SYSTEM. The most important buffer which regulates the pH of blood is *bicarbonate-carbonic acid system* followed by *intracellular buffering action of haemoglobin* and *carbonic anhydrase* in the red cells.

2. PULMONARY MECHANISM. During respiration, CO_2 is removed by the lungs depending upon the partial pressure of CO_2 in the arterial blood.

3. RENAL MECHANISM. The other route by which H$^+$ ions can be excreted from the body is in the urine by:
- *combining with phosphates* to form phosphoric acid;
- *combining with ammonia* to form ammonium ions; and
- *combining with filtered bicarbonate ions* to form carbonic acid.

PRESSURE GRADIENTS AND FLUID EXCHANGES *(p. 95)*

1. OSMOTIC PRESSURE. This is the pressure exerted by the chemical constituents of the body fluids. Accordingly, osmotic pressure may be of the following types:

- **Crystalloid osmotic pressure** exerted by electrolytes present in the ECF and comprises the major portion of the total osmotic pressure.
- **Colloid osmotic pressure or oncotic pressure** exerted by proteins present in the ECF and constitutes a small part of the total osmotic pressure but is more significant physiologically. Since the protein content of the plasma is higher than that of interstitial fluid, oncotic pressure of plasma is higher (average 25 mmHg) than that of interstitial fluid (average 8 mmHg).
- **Effective oncotic pressure** is the difference between the higher oncotic pressure of plasma and the lower oncotic pressure of interstitial fluid and is *the force that tends to draw fluid into the vessels.*

2. HYDROSTATIC PRESSURE. This is the capillary blood pressure.

There is considerable *pressure gradient* at the two ends of capillary loop—being higher at the arteriolar end (average 32 mmHg) than at the venular end (average 12 mmHg).

- **Tissue tension** is the hydrostatic pressure of interstitial fluid and is lower than the hydrostatic pressure in the capillary at either end (average 4 mmHg).
- **Effective hydrostatic pressure** is the difference between the higher hydrostatic pressure in the capillary and the lower tissue tension; it is *the force that drives fluid through the capillary wall into the interstitial space.*

Normally, the fluid exchanges between the body compartments take place as under:

- *At the arteriolar end of the capillary,* the balance between the hydrostatic pressure (32 mmHg) and plasma oncotic pressure (25 mmHg) is the hydrostatic pressure of 7 mmHg which is the outward-driving force so that a small quantity of fluid and solutes leave the vessel to enter the interstitial space.
- *At the venular end of the capillary,* the balance between the hydrostatic pressure (12 mmHg) and plasma oncotic pressure (25 mmHg) is the oncotic pressure of 13 mmHg which is the inward-driving force so that the fluid and solutes re-enter the plasma.
- *The tissue fluid* left after exchanges across the capillary wall escapes into the lymphatics from where it is finally drained into venous circulation.
- *Tissue factors* i.e. oncotic pressure of interstitial fluid and tissue tension, are normally small and insignificant forces opposing the plasma hydrostatic pressure and capillary hydrostatic pressure, respectively.

DISTURBANCES OF BODY FLUIDS AND ELECTROLYTES *(p. 97)*

OEDEMA *(p. 97)*

Oedema may be defined as abnormal and excessive accumulation of fluid in the interstitial tissue spaces and serous cavities. The oedema may be of 2 main types:

1. *Localised* in the organ or limb; and
2. *Generalised (anasarca or dropsy)* when it is systemic in distribution, particularly noticeable in the subcutaneous tissues.

Chapter Five

In the case of oedema in the subcutaneous tissues, momentary pressure of finger produces a depression known as *pitting oedema*. The other variety is *non-pitting* or *solid oedema* in which no pitting is produced on pressure e.g. in myxoedema, elephantiasis. Oedema fluid may be:

■ *transudate* which is more often the case, such as in oedema of cardiac and renal disease; or

■ *exudate* such as in inflammatory oedema.

The differences between transudate and exudate are tabulated in Table 5.1.

TABLE 5.1: Differences between Transudate and Exudate.

FEATURE	TRANSUDATE	EXUDATE
1. *Definition*	Filtrate of blood plasma without changes in endothelial permeability	Oedema of inflamed tissue associated with increased vascular permeability
2. *Character*	Non-inflammatory oedema	Inflammatory oedema
3. *Protein content*	Low (less than 1 g/dl); mainly albumin, low fibrinogen; hence no tendency to coagulate	High (2.5-3.5 g/dl), readily coagulates due to high content of fibrinogen and other coagulation factors
4. *Glucose content*	Same as in plasma	Low (less than 60 mg/dl)
5. *Specific gravity*	Low (less than 1.015)	High (more than 1.018)
6. *pH*	> 7.3	< 7.3
7. *LDH*	Low	High
8. *Effusion LDH/ Serum LDH ratio*	< 0.6	> 0.6
9. *Cells*	Few cells, mainly mesothelial cells and cellular debris	Many cells, inflammatory as well as parenchymal
10. *Examples*	Oedema in congestive cardiac failure	Purulent exudate such as pus

PATHOGENESIS OF OEDEMA *(p. 97)*

The following six mechanisms may be operating singly or in combination to produce oedema:

1. DECREASED PLASMA ONCOTIC PRESSURE. A fall in the total plasma protein level (hypoproteinaemia of less than 5 g/dl), results in lowering of plasma oncotic pressure in a way that it can no longer counteract the effect of hydrostatic pressure of blood. This results in increased outward movement of fluid from the capillary wall and decreased inward movement of fluid from the interstitial space causing oedema. Hypoproteinaemia usually produces generalised oedema (anasarca). Out of the various plasma proteins, albumin has four times higher plasma oncotic pressure than globulin.

The **examples** of oedema by this mechanism are:

i) Oedema of renal disease

ii) Ascites of liver disease

iii) Oedema due to other causes of hypoproteinaemia.

2. INCREASED CAPILLARY HYDROSTATIC PRESSURE. The hydrostatic pressure of the capillary is the force that normally tends to drive fluid through the capillary wall into the interstitial space by counteracting the force of plasma oncotic pressure. A rise in the hydrostatic pressure at the venular end of the capillary which is normally low (average 12 mmHg) to a level more than the plasma oncotic pressure results in minimal or no reabsorption of fluid at the venular end, consequently leading to oedema.

The **examples** of oedema by this mechanism are:

i) *Oedema of cardiac disease* e.g. in congestive cardiac failure, constrictive pericarditis.

ii) *Ascites of liver disease* e.g. in cirrhosis of liver.

iii) *Passive congestion* e.g. in mechanical obstruction due to thrombosis of veins of the lower legs, varicosities, pressure by pregnant uterus, tumours etc.

iv) *Postural oedema.*

3. LYMPHATIC OBSTRUCTION. Normally the interstitial fluid in the tissue spaces escapes by way of lymphatics so that obstruction to outflow of these channels causes localised oedema, known as lymphoedema.

The **examples** of lymphoedema are:

i) Removal of axillary lymph nodes in radical mastectomy for carcinoma of the breast.

ii) Pressure from outside on the main abdominal or thoracic duct such as due to tumours.

iii) Inflammation of the lymphatics as seen in filariasis.

iv) Occlusion of lymphatic channels by malignant cells.

v) Milroy's disease or hereditary lymphoedema.

4. TISSUE FACTORS. The forces acting in the interstitial space—oncotic pressure of the interstitial space and tissue tension, in combination with other mechanisms play a role in causation of oedema.

5. INCREASED CAPILLARY PERMEABILITY. When the capillary endothelium is injured by various 'capillary poisons' such as toxins and their products, histamine, anoxia, venoms, certain drugs and chemicals, the capillary permeability to plasma proteins is enhanced due to development of gaps between the endothelial cells. This, in turn, causes reduced plasma oncotic pressure and elevated oncotic pressure of interstitial fluid which consequently produces oedema.

The **examples** of oedema by this mechanism are:

i) *Generalised oedema* due to increased vascular permeability may occur in systemic infections, poisonings, certain drugs and chemicals, anaphylactic reactions and anoxia.

ii) *Localised oedema* such as *inflammatory oedema, angioneurotic oedema*.

6. SODIUM AND WATER RETENTION. Excessive retention of sodium and water and their decreased renal excretion occur in response to hypovolaemia and lowered concentration of sodium in the renal tubules via stimulation of intrinsic renal and extra-renal mechanisms as well as via release of ADH.

The **examples** of oedema by these mechanism are:

i) *Oedema of cardiac disease* e.g. in congestive cardiac failure.

ii) *Ascites of liver disease* e.g. in cirrhosis of liver.

iii) *Oedema of renal disease* e.g. in nephrotic syndrome, glomerulonephritis.

PATHOGENESIS AND MORPHOLOGY OF
IMPORTANT TYPES OF OEDEMA *(p. 99)*

Renal Oedema *(p. 99)*

1. Oedema in nephrotic syndrome. Since there is persistent and heavy proteinuria (albuminuria) in nephrotic syndrome, there is hypoalbuminaemia causing decreased plasma oncotic pressure resulting in severe generalised oedema *(nephrotic oedema)*. The hypoalbuminaemia causes fall in the plasma volume activating renin-angiotensin-aldosterone mechanism which results in retention of sodium and water.

2. Oedema in glomerulonephritis. Oedema occurs in conditions with diffuse glomerular disease such as in acute diffuse glomerulonephritis and rapidly progressive glomerulonephritis *(nephritic oedema)*. In contrast to nephrotic oedema, nephritic oedema is not due to hypoproteinaemia but is due to excessive reabsorption of sodium and water in the renal tubules via renin-angiotensin-aldosterone mechanism. The protein content of oedema fluid in glomerulonephritis is quite low (less than 0.5 g/dl).

The salient differences between the nephrotic and nephritic oedema are outlined in Table 5.2.

TABLE 5.2: Differences between Nephrotic and Nephritic Oedema.

FEATURE	NEPHROTIC OEDEMA	NEPHRITIC OEDEMA
1. *Cause*	Nephrotic syndrome	Glomerulonephritis (acute, rapidly progressive)
2. *Proteinuria*	Heavy	Moderate
3. *Mechanism*	↓ Plasma oncotic pressure, Na⁺ and water retention	Na⁺ and water retention
4. *Degree of oedema*	Severe, generalised	Mild
5. *Distribution*	Subcutaneous tissues as well as visceral organs	Loose tissues mainly (face, eyes, ankles, genitalia)

3. Oedema in acute tubular injury. Acute tubular injury following shock or toxic chemicals results in gross oedema of the body. The damaged tubules lose their capacity for selective reabsorption and concentration of the glomerular filtrate resulting in increased reabsorption and oliguria.

Cardiac Oedema *(p. 101)*

Generalised oedema develops in right-sided and congestive cardiac failure. Pathogenesis of cardiac oedema is explained on the basis of the following hypotheses:

1. Reduced cardiac output causes hypovolaemia which stimulates intrinsic-renal and extra-renal hormonal (renin-angiotensin-aldosterone) mechanisms as well as ADH secretion resulting in sodium and water retention and consequent oedema.

2. Due to heart failure, there is elevated central venous pressure which is transmitted backward to the venous end of the capillaries, raising the capillary hydrostatic pressure and consequent transudation.

3. Chronic hypoxia may injure the capillary wall causing increased capillary permeability and result in oedema.

In left heart failure, the changes are, however, different. There is venous congestion, particularly in the lungs, so that pulmonary oedema develops rather than generalised oedema.

Cardiac oedema is influenced by gravity and is thus characteristically *dependent oedema* i.e. in an ambulatory patient it is on the lower extremities, while in a bed-ridden patient oedema appears on the sacral and genital areas.

Pulmonary Oedema *(p. 102)*

Acute pulmonary oedema is the most important form of local oedema as it causes serious functional impairment but has special features.

ETIOPATHOGENESIS. The hydrostatic pressure in the pulmonary capillaries is much lower (average 10 mmHg). Normally the plasma oncotic pressure is adequate to prevent the escape of fluid into the interstitial space and hence lungs are normally free of oedema. Pulmonary oedema can result from either the elevation of pulmonary hydrostatic pressure or the increased capillary permeability.

1. Elevation in pulmonary hydrostatic pressure (Haemodynamic oedema). In heart failure, there is increase in the pressure in pulmonary veins which is transmitted to pulmonary capillaries. This results in imbalance between pulmonary hydrostatic pressure and the plasma oncotic pressure so that excessive fluid moves out of pulmonary capillaries into the interstitium of the lungs. Simultaneously, endothelium of the pulmonary capillaries develops fenestrations permitting passage of plasma proteins and fluid into the inter-stitium. As the capacity of the lymphatics to drain the fluid is exceeded (about ten-fold increase in fluid), the excess fluid starts accumulating in the interstitium (*interstitial oedema*). Next follows the thickening of the alveolar walls because of the interstitial oedema. However, prolonged elevation of hydrostatic pressure and due to high pressure of interstitial oedema, the alveolar lining cells break and the alveolar air spaces are flooded with fluid (*alveolar oedema*) driving the air out of alveolus, thus seriously hampering the lung function.

Pulmonary oedema by this mechanism is seen in left heart failure, mitral stenosis, pulmonary vein obstruction, thyrotoxicosis.

2. Increased vascular permeability (Irritant oedema). The vascular endothelium as well as the alveolar epithelial cells (alveolo-capillary membrane) may be damaged causing increased vascular permeability so that excessive fluid and plasma proteins leak out, initially into the interstitium and subsequently into the alveoli.

This mechanism explains pulmonary oedema in fulminant pulmonary and extrapulmonary infections, inhalation of toxic substances, aspiration, shock, radiation injury, hypersensitivity to drugs or antisera, uraemia and adult respiratory distress syndrome (ARDS).

3. Acute high altitude oedema. Individuals climbing to high altitude suddenly without halts and without waiting for acclimatisation to set in, suffer from serious circulatory and respiratory ill-effects. Commonly, the deleterious effects begin to appear after an altitude of 2500 metres is reached. These changes include: appearance of oedema fluid in the lungs, congestion and widespread minute haemorrhages. The underlying mechanism appears to be anoxic damage to the pulmonary vessels.

G/A The lungs in pulmonary oedema are heavy, moist and subcrepitant. Cut surface exudes frothy fluid (mixture of air and fluid).

M/E The alveolar capillaries are congested. Initially the excess fluid collects in the interstitial lung spaces (interstitial oedema) but later the fluid fills the alveolar spaces (alveolar oedema). The interstitium as well as the alveolar spaces thus contain an eosinophilic, granular and pink proteinaceous material, often admixed with some RBCs and macrophages.

In chronically elevated venous pressure, known as chronic passive congestion of lung or *brown induration*, the lungs are firm and heavy. The sectioned surface is rusty brown in colour. *Microscopically*, the alveolar septa are widened and the alveolar spaces contain numerous haemosiderin-laden macrophages (heart failure cells).

Cerebral Oedema (p. 103)

The mechanism of fluid exchange in the brain differs from elsewhere in the body since there are no draining lymphatics in the brain but instead, the function of fluid-electrolyte exchange is performed by the blood-brain barrier located at the endothelial cells of the capillaries.

Chapter Five

Cerebral oedema can be of 3 types:

1. VASOGENIC OEDEMA. This is the most common type and corresponds to oedema elsewhere resulting from increased filtration pressure or increased capillary permeability. Vasogenic oedema is prominent around cerebral contusions, infarcts, brain abscess and some tumours.

2. CYTOTOXIC OEDEMA. In this type, the blood-brain barrier is intact and the fluid accumulation is intracellular. The underlying mechanism is disturbance in the cellular osmoregulation as occurs in some metabolic derangements, acute hypoxia and with some toxic chemicals.

3. INTERSTITIAL OEDEMA. This type of cerebral oedema occurs when the excessive fluid crosses the ependymal lining of the ventricles and accumulates in the periventricular white matter. This mechanism is responsible for oedema in non-communicating hydrocephalus.

OVERHYDRATION *(p. 104)*

Overhydration is a state of pure water excess or water intoxication. Overhydration is encountered in the following conditions:

1. Acute and chronic renal disease
2. Severe congestive heart failure
3. Addison's disease
4. Cirrhosis of the liver
5. Tumours producing ADH e.g. bronchogenic carcinoma
6. Early postoperative period when patient is on infusion of glucose solution but is incapable of diluting the urine due to liberation of vasopressin (ADH) by the stress of surgery.

DEHYDRATION *(p. 104)*

Dehydration or pure water deficiency is a state of deprivation of water without corresponding loss of electrolytes. Pure water deficiency is less common than salt depletion but can occur in the following conditions:

1. Deficient water intake e.g. in dysphagia, obstructive lesion in oesophagus, starvation, intense weakness, coma.

2. Excessive loss of water e.g. in diabetes insipidus, hyperparathyroidism, pyrexia, hyperapnoea.

DISTURBANCES OF ELECTROLYTES *(p. 104)*

COMBINED SODIUM AND WATER DEFICIENCY *(p. 104)*

Combined sodium and water deficiency is more common than deficiency of either component separately. It is commonly called salt depletion because both sodium and chloride are lost equally. Loss of sodium and water can occur in the following conditions:

1. Gastrointestinal disorders e.g. severe vomitings, diarrhoea.
2. Excess loss via the sweat.
3. Excess loss via urine e.g. in patients of heart failure on diuretics, Addison's disease, advanced diabetes mellitus.
4. Excess loss via blood and plasma e.g. in severe haemorrhage, extensive burns.

ABNORMALITIES OF THE pH OF BLOOD *(p. 105)*

The pH of blood depends upon 2 principal factors:
■ the *concentration of bicarbonate;* and
■ the *partial pressure of CO_2* that determines the concentration of carbonic acid.

Accordingly, the disorders of the pH of the blood can be of 2 types:

1. *alterations in the blood bicarbonate* levels (metabolic acidosis and alkalosis); and

2. *alteration in* Pco_2 which depends upon the ventilatory function of the lungs (respiratory acidosis and alkalosis).

HAEMODYNAMIC DISTURBANCES *(p. 106)*

Derangements of blood flow or haemodynamic disturbances are considered under 2 broad headings:

I. *Disturbances in the volume of the circulating blood.* These include: hyperaemia and congestion, haemorrhage and shock.

II. *Circulatory disturbances of obstructive nature.* These are: thrombosis, embolism, ischaemia and infarction.

HYPERAEMIA AND CONGESTION *(p. 106)*

Hyperaemia and congestion are the terms used for increased volume of blood within dilated vessels of an organ or tissue; the increased volume from arterial and arteriolar dilatation being referred to as *hyperaemia or active hyperaemia*, whereas the impaired venous drainage is called *venous congestion or passive hyperaemia*.

Active Hyperaemia *(p. 106)*

The dilatation of arteries, arterioles and capillaries is effected either through sympathetic neurogenic mechanism or via the release of vasoactive substances. The affected tissue or organ is pink or red in appearance (erythema).

The **examples** of active hyperaemia are:

- Inflammation e.g. congested vessels in the walls of alveoli in pneumonia.
- Blushing i.e. flushing of the skin of face in response to emotions.
- Menopausal flush.
- Muscular exercise.
- High grade fever.

Passive Hyperaemia (Venous Congestion) *(p. 106)*

The dilatation of veins and capillaries due to impaired venous drainage results in passive hyperaemia or venous congestion, commonly referred to as *congestion*. Congestion may be acute or chronic, the latter being more common and called *chronic venous congestion* (CVC). The affected tissue or organ is bluish in colour due to accumulation of venous blood (cyanosis). Venous congestion is of 2 types:

- *Local venous congestion* results from obstruction to the venous outflow from an organ or part of the body e.g. portal venous obstruction in cirrhosis of the liver, outside pressure on the vessel wall as occurs in tight bandage, plasters, tumours, pregnancy, hernia etc, or intraluminal occlusion by thrombosis.

- *Systemic (General) venous congestion* is engorgement of systemic veins e.g. in left-sided and right-sided heart failure and diseases of the lungs which interfere with pulmonary blood flow like pulmonary fibrosis, emphysema etc. Usually the fluid accumulates upstream to the specific chamber of the heart which is initially affected. For example, in *left-sided heart failure* (such as due to mechanical overload in aortic stenosis, or due to weakened left ventricular wall as in myocardial infarction) pulmonary congestion results, whereas in *right-sided heart failure* (such as due to pulmonary stenosis or pulmonary hypertension) systemic venous congestion results.

MORPHOLOGY OF CVC OF ORGANS *(p. 107)*

CVC Lung *(p. 107)*

Chronic venous congestion of lung occurs in left heart failure, especially in rheumatic mitral stenosis so that there is consequent rise in pulmonary venous pressure.

G/A The lungs are heavy and firm in consistency. The sectioned surface is dark brown in colour referred to as *brown induration* of the lungs.

M/E The alveolar septa are widened due to the presence of interstitial oedema as well as due to dilated and congested capillaries. The septa are mildly thickened due to slight increase in fibrous connective tissue. Rupture of dilated and congested capillaries may result in minute intra-alveolar haemorrhages. The breakdown of erythrocytes liberates haemosiderin pigment which is taken up by alveolar macrophages, so called *heart failure cells,* present in the alveolar lumina.

CVC Liver *(p. 107)*

Chronic venous congestion of the liver occurs in right heart failure and sometimes due to occlusion of inferior vena cava and hepatic vein.

G/A The liver is enlarged and tender and the capsule is tense. Cut surface shows characteristic *nutmeg* liver due to red and yellow mottled appearance.

M/E The changes of congestion are more marked in the centrilobular zone due to severe hypoxia than in the peripheral zone. The central veins as well as the adjacent sinusoids are distended and filled with blood. The centrilobular hepatocytes undergo degenerative changes, and eventually *centrilobular haemorrhagic necrosis* may be seen. Long-standing cases may show fine centrilobular fibrosis and regeneration of hepatocytes, resulting in cardiac cirrhosis. The peripheral zone of the lobule is less severely affected by chronic hypoxia and shows some *fatty change* in the hepatocytes.

CVC Spleen *(p. 108)*

Chronic venous congestion of the spleen occurs in right heart failure and in portal hypertension from cirrhosis of liver.

G/A The spleen in early stage is slightly to moderately enlarged (upto 250 g as compared to normal 150 g), while in long-standing cases there is progressive enlargement and may weigh upto 500 to 1000 g.

M/E The red pulp shows congestion and marked sinusoidal dilatation with areas of recent and old haemorrhages. These haemorrhages may get organised and form Gamna-Gandy bodies or siderofibrotic nodules which are deposits of haemosiderin pigment and calcium salts on fibrous connective tissue and elastic fibres. The reticulin-network as well as fibrous trabeculae are thickened. The advanced stage seen more commonly in hepatic cirrhosis is called *congestive splenomegaly* and is the commonest cause of hypersplenism.

HAEMORRHAGE *(p. 109)*

Haemorrhage is the escape of blood from a blood vessel. The bleeding may occur *externally, or internally* into the serous cavities (e.g. haemothorax, haemoperitoneum, haemopericardium) or into a hollow viscus. Extravasation of blood into the tissues with resultant swelling is known as *haematoma.* Large extravasations of blood into the skin and mucous membranes are called *ecchymoses. Purpuras* are small areas of haemorrhages (upto 1 cm) into the skin and mucous membrane, whereas *petechiae* are minute pinhead-sized haemorrhages. Microscopic escape of erythrocytes into loose tissues may occur following marked congestion and is known as *diapedesis.*

The various causes of haemorrhage are:

1. *Trauma* to the vessel wall
2. *Spontaneous haemorrhage* e.g. rupture of an aneurysm
3. *Inflammatory lesions of the vessel wall*
4. *Neoplastic invasion*
5. *Vascular diseases* e.g. atherosclerosis
6. *Elevated pressure within the vessels* e.g. cerebral and retinal haemorrhage in systemic hypertension.

The effects of blood loss depend upon 3 main factors:

- the amount of blood loss;
- the speed of blood loss; and
- the site of the haemorrhage.

A sudden loss of 33% of blood volume may cause death, while loss of upto 50% of blood volume over a period of 24 hours may not be necessarily fatal. However, chronic blood loss generally produces an iron deficiency anaemia, whereas acute haemorrhage may lead to serious immediate consequences such as hypovolaemic shock.

SHOCK *(p. 109)*

Shock is defined as a clinical state of cardiovascular collapse characterised by:

- an acute reduction of effective circulating blood volume; and
- an inadequate perfusion of cells and tissues.

The end result is hypotension and cellular hypoxia and, if uncompensated, may lead to impaired cellular metabolism and death. Shock may be of 2 main types:

PRIMARY OR INITIAL SHOCK. It is transient and usually a benign vasovagal attack resulting from sudden reduction of venous return to the heart caused by neurogenic vasodilatation and consequent peripheral pooling of blood. The attack usually lasts for a few seconds or minutes.

SECONDARY OR TRUE SHOCK. This is the form of shock which occurs due to haemodynamic derangements with hypoperfusion of the cells. This type of shock is the true shock which is commonly referred to as 'shock' if not specified.

Etiology and Classification *(p. 110)*

Shock is classified into 3 main etiologic forms:

1. HYPOVOLAEMIC SHOCK. Reduction in blood volume induces hypovolaemic shock. The causes of hypovolaemia include the following:

i) *Severe haemorrhage* (external or internal) e.g. in trauma, surgery.

ii) *Fluid loss* e.g. in severe burns, crush injury to a limb, persistent vomitings and severe diarrhoea causing dehydration.

2. SEPTIC SHOCK. Severe bacterial infections or septicaemia induce septic shock. The predominant causes are as under:

i) **Gram-negative septicaemia (endotoxic shock)** e.g. infection with *E. coli, Proteus, Klebsiella, Pseudomonas* and bacteroides. Endotoxins of gram-negative bacilli have been implicated as the most important mediator of septic shock.

ii) **Gram-positive septicaemia (exotoxic shock)** is less common e.g. infection with streptococci, pneumococci.

Lysis of gram-negative bacteria releases endotoxin, a lipopolysaccharide (LPS), into circulation where it binds to lipopolysaccharide-binding protein (LBP). The complex of LPS-LBP binds to CD14 molecule on the surface of the monocyte/macrophage which in turn is stimulated to elaborate tumour necrosis factor-α (TNF-α). TNF-α induces septic shock by endothelial cell injury.

3. CARDIOGENIC SHOCK. Acute circulatory failure with sudden fall in cardiac output from acute diseases of the heart without actual reduction of blood volume (normovolaemia) results in cardiogenic shock. The causes are:

i) Deficient emptying e.g. myocardial infarction, rupture of the heart, cardiac arrhythmias

ii) Deficient filling e.g. cardiac tamponade from haemopericardium

iii) Obstruction to the outflow e.g. pulmonary embolism, ball valve thrombus.

Pathogenesis *(p. 111)*

There are 2 basic features in the pathogenesis of shock:

1. REDUCED EFFECTIVE CIRCULATING VOLUME. It may result by either of the following mechanisms:

i) by actual loss of blood volume as occurs in hypovolaemic shock; or

ii) by decreased cardiac output without actual loss of blood (normovolaemia) as occurs in cardiogenic shock and septic shock.

2. TISSUE ANOXIA. Following reduction in the effective circulating blood volume from either of the above two mechanisms and from any of the etiologic agents, there is decreased venous return to the heart resulting in decreased cardiac output. This consequently causes reduced supply of oxygen to the organs and tissues and hence tissue anoxia, and shock ensues.

In contrast to hypovolaemic and cardiogenic shock, patients in septic shock have hyperdynamic circulation due to peripheral vasodilatation and pooling of blood, as well as there is increased vascular permeability. This results in reduction of effective circulating blood volume, lowered cardiac output, reduced blood flow (hypotension) and inadequate perfusion of cells and tissues. Disseminated intravascular coagulation (DIC) is prone to develop in septic shock due to endothelial cell injury by toxins.

Stages of Shock *(p. 112)*

Deterioration of the circulation in shock is a progressive phenomenon and can be divided arbitrarily into 3 stages:

1. NON-PROGRESSIVE (INITIAL, COMPENSATED REVERSIBLE) SHOCK. In the early stage of shock, an attempt is made to maintain adequate cerebral and coronary blood supply by redistribution of blood so that the vital organs (brain and heart) are adequately perfused and oxygenated. This is achieved by activation of various neurohormonal mechanisms causing *widespread vasoconstriction* and by *fluid conservation by the kidney.* If the condition that caused the shock is adequately treated, the compensatory mechanism may be able to bring about recovery and re-establish the normal circulation.

2. PROGRESSIVE DECOMPENSATED SHOCK. This is a stage when the patient suffers from some other stress or risk factors (e.g. pre-existing cardiovascular and lung disease) besides persistence of the shock so that there is progressive deterioration. The effects of progressive decompensated shock due to tissue hypoperfusion are as under:

a) Pulmonary hypoperfusion with resultant tachypnoea and adult respiratory distress syndrome.

b) Tissue anoxia causing anaerobic glycolysis results in metabolic lactic acidosis. Lactic acidosis lowers the tissue pH which in turn makes the vasomotor response ineffective. This results in vasodilation and peripheral pooling of blood.

3. DECOMPENSATED (IRREVERSIBLE) SHOCK. When the shock is so severe that in spite of compensatory mechanisms and despite therapy and control of etiologic agent which caused the shock, no recovery takes place, it is called decompensated or irreversible shock. Its effects due to widespread cell injury include the following:

a) Progressive fall in the blood pressure due to deterioration in cardiac output attributed to release of myocardial depressant factor (MDF).

b) Severe metabolic acidosis due to anaerobic glycolysis.

c) Respiratory distress due to pulmonary oedema, tachypnoea and adult respiratory distress syndrome (ARDS).

d) Ischaemic cell death of brain, heart and kidneys due to reduced blood supply to these organs.

Clinically, at this stage the patient has features of coma, worsened heart function and progressive renal failure due to acute tubular necrosis.

A number of hypotheses or factors have been described in irreversibility of shock, with tissue anoxia occupying the central role. These are as under:

i)   Persistence of widespread vasoconstriction.

ii) Vasodilatation and increased vascular permeability.

iii) Myocardial ischaemia.

iv) Cerebral ischaemia.

v)   Vasodepressor material (VDM).

vi) Tumour necrosis factor (TNF).

vii) Intestinal factor.

viii) Bacterial factor.

ix) Hypercoagulability of blood.

Morphologic Complications in Shock *(p. 114)*

Eventually, shock is characterised by multisystem failure. The morphologic changes in shock are due to hypoxia resulting in degeneration and necrosis in various organs.

1. HYPOXIC ENCEPHALOPATHY. Cerebral ischaemia in compensated shock may produce altered state of consciousness. However, if the blood pressure falls below 50 mmHg as occurs in systemic hypotension in prolonged shock and cardiac arrest, brain suffers from serious ischaemic damage with loss of cortical functions, coma, and a vegetative state.

2. HEART IN SHOCK. Heart is more vulnerable to the effects of hypoxia than any other organ. Heart is affected in cardiogenic as well as in other forms of shock. There are 2 types of morphologic changes in heart in all types of shock:

i) Haemorrhages and necrosis.

ii) Zonal lesions.

3. SHOCK LUNG. Lungs due to dual blood supply are generally not affected by hypovolaemic shock but in septic shock the morphologic changes in lungs are quite prominent termed 'shock lung'.

4. SHOCK KIDNEY. One of the important complications of shock is irreversible renal injury, first noted in persons who sustained crush injuries in building collapses in air raids in World War II. The renal ischaemia following systemic hypotension is considered responsible for renal changes in shock. The end-result is generally anuria and death.

5. ADRENALS IN SHOCK. The adrenals show stress response in shock. This includes release of aldosterone in response to hypoxic kidney, release of glucocorticoids from adrenal cortex and catecholamines like adrenaline from adrenal medulla. In severe shock, adrenal haemorrhages may occur.

6. HAEMORRHAGIC GASTROENTEROPATHY. The hypoperfusion of the alimentary tract in conditions such as shock and cardiac failure may result in mucosal and mural infarction called haemorrhagic gastroenteropathy.

Clinical Features *(p. 115)*

The classical features of decompensated shock are characterised by *depression of 4 vital processes:*

- Very low blood pressure
- Subnormal temperature
- Feeble and irregular pulse
- Shallow and sighing respiration

In addition, the patients in shock have pale face, sunken eyes, weakness, cold and clammy skin. Renal dysfunction in shock is clinically characterised by a phase of oliguria due to ATN and a later phase of diuresis due to regeneration of tubular epithelium. Haemoconcentration is present in early oliguric phase while marked electrolyte imbalance occurs in diuretic phase. With progression of the condition, the patient may develop stupor, coma and death.

THROMBOSIS *(p. 115)*

Thrombosis is the process of formation of solid mass in circulation from the constituents of flowing blood; the mass itself is called a *thrombus*. A *blood clot* is the mass of coagulated blood formed *in vitro* e.g. in a test tube. *Haematoma* is the extravascular accumulation of blood clot e.g. into the tissues. *Haemostatic plugs* are the blood clots formed in healthy individuals at the site of bleeding e.g. in injury to the blood vessel. Thrombi developing in the unruptured cardiovascular system may be life-threatening by causing one of the following harmful effects:

1. Ischaemic injury. Thrombi may decrease or stop the blood supply to part of an organ or tissue and cause ischaemia which may subsequently result in infarction.

2. Thromboembolism. The thrombus or its part may get dislodged and be carried along in the bloodstream as embolus to lodge in a distant vessel.

Pathophysiology *(p. 115)*

Since the protective haemostatic plug formed as a result of normal haemostasis is an example of thrombosis, it is essential to describe *thrombogenesis* in relation to the normal haemostatic mechanism.

Virchow described three primary events which predispose to thrombus formation *(Virchow's triad):* endothelial injury, alteration in flow of blood, and hypercoagulability of blood. These events are discussed below:

1. ROLE OF BLOOD VESSEL WALL. The integrity of blood vessel wall is important for maintaining normal blood flow. An intact endothelium has the following functions:

i) It *protects* the flowing blood from the thrombogenic influence of subendothelium.

ii) It elaborates a few *anti-thrombotic* factors (thrombosis inhibitory factors).

iii) It can release a few *prothrombotic factors* which have procoagulant properties (thrombosis favouring factors).

Vascular injury exposes the subendothelial connective tissue (e.g. collagen, elastin, fibronectin, laminin and glycosaminoglycans) which are thrombogenic and thus plays important role in initiating haemostasis as well as thrombosis. A number of factors and conditions may cause vascular injury and predispose to the formation of thrombi:

i) Endocardial injury in myocardial infarction, myocarditis, cardiac surgery, prosthetic valves.

ii) Ulcerated plaques in advanced atherosclerosis.

iii) Haemodynamic stress in hypertension.

iv) Arterial diseases.

v) Diabetes mellitus.

vi) Endogenous chemical agents such as hypercholesterolaemia, endotoxins.

vii) Exogenous chemical agents such as cigarette smoke.

2. ROLE OF PLATELETS. Following endothelial cell injury, platelets come to play a central role in normal haemostasis as well as in thrombosis. The sequence of events is as under:

i) Platelet adhesion. The platelets in circulation recognise the site of endothelial injury and adhere to exposed subendothelial collagen *(primary aggregation)*, von Willebrand's factor is required for such adhesion between platelets and collagen.

ii) Platelet release reaction. The activated platelets then undergo release reaction by which the platelet granules are released to the exterior. Two main types of platelet granules are released:

a) *Alpha granules* containing fibrinogen, fibronectin, platelet-derived growth factor, platelet factor 4 (an antiheparin) and cationic proteins.

b) *Dense bodies* containing ADP (adenosine diphosphate), ionic calcium, 5-HT (serotonin), histamine and epinephrine.

iii) Platelet aggregation. Following release of ADP, a potent platelet aggregating agent, aggregation of additional platelets takes place *(secondary aggregation)*. This results in formation of temporary haemostatic plug. However, stable haemostatic plug is formed by the action of fibrin, thrombin and thromboxane A_2.

3. ROLE OF COAGULATION SYSTEM. Coagulation mechanism is the conversion of the plasma fibrinogen into solid mass of fibrin. The coagulation system is involved in both haemostatic process and thrombus formation.

4. HYPERCOAGULABILITY OF BLOOD. The occurrence of thrombosis in some conditions such as in nephrotic syndrome, advanced cancers, extensive trauma, burns and during puerperium is explained on the basis of hypercoagulability of blood. The effect of hypercoagulability on thrombosis is favoured by advancing age, smoking, use of oral contraceptives and obesity. Hypercoagulability may occur by the following changes in the composition of blood:

i) *Increase in coagulation factors* e.g. fibrinogen, prothrombin, factor VIIa, VIIIa and Xa.

ii) Increase in *platelet count* and their adhesiveness.

iii) Decreased levels of *coagulation inhibitors* e.g. antithrombin III, fibrin split products.

5. ALTERATION OF BLOOD FLOW. Formation of arterial and cardiac thrombi is facilitated by turbulence in the blood flow, while stasis initiates the venous thrombi even without evidence of endothelial injury.

Morphology of Various Types *(p. 118)*

G/A Thrombi may be of various shapes, sizes and composition depending upon the site of origin. Arterial thrombi tend to be white and mural while the venous thrombi are red and occlusive. Mixed or laminated thrombi are also common and consist of alternate white and red layers called lines of Zahn. Red thrombi are soft, red and gelatinous whereas white thrombi are firm and pale.

M/E The composition of thrombus is determined by the rate of flow of blood i.e. whether it is formed in the rapid arterial and cardiac circulation, or in the slow moving flow in veins. The lines of Zahn are formed by alternate layers of light-staining aggregated platelets admixed with fibrin meshwork and dark-staining layer of red cells. Red (venous) thrombi have more abundant red cells, leucocytes and platelets entrapped in fibrin meshwork. Thus, red thrombi closely resemble blood clots *in vitro*.

Chapter Five

Cardiac Thrombi. Thrombi may form in any of the chambers of heart and on the valve cusps. They are more common in the atrial appendages, especially of the right atrium, and on mitral and aortic valves called vegetations which may be seen in infective endocarditis and non-bacterial thrombotic endocarditis. Cardiac thrombi are mural (non-occlusive) as are the mural thrombi encountered in the aorta in atherosclerosis and in aneurysmal dilatations. Rarely, large round thrombus may form and obstruct the mitral valve and is called *ball-valve thrombus*. *Agonal thrombi* are formed shortly before death and may occur in either or both the ventricles. They are composed mainly of fibrin.

ARTERIAL THROMBI. These are:

i) Aorta: aneurysms, arteritis.
ii) Coronary arteries: atherosclerosis.
iii) Mesenteric artery: atherosclerosis, arteritis.
iv) Arteries of limbs: atherosclerosis, diabetes mellitus, Buerger's disease, Raynaud's disease.
v) Renal artery: atherosclerosis, arteritis.
vi) Cerebral artery: atherosclerosis, vasculitis.

VENOUS THROMBI. For example:

i) Veins of lower limbs: deep veins of legs, varicose veins.
ii) Popliteal, femoral and iliac veins: postoperative stage, postpartum.
iii) Pulmonary veins: CHF, pulmonary hypertension.
iv) Hepatic and portal vein: portal hypertension.
v) Superior vena cava: infections in head and neck.
vi) Inferior vena cava: extension of thrombus from hepatic vein.
vii) Mesenteric veins: volvulus, intestinal obstruction.
viii) Renal vein: renal amyloidosis.

Distinguishing features between thrombi formed in rapidly-flowing arterial circulation and slow-moving venous blood are given in Table 5.3.

TABLE 5.3: Distinguishing Features of Arterial and Venous Thrombi.

	FEATURE	ARTERIAL THROMBI	VENOUS THROMBI
1.	**Blood flow**	Formed in rapidly-flowing blood of arteries and heart	Formed in slow-moving blood in veins
2.	**Sites**	Common in aorta, coronary, cerebral, iliac, femoral, renal and mesenteric arteries	Common in superficial varicose veins, deep leg veins, popliteal, femoral and iliac veins
3.	**Thrombogenesis**	Formed following endothelial cell injury e.g. in atherosclerosis	Formed following venous stasis e.g. in abdominal operations, child-birth
4.	**Development**	Usually mural, not occluding the lumen completely, may propagate	Usually occlusive, take the cast of the vessel in which formed, may propagate in both directions
5.	**Macroscopy**	Grey-white, friable with lines of Zahn on surface	Red-blue with fibrin strands and lines of Zahn
6.	**Microscopy**	Distinct lines of Zahn composed of platelets, fibrin with entangled red and white blood cells	Lines of Zahn with more abundant red cells
7.	**Effects**	Ischaemia leading to infarcts e.g. in the heart, brain etc	Thromboembolism, oedema, skin ulcers, poor wound healing

CAPILLARY THROMBI. Minute thrombi composed mainly of packed red cells are formed in the capillaries in acute inflammatory lesions, vasculitis and in disseminated intravascular coagulation (DIC).

Fate of Thrombus *(p. 120)*

The possible fate of thrombi is as under:

1. RESOLUTION. Thrombus activates the fibrinolytic system with consequent release of plasmin which may dissolve the thrombus completely resulting in resolution.

2. ORGANISATION. If the thrombus is not removed, it starts getting organised. Phagocytic cells (neutrophils and macrophages) appear and begin to phagocytose fibrin and cell debris. Capillaries grow into the thrombus from the site of its attachment and fibroblasts start invading the thrombus. Thus, fibro-vascular granulation tissue is formed which subsequently becomes dense and less vascular and is covered over by endothelial cells.

3. PROPAGATION. The thrombus may enlarge in size due to more and more deposition from the constituents of flowing blood. In this way, it may ultimately cause obstruction of some important vessel.

4. THROMBOEMBOLISM. The thrombi in early stage and infected thrombi are quite friable and may get detached from the vessel wall. These are released in part or completely in bloodstream as emboli which produce ill-effects at the site of their lodgement.

Clinical Effects of Thrombosis *(p. 121)*

These depend upon the site of thrombi, rapidity of formation, and nature of thrombi.

1. Cardiac thrombi. Large thrombi in the heart may cause sudden death by mechanical obstruction of blood flow or through thromboembolism to vital organs.

2. Arterial thrombi. These cause ischaemic necrosis of the deprived part (infarct) which may lead to gangrene. Sudden death may occur following thrombosis of coronary artery.

3. Venous thrombi (Phlebothrombosis). These may cause various effects such as:

i)   Thromboembolism

ii) Oedema of area drained

iii) Poor wound healing

iv) Skin ulcer

v)   Painful thrombosed veins (thrombophlebitis)

vi) Painful white leg (phlegmasia alba dolens) due to ileofemoral venous thrombosis in postpartum cases

vii) Thrombophlebitis migrans in cancer.

4. Capillary thrombi. Microthrombi in microcirculation may give rise to disseminated intravascular coagulation (DIC).

EMBOLISM *(p. 121)*

Embolism is the process of partial or complete obstruction of some part of the cardiovascular system by any mass carried in the circulation; the transported intravascular mass detached from its site of origin is called an *embolus*. Most usual forms of emboli (90%) are thromboemboli i.e. originating from thrombi or their parts detached from the vessel wall.

Emboli may be of various types:

A. Depending upon the matter in the emboli, they can be:

i) *Solid* e.g. detached thrombi (thromboemboli), atheromatous material, tumour cell clumps, tissue fragments, parasites, bacterial clumps, foreign bodies.

ii) *Liquid* e.g. fat globules, amniotic fluid, bone marrow.

iii) *Gaseous* e.g. air, other gases.

B. Depending upon whether infected or not, they are called:

i) *Bland,* when sterile.

ii) *Septic,* when infected.

C. Depending upon the source of the emboli, they are classified as:

i) *Cardiac emboli* from left side of heart e.g. emboli originating from atrium and atrial appendages, infarct in the left ventricle, vegetations of endocarditis.

ii) *Arterial emboli* e.g. in systemic arteries in the brain, spleen, kidney, intestine.

iii) *Venous emboli* e.g. in pulmonary arteries.

iv) *Lymphatic emboli* can also occur.

D. Depending upon the flow of blood, two special types of emboli are mentioned:

i) *Paradoxical embolus.* An embolus which is carried from the venous side of circulation to the arterial side or vice versa is called paradoxical or crossed embolus e.g. through arteriovenous communication such as in patent foramen ovale, septal defect of the heart, and arteriovenous shunts in the lungs.

ii) *Retrograde embolus.* An embolus which travels against the flow of blood is called retrograde embolus e.g. metastatic deposits in the spine from carcinoma prostate. The spread occurs by retrograde embolism through intraspinal veins which carry tumour emboli from large thoracic and abdominal veins due to increased pressure in body cavities e.g. during coughing or straining.

Some of the important types of embolism are tabulated in Table 5.4.

TABLE 5.4: Important Types of Embolism.

	TYPE	COMMON ORIGIN
1.	*Pulmonary embolism*	Veins of lower legs
2.	*Systemic embolism*	Left ventricle (arterial)
3.	*Fat embolism*	Trauma to bones/soft tissues
4.	*Air embolism*	Venous: head & neck operations, obstetrical trauma Arterial: cardiothoracic surgery, angiography
5.	*Decompression sickness*	Descent: divers Ascent: unpressurised flight
6.	*Amniotic fluid embolism*	Components of amniotic fluid
7.	*Atheroembolism*	Atheromatous plaques
8.	*Tumour embolism*	Tumour fragments

Thromboembolism *(p. 122)*

A detached thrombus or part of thrombus constitutes the most common type of embolism. These may arise in the arterial or venous circulation:

Arterial (systemic) thromboembolism:

A. *Causes within the heart* (80-85%): These are mural thrombi in the left atrium or left ventricle, vegetations on the mitral or aortic valves, prosthetic heart valves and cardiomyopathy.

B. *Causes within the arteries:* These include emboli developing in relation to atherosclerotic plaques, aortic aneurysms, pulmonary veins and paradoxical arterial emboli from the systemic venous circulation.

The *effects* of arterial emboli depend upon their size, site of lodgement, and adequacy of collateral circulation. If the vascular occlusion occurs, the following ill-effects may result:

i) *Infarction* of the organ or its affected part e.g. ischaemic necrosis in the lower limbs (70-75%), spleen, kidneys, brain, intestine.

ii) *Gangrene* following infarction in the lower limbs if the collateral circulation is inadequate.

iii) *Arteritis and mycotic aneurysm* formation from bacterial endocarditis.

iv) *Myocardial infarction* may occur following coronary embolism.

v) *Sudden death* may result from coronary embolism or embolism in the middle cerebral artery.

Venous thromboembolism:

i) Thrombi in the veins of the lower legs are the most common cause of venous emboli.

ii) Thrombi in the pelvic veins.

iii) Thrombi in the veins of the upper limbs.

iv) Thrombosis in cavernous sinus of the brain.

v) Thrombi in the right side of heart.

The most significant *effect* of venous embolism is obstruction of pulmonary arterial circulation leading to pulmonary embolism described below.

Pulmonary Thromboembolism *(p. 122)*

Pulmonary embolism is the most common and fatal form of venous thromboembolism in which there is occlusion of pulmonary arterial tree by thromboemboli. Pulmonary thrombosis as such is uncommon and may occur in pulmonary atherosclerosis and pulmonary hypertension. Differentiation of pulmonary thrombosis from pulmonary thromboembolism is tabulated in Table 5.5.

TABLE 5.5: Contrasting Features of Pulmonary Thrombosis and Pulmonary Thromboembolism.

FEATURE	PUL. THROMBOSIS	PUL. THROMBOEMBOLISM
1. *Pathogenesis*	Locally formed	Travelled from distance
2. *Location*	In small arteries and branches	In major arteries and branches
3. *Attachment to vessel wall*	Firmly adherent	Loosely attached or lying free
4. *Gross appearance*	Head pale, tail red	No distinction in head and tail; smooth surface dry dull surface
5. *Microscopy*	Platelets and fibrin in layers, Lines of Zahn seen	Mixed with blood clot, lines of Zahn rare

ETIOLOGY. Pulmonary emboli are more common in hospitalised or bed-ridden patients, though they can occur in ambulatory patients as well. The causes are:

i) Thrombi originating from large veins of lower legs (such as popliteal, femoral and iliac) are the cause in 95% of pulmonary emboli.

ii) Less common sources include thrombi in varicosities of superficial veins of the legs, and pelvic veins such as peri-prostatic, periovarian, uterine and broad ligament veins.

PATHOGENESIS. Detachment of thrombi from any of the above-mentioned sites produces a thrombo-embolus that flows through venous drainage into the larger veins draining into right side of the heart.

■ If the thrombus is large, it is impacted at the bifurcation of the main pulmonary artery *(saddle embolus),* or may be found in the right ventricle or its outflow tract.

■ More commonly, there are *multiple emboli,* or a large embolus may be fragmented into many smaller emboli which are then impacted in a number of vessels, particularly affecting the lower lobes of lungs.

■ Rarely, *paradoxical embolism* may occur by passage of an embolus from right heart into the left heart through atrial or ventricular septal defect. In this way, pulmonary emboli may reach systemic circulation.

CONSEQUENCES OF PULMONARY EMBOLISM. Pulmonary embolism occurs more commonly as a complication in patients of acute or chronic debilitating diseases who are immobilised for a long duration. Women in their reproductive period are at higher risk such as in late pregnancy, following delivery and with use of contraceptive pills. The effects of pulmonary embolism depend mainly on the size of the occluded vessel, the number of emboli, and on the cardiovascular status of the patient. The following consequences can result:

i) Sudden death.
ii) Acute cor pulmonale.
iii) Pulmonary infarction.
iv) Pulmonary haemorrhage.
v) Resolution.
vi) Pulmonary hypertension, chronic cor pulmonale and pulmonary arteriosclerosis.

Systemic Embolism *(p. 124)*

This is the type of arterial embolism that originates commonly from thrombi in the diseased heart, especially in the left ventricle. These diseases of heart include myocardial infarction, cardiomyopathy, RHD, congenital heart disease, infective endocarditis, and prosthetic cardiac valves. These arterial emboli invariably cause infarction at the sites of lodgement which include, in descending order of frequency, lower extremity, brain, and internal visceral organs (spleen, kidneys, intestines). *Thus, the effects and sites of arterial emboli are in striking contrast to venous emboli* which are often lodged in the lungs.

Fat Embolism *(p. 124)*

Obstruction of arterioles and capillaries by fat globules constitutes fat embolism. If the obstruction in the circulation is by fragments of adipose tissue, it is called fat-tissue embolism. Following are the important causes of fat embolism:

i) Traumatic causes:
■ *Trauma to bones* e.g. in fractures of long bones leading to passage of fatty marrow in circulation, concussions of bones, after orthopaedic surgical procedures etc.

■ *Trauma to soft tissue* e.g. laceration of adipose tissue and in puerperium due to injury to pelvic fatty tissue.

ii) Non-traumatic causes: Extensive burns, diabetes mellitus, fatty liver, pancreatitis, sickle cell anaemia, decompression sickness, inflammation of bones and soft tissues, extrinsic fat or oils introduced into the body.

PATHOGENESIS. The following mechanisms may be acting singly or in combination.

i) Mechanical theory. Mobilisation of fluid fat may occur following trauma to the bone or soft tissues. The fat globules released from the injured area may enter venous circulation and finally most of the fat is arrested in the small vessels in the lungs.

ii) Emulsion instability theory. This theory explains the pathogenesis of fat embolism in non-traumatic cases. According to this theory, fat emboli are formed by aggregation of plasma lipids (chylomicrons and fatty acids) due to disturbance in natural emulsification of fat.

iii) Intravascular coagulation theory. In stress, release of some factor activates disseminated intravascular coagulation (DIC) and aggregation of fat emboli.

iv) Toxic injury theory. According to this theory, the small blood vessels of lungs are chemically injured by high plasma levels of free fatty acid, resulting in increased vascular permeability and consequent pulmonary oedema.

CONSEQUENCES OF FAT EMBOLISM. The effects of fat embolism depend upon the size and quantity of fat globules, and whether or not the emboli pass through the lungs into the systemic circulation.

i) Pulmonary fat embolism. *M/E* The lungs show hyperaemia, oedema, petechial haemorrhages and changes of adult respiratory distress syndrome (ARDS). In routine stains, the fat globules in the pulmonary arteries, capillaries and alveolar spaces appear as vacuoles. Frozen section is essential for confirmation of globules by fat stains such as Sudan dyes (Sudan black, Sudan III and IV), oil red O and osmic acid.

ii) Systemic fat embolism. Some of the fat globules may pass through the pulmonary circulation such as via patent foramen ovale, arteriovenous shunts in the lungs and vertebral venous plexuses, and get lodged in the capillaries of organs like the brain, kidney, skin etc.

Air Embolism (p. 125)

Air embolism occurs when air is introduced into venous or arterial circulation.

VENOUS AIR EMBOLISM. Air may be sucked into systemic veins under the following circumstances:

i)   Operations on head and neck, and trauma.

ii) Obstetrical operations and trauma.

iii) Intravenous infusion of blood and fluid.

iv) Angiography.

The **effects** of venous air embolism depend upon the following factors:

i) Amount of air introduced into the circulation. The volume of air necessary to cause death is variable but usually 100-150 ml of air entry is considered fatal.

ii) Rapidity of entry of a smaller volume of air is important determinant of a fatal outcome.

iii) Position of the patient during or soon after entry of air is another factor. The air bubbles may ascend into the superior vena cava if the position of head is higher than the trunk (e.g. in upright position) and reach the brain.

iv) General condition of the patient e.g. in severely ill patients, as little as 40 ml of air may have serious results.

The mechanism of death is by entrapment of air emboli in the pulmonary arterial trunk in the right heart. If bubbles of air in the form of froth pass further out into pulmonary arterioles, they cause widespread vascular occlusions. If death from pulmonary air embolism is suspected, the heart and pulmonary artery should be opened *in situ* under water so that escaping froth or foam formed by mixture of air and blood can be detected.

ARTERIAL AIR EMBOLISM. Entry of air into pulmonary vein or its tributaries may occur in the following conditions:

Chapter Five

i)   Cardiothoracic surgery and trauma.

ii) Paradoxical air embolism.

iii) Arteriography.

The **effects** of arterial air embolism are in the form of certain characteristic features:

i)   Marble skin due to blockage of cutaneous vessels.

ii) Air bubbles in the retinal vessels seen ophthalmoscopically.

iii) Pallor of the tongue due to occlusion of a branch of lingual artery.

iv) Coronary or cerebral arterial air embolism may cause sudden death by much smaller amounts of air than in the venous air embolism.

Decompression Sickness (p. 126)

This is a specialised form of gas embolism known by various names such as caisson's disease, divers' palsy or aeroembolism.

Decompression sickness is produced when the individual decompresses suddenly, either from high atmospheric pressure to normal level, or from normal pressure to low atmospheric pressure.

The effects of decompression sickness depend upon:

- depth or altitude reached
- duration of exposure to altered pressure
- rate of ascent or descent
- general condition of the individual

The pathologic changes are more pronounced in sudden decompression from high pressure to normal levels than in those who decompress from low pressure to normal levels. The changes are more serious in obese persons as nitrogen gas is more soluble in fat than in body fluids.

Clinical effects of decompression sickness are of 2 types:

- **Acute form** occurs due to acute obstruction of small blood vessels in the vicinity of joints and skeletal muscles. The condition is clinically characterised by the following:

i)   'The bends', as the patient doubles up in bed due to acute pain in joints, ligaments and tendons.

ii) 'The chokes' occur due to accumulation of bubbles in the lungs, resulting in acute respiratory distress.

iii) Cerebral effects may manifest in the form of vertigo, coma, and sometimes death.

- **Chronic form** is due to foci of ischaemic necrosis throughout body, especially the skeletal system.

i)   Avascular necrosis of bones e.g. head of femur, tibia, humerus.

ii) Neurological symptoms may occur due to ischaemic necrosis in the central nervous system. These include paraesthesias and paraplegia.

iii) Lung involvement in the form of haemorrhage, oedema, emphysema and atelactasis may be seen. These result in dyspnoea, nonproductive cough and chest pain.

iv) Skin manifestations include itching, patchy erythema, cyanosis and oedema.

v)   Other organs like parenchymal cells of the liver and pancreas may show lipid vacuoles.

Amniotic Fluid Embolism (p. 127)

This is the most serious, unpredictable and unpreventible cause of maternal mortality. During labour and in the immediate postpartum period, the contents of amniotic fluid may enter the uterine veins and reach right side of the heart resulting in fatal complications. The amniotic fluid components which may be found in uterine veins, pulmonary artery and vessels of other organs are: epithelial squames, vernix caseosa, lanugo hair, bile from meconium, and mucus. The mechanism by which these amniotic fluid contents enter the maternal circulation is not clear. Possibly, they gain entry either through tears in the myometrium and endocervix, or the amniotic fluid is forced into uterine sinusoids by vigorous uterine contractions.

G/A Notable changes are seen in the lungs such as haemorrhages, congestion, oedema and changes of ARDS, and dilatation of right side of the heart.

These changes are associated with identifiable amniotic fluid contents within the pulmonary microcirculation.

The *clinical syndrome* is characterised by the following features:
- Sudden respiratory distress and dyspnoea
- Deep cyanosis
- Cardiovascular shock
- Convulsions
- Coma
- Unexpected death

The *cause of death* may not be obvious but can occur as a result of the following mechanisms:

i)   Mechanical blockage of the pulmonary circulation in extensive embolism.

ii) Anaphylactoid reaction to amniotic fluid components.

iii) Disseminated intravascular coagulation (DIC) due to liberation of thromboplastin by amniotic fluid.

iv) Haemorrhagic manifestations due to thrombocytopenia and afibrinogenaemia.

Atheroembolism *(p. 127)*

Atheromatous plaques, especially from aorta, may get eroded to form atherosclerotic emboli which are then lodged in medium-sized and small arteries.

Tumour Embolism *(p. 127)*

Malignant tumour cells invade the local blood vessels and may form tumour emboli to be lodged elsewhere, producing metastatic tumour deposits.

ISCHAEMIA *(p. 128)*

Ischaemia is defined as deficient blood supply to part of a tissue. The cessation of blood supply may be complete (complete ischaemia) or partial (partial ischaemia). The harmful effects of ischaemia may result from 3 ways:

1. Hypoxia due to deprivation of oxygen to tissues.

2. Inadequate supply of nutrients to the tissue such as glucose and amino acids.

3. Inadequate clearance of metabolites resulting in accumulation of metabolic waste-products in the affected tissue.

ETIOLOGY. A number of causes may produce ischaemia.

1. Causes in the heart. Inadequate cardiac output resulting from heart block, ventricular arrest and fibrillation may cause hypoxic injury to brain.
- If the arrest continues for 15 seconds, consciousness is lost.
- If the condition lasts for more than 4 minutes, irreversible ischaemic damage to brain occurs.
- If it is prolonged for more than 8 minutes, death is inevitable.

2. Causes in the arteries. The commonest and most important causes of ischaemia are due to obstruction in arterial blood supply. These are:

Chapter Five

i) Luminal occlusion such as due to: thrombosis, embolism

ii) Causes in the arterial wall such as: vasospasm (e.g. in Raynaud's disease), hypothermia, ergotism, arteriosclerosis, polyarteritis nodosa, thromboangiitis obliterans (Buerger's disease), severed vessel wall

iii) Outside pressure on an artery such as: ligature, tourniquet, tight plaster, bandages, torsion.

3. Causes in the veins. Blockage of venous drainage may lead to engorgement and obstruction to arterial blood supply resulting in ischaemia. The examples include the following:

i) Luminal occlusion such as in: thrombosis of mesenteric veins, cavernous sinus thrombosis

ii) Causes in the vessel wall such as in: varicose veins of the legs

iii) Outside pressure on a vein as in: strangulated hernia, intussusception, volvulus

4. Causes in the microcirculation. Ischaemia may result from occlusion of arterioles, capillaries and venules. The causes are as under:

i) Luminal occlusion such as: by red cells (e.g. in sickle cell anaemia, red cells parasitised by malaria, acquired haemolytic anaemia, sludging of the blood), by white cells (e.g. in chronic myeloid leukaemia), by fibrin (e.g. defibrination syndrome), by precipitated cryoglobulins, by fat embolism, and in decompression sickness.

ii) Causes in the microvasculature wall such as: vasculitis e.g. in polyarteritis nodosa, Henoch-Schönlein purpura, Arthus reaction, septicaemia. Frost-bite injuring the wall of small blood vessels.

iii) Outside pressure on microvasculature as in: bedsores.

FACTORS DETERMINING THE SEVERITY OF ISCHAEMIC INJURY. The extent of damage produced by ischaemia due to occlusion of arterial or venous blood vessels depends upon a number of factors.

1. Anatomic pattern. There are 4 different patterns of arterial blood supply:

i) Single arterial supply without anastomosis. Occlusion of such vessels invariably results in ischaemic necrosis e.g.
■ Central artery of the retina
■ Interlobular arteries of the kidneys

ii) Single arterial supply with rich anastomosis. Arterial supply to some organs has rich interarterial anastomoses so that blockage of one vessel can re-establish blood supply bypassing the blocked arterial branch, and hence the infarction is less common in such circumstances e.g.
■ Superior mesenteric artery
■ Inferior mesenteric artery
■ Arterial supply to the stomach by 3 separate vessels
■ Interarterial anastomoses in the 3 main trunks of the coronary arterial system.

iii) Parallel arterial supply. Blood supply to some organs and tissues is such that the vitality of the tissue is maintained by alternative blood supply in case of occlusion of one e.g.
■ Blood supply to brain in the region of circle of Willis.
■ Arterial supply to forearm by radial and ulnar arteries.

iv) Double blood supply. The effect of occlusion of one set of vessels is modified if an organ has dual blood supply e.g.
■ Lungs are perfused by bronchial circulation as well as by pulmonary arterial branches.
■ Liver is supplied by both portal circulation and hepatic arterial flow.

2. General and cardiovascular status. Some of the factors which render the tissues more vulnerable to the effects of ischaemia are:

i) Anaemias (sickle cell anaemia, in particular)

ii) Lowered oxygenation of blood (hypoxaemia)

iii) Senility with marked coronary atherosclerosis

iv) Cardiac failure

v) Blood loss

vi) Shock.

3. Type of tissue affected. The mesenchymal tissues are quite resistant to the effect of ischaemia as compared to parenchymal cells of the organs. The following tissues are more vulnerable to ischaemia:

i) Brain (cerebral cortical neurons, in particular).

ii) Heart (myocardial cells).

iii) Kidney (especially epithelial cells of proximal convoluted tubules).

4. Rapidity of development. Sudden vascular obstruction results in more severe effects of ischaemia than if it is gradual since there is less time for collaterals to develop.

5. Degree of vascular occlusion. Complete vascular obstruction results in more severe ischaemic injury than the partial occlusion.

EFFECTS. The effects of ischaemia are variable and range from 'no change' to 'sudden death'.

1. No effects on the tissues, if the collateral channels develop adequately.

2. Functional disturbances. These result when collateral channels are able to supply blood during normal activity but the supply is not adequate to withstand the effect of exertion. The examples are angina pectoris and intermittent claudication.

3. Cellular changes. Partial ischaemia may produce cellular changes such as cloudy swelling, fatty change, atrophy and replacement fibrosis. Infarction results when the deprivation of blood supply is complete so as to cause necrosis of tissue affected.

4. Sudden death from ischaemia is usually myocardial and cerebral infarction.

INFARCTION *(p. 129)*

Infarction is the process of tissue necrosis resulting from some form of circulatory insufficiency; the localised area of necrosis so developed is called an *infarct*. All the causes of ischaemia discussed above can cause infarction. There are a few other note-worthy features in infarcts:

■ Most commonly, infarcts are caused by interrupted arterial blood supply, called *ischaemic necrosis*.

■ Less commonly, venous obstruction can produce infarcts termed *stagnant hypoxia*.

■ Generally, *sudden, complete, and continuous occlusion* by thrombosis or embolism produces infarcts.

■ Infarcts may be produced by *nonocclusive circulatory insufficiency* as well e.g. incomplete atherosclerotic narrowing of coronary arteries may produce myocardial infarction due to acute coronary insufficiency.

TYPES OF INFARCTS. Infarcts are classified depending upon different features:

1. According to their colour, infarcts may be:

■ *Pale or anaemic,* due to arterial occlusion e.g. in the kidneys, heart, spleen.

■ *Red or haemorrhagic,* seen in soft loose tissues and are caused either by pulmonary arterial obstruction (e.g. in the lungs) or by arterial or venous occlusion (e.g. in the intestines).

2. According to their age, infarcts are classified as: *recent or fresh, old or healed*

Chapter Five

3. According to presence or absence of infection, they may be: *bland*, when free of bacterial contamination, *septic*, when infected.

PATHOGENESIS. The process of infarction takes place as follows:

i) Localised *hyperaemia* due to local anoxaemia.

ii) Within a few hours, the affected part becomes swollen due to *oedema and haemorrhage.*

iii) Cellular changes such as cloudy swelling and degeneration appear early, while death of the cells or necrosis occurs in 12-48 hours.

iv) There is progressive *autolysis* of the necrotic tissue and haemolysis of the red cells.

v) An *acute inflammatory reaction* and *hyperaemia* appear at the same time in the surrounding tissues in response to products of autolysis.

vi) Blood pigments, haematoidin and haemosiderin, liberated by haemolysis are deposited in the infarct.

vii) There is progressive *ingrowth of granulation tissue* from the margin of the infarct so that eventually the infarct is replaced by a fibrous scar.

Infarcts of Different Organs (p. 130)

Table 5.6 summarises the gross appearance and the usual outcome of the common types of infarction.

TABLE 5.6: Infarcts of Most Commonly Affected Organs.

	LOCATION	GROSS APPEARANCE	OUTCOME
1.	*Myocardial infarction*	Pale	Frequently lethal
2.	*Pulmonary infarction*	Haemorrhagic	Less commonly fatal
3.	*Cerebral infarction*	Haemorrhagic or pale	Fatal if massive
4.	*Intestinal infarction*	Haemorrhagic	Frequently lethal
5.	*Renal infarction*	Pale	Not lethal unless massive and bilateral
6.	*Infarct spleen*	Pale	Not lethal
7.	*Infarct liver*	Pale	Not lethal
8.	*Infarcts lower extremity*	Pale	Not lethal

INFARCT LUNG. Embolism of the pulmonary arteries may produce pulmonary infarction, though not always. This is because lungs receive blood supply from bronchial arteries as well, and thus occlusion of pulmonary artery ordinarily does not produce infarcts.

G/A The pulmonary infarcts are classically wedge-shaped with base on the pleura, haemorrhagic, variable in size, and most often in the lower lobes. Fibrinous pleuritis usually covers the area of infarct.

M/E The characteristic histologic feature is coagulative necrosis of the alveolar walls. Initially, there is infiltration by neutrophils and intense alveolar capillary congestion, but later their place is taken by haemosiderin, phagocytes and granulation tissue.

INFARCT KIDNEY. Renal infarction is common, found in upto 5% of autopsies. Majority of them are caused by thromboemboli, most commonly originating from the heart such as in mural thrombi in the left atrium, myocardial infarction, vegetative endocarditis and aortic aneurysm.

G/A Renal infarcts are often multiple and may be bilateral. Characteristically, they are pale or anaemic and wedge-shaped with base resting under the capsule and apex pointing towards the medulla. Generally, a narrow rim of preserved renal tissue under the capsule is spared because it draws its blood supply from the capsular vessels.

M/E The affected area shows characteristic coagulative necrosis of renal parenchyma i.e. there are ghosts of renal tubules and glomeruli without intact nuclei and cytoplasmic content. The margin of the infarct shows inflammatory reaction—initially acute but later macrophages and fibrous tissue predominate.

INFARCT SPLEEN. Spleen is one of the common sites for infarction. Splenic infarction results from occlusion of the splenic artery or its branches. Occlusion is caused most commonly by thromboemboli arising in the heart (e.g. in mural thrombi in the left atrium, vegetative endocarditis, myocardial infarction), and less frequently by obstruction of microcirculation (e.g. in myeloproliferative diseases, sickle cell anaemia, arteritis, Hodgkin's disease, bacterial infections).

G/A Splenic infarcts are often multiple. They are characteristically pale or anaemic and wedge-shaped with their base at the periphery and apex pointing towards hilum.

M/E The features are similar to those found in anaemic infarcts in kidney. Coagulative necrosis and inflammatory reaction are seen. Later, the necrotic tissue is replaced by shrunken fibrous scar.

INFARCT LIVER. Just as in lungs, infarcts in the liver are uncommon due to dual blood supply—from portal vein and from hepatic artery. Obstruction of the portal vein is usually secondary to other diseases such as hepatic cirrhosis, intravenous invasion of primary carcinoma of the liver, carcinoma of the pancreas and pylephlebitis. Occlusion of portal vein or its branches generally does not produce ischaemic infarction but instead reduced blood supply to hepatic parenchyma causes non-ischaemic infarct called *infarct of Zahn.* Obstruction of the hepatic artery or its branches, on the other hand, caused by arteritis, arteriosclerosis, bland or septic emboli, results in ischaemic infarcts of the liver.

G/A Ischaemic infarcts of the liver are usually anaemic but sometimes may be haemorrhagic due to stuffing of the site by blood from the portal vein. Infarcts of Zahn (non-ischaemic infarcts) produce sharply defined red-blue area in liver parenchyma.

M/E Ischaemic infarcts show characteristics of pale or anaemic infarcts as in kidney or spleen.

■ SELF ASSESSMENT

1. **The essential difference between plasma and interstitial fluid compartment is:**
   A. Glucose is higher in the former
   B. Urea is higher in the former
   C. Protein content is higher in the former
   D. Potassium is higher in the former

2. **Osmotic pressure exerted by the chemical constituents of the body fluids has the following features *except*:**
   A. Crystalloid osmotic pressure comprises minor portion of total osmotic pressure
   B. Oncotic pressure constitutes minor portion of total osmotic pressure
   C. Oncotic pressure of plasma is higher
   D. Oncotic pressure of interstitial fluid is lower

Chapter Five

3. **For causation of oedema by decreased osmotic pressure, the following factor is most important:**
   A. Fall in albumin as well as globulin
   B. Fall in globulin level
   C. Fall in albumin level
   D. Fall in fibrinogen level

4. **Transudate differs from exudate in having the following *except*:**
   A. No inflammatory cells
   B. Low glucose content
   C. Low protein content
   D. Low specific gravity

5. **Nephritic oedema differs from nephrotic oedema in having the following *except*:**
   A. Mild oedema
   B. Distributed on face, eyes
   C. Heavy proteinuria
   D. Occurs in acute glomerulonephritis

6. **The following type of oedema is characteristically dependent oedema:**
   A. Nephrotic oedema
   B. Nephritic oedema
   C. Pulmonary oedema
   D. Cardiac oedema

7. **Pulmonary oedema appears due to elevated pulmonary hydrostatic pressure when the fluid accumulation is:**
   A. Two fold
   B. Four fold
   C. Eight fold
   D. Ten fold

8. **Active hyperaemia is the result of:**
   A. Dilatation of capillaries
   B. Dilatation of arterioles
   C. Venous engorgement
   D. Lymphatic obstruction

9. **Sectioned surface of lung shows brown induration in:**
   A. Pulmonary embolism
   B. Pulmonary haemorrhage
   C. Pulmonary infarction
   D. CVC lung

10. **In septic shock, pathogenesis of endothelial cell injury involves the following mechanisms *except*:**
    A. Lipopolysaccharide from lysed bacteria injures the endothelium
    B. Interleukin-1 causes endothelial cell injury
    C. TNF-α causes direct cytotoxicity
    D. Adherence of PMNs to endothelium causes endothelial cell injury

11. **An intact endothelium elaborates the following anti-thrombotic factors *except*:**
    A. Thrombomodulin
    B. ADPase
    C. Tissue plasminogen activator
    D. Thromboplastin

12. **The most common cause of arterial thromboemboli is:**
    A. Cardiac thrombi
    B. Aortic aneurysm
    C. Pulmonary veins
    D. Aortic atherosclerotic plaques

13. **Venous emboli are most often lodged in:**
    A. Intestines
    B. Kidneys
    C. Lungs
    D. Heart

14. **Pathologic changes between sudden decompression from high pressure to normal levels and decompression from low pressure to normal levels are:**
    A. More marked in the former
    B. More marked in the latter
    C. No difference between the two
    D. Acute form is more marked in the latter

15. **The infarct of following organ is invariably haemorrhagic:**
    A. Infarct kidney
    B. Infarct spleen
    C. Infarct lung
    D. Infarct heart

KEY

1 = C	2 = A	3 = C	4 = B	5 = C	6 = D
7 = D	8 = B	9 = D	10 = A	11 = D	12 = A
13 = C	14 = A	15 = C			

6

Inflammation and Healing

INFLAMMATION *(p. 133)*

Inflammation is defined as the local response of living mammalian tissues to injury due to any agent. It is a body defense reaction in order to eliminate or limit the spread of injurious agent as well as to remove the consequent necrosed cells and tissues.

The agents causing inflammation may be as under:

1. *Physical agents* like heat, cold, radiation, mechanical trauma.
2. *Chemical agents* like organic and inorganic poisons.
3. *Infective agents* like bacteria, viruses and their toxins.
4. *Immunological agents* like cell-mediated and antigen-antibody reactions.

Inflammation involves 2 basic processes with some overlapping, viz. early *inflammatory response* and later followed by *healing*.

SIGNS OF INFLAMMATION. The Roman writer Celsus in 1st century A.D. named the famous 4 *cardinal signs of inflammation* as: *rubor* (redness); *tumor* (swelling); *calor* (heat); and *dolor* (pain).

To these, fifth sign *functio laesa* (loss of function) was later added by Virchow.

TYPES OF INFLAMMATION. Depending upon the defense capacity of the host and duration of response, inflammation can be classified as acute and chronic.

I. *Acute inflammation* is of short duration and represents the early body reaction and is usually followed by repair.

II. *Chronic inflammation* is of longer duration and occurs either after the causative agent of acute inflammation persists for a long time, or the stimulus is such that it induces chronic inflammation from the beginning.

ACUTE INFLAMMATION *(p. 134)*

The changes in acute inflammation can be conveniently described under 2 headings:

I. VASCULAR EVENTS *(p. 134)*

These alterations include: haemodynamic changes and changes in vascular permeability.

Haemodynamic Changes *(p. 134)*

The sequence of these changes is as under:

1. Immediate vascular response is of **transient vasoconstriction** of arterioles.
2. Next follows **persistent progressive vasodilatation** which involves mainly the arterioles.
3. Progressive vasodilatation, in turn, may elevate the **local hydrostatic pressure** resulting in transudation of fluid into the extracellular space.
4. **Slowing or stasis** of microcirculation occurs next.
5. Stasis or slowing is followed by **leucocytic margination** or peripheral orientation of leucocytes (mainly neutrophils) along the vascular endothelium.

The features of haemodynamic changes in inflammation are best demonstrated by the **Lewis experiment.** Lewis induced the changes in the skin of inner aspect of forearm by firm stroking with a blunt point. The reaction so elicited is known as *triple response* or *red line response* consisting of *red line, flare, wheal*.

These features, elicit the classical signs of inflammation—redness, heat, swelling and pain.

Altered Vascular Permeability *(p. 135)*

In acute inflammation, normally non-permeable endothelial layer of microvasculature becomes leaky. This is explained by one or more of the mechanisms which are summarised in Table 6.1.

II. CELLULAR EVENTS *(p. 137)*

The cellular phase of inflammation consists of 2 processes: exudation and phagocytosis.

Exudation of Leucocytes *(p. 137)*

The escape of leucocytes from the lumen of microvasculature to the interstitial tissue is the most important feature of inflammatory response. In acute inflammation, polymorphonuclear neutrophils (PMNs) comprise the first line of body defense, followed later by monocytes and macrophages.

The changes leading to migration of leucocytes are as follows:

1. CHANGES IN THE FORMED ELEMENTS OF BLOOD. In the early stage of inflammation, the rate of flow of blood is increased due to vasodilatation. But subsequently, there is slowing or stasis of bloodstream. Due to slowing and stasis, the central stream of cells widens and peripheral plasma zone becomes narrower because of loss of plasma by exudation. This phenomenon is known as *margination*. As a result of this redistribution, the neutrophils of the central column come close to the vessel wall; this is known as *pavementing*.

2. ROLLING AND ADHESION. Peripherally marginated and pavemented neutrophils slowly roll over the endothelial cells lining the vessel wall *(rolling phase)*. This is followed by the transient bond between the leucocytes and endothelial cells becoming firmer *(adhesion phase)*. The following adhesion molecules bring about rolling and adhesion phases:

i) **Selectins:** *P-selectin* (preformed and stored in endothelial cells and platelets), *E-selectin* (synthesised by cytokine-activated endothelial cells) and *L-selectin* (expressed on the surface of *lymphocytes* and neutrophils).

ii) **Integrins** on the endothelial cell surface are activated during the process of loose and transient adhesions between endothelial cells and leucocytes.

iii) **Immunoglobulin superfamily adhesion molecule** such as intercellular adhesion molecule (ICAM-1, 2) help in localising leucocytes to the site of tissue injury and thus help in transmigration of PMNs.

3. EMIGRATION. After sticking of neutrophils to endothelium, the former move along the endothelial surface till a suitable site between the endothelial cells is found where the neutrophils throw out cytoplasmic pseudopods.

Simultaneous to emigration of leucocytes, escape of red cells through gaps between the endothelial cells, *diapedesis*, takes place.

4. CHEMOTAXIS. The chemotactic factor-mediated transmigration of leucocytes after crossing several barriers (endothelium, basement membrane, perivascular myofibroblasts and matrix) to reach the interstitial tissues is called chemotaxis. The concept of chemotaxis is well illustrated by *Boyden's chamber experiment*.

The agents acting as potent chemotactic substances for different leucocytes called *chemokines* are as follows:

i) Leukotriene B_4 (LT-B_4)

TABLE 6.1: Mechanisms of Increased Vascular Permeability.

MECHANISM	MICROVASCULATURE	RESPONSE TYPE	PATHOGENESIS	EXAMPLES
1. Endothelial cell contraction	Venules	Immediate transient (15-30 min)	Histamine, bradykinin, others	Mild thermal injury
2. Endothelial cell retraction	Venules	Somewhat delayed (4-6 hrs) prolonged (24 hrs or more)	IL-1, TNF	In vitro only
3. Direct endothelial cell injury	Arterioles, venules, capillaries	Immediate prolonged (hrs to days), or delayed (2-12 hrs) prolonged (hrs to days)	Cell necrosis and detachment	Moderate to severe burns, severe bacterial infection, radiation injury
4. Leucocyte-mediated endothelial injury	Venules, capillaries	Delayed, prolonged	Leucocyte activation	Pulmonary venules and capillaries
5. Neovascularisation	All levels	Any type	Angiogenesis, VEGF	Healing, tumours

Chapter Six

ii) Platelet factor 4 (PF_4)

iii) Components of complement system (C_3, C_5 in particular)

iv) Cytokines (Interleukins IL-1, IL-5, IL-6)

v) Soluble bacterial products (such as formylated peptides)

vi) Monocyte chemoattractant protein (MCP-1)

vii) Chemotactic factor for CD_4+T cells

viii) Eotaxin chemotactic for eosinophils.

There are specific receptors for each of the chemoattractants listed above.

Phagocytosis (p. 138)

Phagocytosis is defined as the process of engulfment of solid particulate material by the cells (cell-eating). The cells performing this function are called *phagocytes*. There are 2 main types of phagocytic cells:

i) Polymorphonuclear neutrophils (PMNs) which appear early in acute inflammatory response, also called as *microphages*.

ii) Circulating monocytes and fixed tissue mononuclear phagocytes called as *macrophages*.

The process of phagocytosis is similar for both polymorphs and macrophages and involves the following 4 steps:

1. RECOGNITION AND ATTACHMENT STAGE. The phagocytic cells are recognised and attracted to bacteria by chemotatic factors released by bacterial products as well as by tissue proteins. In order to establish a bond between bacteria and the cell membrane of phagocytic cell, the micro-organisms get coated with *opsonins* which are naturally-occurring factors in the serum.

i) *IgG opsonin* is the Fc fragment of immunoglobulin G;

ii) C_{3b} *opsonin* is the fragment of complement;

iii) *Lectins* are carbohydrate-binding proteins in the plasma.

2. ENGULFMENT STAGE. The opsonised particle bound to the surface of phagocyte is ready to be engulfed. This is accomplished by formation of cytoplasmic pseudopods around the particle due to activation of actin filaments beneath cell wall, enveloping it in a phagocytic vacuole.

3. DEGRANULATION STAGE. During this process, the preformed granule-stored products of PMNs are discharged or secreted into the phagosome and the extracellular environment. In particular, the specific or secondary granules of PMNs are discharged (e.g. lysosomes) while the azurophilic granules are fused with phagosomes.

4. KILLING OR DEGRADATION STAGE. Next comes the stage of killing and digestion of micro-organism completing the role of phagocytes as scavanger cells. The micro-organisms after being killed by antibacterial substances are degraded by hydrolytic enzymes. However, this mechanism fails to kill and degrade some bacteria like tubercle bacilli.

The antimicrobial agents act by either of the following mechanisms:

i) **Oxygen-dependent bactericidal mechanism.** An important mechanism of microbicidal killing is by the production of reactive oxygen metabolites (O'_2 H_2O_2, OH', HOCl, HOI, HOBr).

This type of bactericidal activity is carried out either via enzyme myeloperoxidase (MPO) present in the granules of neutrophils and monocytes, or independent of enzyme MPO:

ii) **Oxygen-independent bactericidal mechanism.** Some agents released from the granules of phagocytic cells do not require oxygen for bactericidal activity. These include lysosomal hydrolases, permeability increasing factors, defensins and cationic proteins.

iii) **Nitric oxide mechanism.** In addition to oxygen-dependent and oxygen-independent mechanisms, recently role of nitric oxide (NO) in inflammatory reaction has been emphasised. NO is produced by endothelial cells as well as by activated macrophages.

CHEMICAL MEDIATORS OF INFLAMMATION (p. 140)

Also called as permeability factors or endogenous mediators of increased vascular permeability, these are a large and increasing number of endogenous compounds which can enhance vascular permeability.

The substances acting as chemical mediators of inflammation may be released *from the cells, the plasma, or damaged tissue* itself. They are broadly classified into 2 groups: mediators released by cells; and mediators originating from plasma.

Chemical mediators involved in causing increased vascular permeability and consequent oedema of tissues are shown in Fig. 6.1.

I. Cell-derived Mediators (p. 140)

1. VASOACTIVE AMINES. Two important pharmacologically active amines that have role in the early inflammatory response (first one hour) are histamine and 5-hydroxytryptamine (5-HT) or serotonin.

2. ARACHIDONIC ACID METABOLITES (EICOSANOIDS). Arachidonic acid is a fatty acid, eicosatetraenoic acid, and its 2 main sources are:
■ from diet directly; and
■ conversion of essential fatty acid, linoleic acid to arachidonic acid.

Arachidonic acid must be first activated by stimuli or other mediators like C_{5a} so as to form arachidonic acid metabolites by one of the following 2 pathways: via cyclo-oxygenase pathway (Fig. 6.2) and via lipo-oxygenase pathway (Fig. 6.3).

3. LYSOSOMAL COMPONENTS. The inflammatory cells—neutrophils and monocytes, contain lysosomal granules which on release elaborate a variety of mediators of inflammation.

i) Granules of neutrophils. These are of two types: specific or secondary, and azurophil or primary. The specific granules contain lactoferrin, lysozyme, alkaline phosphatase and collagenase while the large azurophil granules have myeloperoxidase, acid hydrolases and neutral proteases such as elastase, collagenase and proteinase.

Acid proteases act within the cell to cause destruction of bacteria in phagolysosome while neutral proteases attack on the extracellular constituents such as basement membrane, collagen, elastin, cartilage etc.

ii) Granules of monocytes and tissue macrophages. These cells on degranulation also release mediators of inflammation like acid proteases, collagenase, elastase and plasminogen activator. However, they are more active in chronic inflammation than acting as mediators of acute inflammation.

4. PLATELET ACTIVATING FACTOR (PAF). It is released from IgE-sensitised basophils or mast cells, other leucocytes, endothelium and platelets. Apart from its action on platelet aggregation and release reaction, the actions of PAF as mediator of inflammation are: increased vascular permeability; vasodilatation in low concentration and vasoconstriction otherwise; bronchoconstriction; adhesion of leucocytes to endothelium; and chemotaxis.

5. CYTOKINES. Cytokines are polypeptide substances produced by activated lymphocytes *(lymphokines)* and activated monocytes *(monokines).* These agents may act on 'self' cells producing them or on other cells. Currently, main cytokines acting as mediators of inflammation are: interleukin-1 (IL-1), tumour necrosis factor (TNF)-α and β, interferon (IF)-γ, and chemokines (IL-8, PF-4).

i) IL-1 and TNF-α, TNF-β induce endothelial effects in the form of increased leucocyte adherence, thrombogenicity, elaboration of other cytokines, fibroblastic proliferation and acute phase reactions.

ii) IF-γ causes activation of macrophages and neutrophils and is associated with synthesis of nitric acid synthase.

Chapter Six

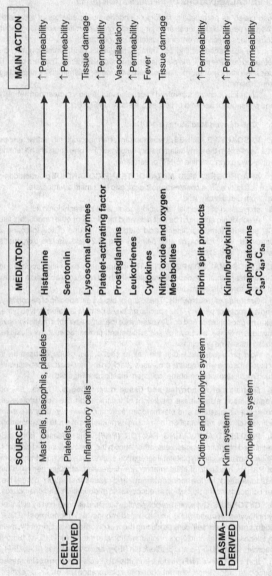

Fig. 6.1: Chemical mediators of inflammation.

SOURCE		MEDIATOR	MAIN ACTION
CELL-DERIVED	Mast cells, basophils, platelets	Histamine	↑ Permeability
	Platelets	Serotonin	↑ Permeability
	Inflammatory cells	Lysosomal enzymes	Tissue damage
		Platelet-activating factor	↑ Permeability
		Prostaglandins	Vasodilatation
		Leukotrienes	↑ Permeability
		Cytokines	Fever
		Nitric oxide and oxygen Metabolites	Tissue damage
PLASMA-DERIVED	Clotting and fibrinolytic system	Fibrin split products	↑ Permeability
	Kinin system	Kinin/bradykinin	↑ Permeability
	Complement system	Anaphylatoxins C_{3a}, C_{4a}, C_{5a}	↑ Permeability

Fig. 6.2: Arachidonic acid metabolites via cyclo-oxygenase pathway.

Fig. 6.3: Arachidonic acid metabolites via lipooxygenase pathway.

iii) **Chemokines** are a family of chemoattractants for inflammatory cells and include: IL-8 chemotactic for neutrophils; platelet factor-4 chemotactic for neutrophils, monocytes and eosinophils; MCP-1 chemotactic for monocytes; and eotaxin chemotactic for eosinophils.

6. NITRIC OXIDE AND OXYGEN METABOLITES. Nitric oxide (NO) was originally described as vascular relaxation factor produced by endothelial cells. It has recently been included as a mediator of inflammatory responses since activated macrophages also produce NO during the oxidation of arginine by the action of enzyme, NO synthase.

II. Plasma-derived Mediators (Plasma Proteases) *(p. 143)*

These include the various products derived from activation and interaction of 4 interlinked systems: kinin, clotting, fibrinolytic and complement (Fig. 6.4).

REGULATION OF INFLAMMATION *(p. 145)*

The onset of inflammatory responses outlined above may have potentially damaging influence on the host tissues as evident in hypersensitivity conditions. Such self-damaging effects are kept in check by the host mechanisms so as to resolve inflammation.

i) **Acute phase reactants.** A variety of acute phase reactant (APR) proteins are released in plasma in response to tissue trauma and infection. These include the following:

Chapter Six

Fig. 6.4: Inter-relationship between clotting, fibrinolytic, kinin and complement systems.

i) *Certain cellular protection factors* (α_1-antitrypsin, α_1-chymotrypsin, α_2-antiplasmin, plasminogen activator inhibitor);

ii) *Some coagulation proteins* (fibrinogen, plasminogen, von Willebrand factor, factor VIII);

iii) *Transport proteins* (ceruloplasmin, haptoglobin);

iv) *Immune agents* (serum amyloid A and P component, C-reactive protein); and

v) *Stress proteins* (heat shock proteins—HSP, ubiquitin).

The APR are synthesised mainly in the liver and to some extent in macrophages. APR combined with systemic features of fever and leucocytosis is termed *'acute phase response'*. Deficient synthesis of APR leads to severe form of disease in chronic and repeated inflammatory responses.

ii) Corticosteroids. The endogenous glucocorticoids act as anti-inflammatory agents. Their levels are raised in infection and trauma by self-regulating mechanism.

iii) Free cytokine receptors. The presence of free receptors for cytokines in the serum correlates directly with disease activity.

iv) Suppressor T cells. A prohibition of suppressor T cells is seen which inhibits the function of T and B cells.

v) Anti-inflammatory chemical mediators. As already described, PGE_2 and prostacyclin have both pro-inflammatory as well as anti-inflammatory actions.

THE INFLAMMATORY CELLS *(p. 146)*

The cells participating in acute and chronic inflammation are circulating leucocytes, plasma cells and tissue macrophages. Summary of their morphology, characteristics and functions is given in Table 6.2.

Mononuclear-Phagocyte System (Reticuloendothelial System) *(p. 147)*

This cell system includes cells derived from 2 sources with common morphology, function and origin. These are as under:

Blood monocytes. These comprise 4-8% of circulating leucocytes.

Tissue macrophages. These include the following cells in different tissues:

   i) Macrophages in inflammation.
   ii) Histiocytes, macrophages present in connective tissues.

TABLE 6.2: Morphology and Functions of Inflammatory Cells.

MORPHOLOGY	FEATURES	MEDIATORS
A, POLYMORPH	i. Initial phagocytosis of bacteria and foreign body ii. Acute inflammatory cell	i. Primary granules (MPO, lysozyme, cationic proteins, acid hydrolases, ii. Secondary granules (elastase lysozyme, alk. phosph, collagenase, lactoferrin) iii. Tertiary granules (gelatinase, cathepsin) iv. Reactive oxygen metabolites
B, MONOCYTE/ MACROPHAGE	i. Bacterial phagocytosis ii. Chronic inflammatory cell iii. Regulates lymphocyte response	i. Acid and neutral hydrolases (lysosomal) ii. Cationic protein iii. Phospholipase iv. Prostaglandins, leukotrienes v. IL-1
C, LYMPHOCYTE	i. Humoral and cell-mediated immune responses ii. Chronic inflammatory cell iii. Regulates macrophage response	i. B cells: antibody production ii. T cells: delayed hypersensitivity, cytotoxicity
D, PLASMA CELL	i. Derived from B cells ii. Chronic inflammatory cell	i. Antibody synthesis ii. Antibody secretion
E, EOSINOPHIL	i. Allergic states ii. Parasitic infestations iii. Chronic inflammatory cell	i. Reactive oxygen metabolites ii. Lysosomal (major basic protein, cationic protein, eosinophil peroxidase, neurotoxin) iii. PGE_2 synthesis
F, BASOPHIL/ MAST CELL	i. Receptor for IgE molecules ii. Electron-dense granules	i. Histamine ii. Leukotrienes iii. Platelet activating factor

iii) Kupffer cells, macrophages of liver cells.
iv) Alveolar macrophages (type II pneumocytes) in lungs.
v) Macrophages/histiocytes of the bone marrow.
vi) Tingible body cells of germinal centres of lymph nodes.

Chapter Six

vii) Littoral cells of splenic sinusoids.
viii) Osteoclasts in the bones.
ix) Microglial cells of the brain.
x) Langerhans' cells/dendritic histiocytes of the skin.
xi) Hoffbauer cells of the placenta.
xii) Mesangial cells of glomerulus.

Role of macrophages in inflammation. The functions of mononuclear-phagocyte cells are as under:

i) *Phagocytosis* (cell eating) and *pinocytosis* (cell drinking).

ii) *Macrophages on activation* by lymphokines released by T lymphocytes or by non-immunologic stimuli elaborate a variety of biologically active substances as under:

a) Proteases like collagenase and elastase which degrade collagen and elastic tissue.
b) Plasminogen activator which activates the fibrinolytic system.
c) Products of complement.
d) Some coagulation factors (factor V and thromboplastin) which convert fibrinogen to fibrin.
e) Chemotactic agents for other leucocytes.
f) Metabolites of arachidonic acid.
g) Growth promoting factors for fibroblasts, blood vessels and granulocytes.
h) Cytokines like interleukin-1 and tumour necrosis factor.
i) Oxygen-derived free radicals.

Giant Cells *(p. 148)*

A few examples of multinucleate giant cells exist in normal tissues (e.g. osteoclasts in the bones, trophoblasts in placenta, megakaryocytes in the bone marrow). However, in chronic inflammation when the macrophages fail to deal with particles to be removed, they fuse together and form multinucleated giant cells. Besides, morphologically distinct giant cells appear in some tumours also.

A. Giant cells in inflammation:

i) Foreign body giant cells. These contain numerous nuclei (up to 100) which are uniform in size and shape and resemble the nuclei of macrophages. These nuclei are scattered throughout the cytoplasm. These are seen in chronic infective granulomas, leprosy and tuberculosis.

ii) Langhans' giant cells. These are seen in tuberculosis and sarcoidosis. Their nuclei are like the nuclei of macrophages and epithelioid cells. These nuclei are arranged either around the periphery in the form of horseshoe or ring or are clustered at the two poles of the giant cell.

iii) Touton giant cells. These multinucleated cells have vacuolated cytoplasm due to lipid content e.g. in xanthoma.

iv) Aschoff giant cells. These multinucleate giant cells are derived from cardiac histiocytes and are seen in rheumatic nodule.

B. Giant cells in tumours:

i) Anaplastic cancer giant cells. These are larger, have numerous nuclei which are hyperchromatic and vary in size and shape.

ii) Reed-Sternberg cells. These are also malignant tumour giant cells which are generally binucleate and are seen in various histologic types of Hodgkin's lymphomas.

iii) Giant cell tumour of bone. This tumour of the bones has uniform distribution of osteoclastic giant cells spread in the stroma.

FACTORS DETERMINING VARIATION IN INFLAMMATORY RESPONSE *(p. 149)*

Although acute inflammation is typically characterised by vascular and cellular events with emigration of neutrophilic leucocytes, not all examples of acute inflammation show infiltration by neutrophils. On the other hand, some chronic inflammatory conditions are characterised by neutrophilic infiltration. For example, *typhoid fever* is an example of acute inflammatory process but the cellular response in it is lymphocytic; *osteomyelitis* is an example of chronic inflammation but the cellular response in this condition is mainly neutrophilic.

The morphologic variation in inflammation depends upon a number of factors and processes. These are discussed below:

1. Factors Involving the Organisms *(p. 149)*

i) Type of injury and infection, ii) virulence, iii) dose, iv) portal of entry, and v) product of organisms.

2. Factors Involving the Host *(p. 149)*

i) General health of host, ii) immune state of host, iii) leukopenia, iv) site or type of tissue involved, and v) local host factors.

3. Type of Exudation *(p. 149)*

i) *Serous*, when the fluid exudate resembles serum or is watery.

ii) *Fibrinous*, when the fibrin content of the fluid exudate is high.

iii) *Purulent or suppurative exudate* is formation of creamy pus as seen in infection with pyogenic bacteria.

iv) *Haemorrhagic*, when there is vascular damage.

v) *Catarrhal*, when the surface inflammation of epithelium produces increased secretion of mucous.

4. Cellular Proliferation *(p. 149)*

i) There is no significant cellular proliferation in *acute bacterial infections* except in typhoid fever in which there is intestinal lymphoid hyperplasia.

ii) *Viral infections* have the ability to stimulate cellular proliferation.

iii) *In rapidly progressive glomerulonephritis*, there is proliferation of glomerular capsular epithelial cells resulting in formation of 'crescents'.

iv) *In chronic inflammation*, cellular proliferation of macrophages, fibroblasts and endothelial cells occurs.

5. Necrosis *(p. 150)*

i) In *gas gangrene*, there is extensive necrosis with discoloured and foul smelling tissues.

ii) In *acute appendicitis*, there is necrosis as a result of vascular obstruction.

iii) In *chronic inflammation* such as tuberculosis, there is characteristic caseous necrosis.

MORPHOLOGY OF ACUTE INFLAMMATION *(p. 150)*

1. PSEUDOMEMBRANOUS INFLAMMATION. It is inflammatory response of mucous surface (oral, respiratory, bowel) to toxins of diphtheria or irritant gases. As a result of denudation of epithelium, plasma exudes on the surface where it coagulates, and together with necrosed epithelium, forms false membrane that gives this type of inflammation its name.

2. ULCER. Ulcers are local defects on the surface of an organ produced by inflammation. Common sites for ulcerations are the stomach, duodenum, intestinal ulcers in typhoid fever, intestinal tuberculosis, bacillary and amoebic dysentery, ulcers of legs due to varicose veins etc.

3. SUPPURATION (ABSCESS FORMATION). When acute bacterial infection is accompanied by intense neutrophilic infiltrate in the inflamed tissue, it results in tissue necrosis. A cavity is formed which is called an abscess and contains purulent exudate or pus and the process of abscess formation is known as suppuration.

4. CELLULITIS. It is a diffuse inflammation of soft tissues resulting from spreading effects of substances like hyaluronidase released by some bacteria.

5. BACTERIAL INFECTION OF THE BLOOD. This includes the following 3 conditions:

i) Bacteraemia is defined as presence of small number of bacteria in the blood which do not multiply significantly. They are commonly not detected by direct microscopy. Blood culture is done for their detection.

ii) Septicaemia means presence of rapidly multiplying, highly pathogenic bacteria in the blood e.g. pyogenic cocci, bacilli of plague etc. Septicaemia is generally accompanied by systemic effects like toxaemia, multiple small haemorrhages, neutrophilic leucocytosis and disseminated intravascular coagulation (DIC).

iii) Pyaemia is the dissemination of small septic thrombi in the blood which cause their effects at the site where they are lodged. This can result in pyaemic abscesses or septic infarcts.

a) *Pyaemic abscesses* are multiple small abscesses in various organs such as in cerebral cortex, myocardium, lungs and renal cortex, resulting from very small emboli fragmented from septic thrombus.

b) *Septic infarcts* result from lodgement of larger fragments of septic thrombi in the arteries with relatively larger foci of necrosis, suppuration and acute inflammation.

SYSTEMIC EFFECTS OF ACUTE INFLAMMATION *(p. 151)*

1. Fever occurs due to bacteraemia. It is thought to be mediated through release of factors like prostaglandins, interleukin-1 and tumour necrosis factor in response to infection.

2. Leucocytosis commonly accompanies the acute inflammatory reactions, usually in the range of 15,000-20,000/μl. When the counts are higher than this with 'shift to left' of myeloid cells, the blood picture is described as leukaemoid reaction. Usually, in bacterial infections there is neutrophilia; in viral infections lymphocytosis; and in parasitic infestations, eosinophilia. Typhoid fever, an example of acute inflammation, however, induces leucopenia with relative lymphocytosis.

3. Lymphangitis-lymphadenitis is one of the important manifestations of localised inflammatory injury. The lymphatics and lymph nodes that drain the inflamed tissue show reactive inflammatory changes in the form of lymphangitis and lymphadenitis. This response represents either a nonspecific reaction to mediators released from inflamed tissue or is an immunologic response to a foreign antigen. The affected lymph nodes may show hyperplasia of lymphoid follicles (follicular hyperplasia) and proliferation of mononuclear phagocytic cells in the sinuses of lymph node (sinus histiocytosis).

4. Shock may occur in severe cases. Massive release of cytokine TNF-α, a mediator of inflammation, in response to severe tissue injury or infection results in profuse systemic vasodilatation, increased vascular permeability and intravascular volume loss. The net effect of these changes is hypotension and shock.

FATE OF ACUTE INFLAMMATION *(p. 152)*

1. Resolution. It means complete return to normal tissue following acute inflammation. This occurs when tissue changes are slight and the cellular changes are reversible e.g. resolution in lobar pneumonia.

2. Healing by scarring. This takes place when the tissue destruction in acute inflammation is extensive so that there is no tissue regeneration but actually there is healing by fibrosis.

3. Suppuration. When the pyogenic bacteria causing acute inflammation result in severe tissue necrosis, the process progresses to suppuration.

4. Chronic inflammation. The acute inflammation may progress to chronic inflammation in which the processes of inflammation and healing proceed side by side.

CHRONIC INFLAMMATION *(p. 152)*

Chronic inflammation is defined as prolonged process in which tissue destruction and inflammation occur at the same time. Chronic inflammation can be caused by one of the following 3 ways:
1. Chronic inflammation following acute inflammation.
2. Recurrent attacks of acute inflammation.
3. Chronic inflammation starting *de novo*.

General Features of Chronic Inflammation *(p. 152)*

1. Mononuclear Cell Infiltration. Chronic inflammatory lesions are infiltrated by mononuclear inflammatory cells like phagocytes and lymphoid cells. Phagocytes are represented by circulating monocytes, tissue macrophages, epithelioid cells and sometimes, multinucleated giant cells. The macrophages comprise the most important cells in chronic inflammation. These may appear at the site of chronic inflammation from:
i) chemotactic factors and adhesion molecules for continued infiltration of macrophages;
ii) local proliferation of macrophages; and
iii) longer survival of macrophages at the site of inflammation.

Other chronic inflammatory cells include lymphocytes, plasma cells, eosinophils and mast cells. In chronic inflammation, lymphocytes and macrophages influence each other and release mediators of inflammation.

2. Tissue Destruction or Necrosis. Tissue destruction and necrosis are central feature of most forms of chronic inflammatory lesions. This is brought about by activated macrophages which release of a variety of biologically active substances e.g. protease, elastase, collagenase, lipase, reactive oxygen radicals, cytokines (IL-1, IL-8, TNF), nitric oxide, angiogenesis growth factor etc.

3. Proliferative Changes. As a result of necrosis, proliferation of small blood vessels and fibroblasts is stimulated resulting in formation of inflammatory granulation tissue. Eventually, healing by fibrosis and collagen laying takes place.

Systemic Effects of Chronic Inflammation *(p. 153)*

1. Fever. Invariably there is mild fever, often with loss of weight and weakness.

2. Anaemia. Chronic inflammation is accompanied by anaemia of varying degree.

3. Leucocytosis. As in acute inflammation, chronic inflammation also has leucocytosis but generally there is relative lymphocytosis in these cases.

4. ESR. ESR is elevated in all cases of chronic inflammation.

Chapter Six

5. Amyloidosis. Long-term cases of chronic suppurative inflammation may develop secondary systemic (AA) amyloidosis.

Types of Chronic Inflammation *(p. 153)*

For a more descriptive classification, histological features are used for classifying chronic inflammation into 2 corresponding types:

1. Chronic non-specific inflammation. It is characterised by non-specific inflammatory cell infiltration e.g. chronic osteomyelitis, lung abscess. A variant of this type of chronic inflammatory response is chronic suppurative inflammation in which infiltration by polymorphs and abscess formation are additional features e.g. actinomycosis.

2. Chronic granulomatous inflammation. It is characterised by formation of granulomas e.g. tuberculosis, leprosy, syphilis, actinomycosis, sarcoidosis etc.

GRANULOMATOUS INFLAMMATION *(p. 153)*

Granuloma is defined as a circumscribed, tiny lesion, about 1 mm in diameter, composed predominantly of collection of modified macrophages called epithelioid cells, and rimmed at the periphery by lymphoid cells.

Epithelioid cells, so called because of their epithelial cell-like appearance, are modified macrophages/ histiocytes which are somewhat elongated, having pale-staining abundant cytoplasm, vesicular and lightly-staining slipper-shaped nucleus, while the cell membrane of adjacent epithelioid cells is closely apposed due to hazy cell outline. Epithelioid cells are weakly phagocytic.

Besides the presence of epithelioid cells and lymphoid cells, granulomas may have giant cells, necrosis and fibrosis:

The following two factors favour the formation of granulomas:

i) *Presence of poorly digestible irritant* which may be organisms like *Mycobacterium tuberculosis*, particles of talc, etc.

ii) *Presence of cell-mediated immunity* to the irritant, implying thereby the role of hypersensitivity in granulomatous inflammation.

The mechanism of evolution of granuloma is graphically depicted in Fig. 6.5.

EXAMPLES OF GRANULOMATOUS INFLAMMATION *(p. 154)*

Granulomatous inflammation is typical of reaction to poorly digestible agents elicited by tuberculosis, leprosy, fungal infections, schistosomiasis, foreign particles etc.

TUBERCULOSIS *(p. 154)*

Tissue response in tuberculosis represents classical example of chronic granulomatous inflammation in humans.

CAUSATIVE ORGANISM. Tubercle bacillus or Koch's bacillus (named after discovery of the organism by Robert Koch in 1882) called *Mycobacterium tuberculosis* causes tuberculosis in the lungs and other tissues of the human body. The *organism is a strict aerobe and thrives best in tissues with high oxygen tension like in the apex of the lung.*

Infection with avium strain *(M. avium-intracellulare)* is common in patients with AIDS.

M. tuberculosis hominis is a slender rod-like bacillus, 4 μm in length, and can be demonstrated by the following methods:

1. Acid fast (Ziehl-Neelsen) staining.
2. Fluorescent dye methods.
3. Culture of the organism in Lowenstein-Jensen (L.J.) medium for 6 weeks.
4. Guinea pig inoculation method.

Fig. 6.5: Mechanism of evolution of a granuloma (IL=interleukin; IFN= interferon).

INCIDENCE. In spite of great advances in chemotherapy and immunology, tuberculosis still continues to be worldwide in distribution, more common in poorer countries of Africa, Latin America and Asia. Other factors contributing to higher incidence of tuberculosis are malnutrition, inadequate medical care, poverty, crowding, chronic debilitating conditions like uncontrolled diabetes, alcoholism and immunocompromised states like AIDS.

MODE OF TRANSMISSION. Human beings acquire infection with tubercle bacilli by one of the following routes:
1. Inhalation.
2. Ingestion.
3. Inoculation of tissue.
4. Transplacental route.

SPREAD OF TUBERCULOSIS. The disease spreads in the body by various routes:
1. Local spread.
2. Lymphatic spread.

3. Haematogenous spread.
4. By the natural passages. Infection may spread from:
i) lung lesions into pleura (tuberculous pleurisy);
ii) transbronchial spread into the adjacent lung segments;
iii) tuberculous salpingitis into peritoneal cavity (tuberculous peritonitis);
iv) infected sputum into larynx (tuberculous laryngitis);
v) swallowing of infected sputum (ileocaecal tuberculosis); and
vi) renal lesions into ureter and down to trigone of bladder.

HYPERSENSITIVITY AND IMMUNITY IN TUBERCULOSIS. Hypersensitivity or allergy, and immunity or resistance, play a major role in the development of lesions in tuberculosis. Tubercle bacilli as such do not produce any toxins. Tissue changes seen in tuberculosis are not the result of any exotoxin or endotoxin but are instead the result of host response to the organism which is in the form of development of cell-mediated hypersensitivity (or type IV hypersensitivity) and immunity. Both these host responses develop as a consequence of several lipids present in the microorganism which include the following:

1. mycosides such as 'cord factor' which are essential for growth and virulence of the organism in the animals; and

2. glycolipids present in the mycobacterial cell wall like *'Wax-D'* which acts as an adjuvant acting along with tuberculoprotein.

1. In the primary infection, intradermal injection of tubercle bacilli into the skin of a healthy guinea pig evokes no visible reaction for 10-14 days. After this period, a nodule develops at the inoculation site which subsequently ulcerates and heals poorly as the guinea pig, unlike human beings, does not possess any natural resistance. The regional lymph nodes also develop tubercles.

2. In the secondary infection, the sequence of changes is different. The tubercle bacilli are injected into the skin of the guinea pig who has been infected with tuberculosis 4-6 weeks earlier. In 1-2 days, the site of inoculation is indurated and dark, attaining a diameter of about 1 cm. The skin lesion ulcerates which heals quickly and the regional lymph nodes are not affected. This is called *Koch's phenomenon* and is indicative of hypersensitivity and immunity in the host.

Similar type of changes can be produced if injection of live tubercle bacilli is replaced with old tuberculin (OT).

Tuberculin (Mantoux) skin test. This test is done by intradermal injection of 0.1 ml of tuberculoprotein, purified protein derivative (PPD). Delayed type of hypersensitivity develops in individuals who are having or have been previously infected with tuberculous infection which is identified as an indurated area of more than 15 mm in 72 hours. However, patients having disseminated tuberculosis may show negative test due to release of large amount of tuberculoproteins from the endogenous lesions masking the hypersensitivity test.

Immunisation against tuberculosis. Protective immunisation against tuberculosis is induced by injection of attenuated strains of bovine type of tubercle bacilli, *Bacilli Calmette Guerin* (BCG). Cell-mediated immunity with consequent delayed hypersensitivity reaction develops with healing of the lesion, but the cell-mediated immunity persists, rendering the host tuberculin-positive and hence immune.

EVOLUTION OF TUBERCLE. The sequence of events which take place when tubercle bacilli are introduced into the tissue are as under:

1. An *initial response of neutrophils* is evoked which are rapidly destroyed by the organisms.

2. After about 12 hours, there is *progressive infiltration by macrophages*. This is due to coating of tubercle bacilli with serum complement factors C_{2a} and C_{3b} which act as opsonins and attract the macrophages.

3. The macrophages start *phagocytosing* the tubercle bacilli and either kill the bacteria or die away themselves.

4. As a part of body's immune response, T and B cells are activated. Activated CD4+T cells develop the cell-mediated *delayed type hypersensitivity reaction*, while B cells result in formation of antibodies which play no role in body's defence against tubercle bacilli.

5. In 2-3 days, the macrophages undergo structural changes as a result of immune mechanisms—the cytoplasm becomes pale and eosinophilic and their nuclei become elongated and vesicular. These modified macrophages resemble epithelial cells and are called *epithelioid cells*.

6. The epithelioid cells in time aggregate into tight clusters or *granulomas*. Release of cytokines in response to sensitised CD4+T cells and some constituents of mycobacterial cell wall play a role in formation of granuloma.

7. Some of the macrophages form *multinucleated giant cells* by fusion of adjacent cells. The giant cells may be Langhans' type having peripherally arranged nuclei in the form of horseshoe or ring, or clustered at the two poles of the giant cell; or they may be foreign body type having centrally-placed nuclei.

8. Around the mass of epithelioid cells and giant cells is a zone of lymphocytes, plasma cells and fibroblasts. The lesion at this stage is called *hard tubercle* due to absence of central necrosis.

9. Within 10-14 days, the centre of the cellular mass begins to undergo caseation necrosis, characterised by cheesy appearance and high lipid content. This stage is called *soft tubercle* which is the hallmark of tuberculous lesions. The development of caseation necrosis is possibly due to interaction of mycobacteria with activated T cells (CD4+ helper T cells via IF-γ and CD8+ suppressor T cells directly) as well as by direct toxicity of mycobacteria on macrophages.

10. The soft tubercle which is a fully-developed granuloma with caseous centre does not favour rapid proliferation of tubercle bacilli. *Acid-fast bacilli* are difficult to find in these lesions and may be demonstrated at the margins of recent necrotic foci and in the walls of the cavities.

The **fate of a granuloma** is variable:

i) The caseous material may undergo liquefaction and extend into surrounding soft tissues, discharging the contents on the surface. This is called *cold abscess* although there are no pus cells in it.

ii) In tuberculosis of tissues like bones, joints, lymph nodes and epididymis, sinuses are formed and the *sinus tracts* are lined by tuberculous granulation tissue.

iii) The adjacent granulomas may *coalesce* together enlarging the lesion which is surrounded by progressive fibrosis.

iv) In the granuloma enclosed by fibrous tissue, calcium salts may get deposited in the caseous material *(dystrophic calcification)* and sometimes the lesion may even get ossified over the years.

TYPES OF TUBERCULOSIS *(p. 159)*

Lung is the main organ affected in tuberculosis. The infection with tubercle bacilli is of 2 main types:

A. Primary tuberculosis; and
B. Secondary tuberculosis.

A. Primary Tuberculosis *(p. 159)*

The infection of an individual who has not been previously infected or immunised is called *primary tuberculosis* or *Ghon's complex* or *childhood tuberculosis*.

Primary complex or Ghon's complex is the lesion produced at the portal of entry with foci in the draining lymphatic vessels and lymph nodes. The most commonly involved tissues for primary complex are lungs and hilar lymph nodes.

The incidence of disseminated form of progressive primary tuberculosis is particularly high in immunocompromised host e.g. in patients of AIDS.

Primary complex or Ghon's complex in lungs consists of 3 components:

1. Pulmonary component. Lesion in the lung is the primary focus or Ghon's focus. It is 1-2 cm solitary area of tuberculous pneumonia located peripherally under a patch of pleurisy, in any part of the lung but more often in subpleural focus in the upper part of lower lobe.

2. Lymphatic vessel component. The lymphatics draining the lung lesion contain phagocytes containing bacilli and may develop beaded, miliary tubercles along the path of hilar lymph nodes.

3. Lymph node component. This consists of enlarged hilar and tracheo-bronchial lymph nodes in the area drained. The affected lymph nodes are matted and show caseation necrosis.

FATE OF PRIMARY TUBERCULOSIS. Primary complex may have one of the following sequelae:

1. Heal by *fibrosis,* and in time undergo *calcification* and even *ossification*.

2. In some cases, the primary focus in the lung continues to grow and the caseous material is disseminated through bronchi to the other parts of the same lung or the opposite lung. This is called *progressive primary tuberculosis*.

3. At times, bacilli may enter the circulation through erosion in a blood vessel and spread to various tissues and organs. This is called *primary miliary tuberculosis* and the lesions are seen in organs like liver, spleen, kidney, brain and bone marrow.

4. In certain circumstances like in lowered resistance and increased hypersensitivity of the host, bacilli lying dormant in acellular caseous material are activated and cause *progressive secondary tuberculosis.*

B. Secondary Tuberculosis *(p. 159)*

The infection of an individual who has been previously infected or sensitised is called *secondary*, or *post-primary* or *reinfection*, or *chronic tuberculosis*.

The infection may be acquired from:

■ *endogenous source* such as reactivation of dormant primary complex; or

■ *exogenous source* such as fresh dose of reinfection by the tubercle bacilli.

Secondary Pulmonary Tuberculosis *(p. 160)*

Secondary tuberculosis occurs most commonly in lungs in the region of apex.

The lesions in secondary pulmonary tuberculosis usually begin as 1-2 cm apical area of consolidation of the lung, which may in time develop a small area of central caseation necrosis and peripheral fibrosis. It occurs by haematogenous spread of infection from primary complex to the apex of the affected lung where the oxygen tension is high and favourable for growth of aerobic tubercle bacilli.

Patients with HIV infection previously exposed to tuberculous infection have particularly high incidence of reactivation of primary tuberculosis and the pattern of lesions in such cases is similar to that of primary tuberculosis. In addition, opportunistic infection with *M. avium-intracellulare* can occur in cases of AIDS.

FATE OF SECONDARY PULMONARY TUBERCULOSIS *(p. 161)*

1. The lesions may *heal* with fibrous scarring and calcification.

2. The lesions may *coalesce* together to form larger area of tuberculous pneumonia and produce progressive secondary pulmonary tuberculosis with the following pulmonary and extrapulmonary involvements:

i) Fibrocaseous tuberculosis
ii) Tuberculous caseous pneumonia
iii) Miliary tuberculosis.

I.   FIBROCASEOUS TUBERCULOSIS. The original area of tuberculous pneumonia undergoes massive central caseation necrosis which may:

■ either break into a bronchus from a cavity *(cavitary or open fibrocaseous tuberculosis)*; or

■ remain, as a soft caseous lesion without drainage into a bronchus or bronchiole to produce a non-cavitary lesion *(chronic fibrocaseous tuberculosis)*.

The cavity provides favourable environment for proliferation of tubercle bacilli due to high oxygen tension. The cavity may communicate with bronchial tree and becomes the source of spread of infection *('open tuberculosis')*. Ingestion of sputum containing tubercle bacilli from endogenous pulmonary lesions may produce *laryngeal and intestinal tuberculosis.*

G/A Tuberculous cavity is spherical with thick fibrous wall, lined by yellowish, caseous, necrotic material and the lumen is traversed by thrombosed blood vessels. Around the wall of cavity are seen foci of consolidation.

M/E The wall of cavity shows eosinophilic, granular, caseous material which may show foci of dystrophic calcification. Widespread coalesced tuberculous granulomas composed of epithelioid cells, Langhans' giant cells and peripheral mantle of lymphocytes and having central caseation necrosis are seen. The outer wall of cavity shows fibrosis.

II.   TUBERCULOUS CASEOUS PNEUMONIA. The caseous material from a case of secondary tuberculosis in an individual with high degree of hypersensitivity may spread to rest of the lung producing caseous pneumonia.

M/E The lesions show exudative reaction with oedema, fibrin, polymorphs and monocytes but numerous tubercle bacilli can be demonstrated in the exudates.

III.   MILIARY TUBERCULOSIS. This is lymphohaematogenous spread of tuberculous infection from primary focus or later stages of tuberculosis. The spread may occur to systemic organs or isolated organ. The spread is either by entry of infection into pulmonary vein producing disseminated or isolated organ lesion in different extra-pulmonary sites (e.g. liver, spleen, kidney, brain and bone marrow) or into pulmonary artery restricting the development of miliary lesions within the lung. The miliary lesions are millet seed-sized (1 mm diameter), yellowish, firm areas without grossly visible caseation necrosis.

Clinical Features of Tuberculosis *(p. 163)*

1.   Referable to lungs—such as productive cough, may be with haemoptysis, pleural effusion, dyspnoea, orthopnoea etc. Chest X-ray may show typical apical changes like pleural effusion, nodularity, and miliary or diffuse infiltrates in the lung parenchyma.

2.   Systemic features—such as fever, night sweats, fatigue, loss of weight and appetite. Long-standing and untreated cases of tuberculosis may develop systemic secondary amyloidosis.

Causes of death in pulmonary tuberculosis are usually pulmonary insufficiency, pulmonary haemorrhage, sepsis due to disseminated miliary tuberculosis, cor pulmonale or secondary amyloidosis.

LEPROSY *(p. 163)*

Leprosy or Hansen's disease (after discovery of the causative organism by Hansen in 1874) is a chronic infectious disease affecting mainly the cooler parts of the body such as the skin, mouth, respiratory tract, eyes, peripheral nerves, superficial lymph nodes and testis.

Chapter Six

Causative Organism *(p. 163)*

The disease is caused by *Mycobacterium leprae* which closely resembles *Mycobacterium tuberculosis* but is less acid-fast. The organisms in tissues appear as compact rounded masses *(globi)* or are arranged in parallel fashion like *cigarettes-in-pack*.

M. leprae can be demonstrated in tissue sections, in split skin smears by splitting the skin, scrapings from cut edges of dermis, and in nasal smears by the following techniques:

1. *Acid-fast (Ziehl-Neelsen) staining.*
2. *Fite-Faraco staining* procedure is a modification of Z.N. procedure.
3. *Gomori methenamine silver (GMS) staining.*

The slit smear technique gives a reasonable quantitative measure of *M. leprae* when stained with Ziehl-Neelsen method and examined under 100x oil objective for determining the density of bacteria in the lesion *(bacterial index, BI)*.

Nine-banded armadillo, a rodent, acts as an experimental animal model as it develops leprosy which is histopathologically and immunologically similar to human leprosy.

Incidence *(p. 164)*

The disease is endemic in areas with hot and moist climates and in poor tropical countries. According to the WHO, five countries—India, Brazil, Indonesia, Myanmar (Burma) and Nigeria, together constitute vast majority of leprosy cases, of which India accounts for about one-third of all registered leprosy cases globally. In India, the disease is seen more commonly in regions like Tamil Nadu, Bihar, Pondicherry, Andhra Pradesh, Orissa, West Bengal and Assam.

Mode of Transmission *(p. 164)*

Leprosy is a slow communicable disease and the incubation period between first exposure and appearance of signs of disease varies from 2 to 20 years (average about 3 years). The infectivity may be from the following sources:

1. *Direct contact* with untreated leprosy patients who shed numerous bacilli from damaged skin, nasal secretions, mucous membrane of mouth and hair follicles.
2. *Materno-foetal transmission* across the placenta.
3. Transmission from *milk* of leprosy patient to infant.

Classification *(p. 164)*

Leprosy is broadly classified into 2 main types (Table 6.3):

- Lepromatous type representing *low resistance*; and
- Tuberculoid type representing *high resistance*.

Since both these types of leprosy represent two opposite poles of host immune response, these are also called *polar forms* of leprosy. Cases not falling into either of the two poles are classified as *borderline* and *indeterminate types.*

Currently, leprosy is classified into 7 groups *(modified Ridley and Jopling's classification)*. These are:

 TT—Tuberculoid Polar *(High resistance)*
 BT—Borderline Tuberculoid
 TI—Tuberculoid Indefinite
 BB—Mid Borderline
 LI—Lepromatous Indefinite
 BL—Borderline Lepromatous
 LL—Lepromatous Polar *(Low resistance)*

TABLE 6.3: Differences between Lepromatous and Tuberculoid Leprosy.

	FEATURE	LEPROMATOUS LEPROSY	TUBERCULOID LEPROSY
1.	*Skin lesions*	Symmetrical, multiple, hypopigmented, erythematous, maculopapular or nodular (leonine facies).	Asymmetrical, single or a few lesions, hypopigmented and erythematous macular.
2.	*Nerve involvement*	Present but sensory disturbance is less severe.	Present with distinct sensory disturbance.
3.	*Histopathology*	Collection of foamy macrophages or lepra cells in the dermis separated from epidermis by a 'clear zone'.	Hard tubercle similar to granulomatous lesion, eroding the basal layer of epidermis; no clear zone.
4.	*Bacteriology*	Lepra cells highly positive for lepra bacilli seen as 'globi' or 'cigarettes-in-pack' appearance.	Lepra bacilli few, seen in destroyed nerves as granular or beaded forms.
5.	*Immunity*	Suppressed (low resistance).	Good immune response (high resistance).
6.	*Lepromin test*	Negative.	Positive.

Reactions in Leprosy *(p. 164)*

There may be two types of lepra reactions: type I (borderline reactions), and type II (erythema nodosum leprosum).

TYPE I: BORDERLINE REACTIONS. The polar forms of leprosy do not undergo any change in clinical and histopathological picture. The borderline groups are unstable and may move across the spectrum in either direction with upgrading or downgrading of patient's immune state. Accordingly, there may be two types of borderline reaction:

1. **Upgrading reaction** is characterised by increased cell-mediated immunity and occurs in patients of borderline lepromatous (BL) type on treatment who upgrade or shift towards tuberculoid type.

2. **Downgrading reaction** is characterised by lowering of cellular immunity and is seen in borderline tuberculoid (BT) type who downgrade or shift towards lepromatous type.

TYPE II: ERYTHEMA NODOSUM LEPROSUM (ENL). ENL occurs in lepromatous patients after treatment. It is characterised by tender cutaneous nodules, fever, iridocyclitis, synovitis and lymph node involvement.

Clinical Features *(p. 165)*

1. Lepromatous Leprosy:

i)   The skin lesions in LL are generally symmetrical, multiple, slightly hypopigmented and erythematous macules, papules, nodules or diffuse infiltrates. The nodular lesions may coalesce to give *leonine facies* appearance.

ii)   The lesions are hypoaesthetic or anaesthetic but the sensory disturbance is not as distinct as in TT.

2. Tuberculoid leprosy:

i)   The skin lesions in TT occur as either single or as a few asymmetrical lesions which are hypopigmented and erythematous macules.

ii)   There is a distinct sensory impairment.

Histopathology of Leprosy *(p. 165)*

In general, for histopathologic evaluation in all suspected cases of leprosy the following broad *guidelines* should be followed:

Chapter Six

- cell type of granuloma;
- nerve involvement; and
- bacterial load.

The main features in various groups are given in Table 6.3.

Immunology of Leprosy *(p. 166)*

Lepromin test is not a diagnostic test but is used for classifying leprosy on the basis of immune response. Intradermal injection of lepromin, an antigenic extract of *M. leprae,* reveals delayed hypersensitivity reaction in patients of tuberculoid leprosy.

- An early positive reaction appearing as an indurated area in 24-48 hours is called *Fernandez reaction.*
- A delayed granulomatous lesion appearing after 3-4 weeks is called *Mitsuda reaction.*

Patients of lepromatous leprosy are negative by the lepromin test.

The test indicates that cell-mediated immunity is greatly suppressed in LL while patients of TT show good immune response. Delayed type of hyper-sensitivity is conferred by T helper cells.

SYPHILIS *(p. 167)*

Syphilis is a venereal (sexually-transmitted) disease caused by spirochaetes, *Treponema pallidum.*

Causative Organism *(p. 167)*

T. pallidum is a coiled spiral filament 10 μm long that moves actively in fresh preparations. The organism cannot be stained by the usual methods and can be demonstrated in the exudates and tissues by:
1. *dark ground illumination (DGI)* in fresh preparation;
2. *fluorescent antibody technique*; and
3. *silver impregnation techniques.*

Immunology *(p. 167)*

T. pallidum does not produce any endotoxin or exotoxin. The pathogenesis of the lesions appears to be due to host immune response.

Treponemal infection is associated with two important antibodies which are immunoglobulins:

1. The Wassermann antibodies. Wassermann described a complement fixing antibody against antigen of human syphilitic tissue. This antigen is used in the Standard Test for Syphilis (STS) as follows:
i) Wassermann complement fixing test; and
ii) Venereal Disease Research Laboratory (VDRL) test.

2. Treponemal antibodies. Treponemal antibodies are produced which react with treponemal protein. The tests employed for detecting these antibodies are:
i) Reiter protein complement fixation (RPCF) test;
ii) Treponema pallidum immobilisation (TPI) test;
iii) Fluorescent treponemal antibody (FTA) test; and
iv) Treponemal passive haemagglutination (TPHA) test.

Mode of Transmission *(p. 167)*

1. *Sexual intercourse* resulting in lesions on glans penis, vulva, vagina and cervix.
2. *Intimate person-to-person contact* with lesions on lips, tongue or fingers.
3. *Transfusion* of infected blood.
4. *Materno-foetal transmission* in congenital syphilis if the mother is infected.

Stages of Acquired Syphilis *(p. 167)*

Acquired syphilis is divided into 3 stages depending upon the period after which the lesions appear and the type of lesions.

1. PRIMARY SYPHILIS. Typical lesion of primary syphilis is *chancre* which appears on genitals or at extra-genital sites in 2-4 *weeks* after exposure to infection.

M/E

i)   Dense infiltrate of lymphocytes, plasma cells and a few macrophages.

ii) Perivascular aggregation of mononuclear cells, particularly plasma cells (periarteritis and endarteritis).

2. SECONDARY SYPHILIS. Inadequately treated patients of primary syphilis develop *mucocutaneous lesions* and painless lymphadenopathy in 2-3 *months* after the exposure. Mucocutaneous lesions may be in the form of the mucous patches on mouth, pharynx and vagina; and generalised skin eruptions and condyloma lata in anogenital region.

3. TERTIARY SYPHILIS. After a latent period of appearance of secondary lesions and about 2-3 *years* following first exposure, tertiary lesions of syphilis appear. Lesions of tertiary syphilis are much less infective than the other two stages and spirochaetes can be demonstrated with great difficulty. These lesions are of 2 main types:

i) Syphilitic gumma. It is a solitary, localised, rubbery lesion with central necrosis, seen in organs like liver, testis, bone and brain. In liver, the gumma is associated with scarring of hepatic parenchyma *(hepar lobatum)*.

ii) Diffuse lesions of tertiary syphilis. The lesions appear following widespread dissemination of spirochaetes in the body. The diffuse lesions are predominantly seen in cardiovascular and nervous systems.

a) *Cardiovascular syphilis* mainly involves thoracic aorta.

b) *Neurosyphilis* may manifest as: meningovascular syphilis affecting chiefly the meninges; tabes dorsalis affecting the spinal cord; and general paresis affecting the brain.

CONGENITAL SYPHILIS. Congenital syphilis may develop in a foetus of more than 16 weeks gestation who is exposed to maternal spirochaetaemia. There can be 3 possibilities:

1. The child born dead. The child is premature, with macerated skin, enlarged spleen and liver, and with syphilitic epiphysitis.

2. The child born alive (Infantile form). The child may show mucocutaneous lesions of acquired secondary syphilis and bony lesions like epiphysitis and periostitis. The bridge of nose may fall due to ulceration and destruction giving the characteristic 'saddle nose' appearance of congenital syphilis.

3. The late type. The lesions appear after some years. The characteristic 'Hutchinson's teeth' seen in this type are small, widely spaced, peg-shaped permanent teeth. Tertiary lesions like gummas and neurosyphilis may also be seen.

ACTINOMYCOSIS *(p. 169)*

Actinomycosis is a chronic suppurative disease caused by anaerobic bacteria, *Actinomycetes israelii*. The organisms are commensals in the oral cavity, alimentary tract and vagina. The infection is always endogeneous in origin and not person-to-person.

Depending upon the anatomic location of lesions, actinomycosis is of 4 types:

1. Cervicofacial actinomycosis. This is the commonest form (60%) and has the best prognosis. The infection enters from tonsils, carious teeth, periodontal disease or trauma following tooth extraction. Initially, a firm swelling

Chapter Six

develops in the lower jaw ('lumpy jaw'). In time, the mass breaks down and abscesses and sinuses are formed. The discharging pus contains typical tiny yellow sulphur granules.

2. Thoracic actinomycosis. The infection in the lungs is due to aspiration of the organism from oral cavity or extension of infection from abdominal or hepatic lesions.

3. Abdominal actinomycosis. This type is common in appendix, caecum and liver. The abdominal infection results from swallowing of organisms from oral cavity or extension from thoracic cavity.

4. Pelvic actinomycosis. Infection in the pelvis occurs as a complication of intrauterine contraceptive devices (IUCDs).

M/E

i)   The inflammatory reaction is a granuloma with central suppuration. There is formation of abscesses in the centre of lesions and at the periphery are seen chronic inflammatory cells, giant cells and fibroblasts.

ii)   The centre of each abscess contains the bacterial colony, 'sulphur granule', characterised by radiating filaments (hence previously known as *ray fungus*) with hyaline, eosinophilic, club-like ends representative of secreted immunoglobulins.

iii)   Bacterial stains reveal the organisms as gram-positive filaments, nonacid-fast, which stain positively with Gomori's methenamine silver (GMS) staining.

SARCOIDOSIS (BOECK'S SARCOID) *(p. 169)*

Sarcoidosis is a systemic disease of unknown etiology. It is worldwide in distribution and affects adults from 20-40 years of age. The disease is characterised by the presence of non-caseating epithelioid cell granulomas ('sarcoid granuloma') in the affected tissues and organs, notably lymph nodes and lungs. Other sites are the skin, spleen, uvea of the eyes, salivary glands, liver and bones of hands and feet.

ETIOLOGY AND PATHOGENESIS. The cause of sarcoidosis remains unknown. The following observations point towards a possible immune origin of sarcoidosis:

1. Just as in tuberculosis, sarcoidosis is characterised by distinctive granulomatous response against *poorly degradable antigen*, but quite unlike tuberculosis, the antigen in sarcoidosis has eluded workers so far. PCR studies on affected pulmonary tissue have given equivocal result as regards presence of mycobacterial antigen.

2. That there are immunologic abnormalities in sarcoidosis is substantiated by *high levels of CD4+T cells* lavaged from lung lesions.There is also elevation in levels of IL-2 receptors in serum and in lavaged fluid from lungs.

3. There is presence of *activated alveolar macrophages* which elaborate cytokines that initiate the formation of non-caseating granulomas.

M/E

1. The diagnostic feature in sarcoidosis of any organ or tissue is the *non-caseating sarcoid granuloma*, composed of epithelioid cells, Langhans' and foreign body giant cells and surrounded peripherally by fibroblasts.

2. Typically, granulomas of sarcoidosis are *'naked'* i.e. either devoid of peripheral rim of lymphocytes or there is paucity of lymphocytes.

3. In late stage, the granuloma is either *enclosed by hyalinised fibrous tissue* or is replaced by hyalinised fibrous mass.

4. The giant cells in sarcoid granulomas contain certain *cytoplasmic inclusions* like:

i)   *Asteroid bodies*

ii)   *Schaumann's bodies or conchoid (conch like) bodies*

iii)   *Birefringent cytoplasmic crystals*

Chapter Six

KVIEM'S TEST. It is a useful intradermal diagnostic test. The antigen prepared from involved lymph node or spleen is injected intradermally. In a positive test, nodular lesion appears in 3-6 weeks at the inoculation site which on microscopic examination shows presence of non-caseating granulomas.

HEALING *(p. 171)*

Healing is the body response to injury in an attempt to restore normal structure and function. The process of healing involves 2 distinct processes:

■ *Regeneration* when healing takes place by proliferation of parenchymal cells and usually results in complete restoration of the original tissues.

■ *Repair* when the healing takes place by proliferation of connective tissue elements resulting in fibrosis and scarring.

REGENERATION *(p. 171)*

Some parenchymal cells are short-lived while others have a longer lifespan. In order to maintain proper structure of tissues, these cells are under the constant regulatory control of their cell cycle. These include growth factors such as: epidermal growth factor, fibroblast growth factor, platelet-derived growth factor, endothelial growth factor, transforming growth factor-β.

Depending upon their capacity to divide, the cells of the body can be divided into 3 groups:

1. Labile cells. These cells continue to multiply throughout life under normal physiologic conditions. These include: surface epithelial cells of epidermis, alimentary tract, respiratory tract, urinary tract, vagina, cervix, uterine endometrium, haematopoietic cells of bone marrow and cells of lymph nodes and spleen.

2. Stable cells. These cells decrease or lose their ability to proliferate after adolescence but retain the capacity to multiply in response to stimuli throughout adult life. These include: parenchymal cells of organs like liver, pancreas, kidneys, adrenal and thyroid; mesenchymal cells like smooth muscle cells, fibroblasts, vascular endothelium, bone and cartilage cells.

3. Permanent cells. These cells lose their ability to proliferate around the time of birth. These include: neurons of nervous system, skeletal muscle and cardiac muscle cells.

Regeneration of any type of parenchymal cells involves the following 2 processes:

i) Proliferation of original cells from the margin of injury with migration so as to cover the gap.

ii) Proliferation of migrated cells with subsequent differentiation and maturation so as to reconstitute the original tissue.

REPAIR *(p. 172)*

Repair is the replacement of injured tissue by fibrous tissue. Two processes are involved in repair:

1. Granulation tissue formation; and
2. Contraction of wounds.

Repair response takes place by participation of mesenchymal cells (consisting of connective tissue stem cells, fibrocytes and histiocytes), endothelial cells, macrophages, platelets, and the parenchymal cells of the injured organ.

Granulation Tissue Formation *(p. 172)*

The term granulation tissue derives its name from slightly granular and pink appearance of the tissue. Each granule corresponds histologically to proliferation of new small blood vessels which are slightly lifted on the surface by thin covering of fibroblasts and young collagen.

The following 3 phases are observed in the formation of granulation tissue:

1. PHASE OF INFLAMMATION. Following trauma, blood clots at the site of injury. There is acute inflammatory response with exudation of plasma, neutrophils and some monocytes within 24 hours.

2. PHASE OF CLEARANCE. Combination of proteolytic enzymes liberated from neutrophils, autolytic enzymes from dead tissues cells, and phagocytic activity of macrophages clear off the necrotic tissue, debris and red blood cells.

3. PHASE OF INGROWTH OF GRANULATION TISSUE. This phase consists of 2 main processes: angiogenesis or neovascularisation, and fibrogenesis.

i) Angiogenesis (neovascularisation). Formation of new blood vessels at the site of injury takes place by proliferation of endothelial cells from the margins of severed blood vessels. Initially, the proliferated endothelial cells are solid buds but within a few hours develop a lumen and start carrying blood. The newly formed blood vessels are more leaky, accounting for the oedematous appearance of new granulation tissue. Soon, these blood vessels differentiate into muscular arterioles, thin-walled venules and true capillaries.

 a) Angiogenesis takes place under the influence of vascular endothelial growth factor (VEGF) elaborated by mesenchymal cells but its receptors are present in endothelial cells only.

 b) Platelet-derived growth factor (PDGF), transforming growth factor-β (TGF-β), basic fibroblast growth factor (bFGF), other cytokines and surface integrins are the factors which are associated with cellular proliferation.

ii) Fibrogenesis. The newly formed blood vessels are present in an amorphous ground substance or matrix. The new fibroblasts originate from fibrocytes as well as by mitotic division of fibroblasts. Some of these fibroblasts have combination of morphologic and functional characteristics of smooth muscle cells (*myofibroblasts*). Collagen fibrils begin to appear by about 6th day. As maturation proceeds, more and more of collagen is formed while the number of active fibroblasts and new blood vessels decreases. This results in formation of inactive looking scar known as *cicatrisation*.

Contraction of Wounds *(p. 173)*

The wound starts contracting after 2-3 days and the process is completed by the 14th day. During this period, the wound is reduced by approximately 80% of its original size.

In order to explain the mechanism of wound contraction, a number of factors have been proposed.

1. *Dehydration* as a result of removal of fluid
2. *Contraction of collagen*
3. Discovery of *myofibroblasts* appearing in active granulation tissue

WOUND HEALING *(p. 174)*

Healing of skin wounds provides a classical example of combination of regeneration and repair described above. This can be accomplished in one of the following two ways:

■ Healing by first intention *(primary union);* and
■ healing by second intention *(secondary union).*

Healing by First Intention (Primary Union) *(p. 174)*

This is defined as healing of a wound which has the following characteristics:
i) clean and uninfected;
ii) surgically incised;

iii) without much loss of cells and tissue; and

iv) edges of wound are approximated by surgical sutures.

The sequence of events in primary union is described below:

1. Initial haemorrhage. Immediately after injury, the space between the approximated surfaces of incised wound is filled with blood which then clots and seals the wound against dehydration and infection.

2. Acute inflammatory response. This occurs within 24 hours with appearance of polymorphs.

3. Epithelial changes. The basal cells of epidermis from both the cut margins start proliferating and migrating towards incisional space in the form of epithelial spurs.

4. Organisation. By 3rd day, fibroblasts also invade the wound area. By 5th day, new collagen fibrils start forming In 4 weeks, the scar tissue with scanty cellular and vascular elements, a few inflammatory cells and epithelialised surface is formed.

5. Suture tracks. Each suture track is a separate wound and incites the same phenomena as in healing of the primary wound.

Healing by Second Intention (Secondary Union) *(p. 175)*

This is defined as healing of a wound having the following characteristics:

i) open with a large tissue defect, at times infected;

ii) having extensive loss of cells and tissues; and

iii) the wound is not approximated by surgical sutures but is left open.

The sequence of events in secondary union is as under:

1. Initial haemorrhage.

2. Inflammatory phase. There is an initial acute inflammatory response followed by appearance of macrophages which clear off the debris as in primary union.

3. Epithelial changes. As in primary healing, the epidermal cells from both the margins of wound proliferate and migrate into the wound in the form of epithelial spurs.

4. Granulation tissue. The main bulk of secondary healing is by granulations. Granulation tissue is formed by proliferation of fibroblasts and neovascularisation from the adjoining viable elements.

5. Wound contraction. Contraction of wound is an important feature of secondary healing, not seen in primary healing.

6. Presence of infection. Bacterial contamination of an open wound delays the process of healing due to release of bacterial toxins that provoke necrosis, suppuration and thrombosis.

Complications ofWound Healing *(p. 176)*

1. Infection
2. Implantation (epidermal) cyst
3. Pigmentation
4. Deficient scar formation
5. Incisional hernia
6. Hypertrophied scars and keloid formation
7. Excessive contraction
8. Neoplasia

EXTRACELLULAR MATRIX (ECM) *(p. 176)*

The wound is strengthened by proliferation of fibroblasts and myofibroblasts which get structural support from the extracellular matrix. ECM has five main components: collagen, adhesive glycoproteins, basement membrane, elastic fibres, and proteoglycans.

1. COLLAGEN. It is the main component of tissues such as fibrous tissue, bone, cartilage, valves of heart, cornea, basement membrane etc. Depending upon the biochemical composition, 18 types of collagen have been identified called collagen *type I to XVIII*, Type I, III and V are *true fibrillar collagen* which form the main portion of the connective tissue during healing of wounds in scars. Other types of collagen are *non-fibrillar* and amorphous material seen as component of the basement membranes.

2. ADHESIVE GLYCOPROTEINS. Various adhesive glycoproteins acting as glue for the ECM and the cells consist of:
i) Fibronectin
ii) Tenascin or cytotactin
iii) Thrombospondin

3. BASEMENT MEMBRANE. Basement membranes are periodic acid-Schiff (PAS)-positive amorphous structures that lie underneath epithelia of different organs and endothelial cells. They consist of collagen type IV and laminin.

4. ELASTIC FIBRES. While the tensile strength in tissue comes from collagen, the ability to recoil is provided by elastic fibres.

5. PROTEOGLYCANS. These are a group of molecules having 2 components—an essential carbohydrate polymer (called polysaccharide or glycosaminoglycan), and a protein bound to it, and hence the name proteoglycan. Various proteoglycans are distributed in different tissues as under:
i) *Chondroitin sulfate*—abundant in cartilage, dermis
ii) *Heparan sulfate*—in basement membranes
iii) *Dermatan sulfate*—in dermis
iv) *Keratan sulfate*—in cartilage
v) *Hyaluronic acid*—in cartilage, dermis.

Factors Influencing Healing *(p. 177)*

Two types of factors influence the wound healing: those acting locally, and those acting in general.

A. Local factors. These are:
1. Infection
2. Poor blood supply
3. Foreign bodies
4. Movement
5. Exposure to ionising radiation
6. Exposure to ultraviolet light
7. Type, size and location of injury

B. Systemic factors. These are:
1. Age
2. Nutrition
3. Systemic infection
4. Administration of glucocorticoids
5. Uncontrolled diabetics
6. Haematologic abnormalities

HEALING IN SPECIALISED TISSUES *(p. 177)*

Fracture Healing *(p. 177)*

Healing of fracture by callus formation depends upon some clinical considerations whether the fracture is:
■ traumatic or pathological
■ complete or incomplete like green-stick fracture; and
■ simple, comminuted or compound.

■ **Primary union of fractures** occurs in a few special situations when the ends of fracture are approximated.

■ **Secondary union** is the more common process of fracture healing. Secondary bone union is described under the following 3 headings:

I. PROCALLUS FORMATION. Steps involved in it are:

1. *Haematoma* forms due to bleeding from torn blood vessels,

2. *Local inflammatory response* occurs at the site of injury with exudation of fibrin, polymorphs and macrophages.

3. *Ingrowth of granulation tissue* begins with neovascularisation and proliferation of mesenchymal cells from periosteum and endosteum.

4. *Callus composed of woven bone and cartilage* starts within the first few days. The cells of inner layer of the periosteum have osteogenic potential and lay down collagen as well as osteoid matrix in the granulation tissue. The osteoid undergoes calcification and is called *woven bone callus.*

This stage is called provisional callus or procallus formation and is arbitrarily divided into *external, intermediate* and *internal procallus*

II. OSSEOUS CALLUS FORMATION. The procallus acts as scaffolding on which osseous callus composed of lamellar bone is formed.

III. REMODELLING. During the formation of lamellar bone, osteoblastic laying and osteoclastic removal are taking place remodelling the united bone ends, which after sometime, is indistinguishable from normal bone.

COMPLICATIONS OF FRACTURE HEALING. These are:

1. *Fibrous union* may result instead of osseous union

2. *Non-union* may result if some soft tissue is interposed between the fractured ends.

3. *Delayed union* may occur from causes of delayed wound healing in general such as infection, inadequate blood supply, poor nutrition, movement and old age.

Healing of Nervous Tissue *(p. 179)*

CENTRAL NERVOUS SYSTEM. The nerve cells of brain, spinal cord and ganglia once destroyed are not replaced. Axons of CNS also do not show any significant regeneration. The damaged neuroglial cells, however, may show proliferation of astrocytes called gliosis.

PERIPHERAL NERVOUS SYSTEM. In contrast to the cells of CNS, the peripheral nerves show regeneration, mainly from proliferation of Schwann cells and fibrils from distal end.

Healing of Muscle *(p. 179)*

SKELETAL MUSCLE. The regeneration of striated muscle is similar to peripheral nerves.

■ If the muscle sheath is intact, sarcolemmal tubes containing histiocytes appear along the endomysial tube which, in about 3 months time, restores properly oriented muscle fibres e.g. in Zenker's degeneration of muscle in typhoid fever.

■ If the muscle sheath is damaged, it forms a disorganised multinucleate mass and scar composed of fibrovascular tissue.

SMOOTH MUSCLE. Non-striated muscle has limited regenerative capacity e.g. appearance of smooth muscle in the arterioles in granulation tissue.

CARDIAC MUSCLE. Destruction of heart muscle is replaced by fibrous tissue.

Chapter Six

■ SELF ASSESSMENT

1. Increased vascular permeability caused by endothelial cell retraction and contraction affect the following level of circulation:
   A. Arterioles
   B. Venules
   C. Capillaries
   D. Lymphatics

2. Killing of *M. tuberculosis* that grows within the macrophage is brought about by the following mechanisms:
   A. By reactive oxygen species
   B. By oxygen-independent bactericidal mechanism
   C. By nitric oxide mechanism
   D. By hydrolytic enzymes

3. Main cytokines acting as mediators of inflammation are as under *except:*
   A. Interleukin-1 (IL-1)
   B. Tumour necrosis factor α (TNF-α)
   C. Nitric oxide (NO)
   D. Interferon-γ(IF-γ)

4. Receptor for IgE is present on:
   A. Polymorphs
   B. Eosinophil
   C. Basophil
   D. Plasma cell

5. Typhoid fever is an example of:
   A. Acute inflammation
   B. Chronic nonspecific inflammation
   C. Chronic granulomatous inflammation
   D. Chronic suppurative inflammation

6. Tubercle bacilli cause lesions by the following mechanisms:
   A. Elaboration of endotoxin
   B. Elaboration of exotoxin
   C. Type IV hypersensitivity
   D. Direct cytotoxicity

7. The following statements are correct for tubercle bacilli *except:*
   A. Tubercle bacilli can be cultured
   B. Tubercle bacilli are anaerobe
   C. Tubercle bacilli thrive best in the apex of lung
   D. *M. smegmatis* is not pathogenic to man

8. Mantoux test is negative in the following conditions *except:*
   A. Sarcoidosis
   B. Hodgkin's disease
   C. Fulminant tuberculosis
   D. Atypical mycobacterial

9. Tubercle bacilli in caseous lesions are best demonstrated in:
   A. Caseous centre
   B. Margin of necrosis with viable tissue
   C. Epithelioid cells
   D. Langhans' giant cells

10. Leprosy bacilli are:
    A. Not acid fast
    B. As acid fast as tubercle bacilli
    C. Less acid fast compared to tubercle bacilli
    D. More acid fast compared to tubercle bacilli

11. Lepromin test is always positive in:
    A. Lepromatous leprosy
    B. Borderline lepromatous leprosy
    C. Tuberculoid leprosy
    D. Indeterminate leprosy

12. Spirochaetes are most difficult to demonstrate in:
    A. Primary syphilis
    B. Secondary syphilis
    C. Tertiary syphilis
    D. Congenital syphilis

13. **Actinomycosis is caused by:**
    - A. Fungus
    - B. Gram-negative bacteria
    - C. Anaerobic bacteria
    - D. Acid fast bacteria
14. **Typically, sarcoid granuloma has the following features** *except:*
    - A. Non caseating granuloma
    - B. Giant cells have cytoplasmic inclusions
    - C. Peripheral mantle of lymphocytes
    - D. Fibroblastic proliferation at the periphery of a granuloma
15. **The following holds true for stable cells in cell cycle:**
    - A. They remain in cell cycle from one mitosis to the next
    - B. They are in resting phase but can be stimulated to enter the cell cycle
    - C. They have left the cell cycle
    - D. They do not have capacity to multiply in response to stimuli throughout adult life
16. **Connective tissue in scar is formed by the following types of fibrillar collagen:**
    - A. Type II, III, IV
    - B. Type I, III, V
    - C. Type I, II, V
    - D. Type III, V, VII
17. **Basement membrane consists of:**
    - A. Type I collagen
    - B. Type II collagen
    - C. Type III collagen
    - D. Type IV collagen
18. **The following adhesion molecules play a significant role in rolling of PMNs over endothelial cells** *except:*
    - A. Selectins
    - B. Integrins
    - C. CD 44
    - D. ICAM

KEY

1 = B	2 = A	3 = C	4 = C
5 = A	6 = C	7 = B	8 = D
9 = B	10 = C	11 = C	12 = C
13 = C	14 = C	15 = B	16 = B
17 = D	18 = C		

7

Infectious and Parasitic Diseases

INTRODUCTION *(p. 180)*

In general, tropical and under-developed countries are specially affected by infectious diseases than the developed countries. Certain *infectious diseases* are not so common in the developed world now but they continue to be major health problems in the under-developed countries e.g. tuberculosis, leprosy, typhoid fever, cholera, measles, pertussis, malaria, amoebiasis, pneumonia etc. *Vaccines* have been successful in controlling or eliminating some diseases e.g. smallpox, poliomyelitis, measles, pertussis etc. Insecticides have helped in controlling malaria to an extent. However, infections still rank very high *as a cause of death* in the world.

Following is the range of *host-organism inter-relationship,* which may vary quite widely:

1. *Symbiosis* i.e. cooperative association between two dissimilar organisms beneficial to both.
2. *Commensalism* i.e. two dissimilar organisms living together benefitting one without harming the other.
3. *True parasitism* i.e. two dissimilar organisms living together benefitting the parasite but harming the host.
4. *Saprophytism* i.e. organisms living on dead tissues.

Besides the microorganisms, more recently a modified host protein present in the mammalian CNS has been identified called *prion protein*. Prions are transmissible agents just as infectious particles but lack nucleic acid. These agents are implicated in the etiology of spongiform encephalopathy, (including kuru), bovine spongiform encephalopathy (or mad cow disease) and Creutzfeldt-Jakob disease (associated with corneal transplantation).

Infectious diseases are the consequence of inter-relationship between disease-producing properties of microorganisms and host-defense capability against the invading organisms.

Factors Relating to Infectious Agents *(p. 181)*

These are as under:

i) Mode of entry. Microorganisms causing infectious disease may gain entry into the body by various routes e.g.

- through ingestion (external route);
- inoculation (parenteral method);
- inhalation (respiration);
- perinatally (vertical transmission);
- by direct contact (contagious infection); and
- by contaminated water, food, soil, environment or from an animal host (zoonotic infections).

ii) Spread of infection. Microorganisms after entering the body may spread further through the phagocytic cells, blood vessels and lymphatics.

iii) Production of toxins. Bacteria liberate toxins which have effects on cell metabolism.

iv) Virulence of organisms. Many species and strains of organisms may have varying virulence e.g. the three strains of *C. diphtheriae (gravis, intermedius and mitis)* produce the same diphtherial exotoxin but in different amounts.

v) **Product of organisms.** Some organisms produce enzymes that help in spread of infections e.g. hyaluronidase by *Cl. welchii*, streptokinase by streptococci, staphylokinase and coagulase by staphylococci.

Factors Relating to Host *(p. 181)*

i) **Physical barrier.** A break in the continuity of the skin and mucous membranes allows the microorganisms to enter the body.

ii) **Chemical barrier.** Mucus secretions of the oral cavity and the alimentary tract and gastric acidity prevent bacterial colonisation.

iii) **Effective drainage.** The natural passages of the hollow organs like respiratory, gastrointestinal, urinary and genital system provide a way to drain the excretions effectively. Obstruction in any of these passages promotes infection.

iv) **Immune defense mechanisms.** These include the phagocytic leucocytes of blood (polymorphs and monocytes), phagocytes of tissues (mononuclear-phagocyte system) and the immune system.

Methods of Identification *(p. 181)*

The organisms causing infections and parasitic diseases may be identified by routine H & E stained sections in many instances. However, confirmation in most cases requires either application of special staining techniques or by molecular biologic methods (Table 7.1).

TABLE 7.1: Methods of Identification of Microorganisms.

1. *Bacteria*
   i. Gram stain: Most bacteria
   ii. Acid fast stain: Mycobacteria, Nocardia
   iii. Giemsa: Campylobacteria
2. *Fungi*
   i. Silver stain: Most fungi
   ii. Periodic acid-Schiff (PAS): Most fungi
   iii. Mucicarmine: Cryptococci
3. *Parasites*
   i. Giemsa: Malaria, Leishmania
   ii. Periodic acid-Schiff: Amoebae
   iii. Silver stain: Pneumocystis
4. *All classes including viruses*
   i. Culture
   ii. *In situ* hybridisation
   iii. DNA analysis
   iv. Polymerase chain reaction (PCR)

Chapter Seven

DISEASES CAUSED BY BACTERIA, SPIROCHAETES AND MYCOBACTERIA *(p. 181)*

A few common and important examples amongst these are discussed below.

PLAGUE *(p. 182)*

Plague is caused by *Yersinia (Pasteurella) pestis* which is a small gram-negative coccobacillus that grows rapidly on most culture media.

Plague is a zoonotic disease and spreads by rodents, primarily by rats, both wild and domestic; others being squirrels and rabbits.

Infection to humans occurs by rat-flea or by inhalation. After the organisms enter the blood stream, they reach the draining lymph nodes where, rather than being phagocytosed by phagocytic cells, they proliferate rapidly giving rise to tender lymphadenopathy. This occurs within 24-48 hours of infection and is accompanied by chills, fever, myalgia, nausea, vomiting and marked prostration. If untreated, death occurs from disseminated intravascular coagulation (DIC) within 1 to 2 days with development of widespread petechiae and ecchymoses leading to gangrene and hence the name *black death*.

Virulence of the organism *Y. pestis* is attributed to the elaboration of plague toxins: pesticin and lipopolysaccharide endotoxin.

Four forms of plague are recognised:

BUBONIC PLAGUE. This form is characterised by rapid appearance of tender, fluctuant and enlarged regional lymph nodes, several centimeters in diameter, and may have discharging sinuses on the skin.

PNEUMONIC PLAGUE. This is the most dreaded form of plague that occurs by inhalation of bacilli from air-borne particles of carcasses of animals or from affected patient's cough. It is characterised by occurrence of bronchopneumonia.

TYPHOIDAL PLAGUE. This form of plague is unassociated with regional lymphadenopathy. The lesions in typhoidal plague are as follows:
- Necrotic foci in visceral lymphoid tissue.
- Necrotic areas in parenchymal visceral organs.
- G.I. manifestations with diarrhoea and pain abdomen.

SEPTICAEMIC PLAGUE. This is a form of progressive, fulminant bacterial infection associated with profound septicaemia in the absence of afferent regional lymphadenitis.

ANTHRAX *(p. 184)*

Anthrax is a bacterial disease of antiquity caused by *Bacillus anthracis* that spreads from animals to man. The disease is widely prevalent in cattle and sheep but human infection is rare. In India, anthrax in animals is endemic in South due to large unprotected and uncontrolled population of live-stock population. But anthrax is also prevalent in human beings in India; in Pondicherry alone 35 cases have been reported.

ETIOPATHOGENESIS. The causative organism, *Bacillus anthracis,* is a gram-positive, aerobic bacillus, 4.5 μm long. It is a spore-forming bacillus and the spores so formed outside the body are quite resistant. The disease occurs as an exogenous infection by contact with soil or animal products contaminated with spores.

Depending upon the portal of entry, three types of human anthrax is known to occur:
i) **Cutaneous form** by direct contact with skin and is most common.
ii) **Pulmonary form** by inhalation, also called as "wool-sorters' disease" and is most fatal.
iii) **Gastrointestinal form** by ingestion and is rare.

The characteristic lesions of anthrax are haemorrhage, oedema and necrosis at the portal of entry.

1. Cutaneous anthrax is the most common and occurs in two forms: one type is characterized by necrotic lesion due to vascular thrombosis, haemorrhage and acellular necrosis, while the other form begins as a pimple at the point of entry of *B. anthracis* into the abraded exposed skin, more often in the region of hands and the head and neck. The bursting of the blister is followed by extensive oedema and black tissue necrosis resulting in formation of severe 'malignant pustule'. Regional lymph nodes are invariably involved alongwith profound septicaemia.

2. Pulmonary anthrax (wool-sorters' disease) occurring from inhalation of spores of *B. anthracis* in infectious aerosols results in rapid development of malignant pustule in the bronchus. This is followed by development of primary extensive necrotising pneumonia.

3. Intestinal anthrax is rare in human beings and is quite similar to that seen in cattle. Septicaemia and death often results in this type too.

LABORATORY DIAGNOSIS. Anthrax can be diagnosed by a few simple techniques:

Smear examination: Gram stained smear shows rod-shaped, spore-forming, gram-positive bacilli.

Culture: Anthrax bacteria grow on sheep blood agar as flat colonies with an irregular margin (medusa head).

WHOOPING COUGH (PERTUSSIS) *(p. 185)*

Whooping cough is a highly communicable acute bacterial disease of childhood caused by *Bordetella pertussis.*

The causative organism, *B. pertussis,* has strong tropism for the brush border of the bronchial epithelium. The organisms proliferate here and stimulate the bronchial epithelium to produce abundant tenacious mucus. Within 7-10 days after exposure, catarrhal stage begins which is the most infectious stage. There is low grade fever, rhinorrhoea, conjunctivitis and excess tear production. Paroxysms of cough occur with characteristic 'whoop'.

The peripheral blood shows marked lymphocytosis upto 90% and enlargement of lymphoid follicles in the bronchial mucosa and peribronchial lymph nodes.

GRANULOMA INGUINALE *(p. 185)*

Granuloma inguinale is a sexually-transmitted disease affecting the genitalia and inguinal and perianal regions caused by *Calymmatobacterium donovani.* The infection is transmitted through vaginal or anal intercourse and by autoinoculation. Depending upon whether the individual is heterosexual or homosexual, the lesions are located on the penis, scrotum, genitocrural folds and inguinal folds, or in the perianal and anal area respectively. Regional lymphadenopathy generally does not occur.

M/E The dermis and subcutaneous tissues are infiltrated by numerous histiocytes containing many bacteria called *Donovan bodies,* and lymphocytes, plasma cells and neutrophils. These organisms are best demonstrated by silver impregnation techniques.

STAPHYLOCOCCAL INFECTIONS *(p. 185)*

Staphylococci are gram-positive cocci which are present everywhere—in the skin, umbilicus, nasal vestibule, stool etc. Three species are pathogenic to human beings: *Staph. aureus, Staph. epidermidis* and *Staph. saprophyticus.* Most staphylococcal infections are caused by *Staph. aureus.* Staphylococcal infections are among the commonest antibiotic-resistant hospital-acquired infection in surgical wounds.

A wide variety of suppurative diseases are caused by *Staph. aureus* which includes the following:

1. Infections of skin. Staphylococcal infections of skin are quite common. The infection begins from lodgement of cocci in the hair root due to poor hygiene and results in obstruction of sweat or sebaceous gland duct. This is termed *folliculitis.* Involvement of adjacent follicles results in larger lesions called *furuncle.* Further spread of infection horizontally under the skin and subcutaneous tissue causes *carbuncle* or *cellulitis. Styes* are staphylococcal infection of the sebaceous glands of Zeis, the glands of Moll and eyelash follicles. *Impetigo* is yet another staphylococcal skin infection common in school children in which there are multiple pustular lesions on face forming honey-yellow crusts. *Breast abscess* may occur following delivery when staphylococci are transmitted from infant having neonatal sepsis or due to stasis of milk.

2. Infections of burns and surgical wounds. These are quite common due to contamination from the patient's own nasal secretions or from hospital staff.

3. Infections of the upper and lower respiratory tract. Small children under 2 years of age get staphylococcal infections of the respiratory tract commonly. These include pharyngitis, bronchopneumonia, staphylococcal pneumonia and its complications.

4. Bacterial arthritis. Septic arthritis in the elderly is caused by *Staph. aureus.*

5. Infection of bone (Osteomyelitis). Young boys having history of trauma or infection may develop acute staphylococcal osteomyelitis.

6. Bacterial endocarditis. Acute and subacute bacterial endocarditis are complications of infection with *Staph. aureus* and *Staph. epidermidis.*

7. Bacterial meningitis. Surgical procedures on central nervous system may lead to staphylococcal meningitis.

8. Septicaemia. Staphylococcal septicaemia may occur in patients with lowered resistance or in patients having underlying staphylococcal infections. Patients present with features of bacteraemia such as shaking chills and fever.

9. Toxic shock syndrome. Toxic shock syndrome is a serious complication of staphylococcal infection characterised by fever, hypotension and exfoliative skin rash.

STREPTOCOCCAL INFECTIONS *(p. 186)*

Streptococci are also gram-positive cocci but unlike staphylococci, they are more known for their non-suppurative autoimmune complications than suppurative inflammatory responses. Streptococcal infections occur throughout the world but their problems are greater in underprivileged populations where antibiotics are not instituted readily.

The following groups and subtypes of streptococci have been identified and implicated in different streptococcal diseases:

1. *Group A or Streptococcus pyogenes,* also called β-haemolytic streptococci, are involved in causing upper respiratory tract infection and cutaneous infections (erysipelas). In addition, beta haemolytic streptococci are involved in autoimmune reactions in the form of rheumatic heart disease (RHD).

2. *Group B or Streptococcus agalactiae* produces infections in the newborn and is involved in non-suppurative post-streptococcal complications such as RHD and acute glomerulonephritis.

3. *Group C and G streptococci* are responsible for respiratory infections.

4. *Group D or Streptococcus faecalis,* also called enterococci are important in causation of urinary tract infection, bacterial endocarditis, septicaemia etc.

5. *Untypable α-haemolytic streptococci* such as *Streptococcus viridans* constitute the normal flora of the mouth and may cause bacterial endocarditis.

6. *Pneumococci or Streptococcus pneumoniae* are etiologic agents for bacterial pneumonias, meningitis and septicaemia.

CLOSTRIDIAL DISEASES *(p. 187)*

Clostridia are gram-positive spore-forming anaerobic microorganisms found in the gastrointestinal tract of herbivorous animals and man. On degeneration of these microorganisms, the plasmids are liberated which produce many toxins responsible for the following clostridial diseases depending upon the species:

GAS GANGRENE. Gas gangrene is a rapidly progressive and fatal illness in which there is myonecrosis of previously healthy skeletal muscle due to elaboration of myotoxins by some species of clostridia. In majority of cases (80-90%), the source of myotoxins is *C. perfringens* Type A; others are *C. novyi* and *C. septicum.* Generally, traumatic wounds and surgical procedures are followed by contamination with clostridia and become the site of myonecrosis.

TETANUS. Tetanus or 'lock jaw' is a severe acute neurologic syndrome caused by tetanus toxin, tetanospasmin, which is a neurotoxic exotoxin elaborated by *C. tetani.* The spores of the microorganism present in the soil enter the body through a penetrating wound. In underdeveloped countries, tetanus in neonates is seen due to application of soil or dung on the umbilical stump. The degenerated microorganisms liberate the tetanus neurotoxin which causes neuronal stimulation and spasm of muscles.

BOTULISM. Botulism is characterised by symmetric paralysis of cranial nerves, limbs and trunk. The condition occurs following ingestion of food contaminated with neurotoxins of *C. botulinum* and less often by contamination of a penetrating wound.

CLOSTRIDIAL FOOD POISONING. Clostridial food poisoning is caused by enterotoxin elaborated by *C. perfringens.* Out of five serotypes of *C. perfringens,* type A and C produce alpha-enterotoxin that causes food poisoning.

NECROTISING ENTEROCOLITIS. Necrotising enterocolitis or 'pig bel' is caused by beta-enterotoxin produced by *C. perfringens* Type C. The condition occurs especially in undernourished children who suddenly indulge in overeating.

DISEASES CAUSED BY FUNGI *(p. 188)*

Many of the human fungal infections are opportunistic i.e. they occur in conditions with impaired host immune mechanisms. Such conditions include defective neutrophil function, administration of corticosteroids, immuno-suppressive therapy and immunodeficiency states (congenital and acquired).

MYCETOMA *(p. 188)*

Mycetoma is a chronic suppurative infection involving a limb, shoulder or other tissues and is characterised by draining sinuses. The material discharged from the sinuses is in the form of grains consisting of colonies of fungi or bacteria. Mycetomas are of 2 main types:

■ *Mycetomas* caused by actinomyces (higher bacteria) comprising about 60% of cases; and

■ *Eumycetomas* caused by true fungi comprising the remaining 40% of the cases.

Most common fungi causative for eumycetoma are *Madurella mycetomatis* or *Madurella grisea,* both causing black granules from discharging sinuses.

CANDIDIASIS *(p. 188)*

Candidiasis is an opportunistic fungal infection caused most commonly by *Candida albicans* and occasionally by *Candida tropicalis.* In human beings, Candida species are present as normal flora of the skin and mucocutaneous areas, intestines and vagina. The organism becomes pathogenic when the balance between the host and the organism is disturbed. Candida produces superficial infections of the skin and mucous membranes, or may invade deeper tissues:

1. **Oral thrush.** This is the commonest form of mucocutaneous candidiasis seen especially in early life.
2. **Candidal vaginitis.** Vaginal candidiasis or monilial vaginitis is characterised clinically by thick, yellow, curdy discharge.
3. **Cutaneous candidiasis.** Candidal involvement of nail folds producing change in the shape of nail plate (paronychia) and colonisation in the intertriginous areas of the skin.
4. **Systemic candidiasis.** Invasive candidiasis is rare and is usually a terminal event of an underlying disorder associated with impaired immune system. The organisms gain entry into the body through an ulcerative lesion on the skin and mucosa or may be introduced by iatrogenic means.

SUPERFICIAL MYCOSIS *(p. 189)*

Dermatophytes are the most important example of cutaneous mycosis caused by *Microsporum, Trichophyton* and *Epidermophyton.* These superficial fungi are spread by direct contact or by fomites and infect tissues such as the skin, hair and nails.

■ *Tinea capitis* characterised by patchy alopecia affecting the scalp and eyebrows.
■ *Tinea barbae* is acute folliculitis of the beard.
■ *Tinea corporis* is dermatitis with formation of erythematous papules.

DISEASES CAUSED BY VIRUSES *(p. 189)*

VIRAL HAEMORRHAGIC FEVERS *(p. 189)*

Viral haemorrhagic fevers are a group of acute viral infections which have common features of causing haemorrhages, shock and sometimes death. Viruses causing haemorrhagic fevers were earlier called *arthropod-borne (or arbo)* viruses since their transmission was considered to be from arthropods to humans. However, now it is known that all such viruses are not transmitted by arthropod vectors alone and hence now such haemorrhagic fevers are classified according to the routes of transmission and other epidemiologic features into 4 groups:

■ Mosquito-borne (e.g. yellow fever, dengue fever, Rift Valley fever)
■ Tick-borne (e.g. Crimean haemorrhagic fever, Kyasanur Forest disease)
■ Zoonotic (e.g. Korean haemorrhagic fever, Lassa fever)
■ Marburg virus disease and Ebola virus disease by unknown route.
    Of these, mosquito-borne viral haemorrhagic fevers in which *Aedes aegypti* mosquitoes are vectors are the most common problem the world over, especially in underdeveloped countries. Two important examples of Aedes mosquito-borne viral haemorrhagic fevers are yellow fever and dengue fever.

Yellow Fever *(p. 190)*

Yellow fever is the oldest known viral haemorrhagic fever restricted to some regions of Africa and South America. Monkeys carry the virus without suffering from illness and the virus is transmitted from them to humans by *Aedes aegypti* as vector.
    Major pathologic changes are seen in the liver and kidneys.

Liver. The characteristic changes include:
i)   midzonal necrosis;
ii)   Councilman bodies; and
iii) microvesicular steatosis.

Kidneys. The kidneys show the following changes:
i)   coagulative necrosis of proximal tubules;
ii)   accumulation of fat in the tubular epithelium; and
iii) haemorrhages.

Patients tend to recover without sequelae and death rate is less than 5%, death resulting from hepatic or renal failure, and petechial haemorrhages in the brain.

Dengue Haemorrhagic Fever (DHF) *(p. 190)*

Dengue is caused by virus transmitted by bites of mosquito *Aedes aegypti;* the transmission being highest during and after rainy season when mosquitos are numerous.

Dengue occurs in two forms:

1. *Dengue fever or break-bone fever* in an uncomplicated way is a self-limited febrile illness affecting muscles and joints with severe back pain due to myalgia (and hence the name 'break-bone' fever).

2. *Dengue haemorrhagic fever (DHF),* on the other hand, is a severe and potentially fatal form of acute febrile illness characterised by cutaneous and intestinal haemorrhages due to thrombocytopenia, haemoconcentration, hypovolaemic shock and neurologic disturbances. DHF is most common in children under 15 years of age.

Dengue virus infects blood monocytes, lymphocytes and endothelial cells. This initiates complement activation and consumptive coagulopathy including thrombocytopenia. The entire process takes place rapidly and may evolve over a period of a few hours. If patient is treated appropriately at this stage, there is rapid and dramatic recovery. But in untreated cases, *dengue shock syndrome* develops and death occurs.

At autopsy, the predominant organ changes observed are as follows:

i) *Brain:* intracranial haemorrhages, cerebral oedema, dengue encephalitis.

ii) *Liver:* enlarged; necrosis of hepatocytes and Kupffer cells, Reye's syndrome in children.

iii) *Kidneys:* petechial haemorrhages and features of renal failure.

iv) *Muscles and joints:* perivascular mononuclear cell infiltrate.

SEVERE ACUTE RESPIRATORY SYNDROME (SARS) *(p. 191)*

Severe acute respiratory syndrome (SARS) is the human form of bird flu or avian influenza having similar symptomatology. Recently, since the beginning of the year 2004, there have been outbreaks in poultry birds resulting in slaughtering of millions of infected chickens. There have been confirmed reports of spread of infection to human beings during this period in South-East Asia (particularly in Hong Kong, Vietnam, Thailand, South Korea, Japan, Indonesia, Taiwan and China) and its rapidly downhill and fatal clinical course; this has sent alarm bells all over world for quarantine.

ETIOPATHOGENESIS. Bird flu is caused by influenza viruses type A and primarily infects the birds, pigs and horses. Though it is not fatal for wild birds, it can kill poultry birds and people. Humans acquire infection through contaminated nasal, respiratory and faecal material from infected birds. An individual who has human flu and also gets infected with bird flu, then the hybrid virus so produced is highly contagious and causes lethal disease.

CLINICOPATHOLOGICAL FEATURES. Typically, the disease begins with influenza-like features such as fever, cough, sore throat, muscle aches and eye infection. Soon, the patient develops viral pneumonia and acute respiratory distress (hence the term SARS), and terminally kidney failure.

VARICELLA ZOSTER VIRUS INFECTION *(p. 191)*

Varicella zoster virus is a member of herpes virus family and causes chickenpox (varicella) in non-immune individuals and herpes zoster (shingles) in those who had chickenpox in the past.

Chapter Seven

HERPES SIMPLEX VIRUS INFECTION *(p. 192)*

Two of the herpes simplex viruses (HSV)—type 1 and 2, cause 'fever blisters' and herpes genitalis respectively.

HSV-1 causes vesicular lesions on the skin, lips and mucous membranes.

HSV-2 causes herpes genitalis characterised by vesicular and necrotising lesions on the cervix, vagina and vulva.

LYMPHOGRANULOMA VENEREUM *(p. 192)*

Lymphogranuloma venereum (LGV) is a sexually-transmitted disease caused by *Chlamydia trachomatis* and is characterised by mucocutaneous lesions and regional lymphadenopathy.

The condition begins as a painless, herpes-like lesion on the cervix, vagina, or penis. The organisms are carried via lymphatics to regional lymph nodes. The involved lymph nodes are tender, fluctuant and may ulcerate and drain pus.

M/E The lymph nodes have characteristic stellate-shaped abscesses surrounded by a zone of epithelioid cells (granuloma).

CAT-SCRATCH DISEASE *(p. 192)*

Another condition related to LGV, cat-scratch disease, is caused by *Bartonella henselae,* an organism linked to rickettsiae but unlike rickettsiae this organism can be grown in culture. The condition occurs more commonly in children (under 18 years of age). There is regional nodal enlargement which appears about 2 weeks after cat-scratch, and sometimes after thorn injury. The lymphadenopathy is self-limited and regresses in 2-4 months.

M/E
i)   Initially, there is formation of non-caseating sarcoid-like granulomas.
ii)   Subsequently, there are neutrophilic abscesses surrounded by pallisaded histiocytes and fibroblasts, an appearance simulating LGV discussed above.

RABIES *(p. 192)*

Rabies is a fatal form of encephalitis in humans caused by rabies virus. The virus is transmitted into the human body by a bite by infected carnivores e.g. dog, wolf, fox and bats.

M/E Shows characteristic Negri bodies which are intracytoplasmic, deeply eosinophilic inclusions present in neurons of the brainstem.

DISEASES CAUSED BY PARASITES *(p. 193)*

AMOEBIASIS *(p. 193)*

Amoebiasis is caused by *Entamoeba histolytica,* named for its lytic action on tissues. It is the most important intestinal infection of man. The condition is particularly more common in tropical and subtropical areas with poor sanitation.

The parasite occurs in 2 forms: a *trophozoite form* which is active adult form seen in the tissues and diarrhoeal stools, and a *cystic form* seen in formed stools but not in the tissues. The trophozoite form can be stained positively with PAS procedure in tissue sections while amoebic cysts having four nuclei can be identified in stools. The cysts are the infective stage of the parasite and are found in contaminated water or food. The trophozoites are formed from the cyst stage in the intestine and colonise in the caecum and large bowel. The trophozoites as well as cysts are passed in stools but the trophozoites fail to survive outside or are destroyed by gastric secretions.

■   **Amoebic colitis,** the most common type of amoebic infection begins as a small area of necrosis of mucosa which may ulcerate. These ulcerative lesions may enlarge, develop undermining of margins of the ulcer due to lytic action of the trophozoite and have necrotic bed. Such chronic amoebic ulcers are described as flask-shaped ulcers due to their shape.

■ **Amoeboma** is the inflammatory thickening of the wall of large bowel resembling carcinoma of the colon.

■ **Amoebic liver abscess** may be formed by invasion of the radicle of the portal vein by trophozoites.

■ **Other sites** where spread of amoebic infection may occur are peritonitis by perforation of amoebic ulcer of colon, extension to the lungs and pleura by rupture of amoebic liver abscess, haematogenous spread to cause amoebic carditis and cerebral lesions, cutaneous amoebiasis via spread of rectal amoebiasis or from anal intercourse.

MALARIA *(p. 194)*

Malaria is a protozoal disease caused by any one or combination of four species of plasmodia: *Plasmodium vivax, Plasmodium falciparum, Plasmodium ovale* and *Plasmodium malariae*. While *Plasmodium falciparum* causes malignant malaria, the other three species produce benign form of illness. These parasites are transmitted by bite of female *Anopheles* mosquito.

P. falciparum differs from other forms of plasmodial species in 4 respects:

i) It does not have exo-erythrocytic stage.

ii) Erythrocytes of any age are parasitised while other plasmodia parasitise juvenile red cells.

iii) One red cell may contain more than one parasite.

iv) The parasitised red cells are sticky causing obstruction of small blood vessels by thrombi, a feature which is responsible for extraordinary virulence of *P. falciparum*.

The main clinical features of malaria are cyclic peaks of high fever accompanied by chills, anaemia and splenomegaly.

Parasitisation and destruction of erythrocytes are responsible for major pathologic changes:

1. Malarial pigment liberated by destroyed red cells accumulates in the phagocytic cells of the reticuloendothelial system resulting in enlargement of the spleen and liver *(hepatosplenomegaly)*.

2. In falciparum malaria, there is massive absorption of haemoglobin by the renal tubules producing *blackwater fever (haemoglobinuric nephrosis)*.

3. At autopsy, *cerebral malaria* is characterised by congestion and petechiae on the white matter.

4. Parasitised erythrocytes in falciparum malaria are sticky and get attached to endothelial cells resulting in obstruction of capillaries of deep organs such as of the brain leading to hypoxia and death. If the patient lives, *microhaemorrhages* and *microinfarcts* may be seen in the brain.

FILARIASIS *(p. 194)*

Wuchereria bancrofti and *Brugia malayi* are responsible for causing Bancroftian and Malayan filariasis in different geographic regions. The lymphatic vessels inhabit the adult worm, especially in the lymph nodes, testis and epididymis. Microfilariae seen in the circulation are produced by the female worm. Symptomatic cases may have two forms of disease—an acute form and a chronic form.

■ *Acute form* of filariasis presents with fever, lymphangitis, lymphadenitis, epididymo-orchitis, urticaria, eosinophilia and microfilaraemia.

■ *Chronic form* of filariasis is characterised by lymphadenopathy, lymphoedema, hydrocele and elephantiasis.

CYSTICERCOSIS *(p. 195)*

Cysticercosis is infection by the larval stage of *Taenia solium*, the pork tapeworm. The adult tape-worm resides in the human intestines. The eggs are passed in human faeces which are ingested by pigs or they infect vegetables. These eggs then develop into larval stages in the host, spread by blood to any site in the body and form cystic larvae termed *cysticercus celluiosae*. Human beings may acquire infection by the larval stage by eating undercooked pork ('measly pork'), by ingesting uncooked contaminated vegetables, and sometimes, by autoinfection.

TORCH COMPLEX *(p. 196)*

TORCH complex refers to development of common complex of symptoms in infants due to infection with different microorganisms that include: *Toxoplasma*, *Rubella*, *Cytomegalovirus*, and *Herpes* simplex virus. The infection may be acquired by the foetus during intrauterine life, or perinatally and damage the foetus or infant. Since the symptoms produced by TORCH group of organisms are indistinguishable from each other, it is a common practice in a suspected pregnant mother or infant to test for all the four main TORCH agents.

The classic features of syndrome produced by TORCH complex are seen in congenital rubella. The features include: ocular defects, cardiac defects, CNS manifestations, sensorineural deafness, thrombocytopenia and hepatosplenomegaly.

■ SELF ASSESSMENT

1. **The causative organisms of plague are:**
   A. Cocci
   B. Bacilli
   C. Coccobacilli
   D. Nocardia
2. **Lymphocytosis in whooping cough occurs due to:**
   A. Endotoxin by the microorganism
   B. Exotoxin by the microorganism
   C. Cytokine
   D. Histamine-sensitising factor
3. **Granuloma inguinale is characterised by the following *except:***
   A. It is caused by Donovan bacilli
   B. It is characterised by lymphadenopathy
   C. It is a sexually transmitted disease
   D. There are neutrophilic abscesses in the dermis
4. **Prion proteins are implicated in the etiology of:**
   A. Spongiform encephalopathy
   B. Viral encephalitis
   C. Perivenous encephalomyelitis
   D. Progressive multifocal leucoencephalopathy
5. **Streptococci are commonly implicated in the etiology of the following *except:***
   A. Rheumatic heart disease
   B. Glomerulonephritis
   C. Breast abscess
   D. Subacute bacterial endocarditis
6. **Clostridia are implicated in the following *except:***
   A. Botulism
   B. Necrotising enterocolitis
   C. Bacillary dysentery
   D. Pseudomembranous colitis
7. **Fungi in general can be identified by the following stains *except:***
   A. Silver stain
   B. Periodic acid Schiff
   C. Giemsa
   D. Mucicarmine
8. **Mosquito-borne viral haemorrhagic fever include the following examples *except:***
   A. Dengue fever
   B. Yellow fever
   C. Rift Valley fever
   D. Kyasanur Forest fever

9. **Dengue haemorrhagic fever is characterised by following labora-tory findings *except:***
   A. Leucopenia
   B. Lymphocytosis
   C. Decreased haematocrit
   D. Thrombocytopenia

10. **Granuloma inguinale and lymphogranuloma venereum are similar in following aspects, *except:***
    A. Both are sexually transmitted diseases
    B. Both are caused by bacteria
    C. Both are characterised by lymphadenopathy
    D. Both begin as lesions on genitals

11. **Necrotic lesions of *Entamoeba histolytica* are due to:**
    A. Cyst stage
    B. Trophozoite stage
    C. Both cyst and trophozoites
    D. Neither cysts nor trophozoites

12. ***P. falciparum* differs from other plasmodia in following aspects *except:***
    A. It does not have exoerythrocytic stage
    B. It parasitises only juvenile red cells
    C. It causes malignant malaria
    D. One red cell may contain more than one parasite

13. **In the case of SARS in human beings, the mode of infection is:**
    A. From mosquito
    B. Person to person
    C. Poultry birds
    D. Domestic dogs

KEY

1 = C	2 = D	3 = B	4 = A
5 = C	6 = C	7 = C	8 = D
9 = C	10 = C	11 = B	12 = B
13 = C			

Chapter Seven

8

Neoplasia

NOMENCLATURE AND CLASSIFICATION *(p. 197)*

INTRODUCTION. The term 'neoplasia' means new growth; the new growth produced is called 'neoplasm' or 'tumour'. However, all 'new growths' are not neoplasms since examples of new growth of tissues and cells also exist in the processes of embryogenesis, regeneration and repair, hyperplasia and hormonal stimulation.

Therefore, satisfactory definition of a neoplasm or tumour is *'a mass of tissue formed as a result of abnormal, excessive, uncoordinated, autonomous and purposeless proliferation of cells'*. Neoplasms may be 'benign' when they are slow-growing and localised without causing much difficulty to the host, or 'malignant' when they proliferate rapidly, spread throughout the body and may eventually cause death of the host. The common term used for all malignant tumours is cancer.

All tumours, benign as well as malignant, have 2 basic components:

■ *'Parenchyma'* comprised by proliferating tumour cells; parenchyma determines the nature and evolution of the tumour.

■ *'Supportive stroma'* composed of fibrous connective tissue and blood vessels; it provides the framework on which the parenchymal tumour cells grow.

The tumours derive their nomenclature on the basis of the parenchymal component comprising them. The suffix *'-oma'* is added to denote benign tumours. Malignant tumours of epithelial origin are called *carcinomas*, while malignant mesenchymal tumours are named *sarcomas* (*sarcos* = fleshy). However, some cancers are composed of highly undifferentiated cells and are referred to as *undifferentiated malignant tumours.*

Some examples contrary to this concept are: *melanoma* for carcinoma of the melanocytes, *hepatoma* for carcinoma of the hepatocytes, *lymphoma* for malignant tumour of the lymphoid tissue, and *seminoma* for malignant tumour of the testis. *Leukaemia* is the term used for cancer of blood forming cells.

SPECIAL CATEGORIES OF TUMOURS. These are as under:

1. Mixed tumours. When two types of tumours are combined in the same tumour, it is called a mixed tumour. For example:

i) Adenosquamous carcinoma is the combination of adenocarcinoma and squamous cell carcinoma in the endometrium.

ii) Adenoacanthoma is the mixture of adenocarcinoma and benign squamous elements in the endometrium.

iii) Carcinosarcoma is the rare combination of malignant tumour of the epithelium (carcinoma) and of mesenchymal tissue (sarcoma) e.g. carcino sarcoma in thyroid.

iv) Collision tumour is the term used for morphologically two different cancers in the same organ which do not mix with each other.

v) Mixed tumour of the salivary gland (or pleomorphic adenoma) is the term used for benign tumour having combination of both epithelial and mesenchymal tissue elements.

2. Teratomas. These tumours are made up of a mixture of various tissue types arising from totipotent cells derived from the three germ cell layers—ectoderm, mesoderm and endoderm. Most common sites for teratomas are ovaries and testis (*gonadal teratomas*). But they occur at *extra-gonadal sites* as well, mainly in the midline of the body such as in the head and neck region, mediastinum, retroperitoneum, sacrococcygeal region etc.

3. Blastomas. Blastomas or embryomas are a group of malignant tumours which arise from embryonal or partially differentiated cells which would normally form blastema of the organs and tissue during embryogenesis. These tumours occur more frequently in infants and children (under 5 years of age) and include some examples of tumours in this age group: neuroblastoma, nephroblastoma (Wilms' tumour), hepatoblastoma, retinoblastoma, medulloblastoma, pulmonary blastoma.

4. Hamartoma. Hamartoma is benign tumour which is made of mature but disorganised cells of tissues indigenous to the particular organ e.g. hamartoma of the lung consists of mature cartilage, mature smooth muscle and epithelium.

5. Choristoma. Choristoma is the name given to the ectopic islands of normal tissue. Thus, choristoma is heterotopia but is not a true tumour.

CLASSIFICATION. The currently used classification of tumours is based on the histogenesis (i.e. cell of origin) and on the anticipated behaviour.

CHARACTERISTICS OF TUMOURS (p. 198)

The characteristics of tumours are described under the following headings:
I.   Rate of growth
II. Clinical and gross features
III. Microscopic features
IV. Local invasion (Direct spread)
V.   Metastasis (Distant spread)

Based on these characteristics, contrasting features of benign and malignant tumours are summarised in Table 8.1.

I. RATE OF GROWTH (p. 198)

The tumour cells generally proliferate more rapidly than the normal cells. In general, benign tumours grow slowly and malignant tumours rapidly. The rate at which the tumour enlarges depends upon 2 main factors:

1. Rate of division and destruction of tumour cells. In general, malignant tumour cells have increased mitotic rate and slower death rate i.e. the cancer cells do not follow normal controls in cell cycle and are immortal. If the rate of cell division is high, it is likely that tumour cells in the centre of the tumour do not receive adequate nourishment and undergo ischaemic necrosis.

2. Degree of differentiation. Secondly, the rate of growth of malignant tumour is directly proportionate to the degree of differentiation. Poorly differentiated tumours show aggressive growth pattern as compared to better differentiated tumours. Some tumours, after a period of slow growth, may suddenly show spurt in their growth due to development of an aggressive clone of malignant cells. On the other hand, some tumours may cease to grow after sometime.

The regulation of tumour growth is under the control of growth factors secreted by the tumour cells:
i)   Epidermal growth factor (EGF)
ii)   Fibroblast growth factor (FGF)
iii) Platelet-derived growth factor (PDGF)
iv)   Colony stimulating factor (CSF)
v)   Transforming growth factors-β (TGF-β)
vi)   Interleukins (IL).

II. CLINICAL AND GROSS FEATURES (p. 200)

Clinically, benign tumours are generally slow growing, and depending upon the location, may remain asymptomatic (e.g. subcutaneous lipoma), or may

TABLE 8.1: Contrasting Features of Benign and Malignant Tumours.

	FEATURES	BENIGN	MALIGNANT
I.	**CLINICAL AND GROSS FEATURES**		
	1. **Boundaries**	Encapsulated or well-circumscribed	Poorly-circumscribed and irregular
	2. **Surrounding tissue**	Often compressed	Usually invaded
	3. **Size**	Usually small	Often larger
	4. **Secondary changes**	Occur less often	Occur more often
II.	**MICROSCOPIC FEATURES**		
	1. **Pattern**	Usually resembles the tissue of origin closely	Often poor resemblance to tissue of origin
	2. **Basal polarity**	Retained	Often lost
	3. **Pleomorphism**	Usually not present	Often present
	4. **Nucleo-cytoplasmic ratio**	Normal	Increased
	5. **Anisonucleosis**	Absent	Generally present
	6. **Hyperchromatism**	Absent	Often present
	7. **Mitoses**	May be present but are always typical mitoses	Mitotic figures increased and are generally atypical and abnormal
	8. **Tumour giant cells**	May be present but without nuclear atypia	Present with nuclear atypia
	9. **Chromosomal abnormalities**	Infrequent	Invariably present
	10. **Function**	Usually well maintained	May be retained, lost or become abnormal
III.	**GROWTH RATE**	Usually slow	Usually rapid
IV.	**LOCAL INVASION**	Often compresses the surrounding tissues without invading or infiltrating them	Usually infiltrates and invades the adjacent tissues
V.	**METASTASIS**	Absent	Frequently present
VI.	**PROGNOSIS**	Local complications	Death by local and metastatic complications

produce serious symptoms (e.g. meningioma in the nervous system). On the other hand, malignant tumours grow rapidly, may ulcerate on the surface, invade locally into deeper tissues, may spread to distant sites (metastasis), and also produce systemic features such as weight loss, anorexia and anaemia. In fact, two of the cardinal clinical features of malignant tumours are: *invasiveness and metastasis*.

The gross appearance of benign and malignant tumours may be quite variable. However, certain distinctive features characterise almost all tumours—they have a different colour, texture and consistency as compared to the surrounding tissue of origin. Gross terms such as papillary, fungating, infiltrating, haemorrhagic, ulcerative and cystic are used to describe the macroscopic appearance of the tumours.

■ *Benign tumours* are generally spherical or ovoid in shape. They are encapsulated or well-circumscribed, freely movable, more often firm and uniform, unless secondary changes like haemorrhage or infarction supervene.

■ *Malignant tumours,* on the other hand, are usually irregular in shape, poorly-circumscribed and extend into the adjacent tissues. Secondary changes like haemorrhage, infarction and ulceration are seen more often. Sarcomas typically have fish-flesh like consistency while carcinomas are generally firm.

III. MICROSCOPIC FEATURES (p. 200)

For recognising and classifying the tumours, the microscopic characteristics of tumour cells are of greatest importance.

1. Microscopic Pattern (p. 202)

The tumour cells may be arranged in a variety of patterns in different tumours as under:

■ The *epithelial tumours* generally consist of acini, sheets, columns or cords of epithelial tumour cells that may be arranged in solid or papillary pattern.

■ The *mesenchymal tumours* have mesenchymal tumour cells arranged as interlacing bundles, fasicles or whorls, lying separated from each other usually by the intercellular matrix substance.

■ Certain tumours have *mixed patterns* e.g. teratoma arising from totipotent cells, pleomorphic adenoma of salivary gland (mixed salivary tumour), fibroadenoma of the breast, carcinosarcoma of the uterus and various other combinations of tumour types.

■ *Haematopoietic tumours* such as leukaemias and lymphomas often have none or little stromal support.

■ Generally, most benign tumours and low grade malignant tumours *reduplicate* the normal structure of origin more closely so that there is little difficulty in identifying and classifying such tumours. However, anaplastic tumours differ greatly from the arrangement in normal tissue of origin of the tumour and may occasionally pose problems in classifying the tumour.

2. Cytomorphology of Neoplastic Cells (Differentiation and Anaplasia) (p. 202)

The neoplastic cell is characterised by morphologic and functional alterations, the most significant of which are *'differentiation'* and *'anaplasia'*.

■ **Differentiation** is defined as the extent of morphological and functional resemblance of parenchymal tumour cells to corresponding normal cells. If the deviation of neoplastic cell in structure and function is minimal as compared to normal cell, the tumour is described as *'well-differentiated'* such as most benign and low-grade malignant tumours. *'Poorly differentiated', 'undifferentiated'* or *'dedifferentiated'* are synonymous terms for poor structural and functional resemblance to corresponding normal cell.

■ **Anaplasia** is lack of differentiation and is a characteristic feature of most malignant tumours. Depending upon the degree of differentiation, the extent of anaplasia is also variable i.e. poorly differentiated malignant tumours have high degree of anaplasia.

As a result of anaplasia, noticeable morphological and functional alterations in the neoplastic cells are observed (Fig. 8.1).

A, NORMAL MORPHOLOGY		B, CYTOMORPHOLOGY IN CANCER
Basal polarity	1	Loss of basal polarity
No pleomorphism	2	Pleomorphism
N:C ratio low	3	N:C ratio high
No anisonucleosis	4	Anisonucleosis
Normal nuclear chromatin	5	Nuclear hyperchromatism
Nucleoli normal	6	Nucleoli prominent
Normal mitotic figures	7	Abnormal mitotic figures
No giant cells	8	Tumour giant cells
Cytoplasm normal	9	Increased mucin
Chromosomal diploidy	10	DNA aneuploidy

Fig. 8.1: Diagrammatic representation of cytomorphologic features of neoplastic cells. Characteristics of cancer (B) in a gland are contrasted with the appearance of a normal mucous gland (A).

3. Tumour Angiogenesis and Stroma *(p. 204)*

TUMOUR ANGIOGENESIS. In order to provide nourishment to growing tumour, new blood vessels are formed from pre-existing ones (angiogenesis).
i) Microvascular density. The new capillaries add to the vascular density of the tumour which has been used as a marker to assess the rate of growth of tumours and hence grade the tumours. This is done by counting microvascular density in the section of the tumour.
ii) Central necrosis. However, if the tumour outgrows its blood supply as occurs in rapidly growing tumours or tumour angiogenesis fails, its core undergoes ischaemic necrosis.

TUMOUR STROMA. The collagenous tissue in the stroma may be scanty or excessive. In the former case, the tumour is soft and fleshy (e.g. in sarcomas, lymphomas), while in the latter case the tumour is hard and gritty (e.g. infiltrating duct carcinoma breast). Growth of fibrous tissue in tumour is stimulated by basic fibroblast growth factor (bFGF) elaborated by tumour cells.

■ If the epithelial tumour is almost entirely composed of parenchymal cells, it is called *medullary* e.g. medullary carcinoma of the breast, medullary carcinoma of the thyroid.

■ If there is excessive connective tissue stroma in the epithelial tumour, it is referred to as *desmoplasia* and the tumour is hard or *scirrhous* e.g. infiltrating duct carcinoma breast, linitis plastica of the stomach.

4. Inflammatory Reaction *(p. 204)*

At times, prominent inflammatory reaction is present in and around the tumours. It could be the result of ulceration in the cancer when there is secondary infection. The inflammatory reaction in such instances may be acute or chronic. However, some tumours show chronic inflammatory reaction, chiefly of lymphocytes, plasma cells and macrophages, and in some instances granulomatous reaction, in the absence of ulceration. This is due to cell-mediated immunologic response by the host in an attempt to destroy the tumour. In some cases, such an immune response improves the prognosis.

The *examples* of such reaction are: seminoma testis, malignant melanoma of the skin, lymphoepithelioma of the throat, medullary carcinoma of the breast, choriocarcinoma, Warthin's tumour of salivary glands etc.

IV. LOCAL INVASION (DIRECT SPREAD) *(p. 204)*

BENIGN TUMOURS. Most benign tumours form encapsulated or circum-scribed masses that *expand and push aside* the surrounding normal tissues without actually invading, infiltrating or metastasising.

MALIGNANT TUMOURS. Malignant tumours also enlarge by expansion and some well-differentiated tumours may be partially encapsulated as well e.g. follicular carcinoma thyroid. But characteristically, they are distinguished from benign tumours by *invasion, infiltration and destruction* of the surrounding tissue, besides distant metastasis. Often, cancers extend through tissue spaces, permeate lymphatics, blood vessels, perineural spaces and may penetrate a bone by growing through nutrient foramina.

V. METASTASIS (DISTANT SPREAD) *(p. 204)*

Metastasis is defined as spread of tumour by invasion in such a way that discontinuous secondary tumour mass/masses are formed at the site of lodgement. *Metastasis and invasiveness are the two most important features to distinguish malignant from benign tumours.* Benign tumours do not metastasise while all the malignant tumours with a few exceptions like gliomas of the central nervous system and basal cell carcinoma of the skin, can metastasise. Generally, larger, more aggressive and rapidly-growing tumours are more likely to metastasise but there are numerous exceptions.

Routes of Metastasis *(p. 205)*

Cancers may spread to distant sites by following pathways:

1. LYMPHATIC SPREAD. *In general, carcinomas metastasise by lymphatic route while sarcomas favour haematogenous route.* However, sarcomas may also spread by lymphatic pathway. The involvement of lymph nodes by malignant cells may be of two forms:

i) Lymphatic permeation. The walls of lymphatics are readily invaded by cancer cells and may form a continuous growth in the lymphatic channels called lymphatic permeation.

ii) Lymphatic emboli. Alternatively, the malignant cells may detach to form tumour emboli so as to be carried along the lymph to the next draining lymph node. The tumour emboli enter the lymph node at its convex surface and are lodged in the subcapsular sinus where they start growing.

■ Generally, regional lymph nodes draining the tumour are invariably involved producing *regional nodal metastasis* e.g. from carcinoma breast to axillary lymph nodes, from carcinoma thyroid to lateral cervical lymph nodes, bronchogenic carcinoma to hilar and para-tracheal lymph nodes etc.

■ However, all regional nodal enlargements are not due to nodal metastasis because necrotic products of tumour and antigens may also incite regional lymphadenitis of *sinus histiocytosis.*

■ Sometimes lymphatic metastases do not develop first in the lymph node nearest to the tumour because of venous-lymphatic anastomoses or due to obliteration of lymphatics by inflammation or radiation, so called *skip metastasis.*

■ Other times, due to obstruction of the lymphatics by tumour cells, the lymph flow is disturbed and tumour cells spread against the flow of lymph causing *retrograde metastases* at unusual sites e.g. metastasis of carcinoma prostate to the supraclavicular lymph nodes, metastatic deposits from bronchogenic carcinoma to the axillary lymph nodes.

■ *Virchow's lymph node* is nodal metastasis preferentially to supraclavicular lymph node from cancers of abdominal organs e.g. cancer stomach, colon, and gall bladder.

It is believed that lymph nodes in the vicinity of tumour perform multiple roles—as initial barrier filter, and in destruction of tumour cells, while later provide fertile soil for growth of tumour cells.

2. HAEMATOGENOUS SPREAD. *Blood-borne metastasis is the common route for sarcomas but certain carcinomas also frequently metastasise by this mode,* especially those of the lung, breast, thyroid, kidney, liver, prostate and ovary. The common sites for blood-borne metastasis are: the liver, lungs, brain, bones, kidney and adrenals, all of which provide 'good soil' for the growth of 'good seeds' *(seed-soil theory).* However, a few organs such as spleen, heart, skeletal muscle do not allow tumour metastasis to grow. Spleen is unfavourable site due to open sinusoidal pattern which does not permit tumour cells to stay there long enough to produce metastasis.

■ *Systemic veins* drain blood into vena cavae from limbs, head and neck and pelvis. Therefore, cancers of these sites more often metastasise to the lungs.

■ *Portal veins* drain blood from the bowel, spleen and pancreas into the liver. Thus, tumours of these organs frequently have secondaries in the liver.

■ *Arterial spread* of tumours is less likely because they are thick-walled and contain elastic tissue which is resistant to invasion. Nevertheless, arterial spread may occur when tumour cells pass through pulmonary capillary bed.

■ *Retrograde spread* by blood route may occur at unusual sites due to retrograde spread after venous obstruction, just as with lymphatic metastases. Important examples are vertebral metastases in cancers of the thyroid and prostate.

G/A Blood-borne metastases in an organ appear as multiple, rounded nodules of varying sizes, scattered throughout the organ. Sometimes, the metastasis may grow bigger than the primary tumour.

Chapter Eight

M/E The secondary deposits generally reproduce the structure of primary tumour. However, the same primary tumour on metastasis at diferent sites may show varying grades of differentiation.

3. SPREAD ALONG BODY CAVITIES AND NATURAL PASSAGES. Uncommonly, some cancers may spread by *seeding* at other surfaces. These routes of distant spread are as under:

i)   Transcoelomic spread. Certain cancers invade through the serosal wall of the coelomic cavity so that tumour fragments or clusters of tumour cells break off to be carried in the coelomic fluid and are implanted elsewhere in the body cavity e.g.

a) carcinoma of the stomach seeding to both ovaries (Krukenberg tumour);

b) carcinoma of the ovary;

c) pseudomyxoma peritonei; and

d) carcinoma of the bronchus and breast seeding to the pleura and pericardium.

ii)   Spread along epithelium-lined surfaces. It is unusual for a malignant tumour to spread along the epithelium-lined surfaces because intact epithelium and mucus coat are quite resistant to penetration by tumour cells. However, exceptionally a malignant tumour may spread through:

a) the fallopian tube from the endometrium to the ovaries or *vice-versa;*

b) through the bronchus into alveoli; and

c) through the ureters from the kidneys into lower urinary tract.

iii) Spread via cerebrospinal fluid. Malignant tumour of the ependyma and leptomeninges may spread by release of tumour fragments and tumour cells into the CSF and produce metastases at other sites in the central nervous system.

iv) Implantation. Rarely, a tumour may spread by implantation by surgeon's scalpel, needles, sutures, or may be implanted by direct contact such as transfer of cancer of the lower lip to the apposing upper lip.

MECHANISM AND BIOLOGY OF INVASION AND METASTASIS *(p. 207)*

The process of local invasion and distant spread (by lymphatic and haematogenous routes) discussed above involves passage through barriers before gaining access to the vascular lumen. This includes making the passage by the cancer cells by dissolution of extracellular matrix (ECM) at three levels— at the basement membrane of tumour itself, at the level of interstitial connective tissue, and at the basement membrane of microvasculature. The following steps are involved at the cell molecular level:

1.   Aggressive clonal proliferation and angiogenesis. Development of rapidly proliferating clone of cancer cells is explained on the basis of *tumour heterogeneity*, i.e. in the population of monoclonal tumour cells, a subpopulation or clone of tumour cells has the right biologic characteristics to complete the steps involved in the development of metastasis. Tumour angiogenesis plays a very significant role in metastasis.

2. Tumour cell loosening. Normal cells remain glued to each other due to presence of cell adhesion molecules (CAMs), E (epithelial)-cadherin. In epithelial cancers there is either loss or inactivation of E-cadherin and also other CAMs of immunoglobulin superfamily.

3. Tumour cell-ECM interaction. Loosened cancer cells now are attached to ECM proteins, mainly *laminin* and *fibronectin*. This attachment is facilitated due to profoundness of receptors on the cancer cells for both these proteins.

4. Degradation of ECM. Tumour cells overexpress *proteases* and matrix-degrading enzymes, *metalloproteinases* that includes collagenases and gelatinase, while the inhibitors of metalloproteinases are decreased. Another protease, cathepsin D, is also increased in certain cancers.

5. Entry of tumour cells into capillary lumen. The tumour cells after degrading the basement membrane are ready to migrate into lumen of capillaries or venules for which the following mechanisms play a role:

i) *Autocrine motility factor (AMF)* is a cytokine derived from tumour cells and stimulates receptor-mediated motility of tumour cells.

ii) *Cleavage products of matrix components* which are formed following degradation of ECM have properties of tumour cell chemotaxis, growth promotion and angiogenesis in the cancer.

6. Thrombus formation. The tumour cells protruding in the lumen of the capillary are now covered with constituents of the circulating blood and form the thrombus. Thrombus provides nourishment to the tumour cells and also protects them from the immune attack by the circulating host cells.

7. Extravasation of tumour cells. Tumour cells in the circulation (capillaries, venules, lymphatics) may mechanically block these vascular channels and attach to vascular endothelium. In this way, the sequence similar to local invasion is repeated and the basement membrane in exposed.

8. Survival and growth of metastatic deposit. The extravasated malignant cells on lodgement in the right environment grow further under the influence of growth factors produced by host tissues, tumour cells and by cleavage products of matrix components. These growth factors in particular include: PDGF, FGF, TGF-β and VEGF.

PROGNOSTIC MARKERS (p. 208)

Recent evidence has shown that in metastatic tumours, survival of host is correlated with some clinical and molecular features of tumours which act as *prognostic markers.*

i) Clinical prognostic markers: Size, grade, vascular invasion and nodal involvement by the tumour.

ii) Molecular prognostic markers: Molecular markers indicative of poor prognosis in certain specific tumours are:

a) expression of an oncogene by tumour cells *(C-met);*

b) CD 44 molecule;

c) oestrogen receptors;

d) epidermal growth factor receptor;

e) angiogenesis factors and degree of neovascularisation; and

f) expression of *metastasis associated gene* or *nucleic acid* (MAGNA) in the DNA fragment in metastasising tumour.

GRADING AND STAGING OF CANCER (p. 208)

'Grading' and 'staging' are the two systems to determine the prognosis and choice of treatment after a malignant tumour is detected. *Grading is defined as the macroscopic and microscopic degree of differentiation of the tumour, while staging means extent of spread of the tumour within the patient.*

Grading (p. 209)

Grading is largely based on 2 important histologic features: *the degree of anaplasia, and the rate of growth.* Based on these features, cancers are categorised from grade I as the most differentiated, to grade III or IV as the most undifferentiated or anaplastic. *Broders' grading* is as under:

Grade I: Well-differentiated (less than 25% anaplastic cells).

Grade II: Moderately-differentiated (25-50% anaplastic cells).

Grade III: Moderately-differentiated (50-75% anaplastic cells).

Grade IV: Poorly-differentiated or anaplastic (more than 75% anaplastic cells).

Staging *(p. 209)*

The extent of spread of cancers can be assessed by 3 ways—by clinical examination, by investigations, and by pathologic examination of the tissue removed. Two important staging systems currently followed are: TNM staging and AJC staging.

TNM staging. (T for primary tumour, N for regional nodal involvement, and M for distant metastases) was developed by the UICC (Union Internationale Contre Cancer, Geneva).

AJC staging. (American Joint Committee staging) divides all cancers into stage 0 to IV, and takes into account all the 3 components of the preceding system (primary tumour, nodal involvement and distant metastases) in each stage.

EPIDEMIOLOGY AND PREDISPOSITION TO NEOPLASIA *(p. 209)*

CANCER INCIDENCE *(p. 209)*

Worldwide, it is estimated that about 20% of all deaths are cancer-related. There have been changing patterns in incidence of cancers in both the sexes and in different geographic locations as outlined below. Table 8.2 shows worldwide incidence (in descending order) of different forms of cancer in men, women, and children. As evident from the Table, some types of cancers are commoner in India while others are more common in the Western populations since etiologic factors are different.

TABLE 8.2: Most Common Malignant Tumours *(In Descending Order).*

	MEN	WOMEN	CHILDREN
1.	Lung (oral cavity in India)	Breast (cervix in India)	Acute leukaemias
2.	Prostate	Lung	CNS tumours
3.	Colon-rectum	Colon-rectum	Lymphomas
4.	Leukaemia-lymphoma	Leukaemia-lymphoma	Neuroblastoma
5.	Liver	Ovary	Bone sarcomas

EPIDEMIOLOGIC FACTORS *(p. 209)*

The pattern and incidence of cancer depends upon the following:
A) A large number of *predisposing epidemiologic factors or cofactors.*
B) *Chronic non-neoplastic (pre-malignant) conditions.*
C) *Role of hormones in cancer.*

A. Predisposing Factors *(p. 209)*

1. FAMILIAL AND GENETIC FACTORS. In general, the risk of developing cancer in relatives of a known cancer patient is almost three times higher as compared to control subjects. The overall estimates suggest that genetic cancers comprise not greater than 5% of all cancers. Some of the common examples are as under:

i) Retinoblastoma. About 40% of retinoblastomas are familial and show an autosomal dominant inheritance. Carriers of such genetic composition have 10,000 times higher risk of developing retinoblastoma which is often bilateral. Such patients are predisposed to develop another primary malignant tumour, notably osteogenic sarcoma. Retinoblastoma susceptibility gene, *RB gene,* located on chromosome 13 was the first cancer-predisposing gene identified.
ii) Familial polyposis coli. This condition has autosomal dominant inheritance. The polypoid adenomas may be seen at birth or in early age. By the age of 50 years, almost 100% cases of familial polyposis coli develop cancer of the colon.

iii) **Multiple endocrine neoplasia (MEN).** A combination of adenomas of pituitary, parathyroid and pancreatic islets (MEN-I) or syndrome of medullary carcinoma thyroid, pheochromocytoma and parathyroid tumour (MEN-II) are encountered in families.

iv) **Neurofibromatosis or von Recklinghausen's disease.** This condition is characterised by multiple neurofibromas and pigmented skin spots (*cafe au lait spots*).

v) **Cancer of the breast.** Female relatives of breast cancer patients have 2 to 3 times higher risk of developing breast cancer.

vi) **DNA-chromosomal instability syndromes.** These are a group of pre-neoplastic conditions having defect in DNA repair mechanism. A classical example is xeroderma pigmentosum, an autosomal recessive disorder, characterised by extreme sensitivity to ultraviolet radiation. The patients may develop various types of skin cancers such as basal cell carcinoma, squamous cell carcinoma and malignant melanoma.

2. RACIAL AND GEOGRAPHIC FACTORS. Differences in racial incidence of some cancers may be partly attributed to the role of genetic composition but are largely due to influence of the environment and geographic differences affecting the whole population such as climate, soil, water, diet, habits, customs etc.

i) **White Europeans and Americans** develop most commonly malignancies of the lung, breast, and colon. Liver cancer is uncommon in these races. Breast cancer is uncommon in Japanese women but is more common in American women.

ii) **Black Africans,** on the other hand, have more commonly cancers of the skin, penis, cervix and liver.

iii) **Japanese** have five times higher incidence of carcinoma of the stomach than the Americans.

iv) **South-East Asians,** especially of Chinese origin have more commonly nasopharyngeal cancer.

v) **Indians** of both sexes have higher incidence of carcinoma of the oral cavity and upper aerodigestive tract, while in females carcinoma of uterine cervix and of breast run parallel in incidence. Cancer of the liver in India is more due to viral hepatitis (HBV and HCV) and subsequent cirrhosis than due to alcoholism.

3. ENVIRONMENTAL AND CULTURAL FACTORS. We are surrounded by an environment of carcinogens which we eat, drink, inhale and touch. Some of the examples are given below:

i) **Cigarette smoking** is the single most important environmental factor implicated in the etiology of cancer of the oral cavity, pharynx, larynx, oesophagus, lungs, pancreas and urinary bladder.

ii) **Alcohol abuse** predisposes to the development of cancer of oropharynx, larynx, oesophagus and liver.

iii) **Alcohol and tobacco together** further accentuate the risk of developing cancer of the upper aerodigestive tract.

iv) **Cancer of the cervix** is linked to a number of factors such as age at first coitus, frequency of coitus, multiplicity of partners, parity etc. Sexual partners of circumcised males have lower incidence of cervical cancer than the partners of uncircumcised males.

v) **Penile cancer** is rare in the Jews and Muslims as they are customarily circumcised.

vi) **Betel nut cancer** of the cheek and tongue is quite common in some parts of India due to habitual practice of keeping the bolus of *paan* in a particular place in mouth for a long time.

vii) A large number of **industrial and environmental substances** are carcinogenic and are occupational hazard for some populations. These include exposure to substances like arsenic, asbestos, benzene, vinyl chloride, naphthylamine etc.

viii) Certain constituents of diet have also been implicated in the causation of cancer. Overweight individuals, deficiency of vitamin A and people consuming diet rich in animal fats and low in fibre content are more at risk of developing certain cancers such as colonic cancer. Diet rich in vitamin E, on the other hand, possibly has some protective influence by its antioxidant action.

4.   AGE. Generally, cancers occur in older individuals past 5th decade of life. Some tumours have two peaks of incidence e.g. acute leukaemias occur in children and in older age group. Besides acute leukaemias, *other tumours in infancy and childhood* are: neuroblastoma, nephroblastoma (Wilms' tumour), retinoblastoma, hepatoblastoma, rhabdomyosarcoma, Ewing's sarcoma, teratoma and CNS tumours.

5.   SEX. Apart from the malignant tumours of organs peculiar to each sex, most tumours are generally more common in men than in women except cancer of the breast, gall bladder, thyroid and hypopharynx. Although there are geographic and racial variations, *cancer of the breast* is the commonest cancer in *women* throughout the world while *lung cancer* is the commonest cancer in *men*.

B.   Chronic Non-neoplastic (Premalignant) Conditions *(p. 211)*

Premalignant lesions are a group of conditions which predispose to the subsequent development of cancer.

Some examples of premalignant lesions are given below:

1.   Carcinoma *in situ* (intraepithelial neoplasia). When the cytological features of malignancy are present but the malignant cells are confined to epithelium without invasion across the basement membrane, it is called as carcinoma *in situ* or intraepithelial neoplasia (CIN). The common sites are:

i)   Uterine cervix at the junction of ecto and endocervix
ii)   Bowen's disease of the skin
iii)   Actinic or solar keratosis
iv)   Oral leukoplakia
v)   Intralobular and intraductal carcinoma of the breast.

The area involved in carcinoma *in situ* may be single and small, or multifocal. As regards the behaviour of CIN, it may regress and return to normal or may develop into invasive cancer.

2.   Some benign tumours. Commonly, benign tumours do not become malignant. However, there are some exceptions e.g.

i)   Multiple villous adenomas of the large intestine have high incidence of developing adenocarcinoma.
ii)   Neurofibromatosis (von Recklinghausen's disease) may develop into sarcoma.

3.   Miscellaneous conditions. Certain inflammatory and hyperplastic conditions are prone to development of cancer, e.g.

i)   Patients of long-standing ulcerative colitis are predisposed to develop colorectal cancer.
ii)   Cirrhosis of the liver has predisposition to develop hepatocellular carcinoma.
iii)   Chronic bronchitis in heavy cigarette smokers may develop cancer of the bronchus.
iv)   Chronic irritation from jagged tooth or ill-fitting denture may lead to cancer of the oral cavity.
v) Squamous cell carcinoma developing in an old burn scar (Marjolin's ulcer).

C.   Hormones and Cancer *(p. 211)*

Cancer is more likely to develop in organs and tissues which undergo proliferation under the influence of excessive hormonal stimulation. On cessation of hormonal stimulation, such tissues become atrophic. Hormone-sensitive tissues developing tumours are the breast, endometrium, myometrium, vagina, thyroid, liver, prostate and testis. Some examples of hormones influencing carcinogenesis in experimental animals and humans are given below:

1. OESTROGEN. Its role in tumours is as under.

i) In experimental animals. Induction of breast cancer in mice by administration of high-dose of oestrogen and reduction of the tumour development following oophorectomy is the most important example. Associated infection with mouse mammary tumour virus (MMTV, *Bittner milk factor*) has an added influence on the development of breast cancer in mice.

ii) In humans. Women receiving oestrogen therapy and women with oestrogen-secreting granulosa cell tumour of the ovary have increased risk of developing endometrial carcinoma. Adenocarcinoma of the vagina is seen with increased frequency in adolescent daughters of mothers who had received oestrogen-therapy during pregnancy.

2. CONTRACEPTIVE HORMONES. The sequential types of oral contraceptives increase the risk of developing breast cancer. Other tumours showing a slightly increased frequency in women receiving contraceptive pills for long durations are benign tumours of the liver.

3. ANABOLIC STEROIDS. Consumption of anabolic steroids by athletes to increase the muscle mass increases the risk of developing benign and malignant tumours of the liver.

4. HORMONE-DEPENDENT TUMOURS. There is tumour regression on removal of the stimulus for excessive hormonal secretion e.g.

i)   *Prostatic cancer* usually responds to the administration of oestrogens.

ii) *Breast cancer* may regress with oophorectomy, hypophysectomy or on administration of male hormones.

iii) *Thyroid cancer* may slow down in growth with administration of thyroxine that suppresses the secretion of TSH by the pituitary.

CARCINOGENESIS:
ETIOLOGY AND PATHOGENESIS OF CANCER *(p. 212)*

There has been ever-increasing list of agents implicated in etiology of cancer. There has been still greater accumulation in volumes of knowledge on pathogenesis of cancer, especially due to tremendous strides made in the field of molecular biology and genetics in the last decade.

The subject of etiology and pathogenesis of cancer is discussed under the following 4 broad headings:

A. Molecular pathogenesis of cancer (genes and cancer)
B. Chemical carcinogens and chemical carcinogenesis
C. Physical carcinogens and radiation carcinogenesis
D. Biologic carcinogens and viral oncogenesis.

A. MOLECULAR PATHOGENESIS OF CANCER
   (GENES AND CANCER) *(p. 212)*

Basic Concept of Molecular Pathogenesis *(p. 212)*

The mechanism as to how a normal cell is transformed to a cancer cell is complex. In the last decade, there has been vast accumulation of literature to explain the pathogenesis of cancer at molecular level.

1. Monoclonality of tumours. There is strong evidence that most human cancers arise from a single clone of cells by genetic transformation or mutation. For example:

i)   In a case of multiple myeloma (a malignant disorder of plasma cells), there is production of a single type of immunoglobulin or its chain as seen by monoclonal spike in serum electrophoresis.

ii) Due to inactivation of one of the two X-chromosomes in females (paternal or maternal derived), women are mosaics with two types of cell populations e.g. for glucose-6-phosphatase dehydrogenase (G6PD) isoenzyme A and B. It is observed that all the tumour cells in benign uterine tumours (leiomyoma) contain either A or B genotype of G6PD (i.e. the tumour cells are derived from a single progenitor clone of cell), while the normal myometrium is mosaic of both types of cells derived from A as well as B isoenzyme.

2. Genetic theory of cancer. Cell growth of normal as well as abnormal types is under genetic control. In cancer, there is either abnormality in the genes of the cell, or there are normal genes with abnormal expression. The abnormality in genetic composition may be from an inherited or induced mutation (induced by etiologic carcinogenic agents namely: chemicals, viruses, radiation). The mutated cells transmit their characters to the next progeny of cells and result in cancer.

3. Genetic regulators of normal and abnormal mitosis. In normal cell growth, regulatory genes control mitosis as well as cell aging, terminating in cell death by apoptosis.

■ **In normal cell growth,** there are 4 regulatory genes:

i) Proto-oncogenes are growth-promoting genes.

ii) Anti-oncogenes are growth-inhibiting or growth suppressor genes.

iii) Apoptosis regulatory genes control the programmed cell death.

iv) DNA repair genes are those normal genes which regulate the repair of DNA damage that has occurred during mitosis.

■ **In cancer,** the transformed cells are produced by abnormal cell growth due to genetic damage to these normal controlling genes. Thus, corresponding abnormalities are genetics, as under:

i) Activation of growth-promoting oncogenes causing transformation of cell (mutant form of normal proto-oncogene in cancer is termed *oncogene*). Gene products of oncogenes are called *oncoproteins*. Oncogenes are considered *dominant* since they appear inspite of presence of normal proto-oncogenes.

ii) Inactivation of cancer-suppressor genes (i.e. inactivation of anti-oncogenes) permitting the cellular proliferation of transformed cells. Anti-oncogenes are active in *recessive* form which mean that they are active only if both alleles are damaged.

iii) Abnormal apoptosis regulatory genes which may act as oncogenes or anti-oncogenes. Accordingly, these genes may be active in dominant or recessive form.

iv) Failure of DNA repair genes and thus inability to repair the DNA damage resulting in mutations.

4. Multi-step process of cancer growth and progression. Carcinogenesis is a gradual multi-step process involving many generations of cells. The various causes may act on the cell one after another (*multi-hit process*). The same process is also involved in further progression of the tumour. Ultimately, the cells so formed are genetically and phenotypically transformed cells having phenotypic features of malignancy—excessive growth, invasiveness and distant metastasis.

CANCER-RELATED GENES AND CELL GROWTH (p. 214)
(Hallmarks of Cancer)

It is apparent from the above discussion that genes control the normal cellular growth, while in cancer these controlling genes are altered, typically by mutation. A large number of such cancer-associated genes have been described, each with a specific function in cell growth. Some of these genes are commonly associated in many tumours (e.g. *p53* or *TP53*), while others are specific to particular tumours. Therefore, it is considered appropriate to discuss the role of cancer-related genes with regard to their functions in cellular growth. Following are the *major genetic properties or hallmarks of cancer:*

1. Excessive and autonomous growth: Growth-promoting oncogenes.
2. Refractoriness to growth inhibition: Growth suppressing anti-oncogenes.
3. Escaping cell death by apoptosis: Genes regulating apoptosis and cancer.
4. Avoiding cellular aging: Telomeres and telomerase in cancer.
5. Continued perfusion of cancer: Cancer angiogenesis.
6. Invasion and distant metastasis: Cancer dissemination.
7. DNA damage and repair system: Mutator genes and cancer.
8. Cancer progression and tumour heterogeneity: Clonal aggressiveness.

1. Excessive and Autonomous Growth: Growth Promoting Oncogenes

Mutated form of normal proto-oncogenes in cancer is called oncogenes. Oncogenes differ from 'normal genes' in following respects:

■ mutation in the structure of gene;

■ lacking the normal growth-promoting signals of proto-oncogenes; and

■ they act by over-expression to promote autonomous and excessive cellular proliferation.

In general, activation of oncogenes in human tumours can occur by following mechanisms:

i) Point mutations and deletion. The most important example is *RAS* oncogene carried in many human tumours such as bladder cancer, pancreatic adenocarcinoma, cholangiocarcinoma.

ii) Chromosomal translocation. Mechanism of transfer of a portion of one chromosome to another is implicated in the pathogenesis of leukaemias and lymphomas e.g.

■ Philadelphia chromosome seen in 95% cases of chronic myelogenous leukaemia in which *c-ABL* proto-oncogene on chromosome 9 is translocated to chromosome 22.

■ In 75% cases of Burkitt's lymphoma, translocation of *c-MYC* proto-oncogene from its site on chromosome 8 to a portion on chromosome 14.

iii) Gene amplification. Chromosomal alterations that result in increase in the number of copies of a gene is found in some examples of solid human tumours e.g.

■ Neuroblastoma having *n-MYC HSR* region.

■ *ERB-B* in breast and ovarian cancer.

The steps in signal transduction for cell proliferation by oncogenes are discussed below in relation to mitosis in normal cell cycle (Table 8.3):

i) Growth factors (GFs). These are polypeptides elaborated by many cells and normally act on another cell than the one which synthesised it to stimulate its proliferation i.e. *paracrine action.* However, a cancer cell may synthesise a GF and respond to it as well; this way cancer cells acquire growth self sufficiency. The examples of such GFs are as under:

a) Platelet-derived growth factor (PDGF) in glioblastoma.

b) Transforming growth factor-α (TGF-α) is over-expressed in sarcomas.

c) Fibroblast growth factor (FGF) in cancer of the bowel and breast.

ii) Receptors for GFs. Many oncogenes encoding for GF receptors have been described which act more commonly by overexpression of normal GF than by mutation. For example:

a) ERB1 is an EGF receptor which acts by overexpression of normal GF receptor in squamous cell carcinoma.

b) HER2, also called *ERB2,* is another EGF receptor which is overexpressed in breast cancer and carcinoma of lungs, ovary, stomach.

TABLE 8.3: Important Oncogenes, their Mechanism of Activation and Associated Human Tumours.

TYPE		ONCOGENE	ASSOCIATED HUMAN TUMOURS
1. **Growth factors (GFs)**			
	i)	*PDGF*	Glioblastoma
	ii)	*TGF-α*	Sarcomas
	iii)	*FGF*	Ca bowel, breast
2. **Receptors for GFs**			
	i)	*ERB B₁*	Squamous cell carcinoma
	ii)	*HER₂ (α ERB₂)*	Ca breast, ovary, stomach, lungs
3. **Signal transduction proteins**		*RAS*	Common in 1/3rd human tumours,
			Ca lung, colon, pancreas
		BCR-ABL	CML, acute leukaemias
4. **Nuclear regulatory molecules (Transcription proteins)**		*MYC* (translocated)	Burkitt's lymphoma
		MYC (amplified)	Ca lungs, breast, colon
5. **Cell cycle regulatory proteins**		*Cyclin D*	Ca breast, liver, mantle cell lymphoma
		CDK4	Glioblastoma, melanoma, sarcomas

PDGF = platelet-derived growth factor; FGF = fibroblast growth factor; TGF-α = Transforming growth factor; CDK = cyclin-dependent kinase

iii) Signal transduction proteins. The normal signal transduction proteins which transduce signal from the GF receptors on the cell surface to the nucleus of the cell is mutated in some cancers e.g.

a) Mutated RAS gene. This is the most common form of oncogene in human tumours. About a third of all human tumours carry mutated *RAS* gene (*RAS* for Rat Sarcoma gene where it was first described), seen in particular in carcinoma colon, lung and pancreas. Normally, the inactive form of *RAS* protein is GDP (guanosine diphosphate)-bound while the activated form is bound to GTP. GDP/GTP are homologous to G proteins and take part in signal transduction in a similar way just as G proteins act as 'on-off switch' for signal transduction. Normally, active *RAS* protein is inactivated by GTPase activity, while mutated *RAS* gene remains unaffected by GTPase and therefore, continues to signal the cell proliferation. Common mode of activation of *RAS* gene is by point mutation.

b) BCR-ABL hybrid gene. ABL gene is a non-GF receptor proto-oncogene having tyrosine kinase activity. *ABL* gene from its normal location on chromosome 9 is translocated to chromosome 22 where it fuses with *BCR* (breakpoint cluster region) gene and forms an *ABL-BCR* hybrid gene which is more potent in signal transduction pathway. *ABL-BCR* hybrid gene is seen in chronic myeloid leukaemia and some acute leukaemias.

iv) Nuclear regulatory molecules. The signal transduction pathway that started with GFs ultimately reaches the nucleus where it regulates DNA transcription. Out of various nuclear regulatory transcription proteins described, the most important is *MYC* gene, seen most commonly in human tumours. Normally *MYC* protein binds to the DNA and regulates the cell cycle by transcriptional activation and its levels fall immediately after cell enters the cell cycle. *MYC* oncogene, on the other hand, is associated with persistent or overexpression of *MYC* oncoproteins which, in turn, causes autonomous cell proliferation. The examples of tumours carrying *MYC* oncogene are:

a) Burkitt's lymphoma in which mutation in *MYC* gene is due to *translocation* t(8;14).

b) In cancer of lung, breast and colon, *MYC* gene is mutated due to *amplification*.

v) Cell cycle regulatory proteins. Normally the cell cycle is under regulatory control of cyclins and cyclin-dependent kinases (CDKs) A, B, E and D. Cyclins are so named since they are cyclically synthesised during different phases of the cell cycle and their degradation is also cyclic. Cyclins activate as well as work together with CDKs, while many inhibitors of CDKs (CDKIs) are also known. Although all steps in the cell cycle are under regulatory controls, G1 → S phase is the most important checkpoint for regulation by oncogenes as well as anti-oncogenes. Mutations in cyclins (in particular cyclin D) and CDKs (in particular CDK4) are most important growth promoting signals in cancers. The examples of tumours having such oncogenes are:

a) *Overexpression of cyclin D* in cancers of breast, liver and mantle cell lymphoma.

b) *Amplification of CDK4* in malignant melanoma, glioblastoma and sarcomas.

2. Refractoriness to Growth Inhibition: Growth Suppressing Anti-oncogenes

The mutation of normal growth suppressor anti-oncogenes results in removal of the brakes for growth; thus the inhibitory effect to cell growth is removed and the abormal growth continues unchecked. In other words, mutated anti-oncogenes behave like growth-promoting oncogenes.

As compared to the signals and signal transduction pathways for oncogenes described above, the steps in mechanisms of action by growth suppressors are not as well understood. In general, the point of action by anti-oncogenes is also G1 → S phase transition and probably act either by inducing the dividing cell from the cell cycle to enter into G0 (resting) phase, or by acting in a way that the cell lies in the post-mitotic pool losing its dividing capability.

Major anti-oncogenes implicated in human cancers are as under (Table 8.4):

TABLE 8.4: Important Tumour-suppressor Genes and Associated Human Tumours.

	GENE	LOCATION	ASSOCIATED HUMAN TUMOURS
1.	*RB*	Nucleus (q13)	Retinoblastoma, osteosarcoma
2.	*TP53 (p53)*	Nucleus (p17)	Most human cancers, common in ca. lung, head and neck, colon, breast
3.	*TGF–β*	Extracellular GF	Ca pancreas, colon, stomach
4.	*APC*	Cytosol	Ca colon
5.	**Others**		
	i) *WT 1 and 2*	Nucleus	Wilms' tumour
	ii) *NF 1 and 2*	Plasma membrane	Neurofibromatosis type 1 and 2
	iii) *BRCA 1 and 2*	Nucleus	Ca breast, ovary

i) *RB* gene. *RB* gene is located on long arm (q) of chromosome 13. This is the first ever tumour suppressor gene identified and thus has been amply studied. Normally, *RB* gene product is a nuclear transcription protein which is virtually present in every human cell. It exists in both an *active* and an *inactive* form. Active *RB* gene protein acts to inhibit the cell cycle at G1 → S phase. Stimulation of the cell by growth factors renders the *RB* gene protein inactive and thus permits the cell to cross G1 → S phase.

The mutant form of *RB* gene is involved in retinoblastoma, the most common intraocular tumour in young children. The tumour occurs in two forms: sporadic and inherited/familial. Besides retinoblastoma, children inheriting mutant *RB* gene have 200 times greater risk of development of other cancers in early adult life, most notably osteosarcoma; others are cancers of breast, colon and lungs.

ii) *TP53* gene (*p53*). Located on the short arm (p) of chromosome 17, *p53* gene (currently termed *TP53*) is normally a growth suppressor anti-oncogene.

The two major functions of *TP53* in the normal cell cycle are as under:

a) In blocking mitotic activity: *TP53* inhibits the cyclins and CDKs and prevents the cell to enter G1 phase transiently. This breathing time in the cell cycle is utilised by the cell to repair the DNA damage.

b) In promoting apoptosis: *TP53* acts together with another anti-oncogene, *RB* gene, and identifies the genes that have damaged DNA which cannot be repaired by inbuilt system. *TP53* directs such cells to apoptosis by activating apoptosis-inducing *BAX* gene, and thus bringing the defective cells to an end.

Because of these significant roles in cell cycle, *TP53* is called as 'protector of the genome'.

In its mutated form, *TP53* stops to act as growth suppressor and instead acts like an oncogene, *c-onc*. Majority of human cancers have either a mutation in *TP53* or its expression is up- or down-regulated. Some common examples of human cancers having defective *TP53* are: cancers of lung, head and neck, colon and breast. Besides, mutated *TP53* is also seen in the sequential development stages of cancer from hyperplasia to carcinoma *in situ* and into invasive carcinoma.

iii) Transforming growth factor-β (*TGF*-β). Normally, *TGF*-β is significant inhibitor of cell proliferation, mainly by its action on G1 phase of cell cycle. Its mutant form impairs the growth inhibiting effect and thus permits cell proliferation. Examples of mutated form of *TGF*-β are seen in cancers of pancreas, colon, stomach etc.

iv) Adenomatous polyposis coli (APC) gene. The *APC* gene is normally inhibitory to mitosis, which is done by a cytoplasmic protein, β-catenin. β-catenin normally blocks the signal to the nucleus for activating mitosis. In colon cancer, APC gene is lost and thus the cancer cells continue to undergo mitosis without the inhibitory influence of β-catenin.

v) Other anti-oncogenes. A few other tumour-suppressor genes having mutated germline in various tumours are as under:

a) Wilms' tumour (WT) gene: *WT* gene normally prevents neoplastic proliferation of cells in embryonic kidney. Mutant form of WT-1 and 2 are seen in hereditary Wilms' tumour.

b) Neurofibroma (NF) gene: *NF* genes normally prevent proliferation of Schwann cells. Two mutant forms are described: *NF1* and *NF2* seen in neurofibromatosis type 1 and type 2.

c) BRCA 1 and BRCA 2 genes: These are breast *(BR)* cancer *(CA)* susceptibility genes, especially in inherited cases of breast cancer.

3. Escaping Cell Death by Apoptosis:
   Genes Regulating Apoptosis and Cancer

Apoptosis in normal cell is guided by cell death receptor, CD95, resulting in DNA damage. Besides, there is role of some other pro-apoptotic factors (*BAD*, *BAX*, *BID* and *TP53*) and apoptosis-inhibitors (*BCL2, BCL-X*).

In cancer cells, the function of apoptosis is interfered due to mutations in the above genes which regulate apoptosis in the normal cell. The examples of tumours by this mechanism are as under:

a) **BCL2 gene** is seen in normal lymphocytes, but its mutant form with characteristic translocation was first described in B-cell lymphoma and hence the name. It is also seen in many other human cancers such as that of breast, thyroid and prostate. Mutation in *BCL2* gene removes the apoptosis-inhibitory control on cancer cells, thus more live cells undergoing mitosis contributing to tumour growth.

b) **CD95** receptors are depleted in hepatocellular carcinoma and hence the tumour cells escape apoptosis.

4. Avoiding Cellular Aging: Telomeres and Telomerase in Cancer

After each mitosis (cell doubling) there is progressive shortening of telomeres which are the terminal tips of chromosomes. Telomerase is the RNA enzyme that helps in repair of such damage to DNA and maintains normal telomere length in successive cell divisions. However, it has been seen that after repetitive mitosis for a maximum of 60 to 70 times, telomeres are lost in normal cells and the cells cease to undergo mitosis. Telomerase is active in normal stem cells but not in normal somatic cells.

Cancer cells in most malignancies have markedly upregulated telomerase enzyme, and hence telomere length is maintained. Thus, cancer cells avoid aging, mitosis does not slow down or cease, thereby immortalising the cancer cells.

5. Continued Perfusion of Cancer: Tumour Angiogenesis

Cancers can only survive and thrive if the cancer cells are adequately nourished and perfused, as otherwise they cannot grow further. Neovascularisation in the cancers not only supplies the tumour with oxygen and nutrients, but the newly formed endothelial cells also elaborate a few growth factors for progression of primary as well as metastatic cancer. The stimulus for angiogenesis is provided by the release of various factors:

i) **Promoters of tumour angiogenesis** include the most important *vascular endothelial growth factor (VEGF)* (released from genes in the parenchymal tumour cells) and *basic fibroblast growth factor (bFGF)*.

ii) **Anti-angiogenesis factors** inhibiting angiogenesis include *thrombospondin-1* (also produced by tumour cells themselves), *angiostatin, endostatin and vasculostatin*.

6. Invasion and Distant Metastasis: Cancer Dissemination

One of the most important characteristic of cancers is invasiveness and metastasis. The mechanisms involved in the biology of invasion and metastasis are discussed already.

7. DNA Damage and Repair System: Mutator Genes and Cancer

Normal cells during complex mitosis suffer from minor damage to the DNA which is detected and repaired before mitosis is completed so that integrity of the genome is maintained. Similarly, small mutational damage to the dividing cell by exogenous factors (e.g. by radiation, chemical carcinogens etc) is also repaired. *TP53* gene is held responsible for detection and repair of DNA damage. However, if this system of DNA repair is defective as happens in some inherited mutations (mutator genes), the defect in DNA is passed to the next progeny of cells and cancer results.

The examples of mutator genes exist in the following inherited disorders associated with increased propensity to cancer:

Chapter Eight

i) Hereditary non-polyposis colon cancer (Lynch syndrome) is characterised by hereditary predisposition to develop colorectal cancer.

ii) Ataxia telangiectasia (AT) has *ATM* (*M* for mutated) gene. These patients have multiple cancers.

iii) Xeroderma pigmentosum is an inherited disorder in which there is defect in DNA repair mechanism. UV radiation damage to DNA cannot be repaired. Thus, such patients are more prone to various forms of skin cancers.

iv) Bloom syndrome is an example of damage by ionising radiation which cannot be repaired due to inherited defect and the patients have increased risk to develop cancers, particularly leukaemia.

v) Hereditary breast cancer patients having mutated *BRCA1* and *BRCA2* genes carrying inherited defect in DNA repair mechanism.

8. Cancer Progression and Heterogeneity: Clonal Aggressiveness

Another feature of note in biology of cancers is that with passage of time they become more aggressive; this property is termed *tumour progression*. Clinical parameters of cancer progression are: increasing size of the tumour, higher histologic grade, areas of tumour necrosis, invasiveness and distant metastasis.

In terms of molecular biology, this attribute of cancer is due to the fact that with passage of time cancer cells acquire more and more *heterogeneity*. This means that though cancer cells remain monoclonal in origin, they acquire more and more mutations which in turn produce multiple-mutated subpopulations of more aggressive clones of cancer cells (i.e. heterogeneous cells) in the growth which have tendency to invade, metastasise and be refractory to hormonal influences.

The above properties of cancer cells are schematically illustrated in Fig. 8.2.

B. CHEMICAL CARCINOGENESIS *(p. 219)*

The first ever evidence of any cause for neoplasia came from the observation of Sir Percival Pott in 1775 that there was higher incidence of cancer of the scrotum in chimney-sweeps in London than in the general population. This invoked wide interest in soot and coal tar as possible carcinogenic agent and the possibility of other occupational cancers. The first successful experimental induction of cancer was produced by two Japanese workers (Yamagiwa and Ichikawa) in 1914 in the rabbit's skin by repeatedly painting with coal tar.

Stages in Chemical Carcinogenesis *(p. 219)*

The induction of cancer by chemical carcinogens occurs after a delay—weeks to months in the case of experimental animals, and often several years in man. Other factors that influence the induction of cancer are the dose and mode of administration of carcinogenic chemical, individual susceptibility and various predisposing factors.

Basic mechanism of chemical carcinogenesis is by induction of mutation in the proto-oncogenes and anti-oncogenes. The phenomena of cellular transformation by chemical carcinogens (as also other carcinogens) is a progressive process involving 2 distinct sequential stages: initiation and promotion.

1. INITIATION OF CARCINOGENESIS

Chemical carcinogens acting as initiators of carcinogenesis can be grouped into 2 categories (Table 8.5):

I. Direct-acting carcinogens. These are a few chemical substances (e.g. alkylating agents, acylating agents) which can induce cellular transformation without undergoing any prior metabolic activation.

Fig. 8.2: Schematic representation of activation-inactivation of cancer-associated genes in cell cycle.

EXTRACELLULAR SPACE

CELL MEMBRANE

CYTOSOL

NUCLEUS

DNA

Growth factors
(PDGF, TGFα, FGF)

Receptors for growth factors
(ERB1, HER2↑)

Signal transduction proteins
(Mutated RAS, overexpressed BCL-ABL)

Apoptosis-associated genes
(BCL2, BAX, TP53, CD95)

Antioncogenes
(TP53, RB)

Transcription proteins
(MYC)

DNA repair gene
(Mutator gene)

Telomerase

Cell cycle activator-inhibitor
(Cyclins, CDK, CDKI)

Chapter Eight

TABLE 8.5: Important Chemical Carcinogens.

CARCINOGEN	TUMOUR
I. DIRECT-ACTING CARCINOGENS	
a) *Alkylating agents*	
• Anti-cancer drugs (e.g. cyclo-phosphamide, chlorambucil, busulfan, melphalan, nitrosourea etc)	
• β-propiolactone	• Lymphomas
• Epoxides	• Leukaemias
b) *Acylating agents*	
• Acetyl imidazole	
• Dimethyl carbamyl chloride	
II. INDIRECT-ACTING CARCINOGENS (PROCARCINOGENS):	
a) *Polycyclic aromatic hydrocarbons* (in tobacco, smoke, fossil fuel, soot, tar, minerals oil, smoked animal foods, industrial and atmospheric pollutants)	• Lung cancer
	• Skin cancer
• Anthracenes (benza-, dibenza-, dimethyl benza-)	• Cancer of oral cavity
• Benzapyrene	• Sarcoma
• Methylcholanthrene	
b) *Aromatic amines and azo-dyes*	
• β-naphthylamine	• Bladder cancer
• Benzidine	
• Azo-dyes (e.g. butter yellow, scarlet red etc)	• Hepatocellular carcinoma
c) *Naturally-occurring products*	
• Aflatoxin B	
• Actinomycin D	
• Mitomycin C	• Hepatocellular carcinoma
• Safrole	
• Betel nuts	
d) *Miscellaneous*	
• Nitrosamines and nitrosamides	• Gastric carcinoma
• Vinyl chloride monomer	• Haemangiosarcoma of liver
• Asbestos	• Bronchogenic carcinoma, mesothelioma
• Arsenical compounds	• Epidermal hyperplasia, basal cell carcinoma
• Metals (e.g. nickel, lead, cobalt, chromium etc)	• Lung cancer
• Insecticides, fungicides (e.g. aldrin, dieldrin, chlordane etc)	• Cancer in experimental animals
• Saccharin and cyclomates	

II. Indirect-acting carcinogens or procarcinogens. These require metabolic conversion within the body so as to become 'ultimate' carcinogens having carcinogenicity e.g. polycyclic aromatic hydrocarbons, aromatic amines, azo dyes, naturally-occurring products and others.

In either case, the following steps are involved in transforming 'the target cell' into 'the initiated cell' (Fig. 8.3):

a) Metabolic activation. Vast majority of chemical carcinogens are indirect-acting or procarcinogens requiring metabolic activation, while direct-acting

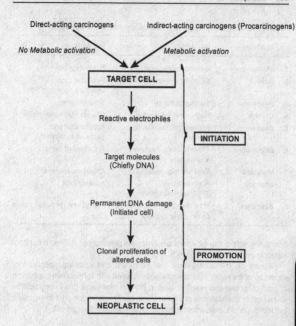

Direct-acting carcinogens   Indirect-acting carcinogens (Procarcinogens)

No Metabolic activation   *Metabolic activation*

TARGET CELL

Reactive electrophiles

INITIATION

Target molecules
(Chiefly DNA)

Permanent DNA damage
(Initiated cell)

Clonal proliferation of
altered cells   **PROMOTION**

NEOPLASTIC CELL

Fig. 8.3: Sequential stages in chemical carcinogenesis.

carcinogens do not require this activation. The indirect-acting carcinogens are activated in the liver by the mono-oxygenases of the cytochrome P-450 system in the endoplasmic reticulum. In some circumstances, the procarcinogen may be detoxified and rendered inactive metabolically.

b) Reactive electrophiles. While direct-acting carcinogens are intrinsically electrophilic, indirect-acting substances become electron-deficient after metabolic activation i.e. reactive electrophiles. Following this step, both types of chemical carcinogens behave alike and their reactive electrophiles bind to electron-rich portions of other molecules of the cell such as DNA, RNA and other proteins.

c) Target molecules. The primary target of electrophiles is DNA, producing mutagenesis. The change in DNA may lead to 'the initiated cell' or some form of cellular enzymes may be able to repair the damage in DNA.

It has been observed that most frequently affected oncogene is *RAS* gene mutation and anti-oncogene (tumour suppressor) is *TP53* gene mutation.

d) The initiated cell. The unrepaired damage produced in the DNA of the cell becomes permanent and fixed only if the altered cell undergoes at least one cycle of proliferation. This results in transferring the change to the next progeny of cells so that the DNA damage becomes *permanent* and *irreversible*, which are the characteristics of the initiated cell.

The stimulus for proliferation may come from regeneration of surviving cells, dietary factors, hormone-induced hyperplasia, viruses etc.

2. PROMOTION OF CARCINOGENESIS

Promotion is the next sequential stage in the chemical carcinogenesis. Promoters of carcinogenesis are substances such as phorbol esters, phenols,

TABLE 8.6: Contrasting Features of Initiator and Promoter Carcinogens.

FEATURE	INITIATOR	PROMOTER
1. *Mechanism*	Induction of mutation	Not mutagenic
2. *Dose*	Single for a short time	Repeated dose exposure, for a long time
3. *Response*	Sudden response	Slow response
4. *Change*	Permanent, irreversible	Change may be reversible
5. *Sequence*	Applied first, followed by promoter	Applied after prior exposure to initiator
6. *Effectivity*	Effective alone if exposed in large dose	Not effective alone
7. *Molecular changes*	Most common mutation of *RAS* oncogene, *TP53* anti-oncogene	Clonal expansion of mutated cells
8. *Examples*	Most chemical carcinogens, radiation	Hormones, phorbol esters

hormones, artificial sweeteners and drugs like phenobarbital. They differ from initiators as outlined in Table 8.6.

It may be mentioned here that persistent and sustained application/ exposure of the cell to initiator alone unassociated with subsequent application of promoter may also result in cancer. But the *vice versa* does not hold true since neither application of promoter alone, nor its application prior to exposure to initiator carcinogen, would result in transformation of target cell.

Tests for Chemical Carcinogenicity *(p. 224)*

There are 2 main methods of testing chemical compound for its carcinogenicity:

1. EXPERIMENTAL INDUCTION. The traditional method is to administer the chemical compound under test to a batch of experimental animals like mice or other rodents by an appropriate route e.g. painting on the skin, giving orally or parenterally, or by inhalation.

2. TESTS FOR MUTAGENICITY (AMES' TEST). A mutagen is a substance that can permanently alter the genetic composition of a cell. Ames' test evaluates the ability of a chemical to induce mutation in the mutant strain of *Salmonella typhimurium* that cannot synthesise histidine. Such strains are incubated with the potential carcinogen to which liver homogenate is added to supply enzymes required to convert procarcinogen to ultimate carcinogen. If the chemical under test is mutagenic, it will induce mutation in the mutant strains of *S. typhimurium* in the form of functional histidine gene, which will be reflected by the number of bacterial colonies growing on histidine-free culture medium.

C. PHYSICAL CARCINOGENESIS *(p. 224)*

Physical agents in carcinogenesis are divided into 2 groups:

1. Radiation Carcinogenesis *(p. 224)*

Ultraviolet (UV) light and ionising radiation are the two main forms of radiation carcinogens which can induce cancer in experimental animals and are implicated in causation of some forms of human cancers. A property common between the two forms of radiation carcinogens is the appearance of mutations followed by a long period of latency after initial exposure, often 10-20 years or even later.

i) ULTRAVIOLET LIGHT. The main source of UV radiation is the sunlight; others are UV lamps and welder's arcs. UV light penetrates the skin for a few millimetres only so that its effect is limited to epidermis. The efficiency of UV light as carcinogen depends upon the extent of light-absorbing protective melanin pigmentation of the skin. In humans, excessive exposure to UV rays can cause various forms of skin cancers—squamous cell carcinoma, basal cell carcinoma and malignant melanoma.

Mechanism. UV radiation may have various effects on the cells. The most important is induction of mutation; others are inhibition of cell division, inactivation of enzymes and sometimes causing cell death. The most important biochemical effect of UV radiation is the formation of pyrimidine dimers in DNA. Such UV-induced DNA damage in normal individuals is repaired, while in the predisposed persons who are excessively exposed to sunlight such damage remain unrepaired.

ii) IONISING RADIATION. Ionising radiation of all kinds like X-rays, α-, β- and γ-rays, radioactive isotopes, protons and neutrons can cause cancer in animals and in man. Most frequently, radiation-induced cancers are all forms of leukaemias (except chronic lymphocytic leukaemia); others are cancers of the thyroid (most commonly papillary carcinoma), skin, breast, ovary, uterus, lung, myeloma, and salivary glands.The risk is increased by higher dose and with high LET (linear energy transfer) such as in neutrons and α-rays than with low LET as in X-rays and γ-rays.

Mechanism. Radiation damages the DNA of the cell by one of the 2 possible mechanisms:

a) It may directly alter the cellular DNA.

b) It may dislodge ions from water and other molecules of the cell and result in formation of highly reactive free radicals that may bring about the damage.

Damage to the DNA resulting in mutagenesis is the most important action of ionising radiation. It may cause chromosomal breakage, translocation, or point mutation.

2. Non-radiation Physical Carcinogenesis *(p. 226)*

Mechanical injury to the tissues such as from stones in the gallbladder, stones in the urinary tract, and healed scars following burns or trauma, has been suggested as the cause of increased risk of carcinoma in these tissues but the evidence is not convincing.

D. BIOLOGIC CARCINOGENESIS *(p. 226)*

The epidemiological studies on different types of cancers indicate the involvement of transmissible biologic agents in their development, chiefly *viruses*. Other biologic agents implicated in carcinogenesis are as follows:

■ **Parasites** e.g. *Schistosoma haematobium* infection of the urinary bladder is associated with high incidence of squamous cell carcinoma of the urinary bladder in some parts of the world such as in Egypt. *Clonorchis sinensis,* the liver fluke, lives in the hepatic duct and is implicated in causation of cholangiocarcinoma.

■ **Fungus** *Aspergillus flavus* grows in stored grains and liberates aflatoxin; its human consumption, especially by those with HBV infection, is associated with development of hepatocellular carcinoma.

■ **Bacteria** *Helicobacter pylori,* a gram-positive spiral-shaped micro-organism, colonises the gastric mucosa and has been found in cases of chronic gastritis and peptic ulcer; its prolonged infection may lead to gastric lymphoma and gastric carcinoma.

However, the role of viruses in the causation of cancer is more significant. It has been estimated that about 20% of all cancers worldwide are virus-associated cancers.

Chapter Eight

VIRAL CARCINOGENESIS *(p. 226)*

Oncogenic viruses can be transmitted by one of the 3 routes:

i) *Vertical transmission,*

ii) *Horizontal transmission,*

iii) *By inoculation.*

Based on their nucleic acid content, oncogenic viruses fall into 2 broad groups:

1. Those containing deoxyribonucleic acid are called *DNA oncogenic viruses.*

2. Those containing ribonucleic acid are termed *RNA oncogenic viruses.*

DNA Oncogenic Viruses *(p. 227)*

DNA oncogenic viruses have direct access to the host cell nucleus and are incorporated into the genome of the host cell. DNA viruses are classified into 5 subgroups, each of which is capable of producing neoplasms in different hosts (Table 8.7). These are: Papovaviruses, Herpesviruses, Adenoviruses, Poxviruses and Hepadna viruses.

TABLE 8.7: DNA Oncogenic Viruses.

	VIRUS	HOST	ASSOCIATED TUMOUR
1.	*PAPOVAVIRUSES*		
	Human papilloma virus	Humans	Cervical cancer and its precursor lesions, squamous cell carcinoma at other sites
			Skin cancer in epidermodysplasia verruciformis
			Papillomas (warts) on skin, larynx, genitals (genital warts)
	Papilloma viruses	Cotton-tail rabbits	Papillomas (Warts)
		Bovine	Alimentary tract cancer
	Polyoma virus	Mice	Various carcinomas, sarcomas
	SV-40 virus	Monkeys	Harmless
		Hamsters	Sarcoma
		Humans	? Mesothelioma
2.	*HERPESVIRUSES*		
	Epstein-Barr virus	Humans	Burkitt's lymphoma
			Nasopharyngeal carcinoma
	Human herpesvirus 8 (Kaposi's sarcoma herpesvirus)	Humans	Kaposi's sarcoma
			B cell lymphoma
	Lucke' frog virus	Frog	Renal cell carcinoma
	Marek's disease virus	Chickens	T-cell leukaemia-lymphoma
3.	*ADENOVIRUSES*	Hamsters	Sarcomas
4.	*POXVIRUSES*	Rabbits	Myxomatosis
		Humans	Molluscum contagiosum, papilloma
5.	*HEPADNAVIRUSES*		
	Hepatitis B virus	Humans	Hepatocellular carcinoma

RNA Oncogenic Viruses *(p. 229)*

RNA oncogenic viruses are retroviruses i.e. they contain the enzyme reverse transcriptase (RT), though all retroviruses are not oncogenic (Table 8.8). The enzyme, reverse transcriptase, is required for reverse transcription of viral RNA to synthesise viral DNA strands i.e. reverse of normal—rather than DNA encoding for RNA synthesis, viral RNA transcripts for the DNA by the enzyme RT present in the RNA viruses. RT is a DNA polymerase and helps to form complementary DNA (cDNA) that moves into host cell nucleus and gets incorporated into it.

TABLE 8.8: RNA Oncogenic Viruses.

VIRUS	HOST	ASSOCIATED TUMOUR
1. ACUTE TRANSFORMING VIRUSES		
Rous sarcoma virus	Chickens	Sarcoma
Leukaemia-sarcoma virus	Avian, feline, bovine, primate	Leukaemias, sarcomas
2. SLOW TRANSFORMING VIRUSES		
	Mice, cats, bovine	Leukaemias, lymphomas
Mouse mammary tumour virus (Bittner milk factor)	Daughter mice	Breast cancer
3. HUMAN T-CELL LYMPHOTROPIC VIRUS (HTLV)		
HTLV-I	**Human**	Adult T-cell leukaemia lymphoma (ATLL)
HTLV-II	**Human**	T-cell variant of hairy cell leukaemia
4. HEPATITIS C VIRUS		
HCV	**Human**	Hepatocellular carcinoma

Based on their activity to transform target cells into neoplastic cells, RNA viruses are divided into 3 subgroups—acute transforming viruses, slow transforming viruses, and human T-cell lymphotropic viruses (HTLV). The former two are implicated in inducing a variety of tumours in animals while HTLV is causative for human T-cell leukaemia and lymphoma.

In general, RNA viruses have 3 genes: *gag* gene (for group antigen), *pol* gene (that codes for polymerase enzyme), and *env* gene (for envelope protein), while acute transforming viruses have a fourth gene *tat* gene that transforms the oncogene in the susceptible cell.

Mechanisms of Viral Oncogenesis *(p. 231)*

1. Mode of DNA viral oncogenesis. Host cells infected by DNA oncogenic viruses may have one of the following 2 results:

i) Replication. The virus may replicate in the host cell with consequent lysis of the infected cell and release of virions.

ii) Integration. The viral DNA may integrate into the host cell DNA.

The latter event (integration) results in neoplastic transformation of the host cell, while the former (replication) brings about cell death but no neoplastic transformation. A feature essential for host cell transformation is the expression of virus-specific T-(transforming protein) antigens immediately after infection of the host cell by DNA oncogenic virus.

2. Mode of RNA viral oncogenesis. As the name suggests, RNA viruses or retroviruses contain two identical strands of RNA and the enzyme, reverse transcriptase. The steps involved in transformation of host cells by RNA oncogenic viruses are as under:

i) Reverse transcriptase is RNA-dependent DNA synthetase that acts as a template to synthesise a *single strand of matching viral* DNA i.e. reverse of the normal in which DNA is transcribed into messenger RNA.

ii) The single strand of viral DNA is then copied by DNA dependent DNA synthetase to form another strand of complementary DNA resulting in *double-stranded viral* DNA or provirus.

iii) The provirus is then integrated into the DNA of the host cell genome and may transform the cell into *neoplastic cell.*

iv) Retroviruses are *replication-competent.* The host cells which allow replication of integrated retrovirus are called permissive cells. Non-permissible cells do not permit replication of the integrated retrovirus.

v) Viral replication begins after integration of the provirus into host cell genome. Integration results in transcription of proviral genes or progenes into messenger RNA which then forms *components of the virus particle*—virion core protein from *gag* gene, reverse transcriptase from *pol* gene, and envelope glycoprotein from *env* gene. The three components of virus particle are then assembled at the plasma membrane of the host cell and the virus particles released by budding off from the plasma membrane, thus completing the process of replication.

VIRUSES AND HUMAN CANCER: A SUMMARY *(p. 231)*

In man, epidemiological as well as circumstantial evidence has been accumulating since the discovery of contagious nature of common human wart (papilloma) in 1907 that cancer may have viral etiology. Presently, about 20% of all human cancers worldwide are believed to have 'virus association'. Aside from experimental evidence, the etiologic role of DNA and RNA viruses in a variety of human neoplasms has already been explained above. Here, a summary of different viruses implicated in human tumours is presented:

Benign tumours. There are 2 conditions which are actually doubtful as tumours in which definite viral etiology is established. These are:
i)   Human wart (papilloma) caused by human papilloma virus; and
ii) Molluscum contagiosum caused by poxvirus.

Malignant tumours. The following 8 human cancers have enough epidemiological, serological, and in some cases genomic evidence that viruses are implicated in their etiology:
i)   *Burkitt's lymphoma* by Epstein-Barr virus.
ii)   *Nasopharyngeal carcinoma* by Epstein-Barr virus.
iii) *Primary hepatocellular carcinoma* by hepatitis B virus and hepatitis C virus.
iv) *Cervical cancer* by high risk human papilloma virus types (HPV 16 and 18).
v)   *Kaposi's sarcoma* by human herpes virus type 8 (HHV 8).
vi) *B cell lymphoma* by HHV8.
vii) *Adult T-cell leukaemia and lymphoma* by HTLV-I.
viii) *T-cell variant of hairy cell leukaemia* by HTLV-II.

CLINICAL ASPECTS OF NEOPLASIA *(p. 232)*

Two major aspects of clinical significance in assessing the course and management of neoplasia are: tumour-host inter-relationship (i.e. the effect of tumour on host and *vice versa*) and laboratory diagnosis of cancer.

EFFECT OF TUMOUR ON HOST *(p. 232)*

Malignant tumours produce more ill-effects than the benign tumours.

1. LOCAL EFFECTS. Both benign and malignant tumours cause local effects on the host due to their size or location. Some of the local effects of tumours are as under:
i) Compression, ii) mechanical obstruction, iii) tissue destruction, and iv) infarction, ulceration, haemorrhage.

2. CANCER CACHEXIA. Patients with advanced and disseminated cancers terminally have asthenia (emaciation), and anorexia, together referred to as cancer cachexia (meaning wasting). Possibly, cachectin or tumour necrosis factor α (TNF-α) and interleukin-1 derived from macrophages play a contributory role in cachexia.

3. FEVER. Fever of unexplained origin may be presenting feature in some malignancies such as in Hodgkin's disease, adenocarcinoma kidney, osteogenic sarcoma and many other tumours.

4. PARANEOPLASTIC SYNDROMES. Paraneoplastic syndromes (PNS) are a group of conditions developing in patients with advanced cancer which are neither explained by direct and distant spread of the tumour, nor by the usual hormone elaboration by the tissue of origin of the tumour. About 10 to 15% of the patients with advanced cancer develop one or more of the syndromes included in the PNS. Rarely, PNS may be the earliest manifestation of a latent cancer.

The various clinical syndromes included in the PNS are as summarised in Table 8.9.

HOST RESPONSE AGAINST TUMOUR
(IMMUNE SURVEILLANCE OF CANCER) *(p. 235)*

It has long been thought that host defense mechanism in the form of immunological response exists so as to counter the growth and spread of cancer. The following observations provide basis for this thinking:

1. Certain cancers evoke significant lymphocytic infiltrates composed of immunocompetent cells and such tumours have somewhat better prognosis e.g. medullary carcinoma breast, seminoma testis.

2. Rarely, a cancer may spontaneously regress partially or completely e.g. malignant melanoma.

3. It is highly unusual to have primary and secondary tumours in the spleen due to its ability to destroy the growth and proliferation of tumour cells.

4. Immune surveillance exists is substantiated by increased frequency of cancers in immunodeficient host e.g. in AIDS patients, or in organ transplant recipients.

1. TUMOUR ANTIGENS. Following two types of tumour antigens encountered by cytotoxic T lymphocytes CTL, also called CD8+T cells:

i) Tumour-specific antigens (TSA) are located on tumour cells but are not present on normal cells. They are unique or specific antigens for particular tumour and not shared by normal cells. Therefore, TSAs are targets of attack by tumour-specific cytotoxic CD8+T lymphocytes. The examples are:

a) Testis specific antigen having MAGE genes.

b) Antigens responsible for mutational change in some tumours e.g. *TP53*, *RAS* gene, β-catenin etc.

c) Overexpressed antigens e.g. *HER2* protein in cancer of the breast, ovary.

d) Antigens from oncogenic viruses e.g. HPV, EBV.

e) Mucins associated antigens e.g. in cancers of the pancreas, breast, ovary.

f) Oncofoetal antigens e.g. α-foetoprotein, carcinoembryonic antigen in cancers of liver, colon.

ii) Tumour associated antigen (TAA) are present on tumour cells as well as on some normal cells. TAA are, thus, antigens shared by tumour cells and normal host cells from where the tumour originated e.g.

a) Tissue specific antigens such as melanocyte specific proteins.

b) Differentiation specific antigens e.g. CD10 in benign prostatic epithelium, prostate specific antigen (PSA) in carcinoma of prostate.

2. IMMUNE RESPONSES. The nature of host immune response to tumours demonstrated in animal studies and in patients with various types of cancers can be categorised as under:

i) Cell-mediated mechanism. This is the main mechanism of destruction of tumour cells by the host.

TABLE 8.9: Summary of Paraneoplastic Syndromes.

CLINICAL SYNDROME	UNDERLYING CANCER	MECHANISM
1. ENDOCRINE SYNDROME:		
i. *Hypercalcaemia*	Lung (sq. cell ca.), kidney, breast, Adult T-cell leukaemia-lymphoma	Parathromone-like protein vitamin D
ii. *Cushing's syndrome*	Lung (small cell carcinoma), pancreas, neural tumours	ACTH or ACTH-like substance
iii. *Inappropriate anti-diuresis*	Lung (small cell ca.), prostate, intracranial tumour	ADH or atrial natriuretic factor
iv. *Hypoglycaemia*	Pancreas (islet cell tumour), mesothelioma, fibrosarcoma	Insulin or insulin-like substance
v. *Carcinoid syndrome*	Bronchial carcinoid tumour, carcinoma pancreas, stomach	Serotonin, bradykinin
vi. *Polycythaemia*	Kidney, liver, cerebellar haemangioma	Erythropoietin
2. NEUROMUSCULAR SYNDROMES:		
i. *Myasthenia gravis*	Thymoma	Immunologic
ii. *Neuromuscular disorders*	Lung (small cell ca.), breast	Immunologic
3. OSSEOUS, JOINT AND SOFT TISSUE:		
i. *Hypertrophic osteoarthropathy*	Lung	Not known
ii. *Clubbing of fingers*	Lung	Not known
4. HAEMATOLOGIC SYNDROMES:		
i. *Thrombophlebitis* (Trousseau's phenomenon)	Pancreas, lung, GIT	Hypercoagulability
ii. *Non-bacterial thrombotic endocarditis*	Advanced cancers	Hypercoagulability
iii. *Disseminated intravascular coagulation (DIC)*	AML, adenocarcinoma phenomena	Chronic thrombotic
iv. *Anaemia*	Thymoma	Unknown
5. GASTROINTESTINAL SYNDROMES:		
i. *Malabsorption*	Lymphoma of small bowel	Hypoalbuminaemia
6. RENAL SYNDROMES:		
i. *Nephrotic syndrome*	Advanced cancers	Renal vein thrombosis, systemic amyloidosis
7. CUTANEOUS SYNDROMES:		
i. *Acanthosis nigricans*	Stomach, large bowel	Immunologic
ii. *Seborrheic keratosis*	Bowel	Immunologic
iii. *Exfoliative dermatitis*	Lymphoma	Immunologic
8. AMYLOIDOSIS:		
i. *Primary*	Multiple myeloma	Immunologic (AL protein)
ii. *Secondary*	Kidney, lymphoma, solid tumours	AA protein

a) *Specifically sensitised cytotoxic T lymphocytes (CTL)* i.e. CD8+ T cells which are directly cytotoxic requiring contact between them and tumour cell. They specifically attack the virally induced cancers e.g. in Burkitt's lymphoma (EBV-induced), invasive squamous cell carcinoma (HPV-induced).

b) *Natural killer (NK) cells* are lymphocytes which destroy tumour cells without sensitisation, either directly or by antibody-dependent cellular cytotoxicity (ADCC).

c) *Macrophages* are activated by interferon-γ secreted by T-cells and NK-cells, and therefore there is close collaboration of these lymphocytes with macrophages. Activated macrophages mediate cytotoxicity by production of oxygen free radicals or by tumour necrosis factor.

ii) Humoral mechanism. Humoral antibodies may act by complement activation or by antibody-dependent cytotoxicity by NK cells.

iii) Inhibitory (Regulatory) mechanism. In spite of host immune responses, most cancers grow relentlessly. This is due to some of the following controlling mechanisms:

a) During progression of the cancer, immunogenic cells may disappear.

b) Cytotoxic T-cells and NK-cells may play a self regulatory role.

c) Immunosuppression mediated by various acquired carcinogenic agents (viruses, chemicals, radiation).

d) Immunoinhibitory role of factors secreted by tumours e.g. transforming growth factor-β.

DIAGNOSIS OF CANCER *(p. 236)*

1. Histological Methods *(p. 236)*

These methods are based on microscopic examination of properly fixed tissue (excised tumour mass or open/needle biopsy from the mass), supported with complete clinical and investigative data. These methods are most valuable in arriving at the accurate diagnosis.

The histological diagnosis by either of these methods is made on the basis that cytological features of *benign tumours* resemble those of normal tissue and that they are unable to invade and metastasise, while *malignant tumours* are identified by lack of differentiation in cancer cells termed 'anaplasia' or 'cellular atypia' and may invade as well as metastasise.

2. Cytological Methods *(p. 236)*

Cytological methods for diagnosis consist of study of cells shed off into body cavities (exfoliative cytology) and study of cells by putting a fine needle introduced under vacuum into the lesion (fine needle aspiration cytology, FNAC).

3. Histochemistry and Cytochemistry *(p. 238)*

Histochemistry and cytochemistry are additional diagnostic tools which help the pathologist in identifying the chemical composition of cells, their constituents and their products by special staining methods.

Though immunohistochemical techniques are more useful for tumour diagnosis (see below), histochemical and cytochemical methods are still employed for this purpose.

4. Immunohistochemistry *(p. 238)*

This is an immunological method of recognising a cell by one or more of its specific components in the cytoplasm, cell membrane or nucleus. These cell components (called antigens) combine with specific antibodies on the formalin-fixed paraffin sections or cytological smears. The complex of antigen-antibody on slide is made visible for light microscopic identification by either fluorescent dyes ('fluorochromes') or by enzyme system ('chromogens').

Though the list of immunohistochemical stains is ever increasing, one important group of such antibody stains is directed against various classes of

TABLE 8.10: Intermediate Filaments and their Significance in Tumour Diagnosis.

INTERMEDIATE FILAMENT	TUMOUR
1. *Keratins*	Carcinomas, mesotheliomas, some germ cells tumours
2. *Vimentin*	Sarcomas, melanomas, lymphomas
3. *Desmin*	Myogenic tumours
4. *Neurofilaments (NF)*	Neural tumours
5. *Glial fibrillary acidic protein (GFAP)*	Glial tumours

intermediate filaments which is useful in classification of poorly-differentiated tumours of epithelial or mesenchymal origin (Table 8.10).

5. Electron Microscopy *(p. 238)*

Ultrastructural examination of tumour cells offers selective role in diagnostic pathology.

i) Cell junctions—their presence and type.

ii) Cell surface, e.g. presence of microvilli.

iii) Cell shape and cytoplasmic extensions.

iv) Shape of the nucleus and features of nuclear membrane.

v) Nucleoli—size and density.

vi) Cytoplasmic organelles—their number is generally reduced.

vii) Dense bodies in the cytoplasm.

viii) Any other secretory product in the cytoplasm e.g. melanosomes in melanoma and membrane-bound granules in endocrine tumours.

6. Tumour Markers (Biochemical Assays) *(p. 239)*

In order to distinguish from the preceding techniques of tumour diagnosis in which 'stains' are imparted on the tumour cells in section or smear, tumour markers are biochemical assays of products elaborated by the tumour cells in blood or other body fluids (Table 8.11). It is, therefore, pertinent to keep in mind that many of these products are produced by normal body cells too, and thus the biochemical estimation of the product in blood reflects the total substance and not by the tumour cells alone. These methods, therefore, lack sensitivity as well as specificity and can only be employed for:

■ *firstly*, as an adjunct to the pathologic diagnosis arrived at by other methods and not for primary diagnosis of cancer; and

■ *secondly*, can be used for prognostic and therapeutic purposes.

7. Modern Aids in Tumour Diagnosis *(p. 239)*

i) **Flow cytometry.** This is a computerised technique by which the detailed characteristics of individual tumour cells are recognised and quantified and the data can be stored for subsequent comparison too.

ii) *In situ* **hybridisation**. This is a molecular technique by which nucleic acid sequences (cellular/viral DNA and RNA) can be localised by specifically-labelled nucleic acid probe directly in the intact cell (*in situ*) rather than by DNA extraction (see below).

iii) **Molecular diagnostic techniques.** The group of molecular biologic methods in the tumour diagnostic laboratory are a variety of DNA/RNA-based molecular techniques in which the DNA/RNA are extracted (compared from *in*

TABLE 8.11: Important Tumour Markers.

	MARKER	CANCER
1.	**Oncofoetal antigens:**	
	i. Alpha-foetoprotein (AFP)	Hepatocellular carcinoma, non-seminomatous germ cell tumours of testis
	ii. Carcino-embryonic antigen (CEA)	Cancer of bowel, pancreas, breast
2.	**Cytoplasmic proteins:**	
	i. Immunoglobulins	Multiple myeloma, other gammopathies
	ii. Prostate specific antigen (PSA)	Prostate carcinoma
3.	**Enzymes:**	
	i. Prostate acid phosphatase (PAP)	Prostatic carcinoma
	ii. Neuron-specific enolase (NSE)	Neuroblastoma, oat cell carcinoma lung
4.	**Hormones:**	
	i. Human chorionic gonadotropin (HCG)	Trophoblastic tumours, non-seminomatous germ cell tumours of testis
	ii. Calcitonin	Medullary carcinoma thyroid
	iii. Catecholamines and vanillyl mandelic acid (VMA)	Neuroblastoma, pheochromocytoma
	iv. Ectopic hormone production	Paraneoplastic syndromes
5.	**Secreted cancer antigens:**	
	i. CA-125	Ovary
	ii. CA-15-3	Breast

situ above) from the cell and then analysed. The molecular methods in tumour diagnosis can be applied in haematologic as well as non-haematologic malig-nancies by:

- analysis of molecular cytogenetic abnormalities;
- mutational analysis;
- antigen receptor gene rearrangement; and
- by study of oncogenic viruses at molecular level.

iv) DNA microarray analysis of tumours. Currently, it is possible to perform molecular profiling of a tumour by use of gene chip technology which allows measurement of levels of expression of several thousand genes (up-regulation or down-regulation) simultaneously.

■ **SELF ASSESSMENT**

1. **Hamartoma refers to:**
   A. Tumour differentiating towards more than one cell line
   B. Tumour arising from totipotent cells
   C. Mass of disorganised but mature cells indigenous to the part
   D. Mass of ectopic rests of normal tissue
2. **Increased number of normal mitoses may be present in the following tissues *except*:**
   A. Bone marrow cells   B. Nails
   C. Hepatocytes   D. Intestinal epithelium

Chapter Eight

3. A tumour is termed medullary when it is almost entirely composed of:
   - A. Amyloid stroma
   - B. Large areas of necrosis
   - C. Abundant lymphoid tissue
   - D. Parenchymal cells

4. All the following malignant tumours metastasise *except:*
   - A. Synovial sarcoma
   - B. Malignant mesothelioma
   - C. Glioma
   - D. Neuroblastoma

5. The following malignant tumours frequently spread through haematogenous route *except:*
   - A. Bronchogenic carcinoma
   - B. Renal cell carcinoma
   - C. Follicular carcinoma thyroid
   - D. Seminoma testis

6. Degradation of ECM is brought about by the following *except:*
   - A. Proteases
   - B. Metalloproteinases
   - C. Free radicals
   - D. Cathepsin D

7. Grading of tumours depends upon the following *except:*
   - A. Degree of anaplasia
   - B. Metastatic spread
   - C. Rate of growth of cells
   - D. Degree of differentiation

8. Patients of xeroderma pigmentosum are prone to develop the following cancers *except*:
   - A. Basal cell carcinoma
   - B. Sweat gland carcinoma
   - C. Malignant melanoma
   - D. Squamous cell carcinoma

9. The primary target of reactive electrophiles is as under:
   - A. Cytochrome P-450
   - B. RNA
   - C. DNA
   - D. Mitochondria

10. Carcinogenic influence of radiation appears after:
    - A. < 2 years
    - B. 2-5 years
    - C. 5-10 years
    - D. > 10 years

11. The following hereditary diseases have higher incidence of cancers due to inherited defect in DNA repair mechanism *except*:
    - A. Ataxia telangiectasia
    - B. Xeroderma pigmentosum
    - C. Familial polyposis coli
    - D. Bloom's syndrome

12. The following form of ionising radiation exposure is associated with highest risk of cancer:
    - A. α-rays
    - B. β-rays
    - C. γ-rays
    - D. X-rays

13. Women receiving oestrogen therapy have an increased risk of developing the following cancers *except*:
    - A. Breast cancer
    - B. Endometrial carcinoma
    - C. Gallbladder cancer
    - D. Hepatocellular carcinoma

14. Important cyclins in cell cycle include the following *except:*
    - A. Cyclin A
    - B. Cyclin B
    - C. Cyclin C
    - D. Cyclin D

15. Bittner milk factor is a transmissible agent belonging to the following category:
    - A. Acute transforming virus
    - B. Slow transforming virus
    - C. HTLV-I
    - D. HTLV-II

16. Important examples of tumour suppressor genes implicated in human cancers include the following *except*:
    - A. RB gene
    - B. *TP53*
    - C. APC
    - D. ERB-B

17. An example of tumour-associated antigen (TAA) is:
    - A. Testis specific antigen (MAGE)
    - B. Alpha-fetoprotein (AFP)
    - C. Carcinoembryonic antigen (CEA)
    - D. Prostate specific antigen (PSA)

18. **Hypercalcaemia as a paraneoplastic syndrome is observed in the following tumours** *except:*
    - A. Squamous cell carcinoma lung
    - B. Small cell carcinoma lung
    - C. Renal cell carcinoma
    - D. Breast cancer

19. **Lymphocytic infiltrate is frequently present in the following tumours indicative of host immune response** *except:*
    - A. Seminoma testis
    - B. Medullary carcinoma breast
    - C. Papillary carcinoma thyroid
    - D. Malignant melanoma

20. **The following antibody-stain is used in immunohistochemistry to identify epithelial cells:**
    - A. Desmin
    - B. Vimentin
    - C. Cytokeratin
    - D. Neurofilaments

KEY

1 = C	2 = B	3 = D	4 = C
5 = D	6 = C	7 = B	8 = B
9 = C	10 = D	11 = C	12 = A
13 = C	14 = C	15 = B	16 = D
17 = D	18 = B	19 = C	20 = C

Chapter Eight

9

Environmental and Nutritional Diseases

INTRODUCTION *(p. 241)*

The subject of environmental hazards to health has assumed great significance in the modern world.

Some of the important factors which have led to the alarming environmental degradation are as under:

1. Population explosion
2. Urbanisation of rural and forest land to accommodate the increasing numbers
3. Accumulation of wastes
4. Unsatisfactory disposal of radioactive waste
5. Industrial effluents and automobile exhausts.

But the above atmospheric pollutants appear relatively minor compared with *voluntary intake of three pollutants*—tobacco smoking, alcohol and intoxicant drugs.

ENVIRONMENTAL POLLUTION *(p. 241)*

AIR POLLUTION *(p. 242)*

A vast variety of pollutants are inhaled daily some of which may cause trivial irritation to the upper respiratory pathways, while others may lead to acute or chronic injury to the lungs, and some are implicated in causation of lung cancer. In highly polluted cities where coal consumption and automobile exhaust accumulate in the atmosphere, the air pollutants become visible as 'smog'.

The adverse effects of air pollutants on lung depend upon a few variables that include:

- longer duration of exposure;
- total dose of exposure;
- impaired ability of the host to clear inhaled particles; and
- particle size of 1-5 μm capable of getting impacted in the distal airways to produce tissue injury.

TOBACCO SMOKING *(p. 242)*

Habits *(p. 242)*

Tobacco smoking is the most prevalent and preventable cause of disease and death. The harmful effects of smoking pipe and cigar are somewhat less. Long-term smokers of filter-tipped cigarettes appear to have 30-50% lower risk of development of cancer due to reduced inhalation of tobacco smoke constituents.

In India, a country of one billion people, a quarter (250 million) are tobacco users in one form or the other. Smoking *bidis* and chewing *pan masala*, *zarda* and *gutka* are more widely practiced than cigarettes. Habit of smoking *chutta* (a kind of indigenous cigar) in which the lighted end is put in mouth is practiced in the Indian state of Andhra Pradesh and is associated with higher incidence of squamous cell carcinoma of hard palate. Another habit prevalent in Indian states of Uttar Pradesh and Bihar and in parts of Sri Lanka is chewing of tabacco alone or mixed with slaked lime as a bolus of *paan* kept in mouth for long hours which is the major cause of cancer of upper aerodigestive tract and oral cavity. *Hookah* smoking, in which tobacco smoke passes through a water-filled chamber which cools the smoke before it is inhaled by the smoker, is believed by some reports to deliver less tar and nicotine than cigarettes and hence fewer tobacco-related health consequences.

Dose and Duration (p. 242)

The harmful effects of smoking are related to a variety of factors, the most important of which is dose of exposure expressed in terms of pack years. For example, one pack of cigarettes daily for 5 years means 5 pack years. It is estimated that a person who smokes 2 packs of cigarettes daily at the age of 30 years reduces his life by 8 years than a non-smoker.

Tobacco-Related Diseases (p. 242)

Some of the important constituents of tobacco smoke with adverse effects are given in Table 9.1.

TABLE 9.1: Major Constituents of Tobacco Smoke with Adverse Effects.

	ADVERSE EFFECT	CONSTITUENTS
1.	*Carcinogenesis*	• Tar
		• Polycyclic aromatic hydrocarbons
		• Nitrosamines
2.	*Tumour promoters*	• Nicotine
		• Phenol
3.	*Irritation and toxicity to respiratory mucosa*	• Formaldehyde
		Nitrogen oxide
4.	*Reduced oxygen transport*	• Carbon monoxide

The major diseases accounting for higher mortality in tobacco smokers include, (in descending order of frequency):

CORONARY HEART DISEASE. Cigarette smoking is one of the four major risk factors for myocardial infarction and acts synergistically with the other three—hypercholesterolaemia, hypertension and diabetes mellitus. There is more severe, extensive and accelerated atherosclerosis of coronary arteries and aorta in smokers, possibly due to increased platelet aggregation and impaired lung function that causes reduced myocardial oxygen supply.

LUNG CANCER. This is the most common cancer in men throughout world and most frequent cancer in women too in the United States exceeding its incidence beyond that of breast cancer in that country. Cigarette smoking is strongly implicated in evolution of lung cancer.

OTHER CANCERS. Besides lung cancer, smokers have higher risk of development of cancer of upper aerodigestive tract (lips, oral cavity, larynx, oesophagus), pancreas, urinary bladder and kidney.

NON-NEOPLASTIC DISEASES. These include the following:
i) Chronic obstructive pulmonary disease (COPD) that includes chronic bronchitis and emphysema as the most common.
ii) Peptic ulcer disease with 70% higher risk in smokers.
iii) Early menopause in smoker women.
iv) In smoking pregnant women, higher risk of lower birth weight of foetus, higher perinatal mortality and intellectual deterioration of newborn.

CHEMICAL AND DRUG INJURY *(p. 243)*

During life, each one of us is exposed to a variety of chemicals and drugs. These are broadly divided into the following three categories:

THERAPEUTIC (IATROGENIC) DRUG INJURY *(p. 244)*

Adverse effects of drugs may appear due to:

- overdose;
- genetic predisposition;
- exaggerated pharmacologic response;
- interaction with other drugs; and
- unknown factors.

NON-THERAPEUTIC TOXIC AGENTS *(p. 244)*

ALCOHOLISM *(p. 244)*

Chronic alcoholism is defined as the regular imbibing of an amount of ethyl alcohol (ethanol) that is sufficient to harm an individual socially, psychologically or physically. Generally, 10 gm of ethanol is present in:

- a can of beer (or half a bottle of beer);
- 120 ml of neat wine; or
- 30 ml of 86° proof 43% liquor (small peg).

A daily consumption of 40 gm of ethanol (4 small pegs or 2 large pegs) is likely to be harmful but intake of 100 gm or more daily is certainly dangerous. Daily and heavy consumption of alcohol is more harmful than moderate social drinking since the liver, where ethanol is metabolised, gets time to heal.

Metabolism *(p. 244)*

Absorption of alcohol begins in the stomach and small intestine and appears in blood shortly after ingestion. Alcohol is then distributed to different organs and body fluids proportionate to the blood levels of alcohol. About 2-10% of absorbed alcohol is excreted via urine, sweat and exhaled through breath. Alcohol is metabolised in the liver by the following 3 pathways:

- By the major rate-limiting pathway of alcohol dehydrogenase (ADH) in the cytosol, especially with low blood alcohol levels.
- Via microsomal P-450 system when the blood alcohol level is high.
- Minor pathway via catalase from peroxisomes.

Effects of Alcoholism *(p. 245)*

A. ACUTE ALCOHOLISM. The acute effects of inebriation are most prominent on the central nervous system but it also injures the stomach and liver.

1. Central nervous system. Alcohol acts as a CNS depressant; the intensity of effects of alcohol on the CNS are related to the quantity consumed and duration over which consumed, which are reflected by blood levels of alcohol.

2. Stomach. Acute alcohol intoxication may cause vomiting, acute gastritis and peptic ulceration.

3. Liver. Acute alcoholic injury to the liver is explained in Chapter 19.

B. CHRONIC ALCOHOLISM. Chronic alcoholism produces widespread injury to organs and systems. Contrary to the earlier belief that chronic alcoholic injury results from nutritional deficiencies, it is now known that most of the alcohol-related injury to different organs is due to toxic effects of alcohol and accumulation of its main toxic metabolite, acetaldehyde, in the blood.

Some of the more important organ effects in chronic alcoholism are as under:

1. Liver. Alcoholic liver disease and cirrhosis.

2. Pancreas. Chronic calcifying pancreatitis and acute pancreatitis.

3. **Gastrointestinal tract.** Gastritis, peptic ulcer and oesophageal varices.

4. **Central nervous system.** Peripheral neuropathies and Wernicke-Korsakoff syndrome, cerebral atrophy, cerebellar degeneration and amblyopia (impaired vision).

5. **Cardiovascular system.** Alcoholic cardiomyopathy and beer-drinkers' myocardiosis.

6. **Endocrine system.** In men, testicular atrophy, feminisation, loss of libido and potency, and gynaecomastia.

7. **Blood.** Haematopoietic dysfunction with secondary megaloblastic anaemia.

8. **Immune system.** Susceptible to various infections.

9. **Cancer.** Higher incidence of cancers of upper aerodigestive tract.

LEAD POISONING *(p. 246)*

Lead poisoning may occur in children or adults due to accidental or occupational ingestion.

In children, the main sources are:

■ Chewing of lead-containing furniture items, toys or pencils.

■ Eating of lead paint flakes from walls.

In adults, the sources are:

■ Occupational exposure to lead during spray painting, recycling of automobile batteries (lead oxide fumes), mining, and extraction of lead.

■ Accidental exposure by contaminated water supply, house freshly coated with lead paint, and sniffing of lead-containing petrol (hence unleaded petrol introduced as fuel).

Lead is absorbed through the gastrointestinal tract or lungs. The absorbed lead is distributed in two types of tissues:

a) *Bones, teeth, nails and hair* representing relatively harmless pool of lead and appears as areas of increased bone densities ('lead lines') on X-ray. Lead lines are also seen in the gingiva.

b) *Brain, liver, kidneys and bone marrow* accumulate the remaining 10% lead which is directly toxic to these organs. It is excreted via kidneys.

Lead toxicity occurs in the following organs predominantly:

1. **Nervous system:**

■ *In children,* lead encephalopathy; oedema of brain, flattening of gyri and compression of ventricles.

■ *In adults,* demyelinating peripheral motor neuropathy.

2. **Haematopoietic system:**

■ *Microcytic hypochromic anaemia*

■ Prominent basophilic stippling of erythrocytes.

3. **Kidneys:** Lead is toxic to proximal tubular cells of the kidney and produces *lead nephropathy.*

4. **Gastrointestinal tract:** Acute abdomen presenting as lead colic.

CARBON MONOXIDE POISONING *(p. 247)*

Carbon monoxide (CO) is a colourless and odourless gas produced by incomplete combustion of carbon. Sources of CO gas are:

■ automobile exhaust;

■ burning of fossil fuel in industries or at home; and

■ tobacco smoke.

CO is an important cause of accidental death due to systemic oxygen deprivation of tissues. This is because haemoglobin has about 200-times higher affinity for CO than for O_2 and thus varying amount of carboxyhaemoglobin is formed depending upon the extent of CO poisoning.

CO poisoning may present in 2 ways:

- **Acute CO poisoning** in which there is sudden development of brain hypoxia characterised by oedema and petechial haemorrhages.
- **Chronic CO poisoning** presents with nonspecific changes of slowly developing hypoxia of the brain.

DRUG ABUSE *(p. 247)*

1. *Marijuana* or *'pot'* is psychoactive substance most widely used. It is obtained from the leaves of the plant *Cannabis sativa* and contains tetrahydrocannabinol (THC). It may be smoked or ingested.
2. *Derivatives of opium* that includes heroin and morphine. Opioids are derived from the poppy plant.
3. *CNS depressants* include barbiturates, tranquilisers and alcohol.
4. *CNS stimulants* e.g. cocaine and amphetamines.
5. *Psychedelic drugs* (meaning enjoyable perception-giving) e.g. LSD.
6. *Inhalants* e.g. glue, paint thinner, nail polish remover, aerosols, amyl nitrite.

A few common drug abuse-related infectious complications are:
1. At the site of injection—cellulitis, abscesses, ulcers, thrombosed veins
2. Thrombophlebitis
3. Bacterial endocarditis
4. High risk for AIDS
5. Viral hepatitis and its complications
6. Focal glomerulonephritis
7. Talc (foreign body) granuloma formation in the lungs.

ENVIRONMENTAL CHEMICALS *(p. 248)*

1. Agriculture chemicals. Modern agriculture thrives on pesticides, fungicides, herbicides and organic fertilisers which may pose a potential acute poisoning as well as long-term hazard. The problem is particularly alarming in developing countries like India, China and Mexico where farmers and their families are unknowingly exposed to these hazardous chemicals during aerial spraying of crops.

- Acute poisoning by organophosphate insecticides is too well known as accidental or suicidal poison by inhibiting acetyl cholinesterase and causing sudden death.
- Chronic human exposure to low level agricultural chemicals is implicated in cancer, chronic degenerative diseases, congenital malformations and impotence but the exact cause-and-effect relationship is lacking.

2. Volatile organic solvents. Such substances include methanol, chloroform, petrol, kerosene, benzene, ethylene glycol, toluene etc.

3. Metals. Pollution by occupational exposure to toxic metals such as mercury, arsenic, cadmium, iron, nickel and aluminium are important hazardous environmental chemicals.

4. Aromatic hydrocarbons. The halogenated aromatic hydrocarbons containing polychlorinated biphenyl which are contaminant in several preservatives, herbicides and antibacterial agents are a chronic health hazard.

5. Cyanide. Cyanide is a very toxic chemical and kills by blocking cellular respiration by binding to mitochondrial cytochrome oxidase.

6. Environmental dusts. These substances cause pneumoconioses and are implicated in cancer.

INJURY BY PHYSICAL AGENTS *(p. 248)*

THERMAL AND ELECTRICAL INJURY *(p. 248)*

Thermal and electrical burns, fall in body temperature below 35°C (hypothermia) and elevation of body temperature above 41°C (hyperthermia), are all associated with tissue injury.

■ **Hypothermia** may cause focal injury as in frostbite, or systemic injury and death as occurs on immersion in cold water for varying time.

■ **Hyperthermia** likewise, may be localised as in cutaneous burns, and systemic as occurs in fevers.

■ **Thermal burns** depending upon severity are categorised into full thickness (third degree) and partial thickness (first and second degree).

■ **Electrical burns** may cause damage by *firstly*, electrical dysfunction of the conduction system of the heart and death by ventricular fibrillation, and *secondly* by heat produced by electrical energy.

INJURY BY RADIATION *(p. 249)*

As discussed in the preceding chapter, the most important form of radiation injury is ionising radiation which has three types of effects on cells:
i) Somatic effects which cause acute cell killing.
ii) Genetic damage by mutations.
iii) Malignant transformation of cells.

Ionising radiation causes damage to the following major organs:
1. *Skin:* radiation dermatitis, cancer.
2. *Lungs:* interstitial pulmonary fibrosis.
3. *Heart:* myocardial fibrosis, constrictive pericarditis.
4. *Kidney:* radiation nephritis.
5. *Gastrointestinal tract:* strictures of small bowel and oesophagus.
6 *Gonads:* testicular atrophy in males and destruction of ovaries.
7. *Haematopoietic tissue:* pancytopenia due to bone marrow depression.
8. *Eyes:* cataract.

Besides ionising radiation, other form of harmful radiation is *solar (u.v.) radiation* which may cause acute skin injury as sunburns, chronic conditions such as solar keratosis and early onset of cataracts in the eyes.

NUTRITIONAL DISEASES *(p. 249)*

ESSENTIAL NUTRIENTS. There are 6 basic groups of essential nutrients.

1. Proteins. Dietary proteins provide the body with amino acids for endogenous protein synthesis and are also a metabolic fuel for energy (1 g of protein provides 4 Kcal). *Eight essential amino acids* (isoleucine, leucine, lysine, methionine, phenylalanine, theonine, tryptophan and valine) as well as histidine must be supplied by dietary intake as these cannot be synthesised in the body.

2. Fats. Fats and fatty acids (in particular linolenic, linoleic and arachidonic acid) should comprise about 35% of diet with an increased ratio of poly-unsaturated to saturated fats so as to minimise the risk of atherosclerosis (1 g of fat yields 9 Kcal).

3. Carbohydrates. Dietary carbohydrates, though not essential, are the major source of dietary calories (1 g of carbohydrate provides 4 Kcal).

4. Vitamins. These are mainly derived from exogenous dietary sources and are essential for maintaining the normal structure and function of cells.

5. Minerals. A number of minerals like iron, calcium, phosphorus and certain trace elements (e.g. zinc, copper, selenium, iodine, chlorine, sodium, potassium, magnesium, manganese, cobalt, molybdenum etc) are essential for health. Their deficiencies result in a variety of lesions and deficiency syndromes.

6. Water. Water intake is essential to cover the losses in faeces, urine, exhalation and insensible loss so as to avoid under- or over-hydration.

NON-ESSENTIAL NUTRIENTS. Dietary fibre composed of cellulose, hemicellulose and pectin, though considered non-essential, are important due to beneficial effects in colonic cancer, diabetes, coronary artery disease, and in lowering the incidence of colonic cancer.

Pathogenesis of Deficiency Diseases *(p. 249)*

1. Primary deficiency. This is due to either the lack or decreased amount of essential nutrients in diet.

2. Secondary or conditioned deficiency. Secondary or conditioned deficiency is malnutrition occurring as a result of the various factors.

i) Interference with ingestion
ii) Interference with absorption
iii) Interference with utilisation
iv) Increased excretion
v) Increased nutritional demand

OBESITY *(p. 250)*

Obesity is defined as an excess of adipose tissue that imparts health risk; a body weight of 20% excess over ideal weight for age, sex and height is considered a health risk.

Obesity results when caloric intake exceeds utilisation. The imbalance of these two components can occur in the following situations:

1. *Inadequate pushing of oneself away from the dining table* causing overeating.
2. *Insufficient pushing of oneself out of the chair* leading to inactivity and sedentary life style.
3. *Genetic predisposition* to develop obesity.
4. *Diets largely derived from carbohydrates* and fats than protein-rich diet.
5. *Secondary obesity* may result following a number of underlying diseases such as hypothyroidism, Cushing's disease, insulinoma and hypothalamic disorders.

SEQUELAE OF OBESITY. These are as under:

1. Hyperinsulinaemia.
2. Non-insulin dependent diabetes.
3. Hypertension.
4. Hyperlipoproteinaemia.
5. Atherosclerosis.
6. Coronary artery disease and stroke.
7. Cholelithiasis.
8. Hypoventilation syndrome (Pickwickian syndrome).
9. Osteoarthritis.
10. Cancer.

STARVATION *(p. 251)*

Starvation is a state of overall deprivation of nutrients. Its causes may be:

i) deliberate fasting—religious or political;
ii) famine conditions in a country or community; or
iii) secondary undernutrition such as due to chronic wasting diseases (infections, inflammatory conditions, liver disease), cancer etc. Cancer results in malignant cachexia as a result of which cytokines are elaborated e.g. tumour necrosis factor-α, elastases, proteases etc.

A starved individual has lax, dry skin, wasted muscles and atrophy of internal organs.

Metabolic Changes

1. Glucose. During fasting state, insulin-independent tissues such as the brain, blood cells and renal medulla continue to utilise glucose while insulin-dependent tissues like muscle stop taking up glucose.

2. Proteins. *Proteins* breakdown to release amino acids which are used as fuel for hepatic gluconeogenesis so as to maintain glucose needs of the brain.

3. Fats. The fatty acids are converted into ketone bodies in the liver which are used by most organs including brain in place of glucose.

PROTEIN-ENERGY MALNUTRITION (p. 251)

The inadequate consumption of protein and energy as a result of primary dietary deficiency or conditioned deficiency may cause loss of body mass and adipose tissue, resulting in protein energy or protein calorie malnutrition (PEM or PCM).

The spectrum of *clinical syndromes* produced as a result of PEM includes the following:
1. *Kwashiorkor* which is related to protein deficiency though calorie intake may be sufficient.
2. *Marasmus* is starvation in infants occurring due to overall lack of calories.

DISORDERS OF VITAMINS (p. 252)

Vitamins are organic substances which can not be synthesised within the body and are essential for maintenance of normal structure and function of cells.

Vitamins are conventionally divided into 2 groups: fat-soluble and water-soluble.

1. Fat-soluble vitamins are vitamin A, D, E and K. They are absorbed from intestine in the presence of bile salts and intact pancreatic function. Their deficiencies occur more readily due to conditioning factors (*secondary deficiency*). Beside the deficiency syndromes of these vitamins, a state of *hypervitaminosis* due to excess of vitamin A and D also occurs.

2. Water-soluble vitamins are vitamin C and B complex group. These vitamins are more readily absorbed from small intestine. Deficiency of these vitamins is mainly due to *primary (dietary) factors*. Being water soluble, these vitamins are more easily lost due to cooking or processing of food.

Table 9.2 sums up the various clinical disorders produced by vitamin deficiencies.

TRACE ELEMENTS (p. 261)

Several minerals in trace amounts are essential for health since they form components of enzymes and cofactors for metabolic functions. Besides *calcium* and *phosphorus* required for vitamin D manufacture, others include: *iron, copper, iodine, zinc, selenium, manganese, nickel, chromium, molybdenum, fluorine.* However, out of these, the dietary deficiency of first five trace elements is associated with deficiency states:
i) *Iron:* Microcytic hypochromic anaemia.
ii) *Copper:* Muscle weakness, neurologic defect.
iii) *Iodine:* Goitre and hyperthyroidism.
iv) *Zinc:* Growth retardation, infertility.
v) *Selenium:* Myopathy, cardiomyopathy.

DIET AND CANCER (p. 262)

There are three possible mechanisms on which the story of this relationship can be built up:
1. Dietary content of exogenous carcinogens:
i) The most important example in this mechanism comes from naturally-occurring carcinogen *aflatoxin* which is strongly associated with high incidence of hepatocellular carcinoma in those consuming grain contaminated with *Aspergillus flavus.*
ii) *Artificial sweeteners* (e.g. saccharine cyclomates), food additives and pesticide contamination of food are implicated as carcinogens derived from diet.

Chapter Nine

TABLE 9.2: Vitamin Deficiencies.

VITAMINS	DEFICIENCY DISORDERS
I. FAT-SOLUBLE VITAMINS	
Vitamin A (Retinol)	Ocular lesions (night blindness, xerophthalmia, keratomalacia, Bitot's spots, blindness)
	Cutaneous lesions (xeroderma)
	Other lesions (squamous metaplasia of respiratory epithelium, urothelium and pancreatic ductal epithelium, subsequent anaplasia; retarded bone growth)
Vitamin D (Calcitriol)	Rickets in growing children
	Osteomalacia in adults
	Hypocalcaemic tetany
Vitamin E	Degeneration of neurons, retinal pigments, axons of peripheral nerves; denervation of muscles
	Reduced red cell life span
	Sterility in male and female animals
Vitamin K	Hypoprothrombinaemia (in haemorrhagic disease of newborn, biliary obstruction, malabsorption, anticoagulant therapy, antibiotic therapy, diffuse liver disease)
II. WATER-SOLUBLE VITAMINS	
Vitamin C (Ascorbic acid)	Scurvy (haemorrhagic diathesis, skeletal lesions, delayed wound healing, anaemia, lesions in teeth and gums)
Vitamin B Complex	
(i) *Thiamine (Vitamin B₁)*	Beriberi ('dry' or peripheral neuritis, 'wet' or cardiac manifestations, 'cerebral' or Wernicke-Korsakoff's syndrome)
(ii) *Riboflavin (Vitamin B₂)*	Ariboflavinosis (ocular lesions, cheilosis, glossitis, dermatitis)
(iii) *Niacin (Nicotinic acid)*	Pellagra (dermatitis, diarrhoea, dementia)
(iv) *Pyridoxine (Vitamin B₆)*	Vague lesions (convulsions in infants, dermatitis, cheilosis, glossitis, sideroblastic anaemia)
(v) *Folate (Folic acid)*	Megaloblastic anaemia
(vi) *Cyanocobalamin (Vitamin B₁₂)*	Megaloblastic anaemia
	Pernicious anaemia

2. Endogenous synthesis of carcinogens or promoters:

i) In the context of etiology of *gastric carcinoma*, nitrites, nitrates and amines from the digested food are transformed in the body to carcinogens—nitrosamines and nitrosamides.

ii) In the etiology of *colon cancer*, low fibre intake and high animal-derived fats are implicated.

iii) In the etiology of *breast cancer*, epidemiologic studies have implicated the role of animal proteins, fats and obesity with as yet unsubstantiated evidence.

3. Inadequate protective factors: As already mentioned, some components of diet such as *vitamin C, A, E, selenium,* and *β-carotenes* have protective role against cancer. These substances in normal amounts in the body act as antioxidants and protect the cells against free radical injury.

■ SELF ASSESSMENT

---

1. **The harmful effects of smoking of following tobacco products are most severe:**
   A. Cigarettes   B. *Bidis*
   C. Cigar   D. Pipe

2. **The major pathway of ethanol metabolism in the liver is via:**
   A. Alcohol dehydrogenase in the SER
   B. Microsomal P-450
   C. Catalase in the peroxisomes
   D. None of the above

3. **Lead poisoning produces the following change in red cells:**
   A. Pappenheimer bodies
   B. Howell-Jolly bodies
   C. Basophilic stippling
   D. Heinz bodies

4. **Between CO and O_2, haemoglobin has:**
   A. Greater affinity for former
   B. Greater affinity for latter
   C. Equal affinity for both
   D. No affinity for the former

5. **1 g of carbohydrate provides:**
   A. 2 Kcal   B. 4 Kcal
   C. 7 Kcal   D. 9 Kcal

6. **Health risk in obesity is due to weight in excess of the following for age and sex:**
   A. 10 %   B. 20 %
   C. 30 %   D. 40 %

7. **Obesity is due to:**
   A. Hyperplasia of adipocytes only
   B. Hypertrophy of adipocytes only
   C. Hyperplasia as well as hypertrophy of adipocytes
   D. Fatty change in liver only

8. **In starvation, first nutrient to be depleted in the body is:**
   A. Fat   B. Carbohydrate
   C. Protein   D. Vitamins

9. **State of hypervitaminosis occurs in:**
   A. Vitamin A and B   B. Vitamin B and C
   C. Vitamin C and D   D. Vitamin A and D

10. **The main function of vitamin E is:**
    A. Immune regulation
    B. Hepatic microsomal carboxylation
    C. Antioxidant activity
    D. Maintenance of structure and function of epithelia

KEY

1 = B	2 = A	3 = C	4 = A
5 = C	6 = B	7 = C	8 = B
9 = D	10 = C		

Chapter Nine

10

Genetic and Paediatric Diseases

GENETIC DISEASES—INTRODUCTION *(p. 263)*

In the western countries, developmental and genetic birth defects constitute about 50% of total mortality in infancy and childhood, while in the developing and underdeveloped countries 95% of infant mortality is attributed to environmental factors such as poor sanitation and undernutrition.

Genetic and paediatric diseases are covered under the following headings:

1. *Developmental defects:* Errors in morphogenesis
2. *Cytogenetic (Karyotypic) defects:* chromosomal abnormalities
3. *Single-gene defects:* Mendelian disorders
4. *Multifactorial inheritance disorders*
5. *Other paediatric diseases*

DEVELOPMENTAL DEFECTS *(p. 263)*

Developmental defects are a group of abnormalities during foetal life due to errors in morphogenesis. The branch of science dealing with the study of developmental anomalies is called *teratology.*

Pathogenesis *(p. 263)*

The teratogens may result in one of the following outcome:

i) intrauterine death;
ii) intrauterine growth retardation;
iii) functional defects; and
iv) malformation.

The **effects** of teratogens in inducing developmental defects are related to the following factors:

■ *Variable individual susceptibility to teratogen*
■ *Intrauterine stage at which patient is exposed to teratogen*
■ *Dose of teratogen*
■ *Specificity of developmental defect for specific teratogen*

Classification *(p. 263)*

Agenesis means the complete absence of an organ e.g. unilateral or bilateral agenesis of kidney.

Aplasia is the absence of development of an organ with presence of rudiment or anlage e.g. aplasia of lung with rudimentary bronchus.

Hypoplasia is incomplete development of an organ not reaching the normal adult size e.g. microglossia.

Atresia refers to incomplete formation of lumen in hollow viscus e.g. oesophageal atresia.

Developmental dysplasia is defective development of cells and tissues resulting in abnormal or primitive histogenetic structures e.g. renal dysplasia.

Dystraphic anomalies are the defects resulting from failure of fusion e.g. spina bifida.

Ectopia or heterotopia refers to abnormal location of tissue at ectopic site e.g. pancreatic heterotopia in the wall of stomach.

Examples of Developmental Defects *(p. 264)*

1. Anencephaly-spina bifida complex.
2. Thalidomide malformations.

3. Foetal hydantoin syndrome.
4. Foetal alcohol syndrome.
5. TORCH complex.
6. Congenital syphilis.

CYTOGENETIC (KARYOTYPIC) ABNORMALITIES *(p. 264)*

Human germ cells (ova and sperms) contain 23 chromosomes (haploid or N) while all the nucleated somatic cells of the human body contain 23 pairs of chromosomes (diploid or 2N)—44 autosomes and 2 sex chromosomes, being XX in females (46, XX) and XY in males (46, XY). The branch of science dealing with the study of human chromosomal abnormalities is called cytogenetics.

In a female, one of the two X chromosomes (paternal or maternal derived) is inactivated during embryogenesis as stated in *Lyon hypothesis.* This inactivation is passed to all the somatic cells while the germ cells in the female remain unaffected i.e. ovary will always have active X chromosome. Such an inactive X chromosome in the somatic cells in females lies condensed in the nucleus and is called as *sex chromatin* seen specifically in the somatic cells in females. *Nuclear sexing* can be done for genetic female testing by preparing and staining the smears of squamous cells scraped from oral cavity, or by identifying the *Barr body* in the circulating neutrophils as drumstick appendage attached to one of the nuclear lobes. A minimum of 30% cells positive for sex chromatin is indicative of genetically female composition.

Though chromosomes can be studied in any human nucleated cells, circulating lymphocytes are more often used for this purpose. The study is done by arresting the dividing cells in metaphase by colchicine and then spreading them on glass slide and staining them with Giemsa stain.

Karyotype is the photographic representation of the stained preparation of chromosomes.

Based on length of chromosomes, they are divided into 7 groups—A to G, called *Denver classification* adopted at a meeting in Denver, Colorado in US.

Chromosomal banding techniques are employed for study of classes of chromosomes. Chromosomal bands are unique alternate dark and light staining patterns. Banding techniques include:

i)   G-banding (Giemsa stain);
ii) Q-banding (quinacrine fluorescence stain);
iii) R-banding (reverse Giemsa staining); and
iv) C-banding (constitutive heterochromatin demonstration).

Numerical Abnormalities *(p. 265)*

1. Polyploidy is the term used for the number of chromosomes which is a multiple of haploid number e.g. triploid or 3 N (69 chromosomes), tetraploid or 4 N (92 chromosomes). Polyploidy occurs normally in megakaryocytes and dividing liver cells. Polyploidy in somatic cells of conceptus results in spontaneous abortions.

2. Aneuploidy is the number of chromosomes which is not an exact multiple of haploid number e.g. hypodiploid or 2N-1 (45 chromosomes) monosomy, hyperdiploid or 2 N+1 (47 chromosomes) trisomy.

The most common mechanism of aneuploidy is **nondisjunction**. Nondisjunction is the failure of chromosomes to separate normally during cell division during first or second stage of meiosis, or in mitosis.

Three clinically important syndromes resulting from numerical aberrations of chromosomes due to nondisjunction are as under.

■ **Down's syndrome.** There is trisomy 21 in about 95% cases of Down's syndrome due to nondisjunction during meiosis in one of the parents. The incidence of producing offspring with Down's syndrome rises in mothers over 35 years of age.

■ **Klinefelter's syndrome.** Klinefelter's syndrome is the most important example of sex chromosome trisomy. About 80% cases have 47, XXY karyotype while others are mosaics. Typically, these patients have testicular dysgenesis.

■ **Turner's syndrome.** Turner's syndrome is an example of monosomy (45, X0) most often due to loss of X chromosome in paternal meiosis.

Structural Abnormalities *(p. 266)*

During cell division (meiosis as well as mitosis), certain structural abnormalities of chromosomes may appear. These may occur during gametogenesis and then transmitted to all somatic cells and cause hereditary transmissible disorders, or may produce somatic cell mutations and result in changes varying from no effect to some forms of cancers. Structural abnormalities may be balanced or unbalanced.

■ *Balanced structural alteration means* no change in total number of genes or genetic material.

■ *Unbalanced structural alteration* refers to gene rearrangement resulting in loss or gain of genetic material.

Some common forms of structural abnormalities are as under:

TRANSLOCATIONS. Translocation means crossing over or exchange of fragment of chromosome which may occur between non-homologous or homologous chromosomes.

■ **Reciprocal translocation** is the exchange of genetic material between two non-homologous (heterologous) chromosomes without involving centromere (acentric).

i) *Balanced reciprocal translocation* is more common and the individual is phenotypically normal e.g. translocation between long arm(q) of chromosomes 22 and long arm(q) of chromosome 9 written as 46, XX, t (9;22). This translocation is termed Philadelphia chromosome seen in most cases of chronic myeloid leukaemia.

ii) *Unbalanced reciprocal translocations* are less common and account for repeated abortions and malformed children.

■ **Robertsonian translocation** is less common than reciprocal translocation. In this, there is fusion of two acrocentric chromosomes (having very short arms) at the centromere (centric fusion) with loss of short arms.

DELETIONS. Loss of genetic material from the chromosome is called deletion. Deletion may be from the terminal or middle portion of the chromosome.

INVERSION. Inversion is a form of rearrangement involving breaks of a single chromosome at two points.

RING CHROMOSOME. A ring of chromosome is formed by a break at both the telomeric (terminal) ends of a chromosome followed by deletion of the broken fragment and then end-to-end fusion.

ISOCHROMOSOME. When centromere rather than dividing parallel to the long axis, instead divides transverse to the long axis of chromosome, it results in either two short arms only or two long arms only called isochromosomes.

SINGLE-GENE DEFECTS (MENDELIAN DISORDERS) *(p. 267)*

Single-gene defects follow the classic mendelian patterns of inheritance and are also called mendelian disorders. These disorders are the result of mutation of a single gene of large effect.

MUTATIONS. The term mutation is applied to permanent change in the DNA of the cell. Mutations affecting germ cells are transmitted to the next progeny producing *inherited diseases,* while the mutations affecting somatic cells give rise to *various cancers* and *congenital malformations*. Presently, following types of mutations have been described:

i)   Point mutation is the result of substitution of a single nucleotide base by a different base i.e. replacement of an amino acid by another.

ii)   Stop codon or nonsense mutation refers to a type of point mutation in which the protein chain is prematurely terminated or truncated.

iii)   Frameshift mutation occurs when there is insertion or deletion of one or two base pairs in the DNA sequence e.g. in cystic fibrosis of pancreas.

iv)   Trinucleotide repeat mutation is characterised by amplification of a sequence of three nucleotides.

The inheritance pattern of genetic abnormalities may be *dominant or recessive, autosomal or sex-linked. A dominant gene* produces its effects, whether combined with similar dominant or recessive gene. *Recessive genes* are effective only if both genes are similar. However, when both alleles of a gene pair are expressed in heterozygote state, it is called *codominant inheritance*. A single gene may express in multiple allelic forms known as *polymorphism*. Genes on Y-chromosome are determinant for testis and are not known to cause any sex-linked disorder. Therefore, all sex-linked disorders are, in fact, X-linked disorders.

STORAGE DISEASES (INBORN ERRORS OF METABOLISM) *(p. 268)*

Storage diseases or inborn errors of metabolism are biochemically distinct groups of disorders occurring due to genetic defect in the metabolism of carbohydrates, lipids, and proteins resulting in intracellular accumulation of metabolites. These substances may collect within the cells throughout the body but most commonly affected organ or site is the one where the stored material is normally found and degraded. Since lysosomes comprise the chief site of intracellular digestion (autophagy as well as heterophagy), the material is naturally stored in the lysosomes, and hence the generic name 'lysosomal storage diseases'. Cells of mononuclear-phagocyte system are particularly rich in lysosomes; therefore, reticuloendothelial organs containing numerous phagocytic cells like the liver and spleen are most commonly involved in storage disease.

Based on the biochemical composition of the accumulated material within the cells, storage diseases are classified into distinct groups, each group containing a number of diseases depending upon the specific enzyme deficiency. A few general comments can be made about all storage diseases:

■ All the storage diseases occur as a result of autosomal recessive, or sex-(X-) linked recessive genetic transmission.

■ Most, but not all, of the storage diseases are lysosomal storage diseases. Out of the glycogen storage diseases, only type II (Pompe's disease) is due to lysosomal enzyme deficiency.

Glycogen Storage Diseases (Glycogenoses) *(p. 269)*

These are a group of inherited disorders in which there is defective glucose metabolism resulting in excessive intracellular accumulation of glycogen in various tissues. Based on specific enzyme deficiencies, glycogen storage diseases are divided into 8 main types designated by Roman numerals I to VIII. However, based on pathophysiology, glycogen storage diseases can be divided into 3 main subgroups:

1.   Hepatic forms are characterised by inherited deficiency of hepatic enzymes required for synthesis of glycogen for storage (e.g. von Gierke's disease or type I glycogenosis) or due to lack of hepatic enzymes necessary for breakdown of glycogen into glucose (e.g. type VI glycogenosis).

Chapter Ten

2. Myopathic forms on the other hand, are those disorders in which there is genetic deficiency of glycolysis to form lactate in the striated muscle resulting in accumulation of glycogen in the muscles (e.g. McArdle's disease or type V glycogenosis, type VII disease).

3. Other forms are those in which glycogen storage does not occur by either hepatic or myopathic mechanisms. In Pompe's disease or type II glycogenosis, there is lysosomal storage of glycogen, while in type IV there is deposition of abnormal metabolites of glycogen in the brain, heart, liver and muscles.

Mucopolysaccharidoses (MPS) *(p. 270)*

Mucopolysaccharidoses are a group of six inherited syndromes numbered from MPS I to MPS VI. Each of these results from deficiency of specific lysosomal enzyme involved in the degradation of mucopolysaccharides or glycosaminoglycans, and are, therefore, a form of lysosomal storage diseases. Mucopolysaccharides which accumulate in the MPS are: chondroitin sulphate, dermatan sulphate, heparan sulphate and keratan sulphate. All these syndromes are autosomal recessive disorders except MPS II (Hunter's syndrome) which has X-linked recessive transmission.

Gaucher's Disease *(p. 270)*

This is an autosomal recessive disorder in which there is deficiency of lysosomal enzyme, glucocerebrosidase, which normally cleaves glucose from ceramide. This results in lysosomal accumulation of glucocerebroside (ceramide-glucose) in phagocytic cells of the body and sometimes in the neurons.

Clinically, 3 subtypes of Gaucher's disease are identified:

■ **Type I or classic form** is the adult form of disease in which there is storage of glucocerebrosides in the phagocytic cells of the body, principally involving the spleen, liver, bone marrow, and lymph nodes.

■ **Type II** is the infantile form in which there is progressive involvement of the central nervous system.

■ **Type III** is the juvenile form of the disease having features in between type I and type II i.e. they have systemic involvement like in type I and progressive involvement of the CNS as in type II.

M/E Shows large number of characteristically distended and enlarged macrophages called *Gaucher cells* which are found in the spleen, liver, bone marrow and lymph nodes, and in the case of neuronal involvement, in the Virchow-Robin space. The cytoplasm of these cells is abundant, granular and fibrillar resembling crumpled tissue paper.

Niemann-Pick Disease *(p. 271)*

This is also an autosomal recessive disorder characterised by accumulation of sphingomyelin and cholesterol. Majority of the cases (about 80%) have deficiency of sphingomyelinase which is required for cleavage of sphingo-myelin, while a few cases probably result from deficiency of an activator protein.

The condition presents in infancy and is characterised by hepatospleno-megaly, lymphadenopathy and physical and mental underdevelopment.

M/E Shows storage of sphingomyelin and cholesterol within the lysosomes, particularly in the cells of mononuclear phagocyte system. The cells of Niemann-Pick disease are somewhat smaller than Gaucher cells and their cytoplasm is not wrinkled but is instead foamy and vacuolated which stains positively with fat stains.

DISORDERS WITH MULTIFACTORIAL INHERITANCE (p. 271)

These are disorders which result from the combined effect of genetic composition and environmental influences. Some normal phenotypic characteristics have also multifactorial inheritance e.g. colour of hair, eye, skin, height and intelligence. Examples of disorders where environmental influences unmask the mutant genes are: Cleft lip and cleft palate; Pyloric stenosis; Diabetes mellitus; Hypertension; Congenital heart disease; Coronary heart disease.

OTHER PAEDIATRIC DISEASES (p. 271)

TUMOURS OF INFANCY AND CHILDHOOD (p. 272)

Tumours of infancy and childhood comprise 2% of all malignant tumours but they are the leading cause of death in this age group exceeded only by accidents. Benign tumours are more common than malignant neoplasms but they are generally of little immediate consequence. Another aspect requiring consideration here is the difficulty in differentiating benign tumours from tumour-like lesions discussed below.

HISTOGENESIS. It is as under:

■ Some tumours have probably evolved *in utero* and are apparent at birth or in immediate postnatal period. Such tumours are termed *developmental tumours.*

■ Many other tumours originate in abnormally developed organs and organ rests; they become apparent subsequently and are termed *embryonic tumours.*

■ In embryonic tumours, proliferation of embryonic cells occurs which *have not reached the differentiation stage* essential for specialised functions i.e. the cells proliferate as *undifferentiated or as partially differentiated* stem cells and an embryonal tumour is formed.

■ Tumours of infancy and childhood have *some features of normal embryonic or foetal cells* in them which proliferate under growth promoting influence of oncogenes and suffer from mutations which make them appear morphologically malignant.

■ Under appropriate conditions, these malignant embryonal cells may *cease to proliferate* and transform into non-proliferating mature differentiated cells e.g. a neonatal neuroblastoma may mature and differentiate into benign ganglioneuroma; foetal sacrococcygeal teratoma matures with age to adult tissues and is assigned better prognosis.

Benign Tumours and Tumour-like Conditions (p. 272)

1. Hamartomas. Hamartomas are focal accumulations of cells normally present in that tissue but are arranged in an abnormal manner i.e. though present at normal site they do not reproduce normal architecture identical to adjacent tissues.

2. Choristoma (heterotopia). Choristoma or heterotopia is collection of normal cells and tissues at aberrant locations e.g. heterotopic pancreatic tissue in the wall of small bowel or stomach.

Malignant Tumours (p. 273)

Cancers of infancy and childhood differ from those in adults in the following respects:

1. Sites. Cancers of this age group more commonly pertain to haematopoietic system, neural tissue and soft tissues compared to malignant tumours in adults at sites such as the lung, breast, prostate, colon and skin.

2. Genetic basis. Many of paediatric malignant tumours have underlying genetic abnormalities.

3. Regression. Foetal and neonatal malignancies have a tendency to regress spontaneously or to mature.

4. Histologic feature. These tumours have unique histologic feature in having primitive or embryonal appearance rather than pleomorphic-anaplastic histologic appearance.

5. Management. Many of paediatric malignant tumours are curable by chemotherapy and/or radiotherapy but may develop second malignancy.

A few *generalisations* can be drawn about these cancers:

■ In infants and children under 4 years of age: the most common malignant tumours are various types of *blastomas*.

■ Children between 5 to 9 years of age: *haematopoietic malignancies* are more common.

■ In the age range of 10-14 years (prepubertal age): *soft tissue and bony sarcomas* are the prominent tumours.

Based on these broad guidelines, classification of common paediatric malignant tumours at different age groups is presented in Table 10.1.

TABLE 10.1: Common Paediatric Malignant Tumours.

SYSTEM	AGE < 4 YRS	AGE 5-9 YRS	AGE 10-14 YRS
1. *Haemato-poietic*	Acute leukaemia —	Acute leukaemia Lymphoma	— Hodgkin's disease
2. *Blastomas*	Neuroblastoma Hepatoblastoma Retinoblastoma Nephroblastoma (Wilms' tumour)	Neuroblastoma Hepatocellular carcinoma	— Hepatocellular carcinoma
3. *Soft tissues*	Rhabdomyo-sarcoma	Soft tissue sarcoma	Soft tissue sarcoma
4. *Bony*	—	Ewing's sarcoma	Osteogenic sarcoma
5. *Neural*	CNS tumours	CNS tumours	—
6. *Others*	Teratoma	—	Thyroid cancer

■ SELF ASSESSMENT

1. **Teratogens are defined as agents which induce:**
   A. Mitosis
   B. Carcinogenesis
   C. Birth defects
   D. Fallot's tetralogy

2. **For chromosomal study, it is best to use the following nucleated cells:**
   A. Polymorphs
   B. Lymphocytes
   C. Epithelial cells
   D. Fibroblasts

3. **For chromosomal study, the dividing cells are arrested by colchicine in the following phase of cell cycle:**
   A. Prophase
   B. Metaphase
   C. Anaphase
   D. Telophase

4. **Denver classification divides chromosomes based on their length into the following groups:**
   A. A to C (3 groups)
   B. A to E (5 groups)
   C. A to G (7 groups)
   D. A to I (9 groups)

5. **Polyploidy is generally not a feature of dividing cells of the following type:**
   A. Megakaryocytes
   B. Hepatocytes
   C. Tubular cells
   D. Conceptus of abortions

6. **Numeric abnormality in chromosome occurs in the following conditions *except*:**
   A. Ph chromosome in CML
   B. Turner's syndrome
   C. Klinefelter's syndrome
   D. Down's syndrome

7. **Mutations affecting germ cells produce:**
   A. Cancers
   B. Inherited diseases
   C. Congenital malformations
   D. Aneuploidy

8. **In lysosomal storage diseases, the following cells are particularly involved:**
   A. Hepatocytes
   B. Skeletal muscle
   C. Macrophages
   D. White pulp of spleen

9. **Out of the following glycogenosis, the following is example of lysosomal storage disease:**
   A. von Gierke's disease
   B. Pompe's disease
   C. Forbe's disease
   D. Anderson's disease

10. **Blastomas are childhood tumours seen more often in the age range of:**
   A. <4 years
   B. 5-9 years
   C. 10-14 years
   D. 14-16 years

KEY

1 = C	2 = B	3 = B	4 = C
5 = C	6 = A	7 = B	8 = C
9 = B	10 = A		

Chapter Ten

11

The Blood Vessels and Lymphatics

ARTERIES *(p. 277)*

NORMAL STRUCTURE *(p. 277)*

Depending upon the calibre and certain histologic features, arteries are divided into 3 types: large (elastic) arteries, medium-sized (muscular) arteries and the smallest arterioles.

M/E All the arteries of the body have 3 layers in their walls: the tunica intima, the tunica media and the tunica adventitia. These layers progressively decrease with diminution in the size of the vessels.

1. Tunica intima. This is the inner coat of the artery. It is composed of the lining endothelium, subendothelial connective tissue and bounded externally by internal elastic lamina.

2. Tunica media. Tunica media is the middle coat of the arterial wall, bounded internally by internal elastic lamina and externally by external elastic lamina. This layer is the thickest and consists mainly of smooth muscle cells and elastic fibres. The *external elastic lamina* consisting of condensed elastic tissue is less well defined than the *internal elastic lamina*.

3. Tunica adventitia. The outer coat of arteries is the tunica adventitia. It consists of loose mesh of connective tissue and some elastic fibres that merge with the adjacent tissues.

As the calibre of the artery decreases, the three layers progressively diminish. Thus, there are structural variations in the three types of arteries:

■ The *large, elastic arteries* such as the aorta, innominate, common carotid, major pulmonary, and common iliac arteries have very high content of elastic tissue in the media and thick elastic laminae and hence the name.

■ The *medium-sized, muscular arteries* are the branches of elastic arteries. All the three layers of arterial wall are thinner than in the elastic arteries.

■ The *arterioles* are the smallest branches with internal diameter 20-100 μm. Structurally, they consist of the three layers as in muscular arteries but are much thinner and cannot be distinguished.

■ Capillaries are about the size of an RBC (7-8 μm) and have a layer of endothelium but no media. Blood from capillaries returns to the heart via *post-capillary venules* and thence into venules and then veins.

ARTERIOSCLEROSIS *(p. 278)*

Arteriosclerosis is a general term used to include all conditions with thickening and hardening of the arterial walls. The following morphologic entities are included under arteriosclerosis.

SENILE ARTERIOSCLEROSIS *(p. 278)*

Senile arteriosclerosis is the thickening of media and intima of the arteries seen due to aging. The changes are non-selective and affect most of the arteries. These are possibly induced by stress and strain on vessel wall during life.

The pathologic changes are as under:

1. Fibroelastosis: The intima and media are thickened due to increase in elastic and collagen tissue.

2. *Elastic reduplication:* The internal elastic lamina is split or reduplicated so that two wavy layers are seen.

HYPERTENSIVE ARTERIOLOSCLEROSIS *(p. 279)*

Arteriolosclerosis is the term used to describe 3 morphologic forms of vascular disease affecting arterioles and small muscular arteries. All the following three types are common in hypertension but may occur due to other causes as well.

Hyaline Arteriolosclerosis *(p. 279)*

Hyaline sclerosis is a common arteriolar lesion that may be seen *physiologically* due to aging, or may occur *pathologically* in hypertensives and in diabetics. The lesions are more severe in patients with hypertension, especially in the kidneys (Chapter 20).

M/E The thickened vessel wall shows structureless, eosinophilic, hyaline material in the intima and media.

Hyperplastic Arteriolosclerosis *(p. 279)*

The hyperplastic or proliferative type of arteriolosclerosis is a characteristic lesion of malignant hypertension; other causes include haemolytic-uraemic syndrome, scleroderma and toxaemia of pregnancy.

M/E The morphologic changes affect mainly the intima, especially of the interlobular arteries in the kidneys. Three types of intimal thickening may occur:
i) *Onion-skin lesion* consists of loosely-placed concentric layers of hyperplastic intimal smooth muscle cells like the bulb of an onion.
ii) *Mucinous intimal thickening* is the deposition of amorphous ground substance, probably proteoglycans, with scanty cells.
iii) *Fibrous intimal thickening* is less common and consists of bundles of collagen, elastic fibres and hyaline deposits in the intima.

Necrotising Arteriolitis *(p. 279)*

In cases of severe hypertension and malignant hypertension, parts of small arteries and arterioles show changes of hyaline sclerosis and parts of these show necrosis, or necrosis may be superimposed on hyaline sclerosis. However, hyaline sclerosis may not be always present in the vessel wall.

MÖNCKEBERG'S ARTERIOSCLEROSIS (MEDIAL CALCIFIC SCLEROSIS) *(p. 279)*

Mönckeberg's arteriosclerosis is calcification of the media of large and medium-sized muscular arteries, especially of the extremities and of the genital tract. The condition occurs as an age-related degenerative process, and therefore, an example of dystrophic calcification, commonly seen in the elderly individuals and has little or no clinical significance. However, medial calcification also occurs in some pathological states like pseudoxanthoma elasticum and in idiopathic arterial calcification of infancy.

M/E Mönckeberg's arteriosclerosis is characterised by deposits of calcium salts in the media without associated inflammatory reaction while the intima and the adventitia are spared. Often, the coexistent changes of atherosclerosis are present altering the histologic appearance.

ATHEROSCLEROSIS *(p. 280)*

Atherosclerosis is a specific form of arteriosclerosis affecting primarily the intima of large and medium-sized muscular arteries and is characterised by fibrofatty plaques or atheromas. Atherosclerosis is the commonest and the most important of the arterial diseases. Though any large and medium-sized artery may be involved in atherosclerosis, the most commonly affected are the aorta, the coronary and the cerebral arterial systems. Therefore, the major clinical syndromes resulting from ischaemia due to atherosclerosis are the myocardial infarcts (*heart attacks*) and the cerebral infarcts (*strokes*); other less common sequelae are peripheral vascular disease, aneurysmal dilatation due to weakened arterial wall, chronic ischaemic heart disease, ischaemic encephalopathy and mesenteric occlusion.

Etiology *(p. 280)*

Atherosclerosis is widely prevalent in industrialised countries. However, majority of the incidences quoted in the literature are based on the major clinical syndromes produced by it, the most important interpretation being that death from myocardial infarction is related to underlying atherosclerosis. Cardiovascular disease, mostly related to atherosclerotic coronary heart disease or ischaemic heart disease (IHD) is the most common cause of death in the developed countries of the world.

Extensive epidemiologic investigations on living populations have revealed a number of **risk factors** which are associated with increased risk of developing clinical atherosclerosis. Often, these risk factors are acting in combination rather than singly. These risk factors are divided into two groups (Table 11.1):

TABLE 11.1: Risk Factors in Atherosclerosis.

I. MAJOR RISK FACTORS	II. MINOR RISK FACTORS
A) Constitutional	1. Environmental influences
1. Age	2. Obesity
2. Sex	3. Hormones:oestrogen deficiency,
3. Genetic factors	oral contraceptives
4. Familial and racial factors	4. Physical inactivity
B) Acquired	5. Stressful life
1. Hyperlipidaemia	6. Infections (*C.pneumoniae*,
2. Hypertension	Herpesvirus, CMV)
3. Diabetes mellitus	7. Homocystinuria
4. Smoking	8. Role of alcohol

I. Major risk factors. These are further considered under 2 headings:

A) *Major constitutional risk factors:* These are non-modifiable major risk factors that includes: increasing age, male sex, genetic abnormalities, and familial and racial predisposition.

B) *Major acquired risk factors*: This includes major risk factors which can be controlled and includes: hyperlipidaemia, hypertension, diabetes mellitus and smoking.

II. Minor risk factors. This includes a host of factors whose role in atherosclerosis is minimal, and in some cases, even uncertain.

Major Constitutional Risk Factors

1. AGE. Atherosclerosis is an age-related disease. Fully-developed atheromatous plaques usually appear in the 4th decade and beyond. Evidence in support comes from the high death rate from IHD in this age group.

2. SEX. The incidence and severity of atherosclerosis are more in men than in women. The prevalence of atherosclerotic IHD is about three times higher in men in 4th decade than in women and the difference slowly declines with age but remains higher at all ages in men. The lower incidence of IHD in women, especially in premenopausal age, is probably due to high levels of oestrogen and high-density lipoproteins, both of which have anti-atherogenic influence.

3. GENETIC FACTORS. Genetic factors play a significant role in atherogenesis. Hereditary genetic derangements of lipoprotein metabolism predispose the individual to high blood lipid level and familial hypercholesterolaemia.

4. FAMILIAL AND RACIAL FACTORS. The familial predisposition to atherosclerosis may be related to other risk factors like diabetes, hypertension and hyperlipoproteinaemia. Racial differences too exist; Blacks have generally less severe atherosclerosis than Whites.

Major Acquired Risk Factors

1. HYPERLIPIDAEMIA. It is now well established that hypercholesterolaemia has directly proportionate relationship with atherosclerosis and IHD. The following evidences are cited in support of this:

i) The atherosclerotic plaques contain cholesterol and cholesterol esters, largely derived from the lipoproteins in the blood.

ii) The lesions of atherosclerosis can be induced in experimental animals by feeding them with diet rich in cholesterol.

iii) Individuals with hypercholesterolaemia due to various causes such as in diabetes mellitus, myxoedema, nephrotic syndrome, von Gierke's disease, xanthomatosis and familial hypercholesterolaemia have increased risk of developing atherosclerosis and IHD.

iv) Populations having hypercholesterolaemia have higher mortality from IHD. Dietary regulation and administration of cholesterol-lowering drugs have beneficial effect on reducing the risk of IHD.

The main lipids in blood are cholesterol (desirable normal 140-200 mg/dl, borderline high 240 mg/dl) and triglycerides (below 160 mg/dl). An elevation of serum cholesterol levels above 260 mg/dl in men and women between 30 and 50 years of age has three times higher risk of developing IHD as compared with people with serum cholesterol levels within normal limits. The lipoproteins are divided into classes according to the density of solvent in which they remain suspended on centrifugation at high speed. The major classes of lipoprotein particles are *chylomicrons, very-low-density lipoproteins (VLDL), low-density lipoproteins (LDL),* and *high-density lipoproteins (HDL).* The major fractions of lipoproteins and their varying effects on atherosclerosis and IHD are as under:

■ *Low-density lipoprotein (LDL)* is richest in cholesterol and has the maximum association with atherosclerosis.

■ *Very-low-density lipoprotein (VLDL)* carries much of the triglycerides and has less marked effect than LDL.

■ *High-density lipoprotein (HDL)* is protective 'good cholesterol' against atherosclerosis.

Aside from lipid-rich diet, high intake of the total number of calories from carbohydrates, proteins, alcohol and sweets has adverse effects.

2. HYPERTENSION. Hypertension is the other major risk factor in the development of atherosclerotic IHD and cerebrovascular disease. It acts probably by mechanical injury to the arterial wall due to increased blood pressure. A systolic pressure of over 160 mmHg or a diastolic pressure of over 95 mmHg is associated with five times higher risk of developing IHD than in people with blood pressure within normal range (140/90 mmHg or less).

3. SMOKING. Cigarette smoking is associated with higher risk of atherosclerotic IHD and sudden cardiac death. Men who smoke a pack of cigarettes a day are 3-5 times more likely to die of IHD than non-smokers. The increased risk and severity of atherosclerosis in smokers is due to reduced level of HDL and accumulation of carbon monoxide in the blood that produces carboxyhaemoglobin and eventually hypoxia in the arterial wall favouring atherosclerosis.

4. DIABETES MELLITUS. Clinical manifestations of atherosclerosis are far more common and develop at an early age in people with both type 1 and 2 diabetes mellitus. The risk of developing IHD is doubled, tendency to develop cerebrovascular disease is high, and frequency to develop gangrene of foot is about 100 times increased.

Pathogenesis *(p. 283)*

As stated above, atherosclerosis is not caused by a single etiologic factor but is a multifactorial disease whose exact pathogenesis is still not known. Currently, pathogenesis of atherosclerosis is explained on the basis of the following two theories:

1. Reaction-to-injury hypothesis, first described in 1973, and modified in 1986 and 1993 by Ross.
2. Monoclonal theory, based on neoplastic proliferation of smooth muscle cells, postulated by Benditt and Benditt in 1973.

1. REACTION-TO-INJURY HYPOTHESIS. This theory is most widely accepted and incorporates aspects of two older historical theories of atherosclerosis—the lipid theory of Virchow and thrombogenic (encrustation) theory of Rokitansky.

■ The *original response to injury theory* was first described in 1973 according to which the initial event in atherogenesis was considered to be endothelial injury followed by smooth muscle cell proliferation so that the early lesions, according to this theory, consist of smooth muscle cells mainly.

■ The *modified response-to-injury hypothesis* described subsequently in 1993 implicates lipoprotein entry into the intima as the initial event followed by lipid accumulation in the macrophages (foam cells now) which according to modified theory, are believed to be the dominant cells in early lesions.

Both these theories—original and modified, have attracted support and criticism. However, following is the generally accepted role of key components involved in atherogenesis:

i) Endothelial injury. It has been known for many years that endothelial injury is the initial triggering event in the development of lesions of atherosclerosis. Actual endothelial denudation is not an essential requirement, but endothelial dysfunction may initiate the sequence of events.

In man, two of the major risk factors which act together to produce endothelial injury are: *haemodynamic stress from hypertension and chronic hyperlipidaemia*. The role of haemodynamic forces in causing endothelial injury is further supported by the distribution of atheromatous plaques at points of bifurcation or branching of blood vessels which are under greatest shear stress.

ii) Intimal smooth muscle cell proliferation. Endothelial injury causes adherence, aggregation and platelet release reaction at the site of exposed subendothelial connective tissue. Proliferation of intimal smooth muscle cells is stimulated by various mitogens released from platelets adherent at the site of endothelial injury and monocytes, the most important of which is platelet-derived growth factor *(PDGF)*; others are fibroblast growth factor *(FGF)*, and transforming growth factor-alpha *(TGF-α)*.

iii) Role of blood monocytes. Though blood monocytes do not possess receptors for normal LDL, LDL does appear in the monocyte cytoplasm to form foam cell. Plasma LDL on entry into the intima undergoes oxidation. The 'oxidised LDL' so formed in the intima performs the following all-important functions on monocytes and endothelium:

■ *For monocytes,* oxidised LDL acts to attract, proliferate, immobilise and activate them as well as is readily taken up by scavenger receptor on the monocyte to transform it to a lipid-laden foam cell.

■ For *endothelium,* oxidised LDL is cytotoxic.

Death of foam cell by apoptosis releases lipid to form lipid core of plaque.

iv) Role of hyperlipidaemia. As stated already, chronic hyperlipidaemia in itself may initiate endothelial injury and dysfunction by causing increased permeability. Secondly, increased serum concentration of LDL and VLDL promotes formation of foam cells, while high serum concentration of HDL has anti-atherogenic effect.

v) Thrombosis. As apparent from the foregoing, endothelial injury exposes subendothelial connective tissue resulting in formation of small platelet aggregates at the site and causing proliferation of smooth muscle cells. This causes mild inflammatory reaction which together with foam cells is incorporated into the atheromatous plaque.

2. MONOCLONAL HYPOTHESIS. This hypothesis is based on the postulate that proliferation of smooth muscle cells is the primary event and that this proliferation is monoclonal in origin similar to cellular proliferation in neoplasms (e.g. in uterine leiomyoma, Chapter 8). The evidence cited in support of monoclonal hypothesis is the observation on proliferated smooth muscle cells in atheromatous plaques which have only one of the two forms of glucose-6-phosphate dehydrogenase (G6PD) isoenzymes, suggesting monoclonality in origin. The monoclonal proliferation of smooth muscle cells in atherosclerosis may be initiated by mutation caused by exogenous chemicals (e.g. cigarette smoke), endogenous metabolites (e.g. lipoproteins) and some viruses.

Morphology

1. FATTY STREAKS AND DOTS. Fatty streaks and dots on the intima by themselves are harmless but may be the precursor lesions of atheromatous plaques. They are seen in all races of the world and begin to appear in the first year of life.

G/A The lesions may appear as flat or slightly elevated and yellow. They may be either in the form of small, multiple dots, about 1 mm in size, or in the form of elongated, beaded streaks.

M/E Fatty streaks lying under the endothelium are composed of closely-packed foam cells, lipid-containing elongated smooth muscle cells and a few lymphoid cells.

2. GELATINOUS LESIONS. Gelatinous lesions develop in the intima of the aorta and other major arteries in the first few months of life. Like fatty streaks, they may also be precursors of plaques.

M/E Gelatinous lesions are foci of increased ground substance in the intima with thinned overlying endothelium.

3. ATHEROMATOUS PLAQUES. A fully developed atherosclerotic lesion is called atheromatous plaque, also called *fibrous plaque, fibrofatty plaque or atheroma.* These lesions may develop from progression of early lesions of the atherosclerosis described above. *Most often and most severely affected is the abdominal aorta,* though smaller lesions may be seen in descending thoracic aorta and aortic arch. The major branches of the aorta around the ostia are often severely involved, especially the iliac, femoral, carotid, coronary, and cerebral arteries.

G/A Atheromatous plaques are white to yellowish-white lesions, varying in diameter from 1-2 cm and raised on the surface by a few millimetres to a centimetre in thickness. Cut section of the plaque reveals the luminal surface as a firm, white *fibrous cap* and a *central core* composed of yellow to yellow-white, soft, porridge-like material and hence the name atheroma.

M/E The appearance of plaque varies depending upon the age of the lesion. However, the following features are invariably present:

■ The superficial luminal part of *fibrous cap* is covered by endothelium, and is composed of smooth muscle cells, dense connective tissue and extra-cellular matrix containing proteoglycans and collagen.

■ The *cellular area* under the fibrous cap is comprised by a mixture of macrophages, foam cells, lymphocytes and a few smooth muscle cells which may contain lipid.

■ The deeper *central soft core* consists of extracellular lipid material, cholesterol clefts, fibrin, necrotic debris and lipid-laden foam cells.

■ In older and *more advanced lesions,* the collagen in the fibrous cap may be dense and hyalinised, smooth muscle cells may be atrophic and foam cells are fewer.

4. COMPLICATED PLAQUES. It is not uncommon to see more than one form of complication in a plaque:

i) Calcification. Calcification occurs more commonly in advanced atheromatous plaques, especially in the aorta and coronaries. The diseased intima cracks like an egg-shell when the vessel is incised and opened.

M/E The calcium salts are deposited in the vicinity of necrotic area and in the soft lipid pool deep in the thickened intima. This form of atherosclerotic *intimal* calcification differs from Mönckeberg's medial calcific arteriosclerosis that affects only the tunica media.

ii) Ulceration. The layers covering the soft pultaceous material of an atheroma may ulcerate as a result of haemodynamic forces or mechanical trauma. This results in discharge of emboli composed of lipid material and debris into the blood stream.

iii) Thrombosis. The ulcerated plaque and the areas of endothelial damage are vulnerable sites for formation of superimposed thrombi. These thrombi may get dislodged to become emboli and lodge elsewhere in the circulation, or may get organised and incorporated into the arterial wall as mural thrombi.

iv) Haemorrhage. Intimal haemorrhage may occur in an atheromatous plaque either from the blood in the vascular lumen through an ulcerated plaque, or from rupture of thin-walled capillaries that vascularise the atheroma from adventitial vasa vasorum. Haemorrhage is particularly a common complication in coronary arteries.

v) Aneurysm formation. Though atherosclerosis is primarily an intimal disease, advanced lesions are associated with secondary changes in the media and adventitia. The changes in media include atrophy and thinning of the media and fragmentation of internal elastic lamina. These changes cause weakening in the arterial wall resulting in aneurysmal dilatation.

Clinical Effects *(p. 288)*

The clinical effects of atherosclerosis depend upon the size and type of arteries affected. In general, the clinical effects result from the following:

1. Slow luminal narrowing causing ischaemia and atrophy.
2. Sudden luminal occlusion causing infarction necrosis.
3. Propagation of plaque by formation of thrombi and emboli.
4. Formation of aneurysmal dilatation and eventual rupture.
   Some of the important effects are listed below:
i) *Aorta*—Aneurysm formation, thrombosis and embolisation to other organs.
ii) *Heart*—Myocardial infarction, ischaemic heart disease.

iii) *Brain*—Chronic ischaemic brain damage, cerebral infarction.
iv) *Small intestine*—Ischaemic bowel disease, infarction.
v) *Lower extremities*—Intermittent claudication, gangrene.

ARTERITIS *(p. 288)*

Arteritis, angiitis and vasculitis are the common terms used for inflammatory process in an artery or an arteriole. It may occur following invasion of the vessel by infectious agents, or may be induced by non-infectious injuries such as chemical, mechanical, immunologic and radiation injury. The non-infectious group is more important than the infectious type.

I. INFECTIOUS ARTERITIS *(p. 288)*

Direct invasion of the artery by infectious agents, especially bacteria and fungi, causes infectious arteritis.

Endarteritis Obliterans *(p. 288)*

Endarteritis obliterans is not a disease entity but a pathologic designation used for non-specific inflammatory response of arteries and arterioles to a variety of irritants. It is commonly seen close to the lesions of peptic ulcers of the stomach and duodenum, tuberculous and chronic abscesses in the lungs, chronic cutaneous ulcers, chronic meningitis, and in post-partum and post-menopausal uterine arteries.

G/A The affected vessels may appear unaltered externally but on cross-section show obliteration of their lumina.

M/E The obliteration of the lumen is due to concentric and symmetric proliferation of cellular fibrous tissue in the intima.

Syphilitic Arteritis *(p. 288)*

Syphilitic or luetic vascular involvement occurs in all stages of syphilis but is more prominent in the tertiary stage. The changes that are found in the syphilitic arteritis are seen within the arterial tissue (*syphilitic endarteritis*) and in the periarterial tissues (*syphilitic periarteritis*). Manifestations of the disease are particularly prominent at two sites—the aorta and the cerebral arteries.

SYPHILITIC AORTITIS. Syphilitic involvement of the ascending aorta and the aortic arch is the commonest manifestation of cardiovascular syphilis. It occurs in about 80% cases of tertiary syphilis. The preferential involvement of arch of aorta may be due to involvement of mediastinal lymph nodes in secondary syphilis through which the treponemes spread to the lymphatics around the aortic arch.

G/A The affected part of the aorta may be dilated, and its wall somewhat thickened and adherent to the neighbouring mediastinal structures. Longitudinally opened vessels show intimal surface studded with pearly-white thickenings, varying from a few millimetres to a centimetre in diametre. These lesions are separated by wrinkled normal intima, giving it characteristic *tree-bark appearance.* Cut section of the lesion shows more firm and fibrous appearance than the atheromatous plaques. However, superimposed atherosclerotic lesions may be present.

M/E
■ Endarteritis and periarteritis of the vasa vasorum located in the media and adventitia.
■ Perivascular accumulation of plasma cells, lymphocytes and macrophages that may form miliary gummas which undergo necrosis and are replaced by scar tissue.

■ Intimal thickenings consist of dense avascular collagen that may undergo hyalinisation and calcification.

The *effects* of syphilitic aortitis may vary from trivial to catastrophic. These are as follows:

a) *Aortic aneurysm* may result from damage to the aortic wall.

b) *Aortic valvular incompetence.*

c) *Stenosis of coronary ostia* is seen in about 20% cases of syphilitic aortitis and may lead to progressive myocardial fibrosis, angina pectoris and sudden death.

The features distinguishing syphilitic aortitis from aortic atheroma are given in Table 11.2.

TABLE 11.2: Contrasting Features of Syphilitic Aortitis and Aortic Atheroma.

FEATURES	SYPHILITIC AORTITIS	AORTIC ATHEROMA
1. *Sites*	Ascending aorta, aortic arch; absent below diaphragm	Progressive increase from the arch to abdominal aorta, more often at the bifurcation
2. *Macroscopy*	Pearly-white intimal lesions resembling tree-bark without fat in the core; ulceration and calcification often not found	Yellowish-white intimal plaques with fat in the core; ulceration and calcification in plaques common
3. *Microscopy*	Endarteritis and periarteritis of vasa vasorum, perivascular infiltrate of plasma cells and lymphocytes	Fibrous cap with deeper core containing foam cells, cholesterol clefts and soft lipid
4. *Effects*	Thoracic aortic aneurysm, incompetence of the aortic valve, stenosis of coronary ostia	Abdominal aortic aneurysm, aortic valve stenosis, stenosis of abdominal branches

CEREBRAL SYPHILITIC ARTERITIS (HEUBNER'S ARTERITIS). Syphilitic involvement of small and medium-sized cerebral arteries occurs during the tertiary syphilis.

G/A The cerebral vessels are white, rigid and thick-walled.

M/E Changes of endarteritis and periarteritis similar to those seen in syphilitic aortitis are found. There is atrophy of muscle in the media and replacement by fibrosis. This results in ischaemic atrophy of the brain.

II. NON-INFECTIOUS ARTERITIS *(p. 290)*

This group consists of most of the important forms of vasculitis, more often affecting arterioles, venules and capillaries, and hence also termed as *small vessel vasculitis*. Their exact etiology is not known but available evidence suggests that many of them have immunologic origin. Serum from many of patients with vasculitis of immunologic origin show the presence of following immunologic features:

1. Anti-neutrophil cytoplasmic antibodies (ANCAs). Patients with immunologic vasculitis have autoantibodies in their serum against the cytoplasmic antigens of the neutrophils, macrophages and endothelial cells; these are called ANCAs. Neutrophil immunofluorescence is used to demonstrate their presence, of which two distinct patterns of ANCAs are seen:

■ *Cytoplasmic ANCA (c-ANCA) pattern* is specific for proteinase-3 (PR-3), a constituent of neutrophilic granules; this is seen in cases with active Wegener's granulomatosis.

■ *Perinuclear ANCA (p-ANCA) pattern* is specific for myeloperoxidase enzyme; this is noted in patients with microscopic polyarteritis nodosa and primary glomerular disease.

2. Anti-endothelial cell antibodies (AECAs). These antibodies are demonstable in cases of SLE, Kawasaki disease and Buerger's disease.

3. Pauci-immune vasculitis. While most cases of immunologic vasculitis have immune complex deposits in the vessel wall, there are some cases which do not have such immune deposits and are termed as cases of pauci-immune vasculitis.

1. Polyarteritis Nodosa *(p. 290)*

Polyarteritis nodosa (PAN) is a necrotising vasculitis involving small and medium-sized muscular arteries of multiple organs and tissues.

The disease occurs more commonly in adult males than females. Most commonly affected organs, in descending order of frequency of involvement, are the kidneys, heart, liver, gastrointestinal tract, muscle, pancreas, testes, nervous system and skin. The syndrome of PAN presents with varied symptoms pertaining to different organs. However, some usual clinical features are fever, malaise, weakness, weight loss, renal manifestations (albuminuria, haematuria and renal failure), vascular lesions in the alimentary tract (abdominal pain and melaena), peripheral neuritis and hypertension. The condition is believed to result from deposition of immune complexes and tumour-related antigens.

G/A The lesions of PAN involve segments of vessels, especially at the bifurcations and branchings, as tiny beaded nodules.

M/E There are 3 sequential stages in the evolution of lesions in PAN:

i) *Acute stage*—There is fibrinoid necrosis in the centre of the nodule located in the media. An acute inflammatory response develops around the focus of fibrinoid necrosis. The inflammatory infiltrate is present in the entire circumference of the affected vessel (periarteritis) and consists chiefly of neutrophils and eosinophils, and some mononuclear cells.

ii) *Healing stage*—This is characterised by marked fibroblastic proliferation producing firm nodularity.

iii) *Healed stage*—In this stage, the affected arterial wall is markedly thickened due to dense fibrosis. The internal elastic lamina is fragmented or lost.

2. Hypersensitivity (Allergic, Leucocytoclastic) Vasculitis *(p. 291)*

Hypersensitivity vasculitis, also called as allergic or leucocytoclastic vasculitis or microscopic polyarteritis, is a group of clinical syndromes differing from PAN in having inflammatory involvement of venules, capillaries and arterioles. The tissues and organs most commonly involved are the skin, mucous membranes, lungs, brain, heart, gastrointestinal tract, kidneys and muscle. The condition results from immunologic response to an identifiable antigen that may be bacteria (e.g. streptococci, staphylococci, mycobacteria), viruses (e.g. hepatitis B virus, influenza virus, CMV), malarial parasite, certain drugs and chemicals. Hypersensitivity vasculitis includes clinicopathologic entities such as serum sickness, Henoch-Schönlein purpura, mixed cryoglobulinaemia, vasculitis associated with malignancy, and vasculitis associated with connective tissue diseases like rheumatoid arthritis and SLE.

M/E The lesions characteristically involve smallest vessels, sparing medium-sized and larger arteries. Two histologic forms are described:

i) *Leucocytoclastic vasculitis,* characterised by fibrinoid necrosis with neutrophilic infiltrate in the vessel wall. Many of the neutrophils are fragmented. This form is found in vasculitis caused by deposits of immune complexes.

ii) *Lymphocytic vasculitis,* in which the involved vessel shows predominant infiltration by lymphocytes. This type is seen in vascular injury due to delayed hypersensitivity or cellular immune reactions.

Chapter Eleven

3. Wegener's Granulomatosis *(p. 291)*

Wegener's granulomatosis is another form of necrotising vasculitis characterised by a *clinicopathologic triad* consisting of the following:

i) Acute necrotising granulomas of the upper and lower respiratory tracts involving nose, sinuses and lungs;

ii) focal necrotising vasculitis, particularly of the lungs and upper airways; and

iii) focal or diffuse necrotising glomerulonephritis.

A *limited form* of Wegener's granulomatosis is the same condition without renal involvement. As with PAN, the condition is more common in adult males and involves multiple organs and tissues. Most commonly involved organs are lungs, paranasal sinuses, nasopharynx and kidneys. The etiology is not known but possibly the lesions occur due to the presence of circulating immune complexes. This is supported by the observation of subepithelial immuno-globulin deposits on the glomerular basement membrane and induction of remission by immunosuppressive therapy. The serum of these patients shows C-ANCA positivity. Disseminated form of Wegener's granulomatosis differs from a related entity, *idiopathic lethal midline granuloma,* in the sense that the latter condition is highly destructive and progressively necrotic disease of the upper airways.

M/E The characteristic feature of Wegener's granulomatosis is the presence of necrotising granulomatous inflammation of the tissues and necrotising vasculitis with or without granulomas.

4. Temporal (Giant Cell) Arteritis *(p. 292)*

This is a form of granulomatous inflammation of medium-sized and large arteries. Preferential sites of involvement are the cranial arteries, especially the temporal, and hence the name. However, the aorta and other major arteries like common carotid, axillary, brachial, femoral and mesenteric arteries are also involved, and therefore, it is preferable to call the entity as *'giant cell arteritis'.* The patients are generally over the age of 70 years with slight female preponderance. The usual clinical manifestations are headache and blindness if ophthalmic artery is involved. The cause of the condition remains unknown though there is suggestion of an T cell mediated immunologic reaction to some component of the arterial wall, especially against the damaged internal elastic lamina.

G/A The affected artery is thickened, cord-like and the lumen is usually reduced to a narrow slit.

M/E i) There is chronic granulomatous reaction, usually around the internal elastic lamina and typically involves the entire circumference of the vessel.

ii) Giant cells of foreign body or Langhans' type are found in two-third of cases.

iii) The internal elastic lamina is often fragmented.

iv) There is eccentric or concentric intimal cellular proliferation causing marked narrowing of the lumen.

5. Takayasu's Arteritis (Pulseless Disease) *(p. 292)*

This is a form of granulomatous vasculitis affecting chiefly the aorta and its major branches and hence is also referred to as *aortic arch syndrome.* The disease affects chiefly young women and is typically characterised by absence of pulse in both arms and presence of ocular manifestations.

G/A The aortic wall is irregularly thickened and intima wrinkled. The branches of major arteries coming off the aortic arch have obliterated lumina.

M/E i)There is severe mononuclear inflammatory infiltrate involving the full thickness of the affected vessel wall.

ii) The inflammatory changes are more severe in the adventitia and media and there is perivascular infiltration of the vasa vasorum.

iii) Granulomatous changes in the media with central necrosis and Langhans' giant cells are found in many cases.

6. Kawasaki's Disease *(p. 292)*

Also known by more descriptive name of '*mucocutaneous lymph node syndrome*', it is an acute and subacute illness affecting mainly young children and infants. Kawasaki's disease is a febrile illness with mucocutaneous symptoms like erosions of oral mucosa and conjunctiva, skin rash and lymphadenopathy.

M/E The picture is of panarteritis resembling PAN, characterised by necrosis and inflammation of the entire thickness of the vessel wall. Therefore, some consider Kawasaki's disease as an infantile form of PAN.

7. Buerger's Disease (Thromboangiitis Obliterans) *(p. 293)*

Buerger's disease is a specific disease entity affecting chiefly small and medium-sized arteries and veins of the extremities and characterised by acute and chronic occlusive inflammatory involvement. The disease affects chiefly men under the age of 35 years who are heavy cigarette smokers. The symptom-complex consists of intermittent claudication due to ischaemia manifested by intense pain affecting the limbs, more commonly the legs. Eventually, gangrene of the affected extremities occurs requiring amputation.

ETIOPATHOGENESIS. Following possible mechanisms have been suggested:

■ There is consistent association with heavy cigarette smoking. This has led to the hypothesis that *tobacco products* cause either direct endothelial damage leading to hypercoagulability and thrombosis. In support is the demonstration of anti-endothelial cell antibodies (AECAs).

■ *Genetic factors* seem to play a role as the disease is has familial occurrence, has HLA association and is seen in individuals with HLA-A9 and HLA-B5 antigens.

G/A The lesions are typically segmental affecting small and medium-sized arteries, especially of the lower extremities. Involvement of the arteries is often accompanied with involvement of adjacent veins and nerves.

M/E i)In *early stage,* there is infiltration by polymorphs in all the layers of vessels and there is invariable presence of mural or occlusive thrombosis of the lumen.

ii) In *advanced stage,* the cellular infiltrate is predominantly mononuclear and may contain an occasional epithelioid cell granuloma with Langhans' giant cells.

8. Miscellaneous Vasculitis *(p. 293)*

Various connective tissue diseases (e.g. rheumatoid arthritis, ankylosing spondylitis and SLE), rheumatic fever, certain malignancies and Henoch-Schönlein purpura are associated with vasculitis. The type of vasculitis is generally of hypersensitivity or allergic angiitis but sometimes may resemble PAN.

Raynaud's Disease and Raynaud's Phenomenon *(p. 293)*

Raynaud's disease is not a vasculitis but is a functional vasospastic disorder affecting chiefly small arteries and arterioles of the extremities, occurring mainly in otherwise young healthy females. The disease affects most commonly the fingers and hands. The ischaemic effect is provoked primarily by cold but other stimuli such as emotions, trauma, hormones and drugs also seem to play a role. Though usually no pathologic changes are observed in the affected vessels, long-standing cases may show endothelial proliferation and intimal thickening.

Raynaud's phenomenon differs from Raynaud's disease in having an underlying cause e.g. secondary to artherosclerosis, connective tissue diseases like scleroderma and SLE, Buerger's disease, multiple myeloma, pulmonary hypertension and ingestion of ergot group of drugs. Raynaud's phenomenon like Raynaud's disease, also shows cold sensitivity but differs from the latter in having structural abnormalities in the affected vessels.

ANEURYSMS (p. 294)

An aneurysm is defined as a permanent abnormal dilatation of a blood vessel occurring due to congenital or acquired weakening or destruction of the vessel wall. Most commonly, aneurysms involve large elastic arteries, especially the aorta and its major branches. Aneurysms can cause various ill-effects such as thrombosis and thromboembolism, alteration in the flow of blood, rupture of the vessel and compression of neighbouring structures.

Classification (p. 294)

A. Depending upon the composition of the wall, these can be:
1. *True aneurysm* composed of all the layers of a normal vessel wall.
2. *False aneurysm* having fibrous wall and occurring often from trauma to the vessel.

B. Depending upon the shape, aneurysms can be of following types:
1. *Saccular* having large spherical outpouching.
2. *Fusiform* having slow spindle-shaped dilatation.
3. *Cylindrical* with a continuous parallel dilatation.
4. *Serpentine or varicose* which tortuous dilatation of the vessel.
5. *Racemose or circoid* having mass of intercommunicating small arteries and veins.

C. Based on pathogenetic mechanisms, aneurysms can be classified as under:
1. *Atherosclerotic (arteriosclerotic) aneurysms* are the most common type,
2. *Syphilitic (luetic) aneurysms* found in the tertiary stage of the syphilis.
3. *Dissecting aneurysms (Dissecting haematoma)* in which the blood enters the separated or dissected wall of the vessel.
4. *Mycotic aneurysms* which result from weakening of the arterial wall by microbial infection.
5. *Berry aneurysms* which are small dilatations especially affecting the circle of Willis in the base of the brain.

Atherosclerotic Aneurysms (p. 295)

Atherosclerotic aneurysms are the most common form of aortic aneurysms. They are seen more commonly in males and the frequency increases after the age of 50 years when the incidence of complicated lesions of advanced atherosclerosis is higher. They are most common in the abdominal aorta, so much so that all forms of aneurysms of abdominal aorta (fusiform, cylindrical and saccular) should be considered atherosclerotic until proved otherwise. Other locations include thoracic aorta (essentially the ascending part and arch of aorta), iliac arteries and other large systemic arteries.

PATHOGENESIS. Obviously, severe atherosclerotic lesions are the basic problem which cause thinning and destruction of the medial elastic tissue resulting in atrophy and weakening of the wall. Since atherosclerotic lesions are most common and severe in abdominal aorta, atherosclerotic aneurysms occur most frequently here. In the thoracic aorta, besides atherosclerotic lesions, medial degeneration is another additional factor implicated in pathogenesis.

G/A Atherosclerotic aneurysms of the abdominal aorta are most frequently infra-renal, above the bifurcation of the aorta but may extend into common iliac arteries. They may be of variable size but are often larger than 5-6 cm in diameter. Atherosclerotic aneurysm is most frequently fusiform in shape and the lumen of aneurysm often contains mural thrombus.

M/E The wall of atherosclerotic aneurysm loses its normal arterial structure. Instead, there is predominance of fibrous tissue in the media and adventitia with mild chronic inflammatory reaction.

EFFECTS 1. Rupture. Rupture of the atherosclerotic aneurysm is the most serious and fatal complication.

2. Compression. The atherosclerotic aneurysm may press upon some adjacent structures such as compression of ureter and erosion on the vertebral bodies.

3. Arterial occlusion. Atherosclerotic aneurysms of the abdominal aorta may occlude the inferior mesenteric artery, or there may be development of occlusive thrombosis.

Syphilitic (Luetic) Aneurysms *(p. 295)*

Cardiovascular syphilis occurs in about 10% cases of syphilis. One of the major complications of syphilitic aortitis is syphilitic or luetic aneurysm that develops in the tertiary stage of syphilis. It usually manifests after the age of 50 years and is more common in men. The predominant site of involvement is thoracic aorta, especially in the ascending part and arch of aorta.

PATHOGENESIS. About 40% cases of syphilitic aortitis develop syphilitic aneurysms. The process begins from inflammatory infiltrate around the vasa vasorum of the adventitia, followed by endarteritis obliterans. This results in ischaemic injury to the media causing destruction of the smooth muscle and elastic tissue of the media and scarring.

G/A Syphilitic aneurysms occurring most often in the ascending part and the arch of aorta are saccular in shape and usually 3-5 cm in diameter. Less often, they are fusiform or cylindrical. The intimal surface is wrinkled and shows *tree-bark appearance.*

M/E The features of healed syphilitic aortitis are seen. The adventitia shows fibrous thickening with endarteritis obliterans of vasa vasorum.

EFFECTS 1. Rupture. Syphilitic aneurysm is likely to rupture causing massive and fatal haemorrhage into the pleural cavity, pericardial sac, trachea and oesophagus.

2. Compression. The aneurysm may press on the adjacent tissues and cause symptoms such as on trachea causing dyspnoea, on oesophagus causing dysphagia, on recurrent laryngeal nerve leading to hoarseness; and erosion of vertebrae, sternum and ribs due to persistent pressure.

3. Cardiac dysfunction. When the aortic root and valve are involved, syphilitic aneurysm produces aortic incompetence and cardiac failure. Narrowing of the coronary ostia may further aggravate cardiac disease.

Dissecting Aneurysms and Cystic Medial Necrosis *(p. 296)*

The term dissecting aneurysm is applied for a dissecting haematoma in which the blood enters the separated (dissected) wall of the vessel and spreads for varying distance longitudinally. The most common site is the aorta and is an acute catastrophic aortic disease. The condition occurs commonly in men in the age range of 50 to 70 years.

PATHOGENESIS i) Hypertensive state. About 90% cases of dissecting aneurysm have hypertension which predisposes such patients to degeneration of the media in some questionable way.

ii) Non-hypertensive cases. These are cases in whom there is some local or systemic connective tissue disorder e.g.

a) *Marfan's syndrome.*
b) Development of *cystic medial necrosis of Erdheim,* especially in old age.
c) *Iatrogenic trauma* during cardiac catheterisation or coronary bypass surgery.
d) *Pregnancy,* for some unknown reasons.

Once medial necrosis has occurred, haemodynamic factors, chiefly hypertension, cause tear in the intima and initiate the dissecting aneurysms. The media is split at its weakest point by the inflowing blood.

G/A Dissecting aneurysm differs from atherosclerotic and syphilitic aneurysms in having no significant dilatation. Therefore, it is currently referred to as *'dissecting haematoma'.* Dissecting aneurysm classically begins in the arch of aorta. In 95% of cases, there is a sharply-incised, transverse or oblique intimal tear, 3-4 cm long, most often located in the ascending part of the aorta. The dissection is seen most characteristically between the outer and middle third of the aortic media so that the column of blood in the dissection separates the *intima and inner two-third of the media* on one side from the *outer one-third of the media and the adventitia* on the other.

In about 10% of dissecting aneurysms, a second intimal tear is seen in the distal part of the dissection so that the blood enters the false lumen through the proximal tear and re-enters the true lumen through the distal tear. If the patient survives, the false lumen may develop endothelial lining and *'double-barrel aorta'* is formed.

M/E The characteristic features of cystic medial necrosis are found:

- Focal separation of the fibromuscular and elastic tissue of the media.
- Numerous cystic spaces in the media containing basophilic ground substance.
- Fragmentation of the elastic tissue.
- Increased fibrosis of the media.

EFFECTS. The classical clinical manifestation of a dissecting aneurysm is excruciating tearing pain in the chest moving downwards. The complications arising from dissecting aneurysms are as under:

1. Rupture. Haemorrhage from rupture of a dissecting aneurysm in the ascending aorta results in mortality in 90% of cases. Most often, haemorrhage occurs into the pericardium.

2. Cardiac disease. Involvement of the aortic valve results in aortic incompetence.

3. Ischaemia. Obstruction of the branches of aorta by dissection results in ischaemia of the tissue supplied.

FIBROMUSCULAR DYSPLASIA*(p. 297)*

Fibromuscular dysplasia first described in 1976, is a non-atherosclerotic and non-inflammatory disease affecting arterial wall, most often renal artery. Though the process may involve intima, media or adventitia, medial fibroplasia is the most common.

G/A The involvement is characteristically segmental—affecting vessel in a bead-like pattern with intervening uninvolved areas.

M/E The beaded areas show collections of smooth muscle cells and connective tissue.

VEINS (p. 298)

NORMAL STRUCTURE (p. 298)

The structure of normal veins is basically similar to that of arteries. The walls of the veins are thinner, the three tunicae (intima, media and adventitia) are less clearly demarcated, the elastic tissue is scanty and not clearly organised into internal and external elastic laminae. All veins, except vena cavae and common iliac veins, have valves best developed in veins of the lower limbs.

VARICOSITIES (p. 298)

Varicosities are abnormally dilated and tortuous veins. The veins of lower extremities are involved most frequently, called *varicose veins*. The veins of other parts of the body which are affected are the lower oesophagus (*oesophageal varices*), the anal region (*haemorrhoids*) and the spermatic cord (*varicocele*).

VARICOSE VEINS (p. 298)

Varicose veins are permanently dilated and tortuous superficial veins of the lower extremities, especially the long saphenous vein and its tributaries. About 10-12% of the general population develops varicose veins of lower legs, with the peak incidence in 4th and 5th decades of life. Adult females are affected more commonly than the males, especially during pregnancy.

ETIOPATHOGENESIS. A number of etiologic and pathogenetic factors are involved in causing varicose veins.
i)   Familial weakness of vein walls and valves is the most common cause.
ii) Increased intraluminal pressure due to prolonged upright posture e.g. in nurses, policemen, surgeons etc.
iii) Compression of iliac veins e.g. during pregnancy, intravascular thrombosis, growing tumour etc.
iv) Hormonal effects on smooth muscle.
v)   Obesity.
vi) Chronic constipation.

G/A The affected veins, especially of the lower extremities, are dilated, tortuous, elongated and nodular. Intraluminal thrombosis and valvular deformities are often found.

M/E There is variable fibromuscular thickening of the wall of the veins due to alternate dilatation and hypertrophy. Degeneration of the medial elastic tissue may occur which may be followed by calcific foci. Mural thrombosis is commonly present which may get organised and hyalinised leading to irregular intimal thickening.

PHLEBOTHROMBOSIS AND THROMBOPHLEBITIS (p. 298)

The terms 'phlebothrombosis' or thrombus formation in veins, and 'thrombophlebitis' or inflammatory changes within the vein wall, are currently used synonymously.

The most common locations for phlebothrombosis and thrombophlebitis are the deep veins of legs accounting for 90% of cases.

G/A The affected veins may appear normal or may be distended and firm. Often, a mural or occlusive thrombus is present.

M/E The thrombus that is attached to the vein wall induces inflammatory-reparative response beginning from the intima and infiltrating into the thrombi. The response consists of mononuclear inflammatory cells and fibroblastic proliferation. In late stage, thrombus is either organised or resolved leading to a thick-walled fibrous vein.

EFFECTS. The clinical effects due to phlebothrombosis and thrombophlebitis may be local or systemic.

Local effects are oedema distal to occlusion, heat, swelling, tenderness, redness and pain.

Systemic effects are more severe and occur due to embolic phenomena, pulmonary thromboembolism being the most common and most important.

Special Types of Phlebothrombosis *(p. 299)*

1. **THROMBOPHLEBITIS MIGRANS.** Thrombophlebitis migrans or migratory thrombophlebitis or Trousseau's syndrome is the term used for multiple venous thrombi that disappear from one site so as to appear at another site. The condition is not a morphologic entity but a clinical one, seen most often in disseminated visceral cancers.

2. **PHLEGMASIA ALBA DOLENS.** This term meaning 'painful white leg' refers to extensive swelling of the leg, occurring most frequently due to iliofemoral venous thrombosis.

3. **PHLEGMASIA CERULEA DOLENS.** This term meaning 'painful blue leg' refers to markedly swollen bluish skin with superficial gangrene.

4. **SUPERIOR VENA CAVAL SYNDROME.** Superior vena caval syndrome refers to obstruction of the superior vena cava. The obstruction results most often from external compression or from thrombosis. Some of the common causes of superior vena caval syndrome are malignancy (especially lung cancer and lymphoma), syphilitic aortic aneurysm and tuberculous mediastinitis.

5. **INFERIOR VENA CAVAL SYNDROME.** Inferior vena caval syndrome is the obstruction of the inferior vena cava. Most often, obstruction results from thrombosis by extension from iliofemoral veins.

LYMPHATICS *(p. 299)*

NORMAL STRUCTURE *(p. 299)*

Lymphatic capillaries, lymphatic vessels and lymph nodes comprise the lymphatic system. Lymphatic capillaries resemble blood capillaries, and larger lymphatics are identical to veins. However, lymphatics lined by a single layer of endothelium have thin muscle in their walls than in veins of the same size and the valves are more numerous.

LYMPHANGITIS *(p. 299)*

Acute lymphangitis occurs in the course of many bacterial infections.

G/A The affected lymphatics are dilated and appear as cutaneous streaks.

M/E The dilated lumen contains acute inflammatory exudate, cell debris and clotted lymph.

Chronic lymphangitis occurs due to persistent and recurrent acute lymphangitis or from chronic infections like tuberculosis, syphilis and actinomycosis.

M/E There is permanent obstruction due to fibrosis of affected lymphatics called chronic lymphoedema.

LYMPHOEDEMA *(p. 300)*

Lymphoedema is swelling of soft tissues due to localised increase in the quantity of lymph. It may be primary (idiopathic) or secondary (obstructive).

I. PRIMARY (IDIOPATHIC) LYMPHOEDEMA. Lymphoedema occurring without underlying secondary cause is called primary or idiopathic lymphoedema. Its various types are as under:

1. Congenital lymphoedema. Congenital lymphoedema has further 2 subtypes.

i)   Milroy's disease is a form of congenital and familial oedema generally affecting one limb but at times may be more extensive and involve the eyelids and lips. The disease is inherited as an autosomal dominant trait and is often associated with other congenital anomalies.

ii)   Simple congenital lymphoedema is non-familial form with unknown etiology. It is often associated with Turner's syndrome and affects one member of the family.

2. Lymphoedema praecox. This is a rare form of lymphoedema affecting chiefly young females. The oedema usually begins in the foot and progresses slowly upwards to involve the whole extremity.

II. SECONDARY (OBSTRUCTIVE) LYMPHOEDEMA. This is the more common form of lymphoedema. The various causes of lymphatic obstruction resulting in lymphoedema are:

i)   Lymphatic invasion by malignant tumour.

ii)   Surgical removal of lymphatics e.g. in radical mastectomy.

iii) Post-irradiation fibrosis.

iv) Parasitic infestations e.g. in filariasis of lymphatics producing elephantiasis.

v)   Lymphangitis causing scarring and obstruction.

TUMOURS AND TUMOUR-LIKE LESIONS *(p. 300)*

Majority of benign vascular tumours are malformations or hamartomas. A hamartoma is a tumour-like lesion made up of tissues indigenous to the part but lacks the true growth potential of true neoplasms. However, there is no clear-cut distinction between vascular hamartomas and true benign tumours and are often described together.

Haemangioma *(p. 300)*

Haemangiomas are quite common lesions, especially in infancy and childhood. The most common site is the skin of the face. Amongst the various clinical and histologic types, three important forms are described below.

CAPILLARY HAEMANGIOMA. These are the most common type. Clinically, they appear as small or large, flat or slightly elevated, red to purple, soft and lobulated lesions, varying in size from a few millimetres to a few centimetres in diametre. They may be present at birth or appear in early childhood. Strawberry birthmarks and 'port-wine mark' are some good examples. The common sites are the skin, subcutaneous tissue and mucous membranes of oral cavity and lips.

M/E Capillary haemangiomas are well-defined but unencapsulated lobules. These lobules are composed of capillary-sized, thin-walled, blood-filled vessels. These vessels are lined by single layer of plump endothelial cells surrounded by a layer of pericytes.

CAVERNOUS HAEMANGIOMA. Cavernous haemangiomas are single or multiple, discrete or diffuse, red to blue, soft and spongy masses. They are often 1 to 2 cm in diameter. They are most common in the skin (especially of the face and neck); other sites are mucosa of the oral cavity.

M/E Cavernous haemangiomas are composed of thin-walled cavernous vascular spaces, filled partly or completely with blood. The vascular spaces are lined by flattened endothelial cells.

GRANULOMA PYOGENICUM. Granuloma pyogenicum is also referred to as *haemangioma of granulation tissue type*. True to its name, it appears as exophytic, red granulation tissue just like a nodule, commonly on the skin and mucosa of gingiva or oral cavity. *Pregnancy tumour* or *granuloma gravidarum* is a variant occurring on the gingiva during pregnancy and regresses after delivery.

M/E It shows proliferating capillaries similar to capillary haemangioma but the capillaries are separated by abundant oedema and inflammatory infiltrate, thus resembling inflammatory granulation tissue.

Lymphangioma *(p. 301)*

Lymphangiomas are lymphatic counterparts of vascular haemangiomas. Lymphangiomas are congenital lesions which are classified as capillary, cavernous and cystic hygroma.

CAPILLARY LYMPHANGIOMA. It is also called as lymphangioma simplex. It is a small, circumscribed, slightly elevated lesion measuring 1 to 2 cm in diameter. The common locations are the skin of head and neck, axilla and mucous membranes.

M/E Capillary lymphangioma is composed of a network of endothelium-lined, capillary-sized spaces containing lymph, separated by lymphoid aggregates.

CAVERNOUS LYMPHANGIOMA. It is more common than the capillary type. The common sites are in the region of head and neck or axilla. A large cystic variety called *cystic hygroma* occurs in the neck producing gross deformity in the neck.

M/E Cavernous lymphangioma consists of large dilated lymphatic spaces lined by flattened endothelial cells and containing lymph. Scanty intervening stromal connective tissue is present.

Glomus Tumour (Glomangioma) *(p. 302)*

Glomus tumour is an uncommon true benign tumour arising from contractile glomus cells that are present in the arteriovenous shunts (Sucquet-Hoyer anastomosis). These tumours are found most often in the dermis of the fingers or toes under a nail. These lesions are characterised by extreme pain.

M/E The tumours are composed of small blood vessels lined by endothelium and surrounded by aggregates, nests and masses of glomus cells. The glomus cells are round to cuboidal cells with scanty cytoplasm.

4. Arteriovenous Malformations *(p. 302)*

An arteriovenous (AV) malformation is a communication between an artery and vein without an intervening capillary bed. It may be congenital or acquired type. Congenital AV malformations have thick-walled vessels with hyalinisation and calcification. Acquired AV malformations reveal mainly changes in the veins which are dilated and thick-walled.

Haemangioendothelioma *(p. 302)*

Haemangioendothelioma is a true tumour of endothelial cells, the behaviour of which is intermediate between a haemangioma and haemangiosarcoma. It is found most often in the skin and subcutaneous tissue in relation to medium-sized and large veins, *Haemangioblastoma* is the term used for similar tumour occurring in the cerebellum.

G/A The tumour is usually well-defined, grey-red, polypoid mass.

M/E There is active proliferation of endothelial cells forming several layers around the blood vessels so that vascular lumina are difficult to identify.

Reticulin stain delineates the pattern of cell proliferation inner to the basement membrane.

Haemangiopericytoma *(p. 303)*

Haemangiopericytoma is an uncommon tumour arising from pericytes. Pericytes are cells present external to the endothelial cells of capillaries and venules.

M/E The tumour is composed of capillaries surrounded by spindle-shaped pericytes outside the capillary basement membrane forming whorled arrangement. Silver impregnation stain (i.e. reticulin stain) is employed to confirm the presence of pericytes outside the basement membrane of capillaries and to distinguish it from haemangioendothelioma.

Angiosarcoma *(p. 303)*

Also known as haemangiosarcoma and malignant haemangioendothelioma, it is a malignant vascular tumour occurring most frequently in the skin, subcutaneous tissue, liver, spleen, bone, lung and retroperitoneal tissues. It can occur in both sexes and at any age. *Hepatic angiosarcomas* are of special interest in view of their association with carcinogens like polyvinyl chloride, arsenical pesticides and radioactive contrast medium, thorotrast.

G/A The tumours are usually bulky, pale grey-white, firm masses with poorly-defined margins. Areas of haemorrhage, necrosis and central softening are frequently present.

M/E The tumours may be well-differentiated masses of proliferating endothelial cells around well-formed vascular channels, to poorly-differentiated lesions composed of plump, anaplastic and pleomorphic cells in solid clusters with poorly identifiable vascular channels.

Kaposi's Sarcoma *(p. 303)*

Kaposi's sarcoma is a malignant angiomatous tumour, first described by Kaposi, Hungarian dermatologist, in 1872. However, the tumour has attracted greater attention more recently due to its frequent occurrence in patients with AIDS. Four forms of Kaposi's sarcoma are described:

1. Classic (European) Kaposi's sarcoma. This is the form which was first described by Kaposi. It is more common in men over 60 years of age of Eastern European descent. The disease is slow and appears as multiple, small, purple, dome-shaped nodules or plaques in the skin, especially on the legs. Involvement of visceral organs occurs in about 10% cases after many years.

2. African (Endemic) Kaposi's sarcoma. This form is common in equatorial Africa. It is so common in Uganda that it comprises 9% of all malignant tumours in men. It is found in younger age, especially in boys and in young men and has a more aggressive course than the classic form.

3. Epidemic (AIDS-associated) Kaposi's sarcoma. This form is seen in about 30% cases of AIDS, especially in young male homosexuals than the other high risk groups. The cutaneous lesions are not localised to lower legs but are more extensively distributed involving mucous membranes, lymph nodes and internal organs early in the course of disease.

4. Kaposi's sarcoma in renal transplant cases. This form is associated with recipients of renal transplants who have been administered immunosuppressive therapy for a long time. The lesions may be localised to the skin or may have widespread systemic involvement.

Chapter Eleven

PATHOGENESIS. The etiology of Kaposi's sarcoma is not clearly known.

■ Epidemiological studies have suggested a *viral association* implicating HIV and human herpesvirus 8 (HSV 8, also called Kaposi's sarcoma HSV). The excessive proliferation of mesenchymal spindle cells of vascular origin occurs due to cooperation between HIV-derived protein and angiogenic cytokines (e.g. oncostatin-M, and basic fibroblast growth factor). Higher incidence of Kaposi's sarcoma in male homosexuals is explained by increased secretion of cytokines by their activated immune system.

■ Defective immunoregulation plays a role in its pathogenesis is further substantiated by observation of *second malignancy* (e.g. leukaemia, lymphoma and myeloma) in about one-third of patients with Kaposi's sarcoma.

■ An *HLA association* with classic type of Kaposi's sarcoma has been observed, implying thereby the role of genetic factors in its etiology.

G/A The lesions in the skin, gut and other organs form prominent, irregular, purple, dome-shaped plaques or nodules.

M/E The changes are nonspecific which evolve through the following 2 stages:

■ In the **early patch stage,** there are irregular vascular spaces separated by interstitial inflammatory cells and extravasated blood and haemosiderin.

■ In the **late nodular stage,** there are slit-like vascular spaces containing red blood cells and separated by spindle-shaped, plump tumour cells. These spindle-shaped tumour cells are probably of endothelial origin.

The clinical course and biologic behaviour of Kaposi's sarcoma is quite variable. The classic form of Kaposi's sarcoma is largely confined to skin and the course is generally slow and insidious with long survival. The endemic (African) and epidemic (AIDS-associated) Kaposi's sarcoma, on the other hand, has a rapidly progressive course, often with widespread cutaneous as well as visceral involvement, and high mortality.

Chapter Eleven

■ SELF ASSESSMENT

1. **Vasa vasora perfuse the vessel wall as follows:**
   A. Whole thickness of vessel wall
   B. Whole of adventitia and media
   C. Adventitia and outer half of media
   D. Adventitia and outer two-third of media

2. **Medial calcification of arteries is seen in the following *except*:**
   A. Mönckeberg's arteriosclerosis
   B. Atherosclerosis
   C. Pseudoxanthoma elasticum
   D. Idiopathic calcification of infancy

3. **Atherosclerosis is predominantly a disease of:**
   A. Intima   B. Media
   C. Adventitia   D. Entire vessel wall

4. **The following lipid has highest association with atherosclerosis:**
   A. Triglycerides
   B. Low-density lipoproteins
   C. Very-low density lipoproteins
   D. High density lipoproteins

5. **Hypertension with systolic pressure of 160 mmHg has greater risk of causing atherosclerosis as under:**
   A. 2-times   B. 3-times
   C. 4-times   D. 5-times

6. **The most important mitogen for smooth muscle proliferation in atherosclerosis is:**
   A Platelet-derived growth factor
   B. Fibroblast growth factor
   C. Epidermal growth factor
   D. Transforming growth factor-α

7. **Cytoplasmic anti-neutrophil cytoplasmic antibodies (C-ANCA) is seen in:**
   A Polyarteritis nodosa
   B. Wegener's granulomatosis
   C. Leucocytoclastic vasculitis
   D. Giant cell arteritis

8. **Biopsy of affected artery in the following condition is not only of diagnostic valve but also cures the main symptom of the patient:**
   A Giant cell arteritis
   B. Takayasu's arteritis
   C. Kawasaki disease
   D. Raynaud's disease

9. **The most common site of involvement of atherosclerotic aneurysm is:**
   A Arch of aorta
   B. Thoracic aorta
   C. Suprarenal abdominal aorta
   D. Infrarenal abdominal aorta

10. **The most common cause of dissecting haematoma is:**
    A. Cystic medial necrosis of Erdheim
    B. Trauma during cardiac catheterisation
    C. Systemic hypertension
    D. Marfan syndrome

11. **Dissecting haematoma causes separation of aortic wall as under:**
    A. Between intima and media
    B. Between inner third of media and outer two-third of media
    C. Between inner two-third of media and outer one-third
    D. Between media and adventitia

12. **In Kaposi's sarcoma, the lesions are more extensively distributed at different body sites and visceral organs in:**
    A. Classic (European) type
    B. African (Endemic) type
    C. AIDS-associated
    D. Renal transplant-associated

KEY

1 = D	2 = B	3 = A	4 = B
5 = D	6 = A	7 = B	8 = A
9 = D	10 = C	11 = C	12 = C

12

The Heart

NORMAL STRUCTURE (p. 305)

ANATOMY AND PHYSIOLOGY. The heart is a muscular pump that ejects blood into the vascular tree with sufficient pressure to maintain optimal circulation. The average weight of heart in an adult male is 300-350 gm while that of an adult female is 250-300 gm. The thickness of the right ventricular wall is 0.3 to 0.5 cm while that of the left ventricular wall is 1.3 to 1.5 cm. The blood in the heart chambers moves in a carefully prescribed pathway: venous blood from systemic circulation → right atrium → right ventricle → pulmonary arteries → lungs → pulmonary veins → left atrium → left ventricle → aorta → systemic arterial supply.

The transport of blood is regulated by cardiac valves: two loose flap-like atrioventricular valves, tricuspid on the right and mitral (bicuspid) on the left; and two semilunar valves with three leaflets each, the pulmonary and aortic valves, guarding the outflow tracts. The normal circumference of the valvular openings measures about 12 cm in tricuspid, 8.5 cm in pulmonary, 10 cm in mitral and 7.5 cm in aortic valve.

The wall of the heart consists mainly of the *myocardium* which is covered externally by thin membrane, the *epicardium* or visceral pericardium, and lined internally by another thin layer, the *endocardium.*

The **myocardium** is the muscle tissue of the heart composed of syncytium of branching and anastomosing, transversely striated muscle fibres arranged in parallel fashion. The space between myocardial fibres contains a rich capillary network and loose connective tissue. The myocardial fibres are connected to each other by irregular joints called as *intercalated* discs. They represent the apposed cell membranes of individual cells which act as tight junctions for free transport of ions and action potentials. The cardiac myocyte is very rich in mitochondria which is the source of large amount of ATP required for cardiac contraction. The cardiac muscle fibre has abundant sarcoplasmic reticulum corresponding to endoplasmic reticulum of other cells. Transverse lines divide each fibre into *sarcomeres* which act as structural and functional subunits. Each sarcomere consists of prominent central *dark A-band* attributed to thick myosin filaments and flanked on either side by *light I-bands* consisting of thin actin filament. The actin bands are in the form of twisted rods overlying protein molecules called *tropomyosin.* These protein molecules are of 3 types: *troponin-I, troponin-T, and troponin-C.* Troponin molecules respond to calcium ions in cyclical contraction-relaxation of myocardial fibres.

The **conduction system** of the heart located in the myocardium is responsible for regulating rate and rhythm of the heart. It is composed of specialised Purkinje fibres which contain some contractile myofilaments and conduct action potentials rapidly. The conduction system consists of 4 major components: 1. The *sinoatrial (SA) node;* 2. The *atrioventricular (AV) bundle;* 3. The *atrioventricular (AV) node;* 4. The *bundle of His.*

The **pericardium** consists of a closely apposed layer, *visceral pericardium or epicardium,* and an outer fibrous sac, the *parietal pericardium.* The two layers enclose a narrow pericardial cavity which is lined by mesothelial cells and normally contains 10-30 ml of clear, watery serous fluid. This fluid functions as lubricant and shock absorbant to the heart.

The **endocardium** is the smooth shiny inner lining of the myocardium that covers all the cardiac chambers, the cardiac valves, the chordae tendineae and the papillary muscles. It is lined by endothelium with connective tissue and elastic fibres in its deeper part.

The **valve cusps and semilunar leaflets** are delicate and translucent structures. The valves are strengthened by collagen and elastic tissue and covered by a layer of endothelium (valvular endocardium).

MYOCARDIAL BLOOD SUPPLY. The cardiac muscle, in order to function properly, must receive adequate supply of oxygen and nutrients. There are three major coronary trunks, each supplying blood to specific segments of the heart:

1. The **anterior descending branch of the left coronary artery** supplies most of the apex of the heart, the anterior surface of the left ventricle, the adjacent third of the anterior wall of the right ventricle, and the anterior two-third of the interventricular septum.

2. The **circumflex branch of the left coronary artery** supplies the left atrium and a small portion of the lateral aspect of the left ventricle.

3. The **right coronary artery** supplies the right atrium, the remainder of the anterior surface of the right ventricle, the adjacent half of the posterior wall of the left ventricle and the posterior third of the interventricular septum.

There are 3 anatomic patterns of distribution of the coronary blood supply, depending upon which of the coronary arteries crosses the crux. *Crux* is the region on the posterior surface of the heart where all the four cardiac chambers and the interatrial and interventricular septa meet. These patterns are as under:

■ **Right coronary artery preponderance** is the most common pattern. In this, right coronary artery supplies blood to the whole of right ventricle, the posterior half of the interventricular septum and a part of the posterior wall of the left ventricle by crossing the crux.

■ **Balanced cardiac circulation** is the next most frequent pattern. In this, the right and left ventricles receive blood supply entirely from right and left coronary arteries respectively. The posterior part of the interventricular septum is supplied by a branch of the right coronary while the anterior part is supplied by a branch of the left coronary artery.

■ **Left coronary preponderance** is the least frequent pattern. In this, the left coronary artery supplies blood to the entire left ventricle, whole of interventricular septum and also supplies blood to a part of the posterior wall of the right ventricle by crossing the crux.

HEART FAILURE *(p. 307)*

Heart failure is defined as the pathophysiologic state in which impaired cardiac function is unable to maintain an adequate circulation for the metabolic needs of the tissues of the body. It may be *acute* or *chronic*. The term congestive heart failure (CHF) is used for the chronic form of heart failure in which the patient has evidence of congestion of peripheral circulation and of lungs. CHF is the end-result of various forms of serious heart diseases.

Etiology *(p. 307)*

1. INTRINSIC PUMP FAILURE. The most common and most important cause of heart failure is weakening of the ventricular muscle due to disease so that the heart fails to act as an efficient pump. The various diseases which may culminate in pump failure by this mechanisms are: i) Ischaemic heart disease ii) Myocarditis iii) Cardiomyopathies iv) Metabolic disorders e.g. beriberi v) Disorders of the rhythm e.g. atrial fibrillation and flutter.

2. INCREASED WORKLOAD ON THE HEART. Increased mechanical load on the heart results in increased myocardial demand resulting in myocardial failure. Increased load on the heart may be in the form of pressure load or volume load.

i) Increased pressure load may occur in the following states:

a) Systemic and pulmonary arterial hypertension.

b) Valvular disease e.g. mitral stenosis, aortic stenosis, pulmonary stenosis.

c) Chronic lung diseases.

ii) Increased volume load occurs when a ventricle is required to eject more than normal volume of the blood resulting in cardiac failure. This is found in the following conditions: a) Valvular insufficiency b) Severe anaemia c) Thyrotoxicosis d) Arteriovenous shunts e) Hypoxia due to lung diseases.

3. IMPAIRED FILLING OF CARDIAC CHAMBERS. Decreased cardiac output and cardiac failure may result from extra-cardiac causes or defect in filling of the heart:

a) Cardiac tamponade e.g. haemopericardium, hydropericardium

b) Constrictive pericarditis.

Types of Heart Failure *(p. 308)*

Heart failure may be acute or chronic, right-sided or left-sided, and forward or backward failure.

ACUTE AND CHRONIC HEART FAILURE. Depending upon whether the heart failure develops rapidly or slowly, it may be acute or chronic.

Acute heart failure. Sudden and rapid development of heart failure occurs in the following conditions: i) Larger myocardial infarction ii) Valve rupture iii) Cardiac tamponade iv) Massive pulmonary embolism v) Acute viral myocarditis vi) Acute bacterial toxaemia.

Chronic heart failure. More often, heart failure develops slowly as observed in the following states: i) Myocardial ischaemia from atherosclerotic coronary artery disease ii) Multivalvular heart disease iii) Systemic arterial hypertension iv) Chronic lung diseases resulting in hypoxia and pulmonary arterial hypertension v) Progression of acute into chronic failure.

LEFT-SIDED AND RIGHT-SIDED HEART FAILURE. Though heart as an organ eventually fails as a whole, but functionally, the left and right heart act as independent units. From clinical point of view, therefore, it is helpful to consider failure of the left and right heart separately. The clinical manifestations of heart failure result from the accumulation of excess fluid *upstream* to the left or right cardiac chamber whichever is initially affected (Fig. 12.1).

Left-sided heart failure. Left-sided heart failure is initiated by stress to the left heart. The major causes are: i) Systemic hypertension ii) Mitral or aortic valve disease (stenosis) iii) Ischaemic heart disease iv) Myocardial diseases e.g. cardiomyopathies, myocarditis v) Restrictive pericarditis.

The clinical manifestations of left-sided heart failure result from accumulation of fluid *upstream* in the lungs and from decreased left ventricular output. Accordingly, the major pathologic changes are as under:

i) Pulmonary congestion and oedema causing dyspnoea and orthopnoea.

ii) Decreased left ventricular output causing hypoperfusion and diminished oxygenation of tissues e.g. in kidneys causing ischaemic acute tubular necrosis, in brain causing hypoxic encephalopathy, and in skeletal muscles causing muscular weakness and fatigue.

Right-sided heart failure. Right-sided heart failure occurs more often as a consequence of left-sided heart failure. However, some conditions affect the right ventricle primarily, producing right-sided heart failure. These are as follows:

i) As a consequence of left ventricular failure.

ii) Cor pulmonale in which right heart failure occurs due to intrinsic lung diseases.

iii) Pulmonary or tricuspid valvular disease.

iv) Pulmonary hypertension secondary to pulmonary thromboembolism.

v) Myocardial disease affecting right side.

vi) Congenital heart disease with left-to-right shunt.

Whatever be the underlying cause, the clinical manifestations of right-sided heart failure are *upstream* of the right heart such as systemic and portal venous congestion, and reduced cardiac output. Accordingly, the pathologic changes are as under:

i) Systemic venous congestion in different tissues and organs e.g. subcutaneous oedema on dependent parts, passive congestion of the liver, spleen, and kidneys, ascites, hydrothorax, congestion of leg veins and neck veins.

ii) Reduced cardiac output resulting in circulatory stagnation causing anoxia, cyanosis and coldness of extremities.

In summary, in early stage the left heart failure manifests with features of pulmonary congestion and decreased left ventricular output, while the right heart failure presents with systemic venous congestion and involvement of the liver and spleen. CHF, however, combines the features of both left and right heart failure. A schematic summary of evolution of CHF is presented in Fig. 12.1.

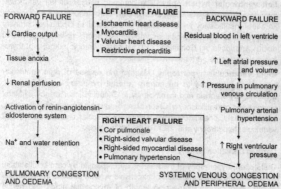

Fig. 12.1: Schematic evolution of congestive heart failure and its effects.

Chapter Twelve

BACKWARD AND FORWARD HEART FAILURE. The mechanism of clinical manifestations resulting from heart failure can be explained on the basis of mutually interdependent backward and forward failure.

Backward heart failure. According to this concept, either of the ventricles fails to eject blood normally, resulting in rise of end-diastolic volume in the ventricle and increase in volume and pressure in the atrium which is transmitted *backward* producing elevated pressure in the veins.

Forward heart failure. According to this hypothesis, clinical manifestations result directly from failure of the heart to pump blood causing diminished flow of blood to the tissues, especially diminished renal perfusion and activation of renin-angiotensin-aldosterone system.

Compensatory Mechanisms: Cardiac Hypertrophy and Dilatation *(p. 310)*

In order to maintain normal cardiac output, several compensatory mechanisms play a role. These include:

■ Compensatory enlargement in the form of *cardiac hypertrophy, cardiac dilatation*, or both.

■ *Tachycardia* (i.e. increased heart rate) due to activation of neurohumoral system e.g. release of norepinephrine and atrial natriouretic peptide, activation of renin-angiotensin-aldosterone mechanism.

Cardiac Hypertrophy *(p. 310)*

Hypertrophy of the heart is defined as an increase in size and weight of the myocardium. It generally results from increased pressure load while increased volume load (e.g. valvular incompetence) results in hypertrophy with dilatation of the affected chamber due to regurgitation of the blood through incompetent valve. The atria may also undergo compensatory changes due to increased workload.

The basic factors that stimulate the hypertrophy of the myocardial fibres are not known. It appears that stretching of myocardial fibres in response to stress induces the cells to increase in length. The elongated fibres receive better nutrition and thus increase in size.

CAUSES. Hypertrophy with or without dilatation may involve predominantly the left or the right heart, or both sides.

Left ventricular hypertrophy. The common causes of left ventricular hypertrophy are: i) Systemic hypertension ii) Aortic stenosis and insufficiency iii) Mitral insufficiency iv) Coarctation of the aorta v) Occlusive coronary artery disease vi) Congenital anomalies like septal defects and patent ductus arteriosus vii) Conditions with increased cardiac output e.g. thyrotoxicosis, anaemia, arteriovenous fistulae.

Right ventricular hypertrophy. Most of the causes of right ventricular hypertrophy are due to pulmonary arterial hypertension. These are: i) Pulmonary stenosis and insufficiency ii) Tricuspid insufficiency iii) Mitral stenosis and/or insufficiency iv) Chronic lung diseases e.g. chronic emphysema, bronchiectasis, pneumoconiosis, pulmonary vascular disease etc. v) Left ventricular hypertrophy and failure of the left ventricle.

Cardiac Dilatation *(p. 311)*

Quite often, hypertrophy of the heart is accompanied by cardiac dilatation. Stress leading to accumulation of excessive volume of blood in a chamber of the heart causes increase in length of myocardial fibres and hence cardiac dilatation as a compensatory mechanism.

CAUSES. Causes of accumulation of excessive volume of blood within the cardiac chambers may result in dilatation of the respective ventricles or both. These are:
i) Valvular insufficiency (mitral and/or aortic insufficiency in left ventricular dilatation, tricuspid and/or pulmonary insufficiency in right ventricular dilatation)
ii) Left-to-right shunts e.g. in VSD
iii) Conditions with high cardiac output e.g. thyrotoxicosis, arteriovenous shunt
iv) Myocardial diseases e.g. cardiomyopathies, myocarditis
v) Systemic hypertension.

G/A Hypertrophy of the myocardium without dilatation is referred to as *concentric,* and when associated with dilatation is called *eccentric.* The weight of the heart is increased above the normal, often over 500 gm. However, excessive epicardial fat is not indicative of true hypertrophy.

The thickness of the left ventricular wall (excluding trabeculae carneae and papillary muscles) above 15 mm is indicative of significant hypertrophy. In concentric hypertrophy, the lumen of the chamber is smaller than usual, while in eccentric hypertrophy the lumen is dilated. In pure hypertrophy, the papillary muscles and trabeculae carneae are rounded and enlarged, while in hypertrophy with dilatation these are flattened.

M/E There is increase in size of individual muscle fibres. There may be multiple minute foci of degenerative changes and necrosis in the hypertrophied myocardium. Ventricular hypertrophy renders the inner part of the myocardium more liable to ischaemia.

EM Reveals increase in the number of myofilaments comprising myofibrils, mitochondrial changes and multiple intercalated discs which are active sites for the formation of new sarcomeres. Besides, the nucleic acid content determinations have shown increase in total RNA and increased ratio of RNA to DNA content of the hypertrophied myocardial fibres.

CONGENITAL HEART DISEASE *(p. 312)*

Congenital heart disease is the abnormality of the heart present from birth. It is the most common and important form of heart disease in the early years of life and is present in about 0.5% of newborn children. The incidence is higher in premature infants.

Congenital anomalies of the heart may be either *shunts* (left-to-right or right-to-left), or defects causing *obstructions* to flow. However, complex anomalies involving *combinations* of shunts and obstructions are also often present. A simple classification of important and common examples of these groups is given in Table 12.1.

TABLE 12.1: Classification of Congenital Heart Diseases.

I.	**MALPOSITIONS OF THE HEART**	
II.	**SHUNTS (CYANOTIC CONGENITAL HEART DISEASE)**	
	A. Left-to-right shunts	
	(Acyanotic or late cyanotic group)	
	1. Ventricular septal defect (VSD)	(25-30%)
	2. Atrial septal defect (ASD)	(10-15%)
	3. Patent ductus arteriosus (PDA)	(10-20%)
	B. Right-to-left shunts (Cyanotic group)	
	1. Tetralogy of Fallot	(6-15%)
	2. Transposition of great arteries	(4-10%)
	3. Persistent truncus arteriosus	(2%)
	4. Tricuspid atresia and stenosis	(1%)
III.	**OBSTRUCTIONS (OBSTRUCTIVE CONGENITAL HEART DISEASE)**	
	1. Coarctation of aorta	(5-7%)
	2. Aortic stenosis and atresia	(4-6%)
	3. Pulmonary stenosis and atresia	(5-7%)

I. MALPOSITIONS OF THE HEART *(p. 312)*

Dextrocardia is the condition when the apex of the heart points to the right side of the chest. It may be accompanied by situs inversus so that all other organs of the body are also transposed in similar way and thus heart is in normal position in relation to them.

II. SHUNTS (CYANOTIC CONGENITAL HEART DISEASE) *(p. 312)*

A shunt may be left-to-right side or right-to-left side of the circulation.

A.   Left-to-Right Shunts (Acyanotic or Late Cyanotic Group) *(p. 312)*

In conditions where there is shunting of blood from left-to-right side of the heart there is volume overload on the right heart producing pulmonary hypertension and right ventricular hypertrophy. At a later stage, the pressure on the right side is higher than on the left side creating late cyanotic heart disease.

1. VENTRICULAR SEPTAL DEFECT (VSD). VSD is the most common congenital anomaly of the heart and comprises about 30% of all congenital heart diseases. The condition is recognised early in life. The smaller defects often close spontaneously, while larger defects remain patent and produce significant effects.

Depending upon the location of the defect, VSD may be of the following types:

1. In 90% of cases, the defect involves *membranous septum* and is very close to the bundle of His.

2. The remaining 10% cases have VSD immediately below the pulmonary valve (*subpulmonic*), below the aortic valve (*subaortic*), or exist in the form of multiple defects in the muscular septum.

The *effects* of VSD are produced due to left-to-right shunt at the ventricular level, increased pulmonary flow and increased volume in the left side of the heart. These effects are:

i)   Volume hypertrophy of the right ventricle.
ii) Enlargement and haemodynamic changes in the tricuspid and pulmonary valves.
iii) Endocardial hypertrophy of the right ventricle.
iv) Pressure hypertrophy of the right atrium.
v)   Volume hypertrophy of the left atrium and left ventricle.

2. ATRIAL SEPTAL DEFECT (ASD). Isolated ASD comprises about 10% of congenital heart diseases. The condition remains unnoticed in infancy and childhood till pulmonary hypertension is induced causing late cyanotic heart disease and right-sided heart failure.

Depending upon the location of the defect, there are 3 types of ASD:

i) Fossa ovalis type or ostium secundum type is the most common form comprising about 90% cases of ASD. The defect is situated in the region of the fossa ovalis.

ii) Ostium primum type comprises about 5% cases of ASD. The defect lies low in the interatrial septum adjacent to atrioventricular valves.

iii) Sinus venosus type accounts for about 5% cases of ASD. The defect is located high in the interatrial septum near the entry of the superior vena cava.

The *effects* of ASD are produced due to left-to-right shunt at the atrial level with increased pulmonary flow. These effects are:

i)   Volume hypertrophy of the right atrium and right ventricle.
ii) Focal or diffuse endocardial hypertrophy of the right atrium and right ventricle.
iii) Volume atrophy of the left atrium and left ventricle.
iv) Small-sized mitral and aortic orifices.

3. PATENT DUCTUS ARTERIOSUS (PDA). The ductus arteriosus is a normal vascular connection between the aorta and the bifurcation of the pulmonary artery. Normally, the ductus closes functionally within the first or second day of life. Its persistence after 3 months of age is considered abnormal.

The *effects* of PDA on heart occur due to left-to-right shunt at the level of ductus resulting in increased pulmonary flow and increased volume in the left heart. These effects are as follows:

i)   Volume hypertrophy of the left atrium and left ventricle.
ii) Enlargement and haemodynamic changes of the mitral and pulmonary valves.
iii) Enlargement of the ascending aorta.

B. Right-to-Left Shunts (Cyanotic Group) *(p. 314)*

In conditions where there is shunting of blood from right side to the left side of the heart, there is entry of poorly-oxygenated blood into systemic circulation resulting in early cyanosis.

1. TETRALOGY OF FALLOT. Tetralogy of Fallot is the most common cyanotic congenital heart disease, found in about 10% of children with anomalies of the heart. The four features of tetralogy are:

i)   Ventricular septal defect (VSD) *('shunt')*.
ii) Displacement of the aorta to right so that it overrides the VSD.
iii) Pulmonary stenosis *('obstruction')*.
iv) Right ventricular hypertrophy.

The severity of the clinical manifestations is related to two factors: extent of pulmonary stenosis and the size of VSD. Accordingly, there are two forms of tetralogy: cyanotic and acyanotic.

In **cyanotic tetralogy,** pulmonary stenosis is greater and the VSD is mild so that there is more resistance to the outflow of blood from right ventricle resulting in right-to-left shunt at the ventricular level and cyanosis. The *effects* on the heart are:

i)   Pressure hypertrophy of the right atrium and right ventricle.
ii) Smaller and abnormal tricuspid valve.
iii) Smaller left atrium and left ventricle.
iv) Enlarged aortic orifice.

In **acyanotic tetralogy,** the VSD is larger and pulmonary stenosis is mild so that there is mainly left-to-right shunt with increased pulmonary flow and increased volume in the left heart but no cyanosis. The *effects* on the heart are:

i)   Pressure hypertrophy of the right ventricle and right atrium.
ii) Volume hypertrophy of the left atrium and left ventricle.
iii) Enlargement of mitral and aortic orifices.

III. OBSTRUCTIONS (OBSTRUCTIVE CONGENITAL HEART DISEASE) *(p. 315)*

Congenital obstruction to blood flow may result from obstruction in the aorta due to narrowing *(coarctation of aorta)*, obstruction to outflow from the left ventricle *(aortic stenosis and atresia)*, and obstruction to outflow from the right ventricle *(pulmonary stenosis and atresia)*.

1. COARCTATION OF AORTA. Coarctation of aorta is localised narrowing in any part of aorta, but the constriction is more often just distal to ductus arteriosus *(postductal or adult)*, or occasionally proximal to the ductus arteriosus *(preductal or infantile type)* in the region of transverse aorta.

i)   In **postductal or adult type,** the obstruction is just distal to the point of entry of ductus arteriosus which is often closed. In the stenotic segment, the aorta is drawn in as if a suture has been tied around it. The aorta is dilated on either side of the constriction. The condition is recognised in adulthood, characterised by hypertension in the upper extremities, weak pulses and low blood pressure in the lower extremities and effects of arterial insufficiency such as claudication and coldness.

ii) In **preductal or infantile type,** the manifestations are produced early in life. The narrowing is proximal to the ductus arteriosus which usually remains patent. The narrowing is generally gradual and involves larger segment of the proximal aorta. There is often associated interatrial septal defect. Preductal coarctation results in right ventricular hypertrophy while the left ventricle is small. Cyanosis develops in the lower half of the body while the upper half remains unaffected.

2. AORTIC STENOSIS AND ATRESIA. The most common congenital anomaly of the aorta is bicuspid aortic valve which does not have much functional significance but predisposes it to calcification. Congenital aortic atresia is rare and incompatible with survival. Aortic stenosis may be acquired (e.g. in rheumatic heart disease, calcific aortic stenosis) or congenital. Congenital aortic stenosis may be of three types:

i) In **valvular stenosis,** the aortic valve cusps are malformed and are irregularly thickened.

ii) In **subvalvular stenosis,** there is thick fibrous ring under the aortic valve causing subaortic stenosis.

iii) In **supravalvular stenosis,** the most uncommon type, there is fibrous constriction above the sinuses of Valsalva.

In all these cases, there is pressure hypertrophy of the left ventricle and left atrium, and dilatation of the aortic root.

3. PULMONARY STENOSIS AND ATRESIA. Pulmonary stenosis is the commonest form of obstructive congenital heart disease comprising about 7% of all congenital heart diseases. It may occur as a component of tetralogy of Fallot or as an isolated defect.

In **pulmonary atresia,** there is no communication between the right ventricle and lungs so that the blood bypasses the right ventricle through an interatrial septal defect. It then enters the lungs via patent ductus arteriosus.

ISCHAEMIC HEART DISEASE *(p. 316)*

Ischaemic heart disease (IHD) is defined as acute or chronic form of cardiac disability arising from imbalance between the myocardial supply and demand for oxygenated blood. Men develop IHD earlier than women and death rates are also slightly higher for men than for women until the menopause.

ETIOPATHOGENESIS *(p. 316)*

IHD is invariably caused by disease affecting the coronary arteries, the most prevalent being atherosclerosis accounting for more than 90% cases, while other causes are responsible for less than 10% cases of IHD.

I. Coronary Atherosclerosis *(p. 316)*

Coronary atherosclerosis resulting in 'fixed' obstruction is the major cause of IHD in more than 90% cases. Here, a brief account of the pathology of lesions in *atherosclerotic coronary artery disease* is presented.

1. Distribution. Atherosclerotic lesions in coronary arteries are distributed in one or more of the three major coronary arterial trunks, the highest incidence being in the anterior descending branch of the left coronary, followed in decreasing frequency, by the right coronary artery and still less in circumflex branch of the left coronary. About one-third of cases have *single-vessel disease*, most often left anterior descending arterial involvement; another one-third have *two-vessel disease,* and the remainder have *three major vessel disease*.

2. Location. Almost all adults show atherosclerotic plaques scattered throughout the coronary arterial system. However, significant stenotic lesions that may produce chronic myocardial ischaemia show more than 75% (three-fourth) reduction in the cross-sectional area of a coronary artery or its branch. The area of severest involvement is about 3 to 4 cm from the coronary ostia, more often at or near the bifurcation of the arteries, suggesting the role of haemodynamic forces in atherogenesis.

3. Fixed atherosclerotic plaques. The atherosclerotic plaques in the coronaries are more often eccentrically located bulging into the lumen from one side. Occasionally, there may be concentric thickening of the wall of the artery. Atherosclerosis produces gradual luminal narrowing that may eventually lead to 'fixed' coronary obstruction.

II. Superadded Changes in Coronary Atherosclerosis *(p. 317)*

The attacks of *acute coronary syndromes,* namely acute myocardial infarction, unstable angina and sudden ischaemic death, are precipitated by certain changes superimposed on a pre-existing fixed coronary atheromatous plaque. These are as under:

1. Acute changes in chronic atheromatous plaque. Though chronic fixed obstructions are the most frequent cause of IHD, acute coronary episodes are often precipitated by sudden changes in chronic plaques such as plaque haemorrhage, fissuring, or ulceration that results in embolisation of atheromatous debris.

2. Coronary artery thrombosis. Transmural acute myocardial infarction is often precipitated by partial or complete coronary thrombosis. The initiation of thrombus occurs due to surface ulceration of fixed chronic atheromatous plaque, ultimately causing complete luminal occlusion. The lipid core of plaque, in particular, is highly thrombogenic.

3. Local platelet aggregation and coronary artery spasm. Some cases of acute coronary episodes are caused by local aggregates of platelets on the atheromatous plaque, short of forming a thrombus. The aggregated platelets release vasospasmic mediators such as thromboxane A_2 which may probably be responsible for coronary vasospasm in the already atherosclerotic vessel.

III. Non-atherosclerotic Causes *(p. 317)*

A number of other lesions may cause IHD in less than 10% of cases. These are as under:
1) Vasospasm. 2) Stenosis of coronary ostia. 3) Arteritis. 4) Embolism. 5) Thrombotic diseases. 6) Trauma. 7) Aneurysms. 8) Compression.

EFFECTS OF MYOCARDIAL ISCHAEMIA *(p. 318)*

Development of lesions in the coronaries is not always accompanied by cardiac disease. Depending upon the suddenness of onset, duration, degree, location and extent of the area affected by myocardial ischaemia, the range of changes and clinical features may vary from an asymptomatic state at one extreme to immediate mortality at another:

A. *Asymptomatic state*
B. Angina pectoris (AP)
C. Acute myocardial infarction (AMI)
D. Chronic ischaemic heart disease (CIHD)/ Ischaemic cardiomyopathy/ Myocardial fibrosis
E. *Sudden cardiac death*

The term *acute coronary syndromes* include a triad of acute myocardial infarction, unstable angina and sudden cardiac death.

ANGINA PECTORIS *(p. 318)*

Angina pectoris is a clinical syndrome of IHD resulting from transient myocardial ischaemia. It is characterised by paroxysmal pain in the substernal or precordial region of the chest which is aggravated by an increase in the demand of the heart and relieved by a decrease in the work of the heart. Often, the pain radiates to the left arm, neck, jaw or right arm.

There are 3 overlapping clinical patterns of angina pectoris with some differences in their pathogenesis:

STABLE OR TYPICAL ANGINA. This is the most common pattern. Stable or typical angina is characterised by attacks of pain following physical exertion or emotional excitement and is relieved by rest. The pathogenesis of condition lies in *chronic stenosing coronary atherosclerosis* that cannot perfuse the myocardium adequately when the workload on the heart increases.

PRINZMETAL'S VARIANT ANGINA. This pattern of angina is characterised by pain at rest and has no relationship with physical activity. The exact pathogenesis of Prinzmetal's angina is not known. It may occur due to *sudden vasospasm* of a coronary trunk induced by coronary atherosclerosis, or may be due to release of humoral vasoconstrictors by mast cells in the coronary adventitia.

UNSTABLE OR CRESCENDO ANGINA. Also referred to as 'pre-infarction angina' or 'acute coronary insufficiency', this is the most serious pattern of angina. It is characterised by more frequent onset of pain of prolonged duration and occurring often at rest. It is thus indicative of an impending myocardial infarction. *Multiple factors* are involved in its pathogenesis which include: stenosing coronary atherosclerosis, complicated coronary plaques (e.g. superimposed thrombosis, haemorrhage, rupture, ulceration etc), platelet thrombi over atherosclerotic plaques and vasospasm of coronary arteries.

ACUTE MYOCARDIAL INFARCTION *(p. 318)*

Acute myocardial infarction (AMI) is the most important consequence of coronary artery disease. Many patients may die within the first few hours of the onset, while remainder suffer from effects of impaired cardiac function. A significant factor that may prevent or diminish the myocardial damage is the development of collateral circulation through anastomotic channels over a period of time. A regular and well-planned exercise programme is likely to encourage good collateral circulation.

INCIDENCE. In industrialised countries, MI accounts for 10-25% of all deaths. Due to the dominant etiologic role of coronary atherosclerosis in MI, the incidence of MI correlates well with the incidence of atherosclerosis in a geographic area.

Age. MI may virtually occur at all ages, though the incidence is higher in the elderly. About 5% of heart attacks occur in young people under the age of 40 years, particularly in those with major risk factors to develop atherosclerosis like hypertension, diabetes mellitus, cigarette smoking, familial hypercholes-terolaemia etc.

Sex. Males throughout their life are at a significantly higher risk of developing MI as compared to females. Women during reproductive period have remarkably low incidence of MI, probably due to the protective influence of oestrogen. The use of oral contraceptives is associated with high risk of developing MI.

ETIOPATHOGENESIS. The etiologic role of severe coronary atherosclerosis (more than 75% compromise of lumen) of one or more of the three major coronary arterial trunks in the pathogenesis of about 90% cases of acute MI is well documented by autopsy studies as well as by coronary angiographic studies. A few notable features in the etiology and pathogenesis of acute MI are considered below:

1. Mechanism of myocardial ischaemia. Myocardial ischaemia is brought about by one or more of the following mechanisms:

i) Diminised coronary blood flow e.g. in coronary artery disease, shock.

ii) Increased myocardial demand e.g. in exercise, emotions.

iii) Hypertrophy of the heart without simultaneous increase of coronary blood flow e.g. in hypertension, valvular heart disease.

2. Role of platelets. Rupture of an atherosclerotic plaque exposes the subendothelial collagen to platelets which undergo aggregation, activation and release reaction. These events contribute to the build-up of the platelet mass that may give rise to emboli or initiate thrombosis.

3. Complicated plaques. Two important complications in coronary atherosclerotic plaques which are frequently encountered are coronary thrombosis and haemorrhage:

i) Superimposed coronary thrombosis is seen in about half the cases of acute MI. Infusion of intracoronary fibrinolysins in the first few hours of development of acute MI in such cases restores blood flow in the blocked vessel in majority of cases.

ii) *Intramural haemorrhage* is found in about one-third cases of acute MI. Haemorrhage and thrombosis may occur together in some cases.

4. Non-atherosclerotic causes. About 10% cases of acute MI are caused by non-atherosclerotic factors such as coronary vasospasm, arteritis, coronary ostial stenosis, embolism, thrombotic diseases, trauma and outside compression.

5. Transmural *versus* subendocardial infarcts. There are some differences in the pathogenesis of the *transmural infarcts* involving the full thickness of ventricular wall and the *subendocardial (laminar) infarcts* affecting the inner subendocardial one-third to half. These are as under (Table 12.2):

TABLE 12.2: Contrasting Features of Subendocardial and Transmural Infarcts.

	FEATURE	TRANSMURAL INFARCT	SUBENDOCARDIAL INFARCT
1.	*Definition*	Full-thickness, solid	Inner third to half, patchy
2.	*Frequency*	Most frequent (95%)	Less frequent
3.	*Distribution*	Specific area of coronary supply	Circumferential
4.	*Pathogenesis*	> 75% coronary stenosis	Hypoperfusion of myocardium
5.	*Coronary thrombosis*	Common	Rare
6.	*Epicarditis*	Common	None

TYPES OF INFARCTS. Infarcts have been classified in a number of ways by the physicians and the pathologists:

1. *According to the anatomic region of the left ventricle involved,* they are called anterior, posterior (inferior), lateral, septal and circumferential, and their combinations like anterolateral, posterolateral (or inferolateral) and anteroseptal.

2. *According to the degree of thickness of the ventricular wall involved,* infarcts are of two types:

i) Full-thickness or transmural, when they involve the entire thickness of the ventricular wall.

ii) Subendocardial or laminar, when they occupy the inner subendocardial half of the myocardium.

3. *According to the age of infarcts,* they are of two types:

i) Newly-formed infarcts are called acute, recent or fresh.

ii) Advanced infarcts are called old, healed or organised.

LOCATION OF INFARCTS. Infarcts are most frequently located in the left ventricle. Right ventricle is less susceptible to infarction due to its thin wall, having less metabolic requirements and is thus adequately nourished by the thebesian vessels. Atrial infarcts, whenever present, are more often in the right atrium, usually accompanying the infarct of the left ventricle. Left atrium is relatively protected from infarction because it is supplied by the oxygenated blood in the left atrial chamber.

The region of infarction depends upon the area of obstructed blood supply by one or more of the three coronary arterial trunks. Accordingly, there are three regions of myocardial infarction:

1. *Stenosis of the left anterior descending coronary artery* is the most common (40-50%). The region of infarction is the anterior part of the left ventricle including the apex and the anterior two-thirds of the interventricular septum.

2. *Stenosis of the right coronary artery* is the next most frequent (30-40%). It involves the posterior part of the left ventricle and the posterior one-third of the interventricular septum.

3. *Stenosis of the left circumflex coronary artery* is seen least frequently (15-20%). Its area of involvement is the lateral wall of the left ventricle.

Early infarcts (3 to 6 hours old) can be detected by histochemical staining for *dehydrogenases* on unfixed slice of the heart. This consists of immersing a slice of unfixed heart in the solution of triphenyltetrazolium chloride (TTC) which imparts red brown colour to the normal heart muscle, while the area of infarcted muscle fails to stain due to lack of dehydrogenases. Another stain for viability of cardiac muscle is nitroblue tetrazolium (NBT) dye which imparts blue colour to unaffected cardiac muscle while infarcted myocardium remains unstained.

A summary of the sequence of gross and microscopic changes in myocardial infarction of varying duration is presented in Table 12.3.

TABLE 12.3: Sequential Pathologic Changes in Myocardial Infarction.

TIME	GROSS CHANGES	LIGHT MICROSCOPY
First week		
0-6 hours	No change or pale; TTC/ NBT test negative in infarcted area	No change; (?) stretching and waviness of fibres
6-12 hours	-do-	Coagulative necrosis begins; neutrophilic infiltration begins; oedema and haemorrhages present
24 hours	Cyanotic red-purple area of haemorrhage	Coagulative necrosis progresses; marginal neutrophilic infiltrate
48-72 hours	Pale, hyperaemic	Coagulative necrosis complete, neutrophilic infiltrate well developed
3-7th day	Hyperaemic border, centre yellow and soft	Neutrophils are necrosed and gradually disappear, beginning of resorption of necrosed fibres by macrophages, onset of fibrovascular response
Second week		
10th day	Red-purple periphery	Most of the necrosed muscle in a small infarct removed; fibrovascular reaction more prominent; pigmented macrophages, eosinophils, lymphocytes, plasma cells present
14th day	—	Necrosed muscle mostly removed; neutrophils disappear; fibrocollagenic tissue at the periphery
Third week	—	Necrosed muscle fibres from larger infarcts removed; more ingrowth of fibrocollagenic tissue
Fourth to sixth week	Thin, grey-white, hard, shrunken fibrous scar	Increased fibrocollagenic tissue, decreased vascularity; fewer pigmented macrophages, lymphocytes and plasma cells

SALVAGE IN EARLY INFARCTS AND REPERFUSION INJURY. In vast majority of cases of AMI, occlusive coronary artery thrombosis has been demonstrated superimposed on fibrofatty plaque. The ischaemic injury to myocardium is reversible if perfusion is restored within the first 20-30 minutes of onset of infarction, failing which irreversible ischaemic necrosis of myocardium sets in. The salvage in early infarcts can be achieved by the following interventions:

1. Institution of *thrombolytic therapy* with thrombolytic agents such as streptokinase and tissue plasminogen activator.
2. *Percutaneous transluminal coronary angioplasty (PTCA).*
3. *Coronary artery stenting.*
4. *Coronary artery bypass surgery.*

However, attempt at reperfusion is fraught with the risk of ischaemic reperfusion injury. Further myonecrosis during reperfusion is possible due to rapid influx of calcium ions and generation of toxic oxygen free radicals.

CHANGES IN EARLY INFARCTS. By special techniques like electron microscopy, chemical and histochemical studies, changes can be demonstrated in early infarcts before detectable light microscopic alterations appear.

1. Electron microscopic changes. Changes by EM examination are evident in less than half an hour of onset of infarction. These changes are:
i) Disappearance of perinuclear glycogen granules within 5 minutes of ischaemia.
ii) Swelling of mitochondria in 20 to 30 minutes.
iii) Disruption of sarcolemma.
iv) Nuclear alterations like peripheral clumping of nuclear chromatin.

2. Chemical and histochemical changes. Analysis of tissues from early infarcts by chemical and histochemical techniques has shown a number of findings. These are:
i) Glycogen depletion in myocardial fibres within 30 to 60 minutes of infarction.
ii) Increase in lactic acid in the myocardial fibres.
iii) Loss of K^+ from the ischaemic fibres.
iv) Increase of Na^+ in the ischaemic cells.
v) Influx of Ca^{++} into the cells causing irreversible cell injury.

Based on the above observations and on leakage of enzymes from the ischaemic myocardium, alterations in the concentrations of various enzymes are detected in the blood of these patients.

DIAGNOSIS. The diagnosis of acute MI is made on the observations of 3 types of features—clinical features, ECG changes, and serum enzyme determinations.

1. Clinical features. Typically, AMI has a sudden onset. i) *Pain;* ii) *Indigestion;* iii) *Apprehension;* iv) *Shock;* v) *Oliguria;* vi) *Low grade fever;* vii) *Acute pulmonary oedema.*

2. ECG changes. The ECG changes are one of the most important parameters. Characteristic ECG changes include ST segment elevation, T wave inversion and appearance of wide deep Q waves.

3. Serum cardiac markers. Certain proteins and enzymes are released into the blood from necrotic heart muscle after MI. Measurement of their levels in serum is helpful in making a diagnosis and plan management. Important myocardial markers in use nowadays are as under:
i) *Creatine phosphokinase (CK) and CK-MB:* CK has three forms—
■ CK-MM derived from skeletal muscle;
■ CK-BB derived from brain and lungs; and
■ CK-MB mainly from cardiac muscles and insignificant amount from extracardiac tissue.

Thus total CK estimation lacks specificity while elevation of CK-MB isoenzyme is considerably specific for myocardial damage. CK-MB has further 2 forms—CK-MB2 is the myocardial form while CK-MB1 is extracardiac form. A ratio of CK-MB2: CK-MB1 above 1.5 is highly sensitive for the diagnosis of acute MI after 4-6 hours of onset of myocardial ischaemia. CK-MB disappears from blood by 48 hours.

ii) *Lactic dehydrogenase (LDH)*. Total LDH estimation also lacks specificity since this enzyme is present in various tissues besides myocardium such as in skeletal muscle, kidneys, liver, lungs and red blood cells. However, like CK, LDH too has two isoforms of which LDH-1 is myocardial-specific. Estimation of ratio of LDH-1: LDH-2 above 1 is reasonably helpful in making a diagnosis. LDH levels begin to rise after 24 hours, reach peak in 3 to 6 days and return to normal in 14 days.

iii) *Cardiac-specific troponins (cTn):* Troponins are contractile muscle proteins present in human cardiac and skeletal muscle but cardiac troponins are specific for myocardium. There are two types of cTn:

■ cardiac troponin T (cTnT); and
■ cardiac troponin I (cTnI).

Both cTnT and cTnI are not found in the blood normally, but after myocardial injury their levels rise very high around the same time when CK-MB is elevated (i.e. after 4-6 hours). Both troponin levels remain high for much longer duration; cTnI for 7-10 days and cTnT for 10-14 days.

iv) *Myoglobin:* Though myoglobin is the first cardiac marker to become elevated after myocardial infarction, it lacks cardiac specificity and is excreted in the urine rapidly. Its levels, thus, return to normal within 24 hours of attack of acute MI.

COMPLICATIONS. Following an attack of acute MI, only 10-20% cases do not develop major complications and recover. The remainder 80-90% cases develop one or more major complications, some of which are fatal. The immediate mortality from acute MI (sudden cardiac death) is about 25%. The important complications which may develop following acute MI are as follows:

1. Arrhythmias. Arrhythmias are the most common form of complications in acute MI.

2. Congestive heart failure. About half the patients with MI develop CHF which may be in the form of right ventricular failure, left ventricular failure or both.

3. Cardiogenic shock. About 10% of patients with acute MI develop cardiogenic shock characterised by hypotension with systolic blood pressure of 80 mmHg or less for many days.

4. Mural thrombosis and thromboembolism. The incidence of thrombo-embolism from intracardiac thrombi and from thrombosis in the leg veins is 15-45% in cases of acute MI and is the major cause of death in 12% cases.

5. Rupture. Rupture of heart occurs in upto 5% cases of acute MI causing death.

6. Cardiac aneurysm. Another 5% of patients of MI develop aneurysm, often of the left ventricle.

7. Pericarditis. Sterile pericarditis appearing on about the second day is common over transmural infarcts.

8. Postmyocardial infarction syndrome. About 3 to 4% of patients who suffered from acute MI develop postmyocardial infarction syndrome or *Dressler's syndrome* subsequently.

CHRONIC ISCHAEMIC HEART DISEASE *(p. 326)*

Chronic ischaemic heart disease, ischaemic cardiomyopathy or myocardial fibrosis are the terms used for focal or diffuse fibrosis in the myocardium

characteristically found in elderly patients of progressive IHD. Such small areas of fibrous scarring are commonly found in the heart of patients who have history of episodes of angina and attacks of MI some years back.

ETIOPATHOGENESIS. The mechanism of development of myocardial fibrosis can be explained by one of the following concepts:

i) Myocardial fibrosis represents healing of minute infarcts.

ii) An alternate concept of development of myocardial fibrosis is healing of minute areas of focal myocytolysis—the myocardial fibres in a small area undergo slow degeneration due to myocardial ischaemia.

G/A The heart may be normal in size or hypertrophied. The left ventricular wall generally shows foci of grey-white fibrosis in brown myocardium. Healed scars of previous MI may be present.

M/E The characteristic features are:

i) There are scattered areas of diffuse myocardial fibrosis, especially around the small blood vessels in the interstitial tissue of the myocardium.

ii) Intervening single fibres and groups of myocardial fibres show variation in fibre size and foci of myocytolysis.

iii) Areas of brown atrophy of the myocardium may also be present.

iv) Coronary arteries show atherosclerotic plaques and may have complicated lesions in the form of superimposed thrombosis.

SUDDEN CARDIAC DEATH *(p. 326)*

Sudden cardiac death is defined as sudden death within 24 hours of the onset of cardiac symptoms. The most important cause is coronary atherosclerosis; less commonly due to coronary vasospasm. The mechanism of sudden death by myocardial ischaemia is almost always by fatal arrhythmias, chiefly ventricular asystole or fibrillation.

At autopsy, such cases reveal most commonly critical atherosclerotic coronary narrowing (more than 75% compromised lumen) in one or more of the three major coronary arterial trunks with superimposed thrombosis or plaque-haemorrhage. Healed and new myocardial infarcts are found in many cases.

Table 12.4 lists the important forms of coronary artery pathology in various types of IHD.

TABLE 12.4: Lesions in Coronary Artery in Various Forms of IHD.

	TYPES OF IHD	CORONARY LESION
1.	*Stable angina*	• Critical coronary narrowing (3/4th)
2.	*Chronic IHD*	• Chronic progressive coronary atherosclerosis
3.	*Unstable (pre-infarction) angina*	• Plaque rupture, haemorrhage, ulceration
		• Mural thrombosis with thromboembolism
4.	*Myocardial infarction*	• Plaque haemorrhage
		• Fissuring and ulceration
		• Complete mural thrombosis
5.	*Sudden ischaemic death*	• Severe multivessel disease
		• Acute changes in plaque
		• Thrombosis with thromboembolism

HYPERTENSIVE HEART DISEASE *(p. 327)*

Hypertensive heart disease or hypertensive cardiomyopathy is the disease of the heart resulting from systemic hypertension of prolonged duration and manifesting by left ventricular hypertrophy. Even mild hypertension (blood pressure higher than 140/90 mm Hg) of sufficient duration may induce

hypertensive heart disease. Amongst the causes of death in hypertensive patients, cardiac decompensation leading to CHF accounts for about one-third of the patients; other causes of death are IHD, cerebrovascular stroke, renal failure following arteriolar nephrosclerosis, and dissecting aneurysm of the aorta.

PATHOGENESIS. Stimulus to hypertrophy of the left ventricle is pressure overload in systemic hypertension. The stress of pressure on the ventricular wall causes increased production of myofilaments, myofibrils, other cell organelles and nuclear enlargement. Since the adult myocardial fibres do not divide, the fibres are hypertrophied. However, the sarcomeres may divide to increase the cell width.

G/A The most significant finding is marked hypertrophy of the heart, chiefly of the left ventricle. The weight of the heart increases to 500 gm or more (normal weight about 300 gm). The thickness of the left ventricular wall increases from its normal 13 to 15 mm upto 20 mm or more. The papillary muscles and trabeculae carneae are rounded and prominent. Initially, there is *concentric hypertrophy* of the left ventricle (without dilatation). But when decompensation and cardiac failure supervene, there is *eccentric hypertrophy (*with dilatation) with thinning of the ventricular wall and there may be dilatation and hypertrophy of right heart as well.

M/E The features are not as prominent as macroscopic appearance. The changes include enlargement and degeneration of myocardial fibres with focal areas of myocardial fibrosis.

COR PULMONALE *(p. 328)*

Cor pulmonale (*cor* = heart; *pulmonale* = lung) or pulmonary heart disease is the disease of right side of the heart resulting from disorders of the lungs. It is characterised by right ventricular dilatation or hypertrophy, or both. Thus, cor pulmonale is the right-sided counterpart of the hypertensive heart disease described above.

Depending upon the rapidity of development, cor pulmonale may be acute or chronic:

■ *Acute cor pulmonale* occurs following massive pulmonary embolism resulting in sudden dilatation of the pulmonary trunk, conus and right ventricle.

■ *Chronic cor pulmonale* is more common and is often preceded by chronic pulmonary hypertension. The various chronic lung diseases causing chronic pulmonary hypertension and subsequent cor pulmonale are: i) chronic emphysema; ii) chronic bronchitis; iii) pulmonary tuberculosis; iv) pneumoconiosis; v) cystic fibrosis; vi) hyperventilation in marked obesity (Pickwickian syndrome); and vii) multiple organised pulmonary emboli.

The sequence of events involved in the pathogenesis of cor pulmonale is summarised in Fig. 12.2.

In *acute cor pulmonale,* there is characteristic ovoid dilatation of the right ventricle, and sometimes of the right atrium. In *chronic cor pulmonale,* there is increase in thickness of the right ventricular wall from its normal 3 to 5 mm upto 10 mm or more. Often, there is dilatation of the right ventricle too.

RHEUMATIC FEVER AND RHEUMATIC HEART DISEASE *(p. 328)*

Rheumatic fever (RF) is a systemic, post-streptococcal, non-suppurative inflammatory disease, principally affecting the heart, joints, central nervous system, skin and subcutaneous tissues. The chronic stage of RF involves all the layers of the heart (pancarditis) causing major cardiac sequelae

Fig. 12.2: Pathogenesis of cor pulmonale
(RVH= right ventricular hypertrophy, RHF= right heart failure).

referred to as rheumatic heart disease (RHD). In spite of its name suggesting an acute arthritis migrating from joint to joint, it is now well known that it is the heart rather than the joints which is first affected. William Boyd years ago gave the dictum *'rheumatism licks the joint, but bites the whole heart'.*

INCIDENCE *(p. 329)*

The disease appears most commonly in children between the age of 5 to 15 years when the streptococcal infection is most frequent and intense. Both the sexes are affected equally, though some investigators have noted a slight female preponderance.

Its incidence has declined in the developed countries as a result of improved living conditions and use of antibiotics in streptococcal infection. But it is still common in the developing countries of the world like in India, Pakistan, some Arab countries, parts of Africa and South America. In India, RHD and RF continue to be a major public health problem. In a multicentric survey in school-going children by the Indian Council of Medical Research, an incidence of 1 to 5.5 per 1000 children has been reported.

ETIOPATHOGENESIS *(p. 329)*

After a long controversy, the etiologic role of preceding throat infection with β-haemolytic streptococci of group A in RF is now generally accepted. However, the mechanism of lesions in the heart, joints and other tissues is not by direct infection but by induction of hypersensitivity or autoimmunity. Thus, there are 2 types of evidences in the etiology and pathogenesis of RF and RHD: the *epidemiologic evidence* and the *immunologic evidence.*

A EPIDEMIOLOGIC EVIDENCE. There is a body of clinical and epidemiological evidence to support the concept that RF occurs following infection of the throat and upper respiratory tract with β-haemolytic streptococci of Lancefield group A. These evidences are as under:
1. There is often a *history* of infection of the pharynx and upper respiratory tract with this microorganism about 2 to 3 weeks prior to the attack of RF.
2. *Subsequent attacks* of streptococcal infection are generally associated with exacerbations of RF.
3. A higher incidence of RF has been observed after outbreaks and *epidemics* of streptococcal infection of throat in children from schools or in young men from training camps.

4. Administration of *antibiotics* leads to lowering of the incidence as well as severity of RF and its recurrences.

5. Cardiac lesions similar to those seen in RHD have been produced in experimental animals by *induction* of repeated infection with β-haemolytic streptococci of group A.

6. Patients with RF have *elevated titres* of antibodies to the antigens of β-haemolytic streptococci of group A such as antistreptolysin O (ASO) and S, antistreptokinase, antistreptohyaluronidase and anti- DNAase B.

7. *Socioeconomic factors* like poverty, poor nutrition, density of population, overcrowding in quarters for sleeping etc are associated with spread of infection, lack of proper medical attention, and hence higher incidence of RF.

8. The *geographic distribution* of the disease, as already pointed out, shows higher frequency and severity of the disease in the developing countries of the world where the living conditions are substandard and medical facilities are insufficient.

9. The incidence of the disease is higher in subtropical and tropical regions with cold, damp climate near the rivers and water-ways which favour the spread of infection.

10. The *individual susceptibility* to RF and familial incidence have been reported.

Despite all these evidences, only a small proportion of patients with streptococcal pharyngeal infection develop RF—the attack rate is less than 3%. There is a suggestion that a *concomitant virus* enhances the effect of streptococci in individuals who develop RF.

B. IMMUNOLOGIC EVIDENCE. It has ben observed that though throat of patients during acute RF contain streptococci, the clinical symptoms of RF appear after a delay of 2-3 weeks and the organisms can not be grown from the lesions in the target tissues. This has led to the concept that lesions are produced as a result of immune response by formation of autoantibodies against bacteria. A number of components of *Streptococcus* identify or cross-react with target human tissues in RHD i.e. cardiac muscle, valves, joints, skin, neurons etc. One such important component is *M-protein* identified as a surface protein of streptococcus which has various antigenic types, and hence corresponding antibodies in humans which target different tissues. The evidences in support are as under:

1. *Cell wall polysaccharide* of group A streptococcus forms antibodies which are reactive against cardiac valves. This is supported by observation of persistently elevated corresponding autoantibodies in patients who have cardiac valvular involvement.

2. *Hyaluronate capsule* of group A streptococcus is identical to human hyaluronate present in joint tissues and thus these tissues are the target of attack.

3. *Membrane antigens* of group A streptococcus react with sarcolemma of smooth and cardiac muscle, dermal fibroblasts and neurons of caudate nucleus.

MORPHOLOGY

RF is generally regarded as an autoimmune focal inflammatory disorder of the connective tissues throughout the body. The *cardiac lesions* of RF in the form of pancarditis, particularly the valvular lesions, are its major manifestations. However, supportive connective tissues at other sites like the synovial membrane, periarticular tissue, skin and subcutaneous tissue, arterial wall, lungs, pleura and the CNS are all affected (*extracardiac lesions*).

A. Cardiac Lesions *(p. 330)*

The pathognomonic feature of pancarditis in RF is the presence of distinctive *Aschoff nodules* or *Aschoff bodies.*

THE ASCHOFF NODULES OR BODIES. The Aschoff nodules or the Aschoff bodies are spheroidal or fusiform distinct tiny structures, 1-2 mm in size, occurring in the interstitium of the heart in RF and may be visible to naked eye. They are especially found in the vicinity of small blood vessels in the myocardium and endocardium and occasionally in the pericardium and the adventitia of the proximal part of the aorta. Lesions similar to the Aschoff nodules may be found in the extracardiac tissues.

Evolution of fully-developed Aschoff bodies involves 3 stages all of which may be found in the same heart at different stages of development. These are as follows:

1.   Early (exudative or degenerative) stage. The earliest sign of injury in the heart in RF is apparent by *about 4th week* of illness. Initially, there is oedema of the connective tissue and increase in acid mucopolysaccharide in the ground substance. This results in separation of the collagen fibres by accumulating ground substance. This change is referred to as *fibrinoid degeneration.*

2.   Intermediate (proliferative or granulomatous) stage. It is this stage of the Aschoff body which is pathognomonic of rheumatic conditions. This stage is apparent in 4th to 13th week of illness. The early stage of fibrinoid change is followed by proliferation of cells that includes infiltration by lymphocytes (mostly T cells), plasma cells, a few neutrophils and the characteristic *cardiac histiocytes (Anitschkow cells)* at the margin of the lesion. Cardiac histiocytes or Anitschkow cells are present in small numbers in normal heart but their number is increased in the Aschoff bodies; therefore they are not characteristic of RHD. These are large mononuclear cells having central round nuclei and contain moderate amount of amphophilic cytoplasm. Some of these modified cardiac histiocytes become multinucleate cells containing 1 to 4 nuclei and are called *Aschoff cells* and are pathognomonic of RHD.

3. Late (healing or fibrous) stage. The stage of healing by fibrosis of the Aschoff nodule occurs in about *12 to 16 weeks* after the illness. The nodule becomes oval or fusiform in shape, about 200 μm wide and 600 μm long. The Anitschkow cells in the nodule become spindle-shaped with diminished cytoplasm and the nuclei stain solidly rather than showing vesicular character. These cells tend to be arranged in a palisaded manner.

RHEUMATIC PANCARDITIS. Although all the three layers of the heart are affected in RF, the intensity of their involvement is variable.

1.   RHEUMATIC ENDOCARDITIS. Endocardial lesions of RF may involve the valvular and mural endocardium, causing *rheumatic valvulitis* and *mural endocarditis,* respectively. Rheumatic valvulitis is chiefly responsible for the major cardiac manifestations in chronic RHD.

RHEUMATIC VALVULITIS. *G/A* The valves in **acute RF** show thickening and loss of translucency of the valve leaflets or cusps. This is followed by the formation of characteristic, small (1 to 3 mm in diameter), multiple, warty *vegetations* or *verrucae,* chiefly along the line of closure of the leaflets and cusps. These tiny vegetations are almost continuous so that the free margin of the cusps or leaflets appears as a rough and irregular ridge. The vegetations in RF appear grey-brown, translucent and are firmly attached so that they are not likely to get detached to form emboli, unlike the friable vegetations of infective endocarditis.

Though all the four heart valves are affected, their frequency and severity of involvement varies: mitral valve alone being the most common site, followed in decreasing order of frequency, by combined mitral and aortic valve. The higher incidence of vegetations on left side of the heart is possibly because of the greater mechanical stresses on the valves of the left heart, especially along the line of closure of the valve cusps.

The **chronic stage of RHD** is characterised by permanent deformity of one or more valves, especially the mitral (in 98% cases alone or along with other valves) and aortic as under:

- Mitral alone = 37% cases.
- Mitral + aortic = 27% cases.
- Mitral + aortic + tricuspid = 22% cases.
- Mitral + tricuspid = 11% cases.
- Aortic alone = 2%.
- Mitral + aortic + tricuspid + pulmonary = less than 1% cases.

Gross appearance of chronic healed mitral valve in RHD is characteristically *'fish mouth'* or *'button hole'* stenosis. Mitral stenosis and insufficiency are commonly combined in chronic RHD; calcific aortic stenosis may also be found.

M/E The inflammatory changes begin in the region of the valve rings (where the leaflets are attached to the fibrous annulus) and then extend throughout the entire leaflet, whereas vegetations are usually located on the free margin of the leaflets and cusps.

i) In the **early (acute) stage,** the histological changes are oedema of the valve leaflet, presence of increased number of capillaries and infiltration with lymphocytes, plasma cells, histiocytes with many Anitschkow cells and a few polymorphs.

ii) In the **healed (chronic) stage,** the vegetations have undergone organisation. The valves show diffuse thickening as a result of fibrous tissue with hyalinisation, and often calcification.

RHEUMATIC MURAL ENDOCARDITIS. Mural endocardium may also show features of rheumatic carditis though the changes are less conspicuous as compared to valvular changes.

G/A The lesions are seen most commonly as *MacCallum's patch* which is the region of endocardial surface in the posterior wall of the left atrium just above the posterior leaflet of the mitral valve. MacCallum's patch appears as a map-like area of thickened, roughened and wrinkled part of the endocardium.

M/E The appearance of MacCallum's patch is similar to that seen in rheumatic valvulitis. The affected area shows oedema, fibrinoid change in the collagen, and cellular infiltrate of lymphocytes, plasma cells and macrophages with many Anitschkow cells.

2. RHEUMATIC MYOCARDITIS. *G/A* In the *early (acute) stage,* the myocardium, especially of the left ventricle, is soft and flabby. In the *intermediate stage,* the interstitial tissue of the myocardium shows small foci of necrosis. Later, tiny pale foci of the Aschoff bodies may be visible throughout the myocardium.

M/E The most characteristic feature of rheumatic myocarditis is the presence of distinctive Aschoff bodies. These diagnostic nodules are scattered throughout the interstitial tissue of the myocardium and are most frequent in the interventricular septum, left ventricle and left atrium.

3. RHEUMATIC PERICARDITIS. *G/A* The usual finding is fibrinous pericarditis in which there is loss of normal shiny pericardial surface due to deposition of fibrin on its surface and accumulation of slight amount of fibrinous exudate in the pericardial sac. If the parietal pericardium is pulled off from the visceral pericardium, the two separated surfaces are shaggy due to thick fibrin covering them. This appearance is often likened to *'bread and butter appearance'* i.e. resembling the buttered surfaces of two slices in a sandwich when they are gently pulled apart.

M/E Fibrin is identified on the surfaces. The subserosal connective tissue is infiltrated by lymphocytes, plasma cells, histiocytes and a few neutrophils. Characteristic Aschoff bodies may be seen which later undergo organisation and fibrosis.

B. Extracardiac Lesions *(p. 333)*

Patients of the syndrome of acute rheumatism develop lesions in connective tissue elsewhere in the body, chiefly the joints, subcutaneous tissue, arteries, brain and lungs.

1. POLYARTHRITIS. Acute and painful inflammation of the synovial membranes of some of the joints, especially the larger joints of the limbs, is seen in about 90% cases of RF in adults and less often in children. As pain and swelling subside in one joint, others tend to get involved, producing the characteristic *'migratory polyarthritis'* involving two or more joints at a time.

M/E The changes are transitory. The synovial membrane and the periarticular connective tissue show hyperaemia, oedema, fibrinoid change and neutrophilic infiltration.

2. SUBCUTANEOUS NODULES. The subcutaneous nodules of RF occur more often in children than in adult. These nodules are small (0.5 to 2 cm in diameter), spherical or ovoid and painless. They are attached to deeper structures like tendons, ligaments, fascia or periosteum and therefore often remain unnoticed by the patient. Characteristic locations are extensor surfaces of the wrists, elbows, ankles and knees.

M/E The subcutaneous nodules of RF are representative of giant Aschoff bodies of the heart. They consist of 3 distinct zones: a central area with fibrinoid changes, surrounded by a zone of histiocytes and fibroblasts forming a palisade arrangement, and the outermost zone of connective tissue which is infiltrated by non-specific chronic inflammatory cells and proliferating blood vessels.

3. ERYTHEMA MARGINATUM. This non-pruritic erythematous rash is characteristic of RF. The lesions occur mainly on the trunk and proximal parts of the extremities.

4. RHEUMATIC ARTERITIS. Arteritis in RF involves not only the coronary arteries and aorta but also occurs in arteries of various other organs such as renal, mesenteric and cerebral arteries.

5. CHOREA MINOR. Chorea minor or Sydenham's chorea or Saint Vitus' dance is a delayed manifestation of RF as a result of involvement of the central nervous system. The condition is characterised by disordered and involuntary jerky movements of the trunk and the extremities accompanied by some degree of emotional instability.

M/E The lesions are located in the cerebral hemispheres, brainstem and the basal ganglia. They consist of small haemorrhages, oedema and perivascular infiltration of lymphocytes.

6. RHEUMATIC PNEUMONITIS AND PLEURITIS. Involvement of the lungs and pleura occurs rarely in RF. Pleuritis is often accompanied with serofibrinous pleural effusion but definite Aschoff bodies are not present. In rheumatic pneumonitis, the lungs are large, firm and rubbery.

Chapter Twelve

CLINICAL FEATURES *(p. 334)*

For diagnosis, the following set of guidelines called *revised Jones' criteria* are followed:

A. Major criteria are: 1) Carditis 2) Polyarthritis 3) Chorea (Sydenham's chorea) 4) Erythema marginatum 5) Subcutaneous nodules

B. Minor criteria are: 1) Fever 2) Arthralgia 3) Previous history of RF 4) Laboratory findings of elevated ESR, raised C-reactive protein, and leucocytosis 5) ECG finding of prolonged PR interval.

C. Supportive evidence of preceding group A streptococcal infection: positive throat culture for group A streptococci, raised titres of streptococcal antibodies (antistreptolysin O and S, antistreptokinase, antistreptohyaluronidase and anti DNAase B).

Clinical diagnosis of RF is made in a case with antecedent laboratory evidence of streptococcal throat infection in the presence of: any two of the major criteria, or occurrence of one major and two minor criteria.

If the heart is spared in a case of acute RF, the patient may have complete recovery without any sequelae. However, once the heart is involved, it is often associated with reactivation and recurrences of the disease. Myocarditis, in particular, is the most life-threatening due to involvement of the conduction system of the heart and results in serious arrhythmias. The long-term sequelae or **stigmata** are the chronic valvular deformities, especially the mitral stenosis. Initially, a state of compensation occurs, while later decompensation of the heart leads to full-blown cardiac failure. Currently, surgical replacement of the damaged valves can alter the clinical course of the disease.

The major **causes of death** in RHD are cardiac failure, bacterial endocarditis and embolism.

NON-RHEUMATIC ENDOCARDITIS *(p. 335)*

Inflammatory involvement of the endocardial layer of the heart is called endocarditis. Though in common usage, if not specified endocarditis would mean inflammation of the valvular endocardium, several workers designate endocarditis on the basis of anatomic area of the involved endocardium such as: *valvular* for valvular endocardium, *mural* for inner lining of the lumina of cardiac chambers, *chordal* for the endocardium of the chordae tendineae, *trabecular* for the endocardium of trabeculae carneae, and *papillary* for the endocardium covering the papillary muscles. Most types of endocarditis are characterised by the presence of 'vegetations' or 'verrucae' which have distinct features. A summary of the distinguishing features of the principal types of vegetations is presented in Table 12.6.

ATYPICAL VERRUCOUS (LIBMAN-SACKS) ENDOCARDITIS *(p. 335)*

Libman and Sacks, two American physicians, described a form of endocarditis in 1924 that is characterised by sterile endocardial vegetations which are distinguishable from the vegetations of RHD and bacterial endocarditis.

ETIOPATHOGENESIS. Atypical verrucous endocarditis is one of the manifestations of 'collagen diseases'. Characteristic lesions of Libman-Sacks endocarditis are seen in *50% cases of acute systemic lupus erythematosus (SLE);* other diseases associated with this form of endocarditis are systemic sclerosis, thrombotic thrombocytopenic purpura (TTP) and other collagen diseases.

G/A Characteristic vegetations occur most frequently on the mitral and tricuspid valves. The vegetations of atypical verrucous endocarditis are small (1 to 4 mm in diameter), granular, multiple and tend to occur on both surfaces of affected valves, in the valve pockets and on the adjoining ventricular and atrial endocardium. The vegetations are sterile unless superimposed by bacterial endocarditis.

M/E The verrucae of Libman-Sacks endocarditis are composed of fibrinoid material with superimposed fibrin and platelet thrombi. The endocardium underlying the verrucae shows characteristic histological changes which include fibrinoid necrosis, proliferation of capillaries and infiltration by histiocytes, plasma cells, lymphocytes, neutrophils and the pathognomonic *haematoxylin bodies of Gross* which are counterparts of LE cells of the blood.

NON-BACTERIAL THROMBOTIC (CACHECTIC, MARANTIC) ENDOCARDITIS (p. 335)

Non-bacterial thrombotic, cachectic, marantic or terminal endocarditis or endocarditis simplex is an involvement of the heart valves by sterile thrombotic vegetations.

ETIOPATHOGENESIS. The exact pathogenesis of lesions in non-bacterial thrombotic endocarditis (NBTE) is not clear. These vegetations are found at autopsy in 0.5 to 5% of cases. The following diseases and conditions are frequently associated with their presence:

1. In patients dying of *chronic debilitating diseases* e.g. advanced cancer (in 50% case of NBTE), chronic tuberculosis, renal failure and chronic sepsis. Hence, the names such as 'cachectic', 'marantic' and 'terminal' endocarditis are used synonymously with NBTE.

2. Occurrence of these lesions in young and well-nourished patients is explained on the basis of *alternative hypothesis* such as allergy, vitamin C deficiency, deep vein thrombosis, and endocardial trauma.

G/A The verrucae of NBTE are located on cardiac valves, chiefly the mitral, and less often aortic and tricuspid. These verrucae are usually small (1 to 5 mm in diameter), single or multiple, brownish and occur along the line of closure of the leaflets but are more friable than the vegetations of RHD. Normal age-related appearance of tag-like appendage at the margin of the valve cusps known as 'Lambl's excrescences' is an example of such healed lesions.

M/E The vegetations in NBTE are composed of fibrin along with entangled RBCs, WBCs and platelets.

BACTERIAL ENDOCARDITIS (p. 336)

Bacterial endocarditis (BE) is serious infection of the valvular and mural endocardium caused by different forms of bacteria (other than tubercle bacilli and non-bacterial microorganisms) and is characterised by typical infected and friable vegetations. Depending upon the severity of infection, BE is subdivided into 2 clinical forms (Table 12.5):

1. **Acute bacterial endocarditis (ABE)** is the fulminant and destructive acute infection of the endocardium by highly virulent bacteria in a previously normal heart and almost invariably runs a rapidly fatal course in a period of 2-6 weeks.

2. **Subacute bacterial endocarditis (SABE) or endocarditis lenta** (*lenta* = slow) is caused by less virulent bacteria in a previously diseased heart and has a gradual downhill course in a period of 6 weeks to a few months and sometimes years.

INCIDENCE. Introduction of antibiotic drugs has helped greatly in lowering the incidence of BE as compared with its incidence in the pre-antibiotic era.

TABLE 12.5: Distinguishing Features of Acute and
Subacute Bacterial Endocarditis.

	FEATURE	ACUTE	SUBACUTE
1.	*Duration*	<6 weeks	>6 weeks
2.	*Most common organisms*	*Staph. aureus,* β-streptococci	*Streptococcus viridans*
3.	*Virulence of organisms*	Highly virulent	Less virulent
4.	*Previous condition of valves*	Usually previously normal	Usually previously damaged
5.	*Lesion on valves*	Invasive, destructive, suppurative	Usually not invasive or suppurative
6.	*Clinical features*	Features of acute infection systemic	Splenomegaly, clubbing of fingers, petechiae

Though BE may occur at any age, most cases of ABE as well as SABE occur over 50 years of age. Males are affected more often than females.

ETIOLOGY. All cases of BE are caused by *infection with microorganisms* in patients having certain predisposing factors.

A. Infective agents. About 90% cases of BE are caused by streptococci and staphylococci.

■ *In ABE,* the most common causative organisms are virulent strains of staphylococci, chiefly *Staphylococcus aureus.* Others are pneumococci, gonococci, β-streptococci and enterococci.

■ *In SABE,* the commonest causative organisms are the streptococci with low virulence, predominantly *Streptococcus viridans,* which forms part of normal flora of the mouth and pharynx. Other less common etiologic agents include other strains of streptococci and staphylococci.

B. Predisposing factors. There are 3 main factors which predispose to the development of both forms of BE:

1. conditions initiating transient bacteraemia, septicaemia and pyaemia;
2. underlying heart disease; and
3. impaired host defenses.

1. *Bacteraemia, septicaemia and pyaemia:* Bacteria gain entrance to the bloodstream causing transient and clinically silent bacteraemia in a variety of day-to-day procedures as well as from other sources of infection. Some of the common examples are:

i) Periodontal infections such as trauma from vigorous brushing of teeth, hard chewing, tooth extraction and other dental procedures.

ii) Infections of the genitourinary tract such as in catheterisation, cystoscopy, obstetrical procedures including normal delivery and abortions.

iii) Infections of gastrointestinal and biliary tract.

iv) Surgery of the bowel, biliary tract and genitourinary tracts.

v) Skin infections such as boils, carbuncles and abscesses.

vi) Upper and lower respiratory tract infections including bacterial pneumonias.

vii) Intravenous drug abuse.

viii) Cardiac catheterisation and cardiac surgery for implantation of prosthetic valves.

2. *Underlying heart disease:* SABE occurs much more frequently in previously diseased heart valves, whereas the ABE is common in previously normal heart. Amongst the commonly associated underlying heart diseases are the following:

i) Chronic rheumatic valvular disease in about 50% cases.

TABLE 12.6: Distinguishing Features of Vegetations in Major Forms of Endocarditis.

FEATURE	RHEUMATIC	LIBMAN-SACKS	NON-BACTERIAL THROMBOTIC	BACTERIAL
1. **Valves commonly affected**	Mitral alone; mitral and aortic combined	Mitral, tricuspid	Mainly mitral; less often aortic and tricuspid	Mitral; aortic; combined mitral and aortic
2. **Location on valve cusps or leaflets**	Occur along the line of closure, atrial surface of atrio-ventricular valves and ventricular surface of semilunar valves	Occur on both surfaces of valve leaflets or cusps, in the valve pockets	Occur along the line of closure	SABE more often on diseased valves: ABE on previously normal valves; location same as in RHD
3. **Macroscopy**	Small, multiple, warty, grey brown, translucent, firmly attached, generally produce permanent valvular deformity	Medium-sized, multiple, generally do not produce significant valvular deformity	Small but larger than those of rheumatic, single or multiple, brownish, firm, but more friable than those of rheumatic	Often large, grey-tawny to greenish, irregular, single or multiple, typically friable
4. **Microscopy**	Composed of fibrin with super-imposed platelet thrombi and no bacteria. Adjacent and underlying endocardium shows oedema, proliferation of capillaries, mononuclear inflammatory infiltrate and occasional Aschoff bodies.	Composed of fibrinoid material with superimposed fibrin and platelet thrombi and no bacteria. The underlying endocardium shows fibrinoid necrosis, proliferation of capillaries and acute and chronic inflammatory infiltrate including the haematoxylin bodies of Gross.	Composed of degenerated valvular tissue, fibrin-platelets thrombi and no bacteria. The underlying valve shows swelling of collagen, fibrinoid change, proliferation of capillaries but no significant inflammatory cell infiltrate.	Composed of outer eosinophilic zone of fibrin and platelets, covering colonies of bacteria and deeper zone of non-specific acute and chronic inflammatory cells. The underlying endocardium may show abscesses in ABE and inflammatory granulation tissue in the SABE.

Chapter Twelve

ii)   Congenital heart diseases in about 20% cases.

iii)   Other causes are syphilitic aortic valve disease, atherosclerotic valvular disease, floppy mitral valve, and prosthetic heart valves.

3.   *Impaired host defenses:* All conditions in which there is depression of specific immunity, deficiency of complement and defective phagocytic function, predispose to BE e.g.

i)   Impaired specific immunity in lymphomas.

ii)   Leukaemias.

iii)   Cytotoxic therapy for various forms of cancers and transplant patients.

iv)   Deficient functions of neutrophils and macrophages.

PATHOGENESIS. There are different hypotheses to explain the occurrence of bacterial implants on the valves:

1.   The circulating bacteria are lodged much more frequently on *previously damaged valves* from diseases, chiefly RHD and congenital heart diseases, than on healthy valves.

2.   Conditions producing *haemodynamic stress* on the valves are liable to cause damage to the endothelium, favouring the formation of platelet thrombi which get infected from circulating bacteria.

3.   Another alternative hypothesis is the occurrence of *non-bacterial thrombotic endocarditis* from prolonged stress which is followed by bacterial contamination.

G/A The lesions are found commonly on the valves of the left heart, most frequently on the mitral, followed in descending frequency, by the aortic, simultaneous involvement of both mitral and aortic valves, and quite rarely on the valves of the right heart. The vegetations in SABE are more often seen on previously diseased valves, whereas the vegetations of ABE are often found on previously normal valves. Like in RHD, the vegetations are often located on the atrial surface of atrioventricular valves and ventricular surface of the semilunar valves. They begin from the contact areas of the valve and may extend along the surface of the valves and on to the adjacent endocardium.

The *vegetations* of BE vary in size from a few millimetres to several centimetres, grey-tawny to greenish, irregular, single or multiple, and typically *friable.* They may appear flat, filiform, fungating or polypoid. The vegetations in ABE tend to be bulkier and globular than those of SABE and are located more often on previously normal valves, may cause ulceration or perforation of the underlying valve leaflet, or may produce myocardial abscesses.

M/E The vegetations of BE consist of 3 zones:

i)   The *outer layer or cap* consists of eosinophilic material composed of fibrin and platelets.

ii)   Underneath this layer is the *basophilic zone* containing colonies of bacteria.

iii)   The *deeper zone* consists of non-specific inflammatory reaction in the cusp itself, and in the case of SABE there may be evidence of repair.

In the acute fulminant form of the disease, the inflammatory cell infiltrate chiefly consists of neutrophils and is accompanied with tissue necrosis and abscesses in the valve rings and in the myocardium. In the subacute form, there is healing by granulation tissue, mononuclear inflammatory cell infiltration and fibroblastic proliferation. Histological evidence of pre-existing valvular disease such as RHD may be present in SABE.

COMPLICATIONS AND SEQUELAE. Most cases of BE present with fever. The acute form of BE is characterised by high grade fever, chills, weakness and malaise while the subacute form of the disease has non-specific manifestations like slight fever, fatigue, loss of weight and flu-like symptoms.

In the early stage, the lesions are confined to the heart, while subsequent progression of the disease leads to involvement of extracardiac organs. In general, severe complications develop early in ABE than in SABE. Complications and sequelae of BE are divided into cardiac and extracardiac:

A. Cardiac complications. These include the following:
i)   Valvular stenosis or insufficiency
ii) Perforation, rupture, and aneurysm of valve leaflets
iii) Abscesses in the valve ring
iv) Myocardial abscesses
v)   Suppurative pericarditis
vi) Cardiac failure from one or more of the foregoing complications.

B. Extracardiac complications. Since the vegetations in BE are typically friable, they tend to get dislodged due to rapid stream of blood and give rise to embolism which is responsible for very common and serious extracardiac complications. These are as under:
i) Emboli originating from the *left side of the heart* and entering the systemic circulation affect organs like the spleen, kidneys, and brain causing infarcts, abscesses and mycotic aneurysms.
ii) Emboli arising from *right side of the heart* enter the pulmonary circulation and produce pulmonary abscesses.
iii) *Petechiae* may be seen in the skin and conjunctiva due to either emboli or toxic damage to the capillaries.
iv) In SABE, there are painful, tender nodules on the finger tips of hands and feet called *Osler's nodes*, while in ABE there is appearance of painless, non-tender subcutaneous maculopapular lesions on the pulp of the fingers called *Janeway's spots*. In either case, their origin is due to toxic or allergic inflammation of the vessel wall.
v) *Focal necrotising glomerulonephritis* is seen more commonly in SABE than in ABE. Occasionally diffuse glomerulonephritis may occur.

The *causes of death* are cardiac failure, persistent infection, embolism to vital organs, renal failure and rupture of mycotic aneurysm of cerebral arteries.

VALVULAR DISEASES AND DEFORMITIES (p. 341)

The valvular deformities may be of 2 types: stenosis and insufficiency. *Stenosis* is the term used for failure of a valve to open completely during diastole resulting in obstruction to the forward flow of the blood. *Insufficiency or incompetence or regurgitation* is the failure of a valve to close completely during systole resulting in back flow or regurgitation of the blood.

MITRAL STENOSIS (p. 341)

Mitral stenosis occurs in approximately 40% of all patients with RHD. About 70% of the patients are women. The latent period between the rheumatic carditis and development of symptomatic mitral stenosis is about two decades.

ETIOLOGY. Mitral stenosis is generally rheumatic in origin. Less common causes include bacterial endocarditis, Libman-Sacks endocarditis, endocardial fibroelastosis and congenital parachute mitral valve.

G/A There are fibrous adhesions of mitral commissures and fusion and shortening of chordae tendineae. In less extensive involvement, the bases of the leaflets of mitral valve are mobile while the free margins have puckered and thickened tissue with narrowed orifice; this is called as *'purse-string puckering'*. The more advanced cases have rigid, fixed and immobile diaphragm-like valve leaflets with narrow, slit-like or oval mitral opening, commonly referred to as *'button-hole'* or *'fish-mouth'* mitral orifice.

EFFECTS 1. Dilatation and hypertrophy of the left atrium.

2. Normal-sized or atrophic left ventricle due to reduced inflow of blood.

3. Pulmonary hypertension resulting from passive backward transmission of elevated left artial pressure which causes:

   i) chronic passive congestion of the lungs;

   ii) hypertrophy and dilatation of the right ventricle; and

   iii) dilatation of the right atrium when right heart failure supervenes.

MITRAL INSUFFICIENCY *(p. 341)*

Mitral insufficiency is caused by RHD in about 50% of patients but in contrast to mitral stenosis, pure mitral insufficiency occurs more often in men (75%).

ETIOLOGY. All the causes of mitral stenosis may produce mitral insufficiency, RHD being the most common cause. In addition, mitral insufficiency may result from non-inflammatory calcification of mitral valve annulus (in the elderly), myxomatous transformation of mitral valve (floppy valve syndrome), rupture of a leaflet or of the chordae tendineae or of a papillary muscle.

G/A The appearance of the mitral valve in insufficiency varies according to the underlying cause.

■ In *myxomatous degeneration* of the mitral valve leaflets (floppy valve syndrome), there is prolapse of one or both leaflets into the left atrium during systole.

■ In *non-inflammatory* calcification of mitral annulus seen in the aged, there is irregular, stony-hard, bead-like thickening in the region of mitral annulus without any associated inflammatory changes.

EFFECTS 1. Dilatation and hypertrophy of the left ventricle.

2. Marked dilatation of the left atrium.

3. Features of pulmonary hypertension such as:

   i) chronic passive congestion of the lungs;

   ii) hypertrophy and dilatation of the right ventricle; and

   iii) dilatation of the right atrium when right heart failure supervenes.

AORTIC STENOSIS *(p. 342)*

Aortic stenosis comprises about one-fourth of all patients with chronic valvular heart disease. About 80% patients of symptomatic aortic stenosis are males. It is of 2 main types:

1. Non-calcific aortic stenosis. The most common cause of non-calcific aortic stenosis is chronic RHD. Other causes are congenital valvular and subaortic stenosis and congenitally bicuspid aortic valve.

2. Calcific aortic stenosis. Calcific aortic stenosis is the more common type. Various causes have been ascribed to it. These include healing by scarring followed by calcification of aortic valve such as in RHD, bacterial endocarditis, *Brucella* endocarditis, Monckeberg's calcific aortic stenosis, healed congenital malformation and familial hypercholesterolaemic xanthomatosis.

G/A The aortic cusps show characteristic fibrous thickening and calcific nodularity of the closing edges. Calcified nodules are often found in the sinuses of Valsalva.

EFFECTS. The major effect of aortic stenosis is obstruction to the outflow resulting in concentric hypertrophy of the left ventricle. Later, when cardiac failure supervenes, there is dilatation as well as hypertrophy of the left ventricle (eccentric hypertrophy).

The *three cardinal symptoms* of aortic stenosis are: exertional dyspnoea, angina pectoris and syncope.

AORTIC INSUFFICIENCY *(p. 342)*

About three-fourth of all patients with aortic insufficiency are males with some having family history of Marfan's syndrome.

ETIOLOGY. In about 75% of patients, the cause is chronic RHD. However, isolated aortic insufficiency is less often due to rheumatic etiology. Other causes include syphilitic valvulitis, infective endocarditis, congenital subaortic stenosis (congenitally bicuspid aortic valve), myxomatous degeneration of aortic valve (floppy valve syndrome), traumatic rupture of the valve cusps, dissecting aneurysm, Marfan's syndrome and ankylosing spondylitis.

G/A. The aortic valve cusps are thickened, deformed and shortened and fail to close. There is generally distension and distortion of the ring.

EFFECTS. There is hypertrophy and dilatation of the left ventricle producing massive cardiac enlargement so that the heart may weigh as much as 1000 gm.

The characteristic physical findings in a patient of aortic insufficiency are awareness of the beatings of the heart, poundings in the head with each heartbeat, low diastolic and high pulse pressure, rapidly rising and collapsing water hammer pulse (Corrigan's pulse), booming 'pistol shot' sound over the femoral artery.

CARCINOID HEART DISEASE *(p. 343)*

ETIOLOGY. Carcinoid syndrome developing in patients with extensive hepatic metastases from a carcinoid tumour is characterised by cardiac manifestations in about half the cases. The lesions are characteristically located in the valves and endocardium of the right side of the heart. The pathogenesis of the cardiac lesions is not certain. But in carcinoid tumour with hepatic metastasis, there is increased blood level of serotonin secreted by the tumour. The increased concentration of serotonin reaches the right side of the heart and causes the lesions but serotonin is inactivated on passage of the blood through the lungs and hence the left heart is relatively spared.

G/A In majority of cases, the lesions are limited to the right side of the heart. Both pulmonary and tricuspid valves as well as the endocardium of the right chambers show characteristic cartilage-like fibrous plaques. Similar plaques may occur on the intima of the great veins, the coronary sinus and the great arteries. Occasionally, the lesions may be found on the left side of the heart.

EFFECTS. The thickening and contraction of the cusps and leaflets of the valves of the outflow tracts of the right heart result mainly in pulmonary stenosis and tricuspid regurgitation, and to a lesser extent, pulmonary regurgitation and tricuspid stenosis.

MYXOMATOUS DEGENERATION OF MITRAL VALVE (MITRAL VALVE PROLAPSE) *(p. 344)*

The condition is also known by other synonyms like 'floppy valve syndrome' or 'mitral valve prolapse'.

ETIOLOGY. Association with Marfan's syndrome has been observed in 90% of patients. Others have noted myxomatous degeneration in cases of Ehlers-Danlos syndrome and in myotonic dystrophy. A rheumatic or congenital etiology has been suggested by a few others.

G/A Any cardiac valve may be involved but mitral valve is affected most frequently. The disease is usually most severe and most common in the posterior leaflet of the mitral valve. The affected leaflet is enlarged, thickened, opaque white, soft and floppy. Cut section of the valve reveals mucoid or myxoid appearance. A significant feature is the ballooning or aneurysmal protrusion of the affected leaflet and hence the name 'mitral valve prolapse' and 'floppy valve syndrome'.

M/E The enlarged cusp shows loose connective tissue with abundant mucoid or myxoid material between stellate cells.

EFFECTS. Usually the condition does not produce any symptoms or significant valvular dysfunction.

MYOCARDIAL DISEASE *(p. 344)*

Involvement of the myocardium occurs in three major forms of diseases already discussed—ischaemic heart disease, hypertensive heart disease and rheumatic heart disease.
I.   *Myocarditis* i.e. inflammatory involvement of the myocardium; and
II. *Cardiomyopathy* i.e. a non-inflammatory myocardial involvement with unknown (primary) or known (secondary) etiology.

MYOCARDITIS *(p. 344)*

Inflammation of the heart muscle is called myocarditis. It is a rather common form of heart disease that can occur at any age. Its exact incidence is difficult to ascertain as the histological examination has been confined to autopsy material only. Reports from different studies have estimated the incidence of myocarditis in 1 to 4% of all autopsies.
    Myocarditis is divided into 4 main etiologic types described below.

I.   INFECTIVE MYOCARDITIS *(p. 344)*

1.   VIRAL MYOCARDITIS. A number of viral infections are associated with myocarditis. Some of the common examples are influenza, poliomyelitis, infectious mononucleosis, hepatitis, smallpox, chickenpox, measles, mumps, rubella, viral pneumonias, coxsackie virus and HIV infections. Cardiac involvement occurs in about 5% of viral infections. Viral myocarditis usually appears after a few days to a few weeks of viral infections elsewhere in the body.

G/A The myocardium is pale and flabby with dilatation of the chambers. There may be focal or patchy areas of necrosis.

M/E There are changes of acute myocarditis. Initially, there is oedema and infiltration of the interstitial tissue by neutrophils and lymphocytes. Later, there is necrosis of individual myocardial fibres and the infiltrate consists of lymphocytes and macrophages.

2.   SUPPURATIVE MYOCARDITIS. Pyogenic bacteria, chiefly *Staphylococcus aureus* or *Streptococcus pyogenes*, which cause septicaemia and pyaemia may produce suppurative myocarditis.

3.   TOXIC MYOCARDITIS. A number of acute bacterial infections produce myocarditis by toxins e.g. in diphtheria, typhoid fever and pneumococcal pneumonia.

4.   INFECTIVE GRANULOMATOUS MYOCARDITIS. Tuberculosis, brucellosis and tularaemia are some examples characterised by granulomatous inflammation in the myocardium. Sarcoidosis, though not a proved bacterial infection, has histological resemblance to other granulomatous myocarditis.

5.   SYPHILITIC MYOCARDITIS. Syphilitic involvement of the myocardium may occur in 2 forms—a *gummatous lesion* consisting of granulomatous inflammation which is more common, and a *primary non-specific myocarditis* which is rare.

6. RICKETTSIAL MYOCARDITIS. Myocarditis occurs quite frequently in scrub typhus (*R. tsutsugamushi*) and Rocky Mountain typhus fever caused by spotted *rickettsii*.

7. PROTOZOAL MYOCARDITIS. Chagas' disease and toxoplasmosis are the two protozoal diseases causing myocarditis.

8. HELMINTHIC MYOCARDITIS. *Echinococcus granulosus* and *Trichinella spiralis* are the two intestinal helminths which may cause myocarditis.

9. FUNGAL MYOCARDITIS. Patients with immunodeficiency, cancer and other chronic debilitating diseases are more prone to develop fungal myocarditis. These include: candidiasis, aspergillosis, blastomycosis, actinomyosis, cryptococcosis, coccidioidomycosis and histoplasmosis.

II. IDIOPATHIC (FIEDLER'S) MYOCARDITIS *(p. 346)*

Idiopathic or Fiedler's myocarditis is an isolated myocarditis unaccompanied by inflammatory changes in the endocardium or pericardium and occurs without the usual apparent causes. The condition is rapidly progressive and causes sudden severe cardiac failure or sudden death.

G/A The heart is soft and flabby. The cardiac chambers are generally dilated and sometimes show hypertrophy.

M/E Two forms of idiopathic myocarditis are described:

i) **Diffuse type** is more common of the two. It is characterised by diffuse non-specific inflammatory infiltrate consisting of lymphocytes, plasma cells, macrophages, eosinophils and a few polymorphs in the interstitial tissue without formation of granulomas.

ii) **Giant cell type or idiopathic granulomatous type** is characterised by formation of non-caseating granulomas consisting of macrophages, lymphocytes, plasma cells and multinucleate giant cells. The giant cells are of foreign body or Langhans' type or of myogenic origin.

III. MYOCARDITIS IN CONNECTIVE TISSUE DISEASES *(p. 346)*

Inflammatory involvement of the myocardium occurs in a number of connective tissue diseases such as rheumatoid arthritis, lupus erythematosus, polyarteritis nodosa, dermatomyositis and scleroderma.

IV. MISCELLANEOUS TYPES OF MYOCARDITIS *(p. 346)*

1. Physical agents. Physical agents like contusion of the myocardium, heatstroke, cardiac surgery and irradiation can initiate non-specific myocarditis.

2. Chemical agents. Toxic chemicals such as arsenic, phosphorus and carbon monoxide cause focal areas of degeneration and necrosis of myocardial fibres and non-specific inflammatory reaction, chiefly consisting of lymphocytes and macrophages.

3. Drugs. Changes similar to those induced by chemical poisons are produced by certain drugs such as phenothiazine compounds, sulfonamides, catecholamines, and cytotoxic compounds.

4. Immunologic agents. Myasthenia gravis, Friedreich's ataxia, and progressive muscular dystrophies initiate a state of autoimmunisation against the myocardium resulting in focal myocardial degeneration and necrosis with secondary inflammatory reaction.

5. Metabolic derangements. Uraemia, hypokalaemia and shock are associated with degeneration and necrosis of the myocardial fibres.

CARDIOMYOPATHY *(p. 347)*

Cardiomyopathy literally means disease of the heart muscle but the term was originally coined to restrict its usage to *myocardial disease of unknown cause*. Cardiomyopathies are classified into two broad groups (Table 12.7):

a)   *primary cardiomyopathy*; and

b)   *secondary cardiomyopathy* i.e. myocardial disease with known underlying cause.

TABLE 12.7: Classification of Cardiomyopathies.

I.   PRIMARY CARDIOMYOPATHY

1.   Idiopathic dilated (or congestive) cardiomyopathy

2.   Idiopathic hypertrophic cardiomyopathy
   i)   Obstructive type
   ii)   Non-obstructive type

3.   Idiopathic restrictive (or obliterative or infiltrative) cardiomyopathy
   i)   Cardiac amyloidosis
   ii)   Endocardial fibroelastosis
   iii) Endomyocardial fibrosis
   iv)   Löeffler's endocarditis (fibroplastic parietal endocarditis with peripheral blood eosinophilia)

II.   SECONDARY CARDIOMYOPATHY

1.   Nutritional disorders (e.g. alcoholic cardiomyopathy, beri-beri heart disease)

2.   Toxic chemicals (e.g. cobalt, arsenic, lithium, hydrocarbons)

3.   Drugs (e.g. emetrine, cyclophosphamide, adriamycin, catecholamines)

4.   Metabolic diseases (e.g. cardiac amyloidosis, haemochromatosis, glycogen storage diseases)

5.   Neuromuscular diseases (e.g. Friedreich's ataxia, muscular dystrophies)

6.   Infiltrations (e.g. leukaemia, carcinomas)

7.   Connective tissue diseases (e.g. rheumatoid arthritis, lupus erythematosus, systemic sclerosis, dermatomyositis)

A.   PRIMARY CARDIOMYOPATHY *(p. 347)*

This is a group of myocardial diseases of unknown cause. It is subdivided into the following 3 pathophysiologic categories:

1.   Idiopathic Dilated (Congestive) Cardiomyopathy *(p. 348)*

This type of cardiomyopathy is characterised by gradually progressive cardiac failure alongwith dilatation of all the four chambers of the heart. Though the etiology is unknown, a few hypotheses based on associations with the following conditions have been proposed:

i)   Possible association of *viral myocarditis* (especially coxsackievirus B).

ii)   Association with *toxic damage* from cobalt and chemotherapy with doxorubicin and other anthracyclines.

iii)   Role of *inherited mutations* has been emphasised lately. Mutations in certain sarcomere proteins such as cardiac troponin-T and β-myosin have been observed.

iv) *Chronic alcoholism* has been found associated with dilated cardiomyopathy. It may be due to thiamine deficiency induced by alcohol and resulting in beri-beri heart disease. This is referred to as 'alcoholic cardiomyopathy' and included by some workers as one of the subtypes of secondary cardiomyopathy.

v)   *Peripartum association*.

G/A The heart is enlarged and increased in weight (upto 1000 gm). The most characteristic feature is prominent dilatation of all the four chambers giving the heart typical globular appearance.

M/E The endomyocardial biopsies or autopsy examination of the heart reveal non-specific and variable changes. There may be hypertrophy of some myocardial fibres and atrophy of others.

2. Idiopathic Hypertrophic Cardiomyopathy *(p. 348)*

This form of cardiomyopathy is known by various synonyms like asymmetrical hypertrophy, hypertrophic subaortic stenosis and Teare's disease. The disease occurs more frequently between the age of 25 and 50 years. Though idiopathic, the following factors have been implicated:

i) *Autosomal dominant inheritance*.

ii) *Inherited mutations* in genes encoding for sarcomere proteins. Particularly implicated are the mutations in heavy and light chains of β-myosin, troponin-I and troponin-T.

iii) *Other contributory factors* are: increased circulating level of catecholamines, myocardial ischaemia as a result of thickened vasculature of the myocardium and abnormally increased fibrous tissue in the myocardium due to hypertrophy.

G/A The characteristic features are cardiac enlargement, increase in weight, normal or small ventricular cavities and myocardial hypertrophy. The hypertrophy of the myocardium is typically asymmetrical and affects the interventricular septum more than the free walls of the ventricles.

M/E The classical feature is the myocardial cell disorganisation in the ventricular septum.

3. Idiopathic Restrictive (Obliterative or Infiltrative) Cardiomyopathy *(p. 349)*

This form of cardiomyopathy is characterised by restriction in ventricular filling due to reduction in the volume of the ventricles. It includes the following entities:

I) CARDIAC AMYLOIDOSIS. Amyloidosis of the heart may occur in any form of systemic amyloidosis or may occur as isolated organ amyloidosis in amyloid of aging and result in subendocardial deposits.

II) ENDOCARDIAL FIBROELASTOSIS. The *infantile form* is clinically characterised by sudden breathlessness, cyanosis, cardiac failure and death whereas the symptoms in the *adult form* last for longer duration. A number of theories have been proposed. These are as under:

a) The infantile form is believed to be congenital in origin occurring due to the effect of intrauterine *endocardial anoxia*.

b) It may occur due to *haemodynamic pressure overload* such as in congenital septal defects and coarctation of the aorta.

c) It may be an expression of *genetic disorder* as noticed in twins, triplets and siblings.

d) Some workers consider this disease a form of *connective tissue disorder*.

e) Certain factors causing *myocardial injury* may initiate the endocardial disease such as in thiamine deficiency (beri-beri heart disease).

f) *Lymphatic obstruction* of the heart has been suggested by some as the causative mechanism.

G/A The characteristic feature is the diffuse or patchy, rigid, pearly-white thickening of the mural endocardium. Left ventricle is predominantly involved, followed in decreasing frequency by left atrium, right ventricle and right atrium.

Chapter Twelve

M/E The typical finding is the proliferation of the collagen and elastic tissue (fibroelastosis) comprising the thickened endocardium.

III) ENDOMYOCARDIAL FIBROSIS. This form of restrictive cardiomyopathy is a tropical condition prevalent in Africa, especially in Uganda and Nigeria, but some cases occur in South India, Sri Lanka, Malaysia and tropical South America. It is seen in children and young adults. The etiology of the condition remains obscure but the geographic distribution suggests the role of certain factors like malnutrition, viral infections and heavy consumption of banana (rich in serotonin).

G/A Endomyocardial fibrosis is characterised by fibrous scarring of the ventricular endocardium that extends to involve the inner third of the myocardium. The atrioventricular valve leaflets are often affected but the semilunar valves are uninvolved.

M/E The endocardium and parts of inner third of the myocardium show destruction of normal tissue and replacement by fibrous tissue.

IV) LÖEFFLER'S ENDOCARDITIS. Also known by the more descriptive term of 'fibroplastic parietal endocarditis with peripheral blood eosinophilia', the condition is considered by some as a variant of the entity described above, endomyocardial fibrosis. However, it differs from the latter in following respects:
a)   There is generally a peripheral blood eosinophilic leucocytosis.
b)   The inflammatory infiltrate in the endocardium and in the part of affected myocardium chiefly consists of eosinophils.
c)   The condition has a worse prognosis.

B.   SECONDARY CARDIOMYOPATHY *(p. 350)*

This is a group of myocardial diseases of known etiologies or having clinical associations.
1.   *Nutritional disorders e.g.* chronic alcoholism, thiamine deficiency causing beri-beri heart disease (Chapter 9).
2.   *Toxic chemicals e.g.* cobalt, arsenic, lithium and hydrocarbons.
3.   *Drugs* e.g. cyclophosphamide, adriamycin, catecholamines.
4.   *Metabolic diseases e.g.* amyloidosis, haemochromatosis, glycogen storage diseases, hypo-and hyperthyroidism, hypo-and hyperkalaemia.
5.   *Neuromuscular diseases e.g.* Friedreich's ataxia, muscular dystrophies.
6.   *Infiltrations* e.g. from leukaemia and carcinoma.
7.   *Connective tissue diseases e.g.* rheumatoid arthritis, systemic sclerosis, dermatomyositis, lupus erythematosus.

PERICARDIAL DISEASE *(p. 350)*

PERICARDIAL FLUID ACCUMULATIONS *(p. 350)*

Accumulation of fluid in the pericardial sac may be watery or pure blood. Accordingly, it is of 2 types:

A.   HYDROPERICARDIUM (PERICARDIAL EFFUSION). Accumulation of fluid in the pericardial cavity due to non-inflammatory causes is called hydropericardium or pericardial effusion. Normally, the pericardial cavity contains 30 to 50 ml of clear watery fluid. Considerable quantities of fluid (upto 1000 ml) can be accommodated in the pericardial cavity without seriously affecting the cardiac function if the accumulation is slow. But sudden accumulation of a smaller volume (upto 250 ml) may produce deficient diastolic filling of the cardiac chambers (cardiac tamponade).
    The various types of effusions and their causes are as follows:

1. Serous effusions. This is the most common type occurring in conditions in which there is generalised oedema e.g. in cardiac (in CHF), renal, nutritional and hepatic causes. The serous effusion is clear, watery, straw-coloured with specific gravity less than 1.015 (transudate).

2. Serosanguineous effusion. This type is found following blunt trauma to chest and cardiopulmonary resuscitation.

3. Chylous effusion. Milky or chylous fluid accumulates in conditions causing lymphatic obstruction.

4. Cholesterol effusion. This is a rare type of fluid accumulation characterised by the presence of cholesterol crystals such as in myxoedema.

B. HAEMOPERICARDIUM. Accumulation of pure blood in the pericardial sac is termed haemopericardium. Massive and sudden bleeding into the sac causes compression of the heart leading to cardiac tamponade. The causes of haemopericardium are:

i)   Rupture of the heart through a myocardial infarct.
ii) Rupture of dissecting aneurysm.
iii) Bleeding diathesis such as in scurvy, acute leukaemias, thrombocytopenia.
iv) Trauma following cardiopulmonary resuscitation or by laceration of a coronary artery.

PERICARDITIS *(p. 350)*

Pericarditis is the inflammation of the pericardial layers and is generally secondary to diseases in the heart or caused by systemic diseases. Pericarditis is classified into acute and chronic types, each of which may have several etiologies.

A. Acute Pericarditis *(p. 350)*

Acute bacterial and non-bacterial pericarditis are the most frequently encountered forms of pericarditis. These may have the following subtypes:

1. SEROUS PERICARDITIS. Acute pericarditis may be accompanied by accumulation of serous effusion which differs from transudate of hydropericardium in having increased protein content and higher specific gravity. Its various causes are as under:

i)   Viral infection e.g. coxsackie A or B viruses, influenza virus, mumps virus, adenovirus and infectious mononucleosis.
ii) Rheumatic fever.
iii) Rheumatoid arthritis.
iv) Systemic lupus erythematosus.
v)   Involvement of the pericardium by malignant tumour in the vicinity e.g. carcinoma lung, mesothelioma and mediastinal tumours.
vi) Tuberculous pericarditis in the early stage.

2. FIBRINOUS AND SEROFIBRINOUS PERICARDITIS. The response of the pericardium by fibrinous exudate is the most common type of pericarditis. Quite often, there is admixture of fibrinous exudate with serous fluid. The various causes of this type of pericarditis are:

i) Uraemia, ii) Myocardial infarction, iii) Rheumatic fever, iv) Trauma such as in cardiac surgery, v) Acute bacterial infections.

3. PURULENT OR FIBRINOPURULENT PERICARDITIS. Purulent or fibrinopurulent pericarditis is mainly caused by pyogenic bacteria (e.g. staphylococci, streptococci and pneumococci) and less frequently by fungi and parasites. The infection may spread to the pericardium by the following routes:

Chapter Twelve

i) By direct extension from neighbouring inflammation e.g. in empyema of the pleural cavity, lobar pneumonia, infective endocarditis and mediastinal infections.

ii) By haematogenous spread.

iii) By lymphatic permeation.

iv) Direct implantation during cardiac surgery.

4. HAEMORRHAGIC PERICARDITIS. Haemorrhagic pericarditis is the one in which the exudate consists of admixture of an inflammatory effusion of one of the foregoing types alongwith blood. The causes are:

i) Neoplastic involvement of the pericardium

ii) Haemorrhagic diathesis with effusion

iii) Tuberculosis

iv) Severe acute infections.

B. Chronic Pericarditis *(p. 351)*

1. TUBERCULOUS PERICARDITIS. The lesions may occur by one of the following mechanisms:

i) Direct extension from an adjacent focus of tuberculosis.

ii) By lymphatic spread e.g. from tracheobronchial lymph nodes, chronic pulmonary tuberculosis or infected pleura.

The exudate is slightly turbid, caseous or blood-stained with sufficient fibrin.

2. CHRONIC ADHESIVE PERICARDITIS. Chronic adhesive pericarditis is the stage of organisation and healing by formation of fibrous adhesions in the pericardium following preceding fibrinous, suppurative or haemorrhagic pericarditis. The process begins by formation of granulation tissue and neovascularisation. Subsequently, fibrous adhesions develop between the parietal and the visceral layers of the pericardium and obliterate the pericardial space. Sometimes, fibrous adhesions develop between the parietal pericardium and the adjacent mediastinum and is termed as *adhesive mediastinopericarditis.* Chronic adhesive pericarditis differs from chronic constrictive pericarditis in not embarrassing the function of the heart.

3. CHRONIC CONSTRICTIVE PERICARDITIS. This is a rare condition characterised by dense fibrous or fibrocalcific thickening of the pericardium resulting in mechanical interference with the function of the heart and reduced cardiac output. The condition usually results from a long-standing preceding causes such as:

i) Tuberculous pericarditis

ii) Purulent pericarditis

iii) Haemopericardium

iv) Concato's disease (polyserositis)

v) Rarely, acute non-specific and viral pericarditis.

4. PERICARDIAL PLAQUES (MILK SPOTS, SOLDIERS' SPOTS). These are opaque, white, shining and well-circumscribed areas of organisation with fibrosis in the pericardium measuring 1 to 3 cm in diameter. They are seen most frequently on the anterior surface of the right ventricle. The exact cause is not known but they are generally believed to arise from healing of preceding pericarditis.

TUMOURS OF THE HEART *(p. 352)*

Tumours of the heart are classified into primary and secondary, the latter being more common than the former.

PRIMARY TUMOURS *(p. 352)*

Primary tumours of the heart are quite rare, found in 0.04% of autopsies. In decreasing order of frequency, the benign tumours encountered in the heart are: myxoma, lipoma, fibroelastoma, rhabdomyoma, haemangioma and lymphangioma. The malignant tumours are still rarer.

MYXOMA. This is the most common primary tumour of the heart comprising about 50% of all primary cardiac tumours. Majority of them occur in the age range of 30 to 60 years. Myxomas may be located in any cardiac chamber or the valves, but 90% of them are situated in the left atrium.

G/A They are often single but may be multiple. They range in size from less than 1 to 10 cm, polypoid, pedunculated, spherical, soft and haemorrhagic masses resembling an organising mural thrombus.

M/E The tumour shows the following features:
i)   There is abundant myxoid or mucoid intercellular stroma positive for mucin.
ii) The cellularity is sparse. The tumour cells are generally stellate-shaped, spindled and polyhedral, scattered in the stroma.
iii) Numerous capillary-sized blood vessels are found and the tumour cells may be aggregated around them.
iv) A few lymphocytes, plasma cells and macrophages are seen.
v)   Foci of haemorrhage and deposits of haemosiderin granules are often present.

SECONDARY TUMOURS *(p. 353)*

Metastatic tumours of the heart are more common than the primary tumours. About 10% cases with disseminated cancer have metastases in the heart. Most of these result from haematogenous or lymphatic spread. In descending order of frequency, primary sites of origin are: carcinoma of the lung, breast, malignant lymphoma, leukaemia and malignant melanoma.

PATHOLOGY OF CARDIAC INTERVENTIONS *(p. 353)*

Nowadays, with the development of surgical and non-surgical therapeutic interventions in coronary artery disease, it has been possible to study the pathology of native as well as grafted vessel and also the mycardium by endomyocardial biopsy.

ENDOMYOCARDIAL BIOPSY *(p. 353)*

Currently, it is possible to perform endomyocardial biopsy (EMB) for making a final histopathologic diagnosis in certain cardiac diseases. The main *indications* for EMB are: myocarditis, cardiac transplant cases, restrictive heart disease, infiltrative heart diseases such as in amyloidosis, storage disorders etc.

BALLOON ANGIOPLASTY *(p. 353)*

Balloon angioplasty is a non-surgical procedure that employs percutaneous insertion and manipulation of a balloon catheter into the occluded coronary artery. The balloon is inflated to dilate the stenotic artery which causes endothelial damage, plaque fracture, medial dissection and haemorrhage in the affected arterial wall. At this stage, unstable angioplasty is liable to be associated with acute coronary syndromes.

CORONARY BYPASS GRAFTING *(p. 354)*

Autologous grafts are used to replace or bypass diseased coronary arteries. Most frequently used is autologous graft of saphenous vein which is reversed (due to valves in the vein) and transplanted, or left internal mammary artery may be used being in the operative area of the heart. Long-term follow-up of bypass surgery has yielded following observations on pathology of grafted vessel:

1. In a reversed saphenous vein graft, long-term luminal patency is 50% after 10 years. Pathologic changes which develop in grafted vein include thrombosis in early stage, intimal thickening and atherosclerosis with or without complicated lesions.

2. Internal mammary artery graft, however, has a patency of more than 90% after 10 years.

3. Atherosclerosis with superimposed complications may develop in native coronary artery distal to the grafted vessel as well as in the grafted vessel.

■ SELF ASSESSMENT

1. **The most common anatomic pattern of distribution of coronary blood supply is:**
   A Left coronary preponderance
   B. Right coronary preponderance
   C. Circumflex preponderance
   D. Balanced circulation

2. **Right heart failure is predominantly characterised by the following** *except:*
   A. Chronic venous congestion liver
   B. Chronic venous congestion spleen
   C. Chronic venous congestion kidney
   D. Pulmonary congestion

3. **The thickness of left ventricular wall in left ventricular hyper-trophy is at least:**
   A. 13 mm   B. 15 mm
   C. 17 mm   D. 19 mm

4. **The features of tetralogy of Fallot are as under** *except:*
   A. VSD
   B. Displacement of aorta to right to override the VSD
   C. Pulmonary stenosis
   D. Left ventricular hypertrophy

5. **Post-ductal coarctation of aorta has following features** *except:*
   A. Hypertension in upper extremities
   B. Weak pulses
   C. High blood pressure in lower extremities
   D. Claudication in lower legs

6. **Non-infarct effects of myocardial ischaemia are as under** *except:*
   A. Sudden cardiac death   B. Angina pectoris
   C. Subendocardial infarcts   D. Chronic ischaemic heart disease

7. **The most thrombogenic constituent of atheroma is:**
   A. Fibrous cap   B. Lipid core
   C. Foam cells   D. Smooth muscle cells

8. **The most important and common complicated atheromatous lesion in coronary artery in acute myocardial infarction is:**
   A. Calcification   B. Coronary thrombosis
   C. Aneurysm   D. Ulceration

9. **Infarcts are least common in:**
   A. Left ventricle   B. Right ventricle
   C. Left atrium   D. Right atrium

10. **The most specific cardiac marker for acute MI is:**
    A. Ratio of CK-MB2: CK-MB1   B. Ratio of LDH1: LDH2
    C. Troponins CTnT and CTnI   D. Myoglobin

11. **Chronic ischaemic heart disease is most often due to:**
    - A. Coronary atherosclerosis
    - B. Repetitive coronary vasospasm
    - C. Embolisation to coronary branches
    - D. Stenosis of coronary ostia

12. **In hypertensive heart disease left ventricular hypertrophy is correlated with:**
    - A Duration of hypertension
    - B. Severity of hypertension
    - C. Cause of hypertension
    - D. Severity of coronary atherosclerosis

13. **In rheumatic heart disease, antibodies against the following streptococcal products are seen in the serum *except:***
    - A. DNAase B
    - B. Streptokinase
    - C. Streptolysin S
    - D. Streptohyaluronidase

14. **Anitschkow cells are believed to be derivative of:**
    - A Cardiac myocyte
    - B. Cardiac histiocyte
    - C. Endocardial smooth muscle cells
    - D. Endothelial cells of lymphatics

15. **In chronic RHD, the most common valvular deformities are:**
    - A. Mitral stenosis and insufficiency
    - B. Mitral stenosis alone
    - C. Mitral insufficiency alone
    - D. Mitral and aortic stenosis combined

16. **MacCallum's patch is region of:**
    - A. Pericardial surface in the posterior wall of left atrium
    - B. Pericardial surface in the posterior wall of left ventricle
    - C. Endocardial surface in the posterior wall of left atrium
    - D. Endocardial surface in the posterior wall of left ventricle

17. **Major criteria in the modified Jones' criteria include the following *except:***
    - A. Carditis
    - B. Polyarthritis
    - C. Raised C-reactive proteins
    - D. Subcutaneous nodules

18. **Haematoxylin bodies of Gross may be seen in vegetations of:**
    - A. Rheumatic valvulitis
    - B. Libman-Sacks endocarditis
    - C. Non-bacterial thrombotic endocarditis
    - D. Subacute bacterial valvulitis

19. **Most frequent underlying heart disease in causation of SABE is:**
    - A Ventricular septal defect
    - B. Chronic rheumatic valvular disease
    - C. Floppy mitral valve
    - D. Atherosclerotic valvular disease

20. **Vegetations of the following types of endocarditis are generally not friable *except* that of:**
    - A Rheumatic endocarditis
    - B. Libman-Sacks endocarditis
    - C. Subacute bacterial endocarditis
    - D. Non-bacterial thrombotic endocarditis

21. **Mitral stenosis causes the following effects on the heart *except:***
    - A Dilatation and hypertrophy of left atrium
    - B. Dilatation and hypertrophy of left ventricle
    - C. Dilatation and hypertrophy of right ventricle
    - D. Dilatation of right atrium

22. **In the following heart disease, there is generally involvement of valves of right heart:**
    A. Heart disease in SLE
    B. Carcinoid heart disease
    C. Non-bacterial thrombotic endocarditis
    D. Subacute bacterial endocarditis

23. **The following type of cardiomyopathy is classically characterised by four chamber dilatation:**
    A. Idiopathic congestive cardiomyopathy
    B. Idiopathic hypertrophic cardiomyopathy
    C. Endomyocardial fibrosis
    D. Loeffler's endocarditis

24. **Heart size may be smaller in:**
    A. Chronic adhesive pericarditis
    B. Chronic constrictive pericarditis
    C. Pericardial plaques
    D. Fibrinopurulent pericarditis

25. **The most common location for myxoma of heart is:**
    A. Left ventricle   B. Right ventricle
    C. Left atrium   D. Interventricular septum

26. **An important protein from bacterial cell surface implicated in pathogenesis of RHD is:**
    A. G-protein   B. M-protein
    C. L-protein   D. X-protein

27. **For endomyocardial biopsy, the safest site for biopsy is:**
    A. Left ventricle   B. Left atrium
    C. Right ventricle   D. Right atrium

KEY

1 = B	2 = D	3 = B	4 = D
5 = C	6 = C	7 = B	8 = B
9 = C	10 = C	11 = A	12 = A
13 = C	14 = B	15 = A	16 = C
17 = C	18 = B	19 = B	20 = C
21 = B	22 = B	23 = A	24 = B
25 = C	26 = B	27 = C	

13

The Haematopoietic System

This section on disorders of the haematopoietic system is concerned with diseases of the blood and bone marrow. The account that follows here is arbitrarily divided into the following subsections for the purpose of convenience of discussion:

(1) bone marrow; (2) red blood cells; (3) white blood cells; (4) platelets and haemorrhagic diathesis; (5) blood groups and blood transfusion.

BONE MARROW (p. 355)

The pluripotent stem cells in the bone marrow give rise to two types of multipotent stem cells: *non-lymphoid stem cells* which differentiate in the bone marrow, and *lymphoid stem cells* which differentiate in the bone marrow and then migrate to the lymphoid tissues. The non-lymphoid stem cells form the circulating erythrocytes, granulocytes, monocytes and platelets. Monocytes on entering the tissues form a variety of phagocytic macrophages, both of which together constitute mononuclear-phagocyte system. Lymphopoietic cells in the marrow undergo differentiation to form B and T lymphocytes of the immune system.

Circulating blood normally contains 3 main types of cells—the red cells (erythrocytes), the white cells (leucocytes) and the platelets (thrombocytes). These blood cells perform their respective physiologic functions: *erythrocytes* are largely concerned with oxygen transport, *leucocytes* play various roles in body defense against infection and tissue injury, while *thrombocytes* are primarily involved in maintaining integrity of blood vessels and in preventing blood loss. The life-span of these cells is variable—neutrophils have the blood life-span of 6-8 hours, followed by platelets with a life-span of 10 days, while the RBCs have the longest life-span of 90-120 days.

HAEMATOPOIESIS (p. 356)

In the human embryo, the *yolk sac* is the main site of haematopoiesis in the first few weeks of gestation. By about 3rd month, however, the *liver and spleen* are the main sites of blood cell formation and continue to do so until about 2 weeks after birth. Haematopoiesis commences in the *bone marrow* by 4th and 5th month and becomes fully active by 7th and 8th month so that at birth practically all the bones contain active marrow. During normal childhood and adult life, therefore, the marrow is the only source of new blood cells. However, during childhood, there is progressive fatty replacement throughout the long bones so that by adult life the haematopoietic marrow is confined to the central skeleton (vertebrae, sternum, ribs, skull, sacrum and pelvis) and proximal ends of femur, tibia and humerus. Even in these haematopoietic areas, about 50% of the marrow consists of fat. Non-haematopoietic marrow in the adult is, however, capable of reverting to active haematopoiesis in certain pathologic conditions. The spleen and liver can also resume their foetal haematopoietic role in certain pathologic conditions and is called *extramedullary haematopoiesis*.

HAEMATOPOIETIC STEM CELLS (p. 356)

The stem cells express a variety of cell surface proteins such as CD34 and adhesion proteins which help the stem cells to "home" to bone marrow when infused. The stem cells have the appearance of small or intermediate-sized lymphocytes and their presence in the marrow can be demonstrated by cell culture techniques by the growth of colony-forming units (CFU) pertaining to different cell lines. The bone marrow provides a suitable environment for growth and development of stem cells. For instance, if haematopoietic stem cells are infused intravenously into a suitably-prepared recipient, they seed the marrow successfully but do not thrive at other sites. This principle forms the basis of bone marrow transplantation performed for various haematologic diseases.

The stem cells, after a series of divisions, differentiate into two types of progenitors—*lymphoid* (immune system) stem cells, and *non-lymphoid or myeloid* (trilineage) stem cells. The former develop into T, B and null lymphocytes while the latter differentiate into 3 types of cell lines—granulocyte-monocyte progenitors (producing neutrophils, eosinophils, basophils and monocytes), erythroid progenitors (producing red cells), and megakaryocytes (as the source of platelets). The differentiation and maturation of these cells from stem cell are regulated by endogenous glycoproteins called as *growth factors, cytokines and hormones.* These are: Erythropoietin, granulocyte colony-stimulating factor (G-CSF), granulocyte-macrophage colony-stimulating factor (GM-CSF), and thrombopoietin.

BONE MARROW EXAMINATION *(p. 357)*

Bone marrow examination may be performed by two methods—*aspiration* and *trephine biopsy*. A comparison of the two methods is summarised in Table 13.1.

TABLE 13.1: Comparison of Bone Marrow Aspiration and Trephine Biopsy.

	FEATURE	ASPIRATION	TREPHINE
1.	*Site*	Sternum, posterior iliac crest; tibial head in infants	Posterior iliac crest
2.	*Instrument*	Salah BM aspiration needle	Jamshidi trephine needle
3.	*Stains*	Romanowsky, Perls' reaction for iron on smears	Haematoxylin and eosin, reticulin on tissue sections
4.	*Time*	Within 1-2 hours	Within 1-7 days
5.	*Morphology*	Better cellular morphology of aspiration smears but marrow architecture is indistinct	Better marrow architectural pattern but cell morphology is not as distinct since tissue sections are examined and not smears
6.	*Indications*	Anaemias, suspected leukaemias, neutropenia thrombocytopenia, polycythaemia, myeloma, lymphomas, carcinomatosis, lipid storage diseases, granulomatous conditions, parasites, fungi, and unexplained enlargements of liver, spleen or lymph nodes.	Additional indications are: myelosclerosis, aplastic anaemia and in cases with 'dry tap' on aspiration.

BONE MARROW ASPIRATION. The method involves suction of marrow via a strong, wide bore, short-bevelled needle fitted with a stylet and an adjustable guard in order to prevent excessive penetration; for instance Salah bone marrow aspiration needle. Smears are prepared immediately from the bone marrow aspirate and are fixed in 95% methanol after air-drying. The usual Romanowsky technique is employed for staining and a stain for iron is performed routinely so as to assess the reticuloendothelial stores of iron.

Estimation of the proportion of cellular components in the marrow, however, can be provided by doing a differential count of at least 500 cells (myelogram, Table 13.2).

TABLE 13.2: Normal Adult Bone Marrow Counts (Myelogram).

Fat/cell ratio : 50:50

Myeloid/erythroid (M/E) ratio : 2-4:1 (mean 3:1)

Myeloid series: 30-45% (37.5%)

* Myeloblasts : 0.1-3.5%
* Promyelocytes: 0.5-5%

Erythroid series: 10-15% (mean 12.5%)

Megakaryocytes: 0.5%

Lymphocytes: 5-20%

Plasma cells: $\leq$ 3%

Reticulum cells: 0.1-2%

TREPHINE BIOPSY. Trephine biopsy is performed by a simple *Jamshidi trephine needle* by which a core of tissue from periosteum to bone marrow cavity is obtained. The tissue is then fixed, decalcified and processed for histological sections and stained with haematoxylin and eosin and for reticulin. Trephine biospy is useful over aspiration since it provides an excellent view of the overall marrow architecture, cellularity, and presence or absence of infiltrates, but is less valuable than aspiration as far as individual cell morphology is concerned.

RED BLOOD CELLS *(p. 358)*

ERYTHROPOIESIS *(p. 358)*

There is a well-defined and readily recognisable lineage of nucleated red cells, the erythroid series, in the marrow.

Erythroid Series *(p. 358)*

1. PRONORMOBLAST. The earliest recognisable cell in the marrow is a pronormoblast or proerythroblast. It is a large cell, 15-20 µm in diameter having deeply basophilic cytoplasm and a large central nucleus containing nucleoli. The deep blue colour of the cytoplasm is due to high content of RNA which is associated with active protein synthesis. Each pronormoblast undergoes 4-5 replications and forms 16-32 mature RBCs.

2. BASOPHILIC (EARLY) NORMOBLAST. It is a round cell having a diameter of 12-16 µm with a large nucleus which is slightly more condensed than the pronormoblast and contains basophilic cytoplasm. Basophilic normoblast undergoes rapid proliferation.

3. POLYCHROMATIC (INTERMEDIATE) NORMOBLAST. Next maturation stage has a diameter of 12-14 µm. The nucleus at this stage is coarse and deeply basophilic. The cytoplasm is characteristically polychromatic i.e. contains admixture of basophilic RNA and acidophilic haemoglobin. The cell at this stage ceases to undergo proliferative activity.

4. ORTHOCHROMATIC (LATE) NORMOBLAST. The final stage in the maturation of nucleated red cells is the orthochromatic or late normoblast. The cell at this stage is smaller, 8-12 µm in diameter, containing a small and pyknotic nucleus with dark nuclear chromatin. The cytoplasm is characteristically acidophilic with diffuse basophilic hue due to the presence of large amounts of haemoglobin.

5. RETICULOCYTE. The nucleus is finally extruded from the late normoblast within the marrow and a reticulocyte results. The reticulocytes are juvenile red cells devoid of nucleus but contain ribosomal RNA so that they are still able to synthesise haemoglobin. A reticulocyte spends 1-2 days in the marrow and circulates for 1-2 days in the peripheral blood before maturing in the spleen, to become a biconcave red cell. The reticulocytes in the peripheral blood are distinguished from mature red cells by slightly basophilic hue in the cytoplasm similar to that of an orthochromatic normoblast. Reticulocytes can be counted in the laboratory by *vital staining* with dyes such as new methylene blue or brilliant cresyl blue. Normal range of reticulocyte count in health is 0.5-2.5% in adults and 2-6% in infants. Their percentage in the peripheral blood is a fairly accurate reflection of erythropoietic activity. Their proportion is increased in conditions of rapid red cell regeneration e.g. after haemorrhage, haemolysis and haematopoietic response of anaemia to treatment.

Erythropoietin *(p. 359)*

Erythropoietic activity is regulated by the hormone, erythropoietin, which is produced in response to anoxia. The principal site of erythropoietin production is the kidney though there is evidence of its extra-renal production in certain unusual circumstances. Its levels are, therefore, lowered in chronic renal diseases, while a case of renal cell carcinoma may be associated with its enhanced production and erythrocytosis.

There is an increased production of erythropoietin in various types of anaemias but in anaemia of chronic diseases (e.g. in infections and neoplastic conditions) there is no such enhancement of erythropoietin. In polycythaemia rubra vera, there is erythrocytosis but depressed production of erythropoietin. This is because of an abnormality of the stem cell class which is not under erythropoietin control.

The Red Cell *(p. 361)*

The mature erythrocytes of the human peripheral blood are non-nucleated cells and lack the usual cell organelles. The normal human erythrocyte is a biconcave disc, 7.2 μm in diameter, and has a thickness of 2.4 μm at the periphery and 1 μm in the centre. The biconcave shape renders the red cells quite flexible so that they can pass through capillaries whose minimum diameter is 3.5 μm. More than 90% of the weight of erythrocyte consist of haemoglobin. The life-span of red cells is 120 days.

NORMAL VALUES AND RED CELL INDICES. Range of *normal red cell count* in health is $5.5 \pm 1.0 \times 10^{12}$/L in men and $4.8 \pm 1.0 \times 10^{12}$/L in women. The *packed cell volume (PCV)* or *haematocrit* is the volume of erythrocytes per litre of whole blood indicating the proportion of plasma and red cells and ranges 0.47 ± 0.07 L/L (40-54%) in men and 0.42 ± 0.05 L/L (37-47%) in women. The *haemoglobin content* in health is 15.5 ± 2.5 g/dl (13-18 g/dl) in men and 14.0 ± 2.5 g/dl (11.5-16.5 g/dl) in women. Based on these normal values, a series of *absolute values* or red cell indices can be derived which have diagnostic importance. These are as under:

1. **Mean corpuscular volume (MCV) =**

    $$\frac{\text{PCV in L/L}}{\text{RBC count/L}}$$

    The normal value is 85 ± 8 fl (77-93 fl)*.

2. **Mean corpuscular haemoglobin (MCH) =**

    $$\frac{\text{Hb/L}}{\text{RBC count/L}}$$

    The normal range is 29.5 ± 2.5 pg (27-32 pg)*.

---

*For conversions, the multiples used are as follows: deci (d) = 10^{-1}, milli (m) = 10^{-3}, micro (μ) = 10^{-6}, nano (n) = 10^{-9}, pico (p) = 10^{-12}, femto (f) = 10^{-15}

SIGNS. 1. Pallor. 2. Hyperdynamic circulation. 3. Attacks of faintness. 4. Retinal haemorrhages. 5. Menstrual disturbances. 6. Mild proteinuria. 7. Anorexia, flatulence.

Investigations of the Anaemic Subject *(p. 365)*

A. HAEMOGLOBIN ESTIMATION. Several methods are available but most reliable and accurate is the cyanmethaemoglobin (HiCN) method employing Drabkin's solution and a spectrophotometer.

B. PERIPHERAL BLOOD FILM EXAMINATION. The blood smear is evaluated in an area where there is neither rouleaux formation nor so thin as to cause red cell distortion. The following abnormalities in erythroid series of cells are particularly looked for in a blood smear:

1. Variation in size (Anisocytosis). Normally, there is slight variation in size.

- *Macrocytes* are classically found in megaloblastic anaemia.
- *Microcytes* are present in iron deficiency anaemia, thalassaemia and spherocytosis.

2. Variation in shape (Poikilocytosis). Poikilocytes are produced in various types of abnormal erythropoiesis e.g. in megaloblastic anaemia, iron deficiency anaemia, thalassaemia, myelosclerosis and microangiopathic haemolytic anaemia.

3. Inadequate haemoglobin formation (Hypochromasia). Increased central pallor is referred to as *hypochromasia*. It may develop either from lowered haemoglobin content (e.g. in iron deficiency anaemia, chronic infections), or due to thinness of the red cells (e.g. in thalassaemia, sideroblastic anaemia).

4. Compensatory erythropoiesis. These changes are:

i) *Polychromasia* is defined as the red cells having more than one type of colour. Polychromatic red cells are slightly larger, and represent reticulocytes and, thus, correlate well with reticulocyte count.

ii) *Normoblastaemia.* A small number of normoblasts (or erythroblasts) may be normally found in cord blood at birth. They are found in large numbers in haemolytic disease of the newborn, other haemolytic disorders and in extramedullary erythropoiesis.

iii) *Punctate basophilia* or *basophilic stippling* is diffuse and uniform basophilic granularity in the cell which does not stain positively with Perls' reaction (in contrast to Pappenheimer bodies which stain positively). Classical punctate basophilia is seen in aplastic anaemia, thalassaemia, myelodysplasia, infections and lead poisoning.

iv) *Howell-Jolly bodies* are purple nuclear remnants, usually found singly, and are larger than basophilic stippling.

5. Miscellaneous changes. Various types of abnormal red cells are as under:

i) *Spherocytosis* is characterised by presence of spheroidal rather than biconcave disc-shaped red cells.

ii) *Schistocytosis* is identified by fragmentation of erythrocytes, found in thalassaemia hereditary elliptocytosis.

iii) *Irregularly contracted red cells* are found in drug and chemical induced haemolytic anaemia.

iv) *Leptocytosis* is the presence of unusually thin red cells, seen in severe iron deficiency and thalassaemia. *Target cell* is a form of leptocyte found in iron deficiency, thalassaemia.

v) *Sickle cells or drepanocytes* are sickle-shaped red cells found in sickle cell disease.

vi) *Crenated red cells* are due to alkaline pH.

vii) *Acanthocytosis* is the presence of coarsely crenated red cells, found in large number in blood film made from splenectomised subjects.

viii) *Burr cells* are cell fragments having one or more spines, found in uraemia.

ix) Stomatocytes have central area having slit-like or mouth-like appearance, found in hereditary stomatocytosis.

x) *Ovalocytosis* or *elliptocytosis* is the oval or elliptical shape of red cells, seen in hereditary ovalocytosis and elliptocytosis.

C. RED CELL INDICES. The abnormalities are:

■ In iron deficiency and thalassaemia, MCV, MCH and MCHC are reduced.

■ In anaemia due to acute blood loss and haemolytic anaemias, MCV, MCH and MCHC are all within normal limits.

■ In megaloblastic anaemias, MCV is raised above the normal range.

D. LEUCOCYTE AND PLATELET COUNT. Measurement of leucocyte and platelet count helps to distinguish pure anaemia from pancytopenia.

E. RETICULOCYTE COUNT. Reticulocyte count (normal 0.5-2.5%) is done in each case of anaemia to assess the marrow erythropoietic activity.

F. ERYTHROCYTE SEDIMENTATION RATE. The ESR is a non-specific test used as a screening test for anaemia.

G. BONE MARROW EXAMINATION. Bone marrow aspiration is done in cases where the cause for anaemia is not obvious.

Classification of Anaemias *(p. 367)*

Several types of classifications of anaemias have been proposed. Two of the widely accepted classifications are based on the pathophysiology and morphology (Table 13.3).

TABLE 13.3: Classification of Anaemias.

A. PATHOPHYSIOLOGIC

    I. Anaemia due to increased blood loss
    a) Acute post-haemorrhagic anaemia
    b) Chronic blood loss

    II. Anaemias due to impaired red cell production
    a) *Cytoplasmic maturation defects*
        1. Deficient haem synthesis:
            Iron deficiency anaemia
        2. Deficient globin synthesis:
            Thalassaemic syndromes
    b) *Nuclear maturation defects*
        Vitamin B_{12} and/or folic acid deficiency:
        Megaloblastic anaemia
    c) *Defect in stem cell proliferation and differentiation*
        1. Aplastic anaemia
        2. Pure red cell aplasia
    d) *Anaemia of chronic disorders*
    e) *Bone marrow infiltration*
    f) *Congenital anaemia*

    III. Anaemias due to increased red cell destruction (Haemolytic anaemias)
        (Details in Table 13.10)
    A. *Extrinsic (extracorpuscular) red cell abnormalities*
    B. *Intrinsic (intracorpuscular) red cell abnormalities*

B. MORPHOLOGIC

    I. Microcytic, hypochromic
    II. Normocytic, normochromic
    III. Macrocytic, normochromic

ANAEMIA OF BLOOD LOSS (p. 368)

Depending upon the rate of blood loss due to haemorrhage, the effects of post-haemorrhagic anaemia appear.

ACUTE BLOOD LOSS. Laboratory Findings are:
i) Normocytic and normochromic anaemia. ii) Low haematocrit. iii) Increased reticulocyte count in peripheral blood (10-15% after one week).

CHRONIC BLOOD LOSS. When the loss of blood is slow and insidious, the effects of anaemia will become apparent only when the rate of loss is more than rate of production and the iron stores are depleted. This results in iron deficiency anaemia.

HYPOCHROMIC ANAEMIA (p. 369)

Iron deficiency is the commonest cause of anaemia the world over. It is estimated that about 20% of women in child-bearing age group are iron deficient, while the overall prevalence in adult males is about 2%. It is the most important, though not the sole, cause of microcytic hypochromic anaemia in which all the three red cell indices (MCV, MCH and MCHC) are reduced and occurs due to defective haemoglobin synthesis. Hypochromic anaemias, therefore, are classified into 2 groups:
I. Hypochromic anaemia due to iron deficiency.
II. Hypochromic anaemias other than iron deficiency.

The latter category includes 3 groups of disorders—sideroblastic anaemia, thalassaemia and anaemia of chronic disorders.

IRON DEFICIENCY ANAEMIA (p. 369)

Iron Metabolism (p. 369)

The amount of iron obtained from the diet should replace the losses from the skin, bowel and genitourinary tract. These losses together are about 1 mg daily in an adult male or in a non-menstruating female, while in a menstruating woman there is an additional iron loss of 0.5-1 mg daily. The iron required for haemoglobin synthesis is derived from 2 primary sources—ingestion of foods containing iron (e.g. leafy vegetables, beans, meats, liver etc) and recycling of iron from senescent red cells.

ABSORPTION. Iron is absorbed mainly in the duodenum and proximal jejunum. *Iron from diet containing haem is better absorbed than non-haem iron.* Absorption of non-haem iron is enhanced by factors such as ascorbic acid (vitamin C), citric acid, amino acids, sugars, gastric secretions and hydrochloric acid. Iron absorption is impaired by factors like medicinal antacids, milk, pancreatic secretions, phytates, phosphates, ethylene diamine tetra-acetic acid (EDTA) and tannates contained in tea.

Non-haem iron is released as ferrous or ferric form but is absorbed almost exclusively as ferrous form; reduction when required takes place at the brush border by *ferrireductase*. Transport across the membrane is accomplished by divalent metal transporter 1 (DMT 1). Once inside the gut cells, ferric iron may be either stored as ferritin or further transported to transferrin by two vehicle proteins—*ferroportin* and *hephaestin*.

DISTRIBUTION. In an adult, iron is distributed in the body as under:
1. **Haemoglobin**—present in the red cells, contains most of the body iron (65%).
2. **Myoglobin**—comprises a small amount of iron in the muscles (3.5%).
3. **Haem and non-haem enzymes**—e.g. cytochrome, catalase, peroxidases, succinic dehydrogenase and flavoproteins constitute a fraction of total body iron (0.5%).

4. Transferrin-bound iron—circulates in the plasma and constitutes another fraction of total body iron (0.5%).

All these forms of iron are in *functional form.*

5. Ferritin and haemosiderin—are the *storage forms* of excess iron (30%). They are stored in the mononuclear-phagocyte cells of the spleen, liver and bone marrow and in the parenchymal cells of the liver.

TRANSPORT. Iron is transported in plasma bound to a β-globulin, transferrin, synthesised in the liver. Transferrin-bound iron is made available to the marrow where the immature red cell precursors utilise iron for haemoglobin synthesis. Transferrin is reutilised after iron is released from it. A small amount of transferrin iron is delivered to other sites such as parenchymal cells of the liver. Normally, transferrin is about one-third saturated.

EXCRETION. The body is unable to regulate its iron content by excretion alone. The amount of iron lost per day is 0.5-1 mg which is independent of iron intake. This loss is nearly twice more (i.e. 1-2 mg/day) in menstruating women. Iron is lost from the body as a result of desquamation of epithelial cells from the gastrointestinal tract, from excretion in the urine and sweat, and loss via hair and nails.

Pathogenesis *(p. 370)*

It is only after the tissue stores of iron are exhausted that the supply of iron to the marrow becomes insufficient for haemoglobin formation so that a state of iron deficiency anaemia develops. The development of iron deficiency depends upon one or more of the following factors:
1. Increased blood loss 2. Increased requirements 3. Inadequate dietary intake 4. Decreased intestinal absorption.

Etiology *(p. 370)*

Etiology of iron deficiency anaemia is summed up in Table 13.4.

1. FEMALES IN REPRODUCTIVE PERIOD OF LIFE. The highest incidence of iron deficiency anaemia is in women during their reproductive period of life. It may be from one or more of the following causes:
i) Blood loss ii) Inadequate intake iii) Increased requirements.

TABLE 13.4: Etiology of Iron Deficiency Anaemia.

I. INCREASED BLOOD LOSS
1. *Uterine* e.g. excessive menstruation in reproductive years, repeated miscarriages, at onset of menarche, post-menopausal uterine bleeding.
2. *Gastrointestinal* e.g. peptic ulcer, haemorrhoids, hookworm infestation, cancer of stomach and large bowel, oesophageal varices, hiatus hernia, chronic aspirin ingestion, ulcerative colitis, diverticulosis.
3. *Renal tract* e.g. haematuria, haemoglobinuria.
4. *Nose* e.g. repeated epistaxis.
5. *Lungs* e.g. haemoptysis.

II. INCREASED REQUIREMENTS
1. Spurts of growth in infancy, childhood and adolescence.
2. Prematurity.
3. Pregnancy and lactation.

III. INADEQUATE DIETARY INTAKE
1. Poor economic status.
2. Anorexia e.g. in pregnancy.
3. Elderly individuals due to poor dentition, apathy and financial constraints.

IV. DECREASED ABSORPTION
1. Partial or total gastrectomy
2. Achlorhydria
3. Intestinal malabsorption such as in coeliac disease.

2. POST-MENOPAUSAL FEMALES. Iron deficiency anaemia may develop in post-menopausal women due to chronic blood loss.

i) Post-menopausal uterine bleeding ii) Bleeding from the alimentary tract.

3. ADULT MALES. It is uncommon for adult males to develop iron deficiency anaemia. The cause may be chronic haemorrhage at one of the following sites:

i) *Gastrointestinal tract* ulcer, haemorrhoids, hookworm infestation, carcinoma of stomach and large bowel, oesophageal varices, hiatus hernia, chronic aspirin ingestion and ulcerative colitis ii) *Urinary tract* iii) *Nose* iv) *Lungs*.

4. INFANTS AND CHILDREN. Iron deficiency anaemia is fairly common during infancy and childhood with a peak incidence at 1-2 years of age. The principal cause for anaemia at this age is increased demand of iron which is not met by the inadequate intake of iron in the diet.

Clinical Features *(p. 372)*

As already mentioned, iron deficiency anaemia is much more common in women between the age of 20 and 45 years than in men; at periods of active growth in infancy, childhood and adolescence; and is also more frequent in premature infants. The clinical consequences of iron deficiency manifest in 2 ways—anaemia itself and epithelial tissue changes.

1. ANAEMIA. The onset of iron deficiency anaemia is generally slow. The usual symptoms are of weakness, fatigue, dyspnoea on exertion, palpitations and pallor of the skin, mucous membranes and sclerae.

2. EPITHELIAL TISSUE CHANGES. Long-standing chronic iron deficiency anaemia causes epithelial tissue changes in some patients. The changes occur in the nails (koilonychia or spoon-shaped nails), tongue (atrophic glossitis), mouth (angular stomatitis), and oesophagus causing dysphagia from development of thin, membranous webs at the postcricoid area (Plummer-Vinson syndrome).

Laboratory Findings *(p. 372)*

1. BLOOD PICTURE AND RED CELL INDICES. These are:

i) **Haemoglobin.** The essential feature is a fall in haemoglobin concentration up to a variable degree.

ii) **Red cells.** The red cells in the blood film are hypochromic and microcytic, and there is anisocytosis and poikilocytosis. Hypochromia generally precedes microcytosis.

iii) **Reticulocyte count.** The reticulocyte count is normal or reduced but may be slightly raised (2-5%) in cases after haemorrhage.

iv) **Absolute values.** The red cell indices reveal a diminished MCV (below 50 fl), diminished. MCH (below 15 pg) and diminished MCHC (below 20 g/dl).

v) **Leucocytes.** The total and differential white cell counts are usually normal.

vi) **Platelets.** Platelet count is usually normal but may be slightly to moderately raised in patients who have had recent bleeding.

2. BONE MARROW FINDINGS. The usual findings are as follows:

i) **Marrow cellularity.** The marrow cellularity is increased due to erythroid hyperplasia (myeloid-erythroid ratio decreased).

ii) **Erythropoiesis.** There is normoblastic erythropoiesis with predominance of small polychromatic normoblasts (micronormoblasts). The *cytoplasmic maturation lags behind* so that the late normoblasts have pyknotic nucleus but persisting polychromatic cytoplasm.

iii) **Other cells.** Myeloid, lymphoid and megakaryocytic cells are normal in number and morphology.

iv) **Marrow iron.** Iron staining (Prussian blue reaction) carried out on bone marrow aspirate smear shows deficient reticuloendothelial iron stores and absence of siderotic iron granules from developing normoblasts.

3. BIOCHEMICAL FINDINGS. The following tests are of additional value:
i) The serum iron level is low ii) Total iron binding capacity (TIBC) is high and rises to give less than 10% saturation iii) The serum ferritin is very low iv) The red cell protoporphyrin is very low.

SIDEROBLASTIC ANAEMIA *(p. 374)*

The sideroblastic anaemias comprise a group of disorders of diverse etiology in which the nucleated erythroid precursors in the bone marrow, show characteristic 'ringed sideroblasts.'

Siderocytes and Sideroblasts *(p. 374)*

Siderocytes and sideroblasts are erythrocytes and normoblasts respectively which contain cytoplasmic granules of iron.

SIDEROCYTES. These are red cells containing granules of non-haem iron. These granules stain positively with Prussian blue reaction as well as stain with Romanowsky dyes when they are referred to as *Pappenheimer bodies*. Siderocytes are normally not present in the human peripheral blood but a small number may appear following splenectomy.

SIDEROBLASTS. These are nucleated red cells (normoblasts) containing siderotic granules which stain positively with Prussian blue reaction.

Normal sideroblasts contain a few fine, scattered cytoplasmic granules representing iron which has not been utilised for haemoglobin synthesis.

Abnormal sideroblasts are further of 2 types:

■ *One type* is a sideroblast containing numerous, diffusely scattered, coarse cytoplasmic granules and are seen in conditions such as dyserythropoiesis and haemolysis.

■ The other type is *ringed sideroblast* in which haem synthesis is disturbed as occurs in sideroblastic anaemias. Ringed sideroblasts contain numerous large granules, often forming a complete or partial ring around the nucleus.

Types of Sideroblastic Anaemias *(p. 375)*

Based on etiology, sideroblastic anaemias are classified into hereditary and acquired types. The acquired type is further divided into primary and secondary forms (Table 13.5).

TABLE 13.5: Classification of Sideroblastic Anaemia.

I.	**HEREDITARY (CONGENITAL) SIDEROBLASTIC ANAEMIA**
II.	**ACQUIRED SIDEROBLASTIC ANAEMIA**
A.	**Primary (idiopathic, refractory) acquired sideroblastic anaemia**
B.	**Secondary acquired sideroblastic anaemia**
1.	*Drugs, chemicals and toxins* e.g. isoniazid, cycloserine, chloramphenicol, cyclophosphamide, alcohol and lead.
2.	*Haematological disorders* e.g. myelofibrosis, polycythaemia vera, acute leukaemia, myeloma, lymphoma and haemolytic anaemia.
3.	*Miscellaneous* e.g. carcinoma, myxoedema, rheumatoid arthritis and SLE.

Laboratory Findings *(p. 375)*

1. There is generally moderate to severe degree of *anaemia*.

2. The *blood picture* shows hypochromic anaemia which may be microcytic, or there may be some normocytic red cells as well (dimorphic).

3. *Absolute values* (MCV, MCH and MCHC) are reduced in hereditary type but MCV is often raised in acquired type.

4. The *bone marrow examination* shows erythroid hyperplasia with usually macronormoblastic erythropoiesis. Marrow iron stores are raised and pathognomonic ring sideroblasts are present.

5. *Serum ferritin* levels are raised.

6. *Serum iron* is usually raised with almost complete saturation of TIBC.

7. There is increased *iron deposition* in the tissue.

Differential diagnosis of various types of hypochromic anaemia by laboratory tests is summarised in Table 13.6.

TABLE 13.6: Laboratory Diagnosis of Hypochromic Anaemias.

TEST	IRON DEFICIENCY	CHRONIC DISORDERS	THALAS-SAEMIA	SIDEROBLASTIC ANAEMIA
1. *MCV, MCH, MCHC*	Reduced	Low normal-to-reduced	Very low	Very low (except MCV raised in aquired type)
2. *Serum iron*	Reduced	Reduced	Normal	Raised
3. *TIBC*	Raised	Reduced	Normal	Normal
4. *Serum ferritin*	Reduced	Raised	Normal	Raised (complete saturation)
5. *Marrow-iron stores*	Absent	Present	Present	Present
6. *Iron in normoblasts*	Absent	Absent	Present	Ring sideroblasts
7. *Hb electro-phoresis*	Normal	Normal	Abnormal	Normal

ANAEMIA OF CHRONIC DISORDERS *(p. 376)*

One of the commonly encountered anaemia is in patients of a variety of chronic systemic diseases in which anaemia develops secondary to disease process but there is no actual invasion of the bone marrow. A list of such chronic systemic diseases is given in Table 13.7.

TABLE 13.7: Anaemias Secondary to Chronic Systemic Disorders.

1. ANAEMIA IN CHRONIC INFECTIONS/INFLAMMATION

a. *Infections* e.g. tuberculosis, lung abscess, pneumonia, osteomyelitis, subacute bacterial endocarditis, pyelonephritis.

b. *Non-infectious inflammations* e.g. rheumatoid arthritis, SLE, vasculitis, dermato-myositis, scleroderma, sarcoidosis, Crohn's disease.

c. *Disseminated malignancies* e.g. Hodgkin's disease, disseminated carcinomas and sarcomas.

2. ANAEMIA OF RENAL DISEASE e.g. uraemia, renal failure.

3. ANAEMIA OF HYPOMETABOLIC STATE e.g. endocrinopathies (myxoedema, Addison's disease, hyperthyroidism, hypopituitarism, Addison's disease), protein malnutrition, scurvy and pregnancy, liver disease.

Pathogenesis *(p. 376)*

A number of factors may contribute to the development of anaemia in chronic systemic disorders, and in many conditions, the anaemia is complicated by other causes such as iron, B_{12} and folate deficiency, hypersplenism, renal failure with consequent reduced erythropoietic activity, endocrine abnormalities etc. However, in general, 2 factors appear to play significant role in the pathogenesis of anaemia in chronic disorders: *defective red cell production* and *reduced red cell life-span*.

Laboratory Findings *(p. 377)*

1. Anaemia is generally mild to moderate.
2. The type of anaemia in these cases is generally normocytic normochromic.
3. Red cell indices indicate that in spite of normocytic normochromic anaemia, MCHC is slightly low.
4. The reticulocyte count is generally low.
5. Measurement of erythrocyte survival generally reveals mild to moderate shortening of their life-span.
6. Examination of the marrow generally reveals normal erythroid maturation. However, the red cell precursors have reduced stainable iron than normal, while the macrophages in the marrow usually contain increased amount of iron.
7. Both serum iron and TIBC are characteristically reduced in this group of anaemias.
8. Serum ferritin levels are increased in these patients.
9. In addition, certain other plasma proteins called 'phase reactants' are raised in patients with chronic inflammation, probably under the stimulus of interleukin-1 released by activated macrophages. These proteins include γ-globulin, C3, haptoglobin, α_1-antitrypsin and fibrinogen.

MEGALOBLASTIC ANAEMIA *(p. 377)*

The megaloblastic anaemias are disorders caused by impaired DNA synthesis and are characterised by a distinctive abnormality in the haematopoietic precursors in the bone marrow in which the *maturation of the nucleus is delayed relative to that of the cytoplasm.* Since cell division is slow but cytoplasmic development progresses normally, the nucleated red cell precursors tend to be larger which Ehrlich in 1880 termed *megaloblasts.* The mature red cells released into the peripheral blood are also abnormal in shape and size, the most prominent abnormality being *macrocytosis.*

The underlying defect for the asynchronous maturation of the nucleus is defective DNA synthesis due to deficiency of vitamin B_{12} (cobalamin) and/or folic acid (folate).

The salient nutritional aspects and metabolic functions of vitamin B_{12} and folic acid are summarised in Table 13.8.

TABLE 13.8: Salient Features of Vitamin B_{12} and Folate Metabolism.

	FEATURE	VITAMIN B_{12}	FOLATE
1.	*Main foods*	Animal proteins only	Green vegetables, meats
2.	*Cooking*	Little effect	Easily destroyed
3.	*Daily requirements*	2-4 μg	100-200 μg
4.	*Daily intake*	5-30 μg	100-500 μg
5.	*Site of absorption*	Ileum	Duodenum and jejunum
6.	*Mechanism of absorption*	Intrinsic factor	Conversion to methyl-THF
7.	*Body stores*	2-3 mg (enough for 2-4 yrs)	10-12 mg (enough for 4 months)

Vitamin B_{12} Metabolism *(p. 377)*

BIOCHEMISTRY. In humans, there are 2 metabolically active forms of cobalamin—methyl-cobalamin and adenosyl-cobalamin, which act as coenzymes.

SOURCES. The only dietary sources of vitamin B_{12} are foods of animal protein origin such as kidney, liver, heart, muscle meats, fish, eggs, cheese and milk.

In contrast to folate, vegetables contain practically no vitamin B_{12}. Cooking has little effect on its activity.

ABSORPTION. After ingestion, vitamin B_{12} in food is released and forms a stable complex with gastric R-binder. R-binder is a form of glycoprotein found in various secretions (e.g. saliva, milk, gastric juice, bile), phagocytes and plasma. On entering the duodenum, the vitamin B_{12}-R-binder complex is digested releasing vitamin B_{12} which then binds to intrinsic factor (IF). The vitamin B_{12}-IF complex, on reaching the distal ileum, binds to the specific receptors on the mucosal brush border, thereby enabling the vitamin to be absorbed. The receptor-bound vitamin B_{12}-IF complex is taken into the ileal mucosal cells where after several hours the IF is destroyed, vitamin B_{12} released and is transferred to another transport protein, transcobalamin (TC) II. The vitamin B_{12}-TC II complex is finally secreted into the portal circulation from where it is taken by the liver, bone marrow and other cells.

TISSUE STORES. Normally, the liver is the principal storage site of vitamin B_{12} and stores about 2 mg of the vitamin, while other tissues like kidney, heart and brain together store about 2 mg. The body stores of vitamin B_{12} are adequate for 2-4 years.

FUNCTIONS. Vitamin B_{12} plays an important role in general cell metabolism, particulary essential for normal haematopoiesis and for maintenance of integrity of the nervous system. Vitamin B_{12} acts as a co-enzyme for 2 main biochemical reactions in the body:

■ *Firstly, as methyl cobalamin (methyl B_{12})* in the methylation of homocysteine to methionine by methyl tetrahydrofolate (THF).

■ *Secondly, as adenosyl cobalamin (adenosyl B_{12})* in propionate metabolism for the conversion of methyl malonyl co-enzyme A to succinyl co-enzyme A.

Lack of adenosyl B_{12} leads to large increase in the level of methyl malonyl CoA and its precursor, propionyl CoA. This results in synthesis of certain fatty acids which are incorporated into the neuronal lipids. This biochemical abnormality may contribute to the neurologic complications of vitamin B_{12} deficiency.

Folate Metabolism *(p. 378)*

BIOCHEMISTRY. Folate or folic acid, a yellow compound, is a member of water-soluble B complex vitamins with the chemical name of *pteroyl glutamic acid (PGA)*.

SOURCES. Folate exists in different plants, bacteria and animal tissues. Its main dietary sources are fresh green leafy vegetables, fruits, liver, kidney, and to a lesser extent, muscle meats, cereals and milk. Folate is labile and is largely destroyed by cooking and canning.

ABSORPTION AND TRANSPORT. Folate is normally absorbed from the duodenum and upper jejunum and to a lesser extent, from the lower jejunum and ileum. However, absorption depends upon the form of folate in the diet.

TISSUE STORES. The liver and red cells are the main storage sites of folate, largely as methyl THF polyglutamate form.

FUNCTIONS. Folate plays an essential role in cellular metabolism. It acts as a co-enzyme for 2 important biochemical reactions involving transfer of 1-carbon units (viz. methyl and formyl groups) to various other compounds. These reactions are as under:

■ *Thymidylate synthetase reaction.* Formation of deoxy thymidylate monophosphate (dTMP) from its precursor form, deoxy uridylate monophosphate (dUMP).

■ *Methylation of homocysteine to methionine.* This reaction is linked to vitamin B_{12} metabolism.

Chapter Thirteen

Biochemical Basis of Megaloblastic Anaemia (p. 380)

The basic biochemical abnormality common to both vitamin B_{12} and folate deficiency is a block in the DNA synthesis pathway and that there is an inter-relationship between vitamin B_{12} and folate metabolism in the methylation reaction of homocysteine to methionine (Fig. 13.2).

Fig. 13.2: Biochemical basis of megaloblastic anaemia (THF = tetrahydrofolate; DHF = dihydrofolate; PGA = pteroyl glutamic acid; dUMP = deoxy uridylate monophosphate; dTMP = deoxy thymidylate monophosphate).

1. Thymidylate synthetase reaction. This reaction involves synthesis of deoxy thymidylate monophosphate (dTMP) from deoxy uridylate mono-phosphate (dUMP). The methyl group of dUMP $\rightarrow$ dTMP reaction is supplied by the co-enzyme, methylene-THF.

2. Homocysteine-methionine reaction. Homocysteine is converted into methionine by transfer of a methyl group from methylene-THF. After transfer of 1-carbon from methylene-THF, THF is produced. This reaction requires the presence of vitamin B_{12} (methyl-B_{12}).

Etiology and Classification of Megaloblastic Anaemia (p. 380)

The etiology of megaloblastic anaemia varies in different parts of the world. As outlined in Table 13.9, megaloblastic anaemia is classified into 3 broad groups: vitamin B_{12} deficiency, folate deficiency, and other causes.

Clinical Features (p. 381)

1. Macrocytic megaloblastic anaemia.
2. Typically, the patient has a smooth, beefy, red tongue.
3. Vitamin B_{12} deficiency, particularly in patients of pernicious anaemia, is associated with significant neurological manifestations in the form of subacute combined, degeneration of the spinal cord and peripheral neuropathy, while folate deficiency may occasionally develop neuropathy only.
4. In addition, patients may have various other symptoms. Mild jaundice, angular stomatitis, purpura, melanin pigmentation, symptoms of malabsorption, weight loss and anorexia.

Chapter Thirteen

TABLE 13.9: Etiologic Classification of Megaloblastic Anaemia.

I.   VITAMIN B$_{12}$ DEFICIENCY

A.   Inadequate dietary intake e.g. strict vegetarians, breast-fed infants.

B.   Malabsorption

1.   *Gastric causes:* pernicious anaemia, gastrectomy, congenital lack of intrinsic factor.

2.   *Intestinal causes:* tropical sprue, ileal resection, Crohn's disease, intestinal blind loop syndrome, fish-tapeworm infestation.

II.   FOLATE DEFICIENCY

A.   Inadequate dietary intake e.g. in alcoholics, teenagers, infants, old age, poverty.

B.   Malabsorption e.g. in tropical sprue, coeliac disease, partial gastrectomy, jejunal resection, Crohn's disease.

C.   Excess demand

1.   *Physiological:* pregnancy, lactation, infancy.

2.   *Pathological:* malignancy, increased haematopoiesis, chronic exfoliative skin disorders, tuberculosis, rheumatoid arthritis.

D.   Excess urinary folate loss e.g. in active liver disease, congestive heart failure.

III.   OTHER CAUSES

A.   Impaired metabolism e.g. inhibitors of dihydrofolate (DHF) reductase such as methotrexate and pyrimethamine; alcohol, congenital enzyme deficiencies.

B.   Unknown etiology e.g. in Di Guglielmo's syndrome, congenital dyserythropoietic anaemia, refractory megaloblastic anaemia.

A. General Laboratory Findings *(p. 381)*

1. BLOOD PICTURE AND RED CELL INDICES. i) The haemoglobin estimation reveals values below the normal range.

ii)   The red blood cell morphology in a blood film shows the characteristic macrocytosis. However, *macrocytosis* can also be seen in several other disorders such as: haemolysis, liver disease, alcoholism, hypothyroidism, aplastic anaemia, myeloproliferative disorders and reticulocytosis. In addition, the blood smear demonstrates marked anisocytosis, poikilocytosis and presence of macroovalocytes.

iii)   The reticulocyte count is generally low to normal in untreated cases.

iv)   The red cell indices reveal an elevated MCV (above 120 fl) proportionate to the severity of macrocytosis, elevated MCH (above 50 pg) and normal or reduced MCHC.

v)   The total white blood cell count may be reduced. Presence of characteristic hypersegmented neutrophils (having more than 5 nuclear lobes) in the blood film should raise the suspicion of megaloblastic anaemia.

vi)   Platelet count may be moderately reduced in severely anaemic patients.

2. BONE MARROW FINDINGS. The bone marrow examination is very helpful in the diagnosis of megaloblastic anaemia.

i)   The marrow is hypercellular with a decreased myeloid-erythroid ratio.

ii)   The erythroid hyperplasia is due to characteristic megaloblastic erythropoiesis. *Megaloblasts* are abnormal, large, nucleated erythroid precursors, having nuclear-cytoplasmic asynchrony i.e. the nuclei are less mature than the development of cytoplasm. The nuclei are large, having fine, reticular and open chromatin that stains lightly, while the haemoglobinisation of the cytoplasm proceeds normally or at a faster rate i.e. *nuclear maturation lags behind that of cytoplasm.*

iii)   Granulocyte precursors are also affected to some extent. Giant forms of metamyelocytes and band cells may be present in the marrow.

iv)   Prussian blue staining for iron in the marrow shows an increase in the number and size of iron granules in the erythroid precursors. Iron in the reticulum cells is increased.

B. Special Tests for Cause of Specific Deficiency *(p. 383)*

TESTS FOR VITAMIN B$_{12}$ DEFICIENCY. Following tests are done to establish the vitamin B$_{12}$ deficiency:

1. SERUM VITAMIN B$_{12}$ ASSAY. Assay of vitamin B$_{12}$ in blood can be done by 2 methods—microbiologic assay and radioassay.

2. SCHILLING TEST (RADIOISOTOPE ABSORPTION TEST). Schilling test is done to detect vitamin B$_{12}$ deficiency as well as to distinguish and detect lack of IF and malabsorption. The results of test also depend upon good renal function and proper urinary collection.

3. SERUM ENZYME LEVELS. Besides Schilling test, another way of distinguishing whether megaloblastic anaemia is due to cobalamine or folate is by serum determination of methylmalonic acid and homocysteine. Both are elevated in cobalamine deficiency, while in folate deficiency there is only elevation of homocysteine and not of methylmalonic acid.

TESTS FOR FOLATE DEFICIENCY. Measurement of *formiminoglutamic acid (FIGLU) urinary excretion* after histidine load was used formerly for assessing folate status but it is less specific and less sensitive than the serum assays. Currently, following tests are used to detect folate deficiency.

1. URINARY EXCRETION OF FIGLU

2. SERUM FOLATE ASSAY. The folate in serum can be estimated by 2 methods—microbiological assay and radioassay.

3. RED CELL FOLATE ASSAY. Red cells contain 20-50 times more folate than the serum and that red cell folate assay is more reliable indicator of tissue stores of folate than serum folate assay. Both microbiological and radioassay methods can be used for estimation of red cell folate.

PERNICIOUS ANAEMIA *(p. 384)*

Pernicious anaemia (PA) was first described by Addison in 1855 as a chronic disorder of middle-aged and elderly individual of either sex in which intrinsic factor secretion ceases owing to atrophy of the gastric mucosa. The condition is, therefore, also termed Addisonian megaloblastic anaemia. The average age at presentation is 60 years.

Pathogenesis *(p. 384)*

There is evidence to suggest that the atrophy of gastric mucosa in PA is caused by an autoimmune reaction against gastric parietal cells. The evidences in support of immunological abnormalities in pernicious anaemia are as under:
1. The incidence of PA is high in patients with *other autoimmune diseases.*
2. Patients with PA have abnormal *circulating autoantibodies* such as anti-parietal cell antibody (90% cases) and anti-intrinsic factor antibody (50% cases).
3. *Relatives* of patients with PA have an increased incidence of the disease or increased presence of autoantibodies.
4. *Corticosteroids* have been reported to be beneficial in curing the disease both pathologically and clinically.
5. PA is more common in patients with *agammaglobulinaemia.*

M/E The most characteristic pathologic finding in PA is gastric atrophy affecting the acid- and pepsin-secreting portion of the stomach and sparing the antrum. Gastric epithelium may show cellular atypia. About 2-3% cases of PA develop carcinoma of the stomach.

Clinical Features *(p. 385)*

The disease has insidious onset and progresses slowly. The clinical manifestations are mainly due to vitamin B$_{12}$ deficiency. These include: anaemia, glossitis, neurological abnormalities (neuropathy, subacute combined degeneration of the spinal cord, retrobulbar neuritis), gastrointestinal manifestations (diarrhoea, anorexia, weight loss, dyspepsia), hepatosplenomegaly, congestive heart failure and haemorrhagic manifestations.

Laboratory Findings *(p. 385)*

1. *Hypergastrinaemia*
2. *Pentagastrinaemia*
3. *Haematologic findings* in blood and bone marrow are similar to those seen in megaloblastic anaemia discussed above.
4. *Biochemical alterations* reveal rise in serum bilirubin, LDH, haptoglobin, ferritin and iron. Serum folate is usually normal but red cell folate is almost always reduced.
5. *Schilling test* is abnormal due to IF deficiency as observed by low 24-hour urinary excretion of labelled vitamin B_{12}.
6. *Chromosomal abnormalities* are frequently present in bone marrow cells which disappear after therapy.

HAEMOLYTIC ANAEMIAS *(p. 385)*

Haemolytic anaemias are defined as anaemias resulting from an increase in the rate of red cell destruction. Normally, effete red cells undergo lysis at the end of their life-span of 90-120 days within the cells of reticuloendothelial (RE) system in the spleen and elsewhere (extravascular haemolysis), and haemoglobin is not liberated into the plasma in appreciable amounts. The red cell life-span is shortened in haemolytic anaemia i.e. there is accelerated haemolysis.

The premature destruction of red cells in haemolytic anaemia may occur by 2 mechanisms:

■ **Firstly,** the red cells undergo lysis in the circulation and release their contents into plasma *(intravascular haemolysis)*. In these cases the plasma haemoglobin rises substantially and part of it may be excreted in the urine *(haemoglobinuria)*.

■ **Secondly,** the red cells are taken up by cells of the RE system where they are destroyed and digested *(extravascular haemolysis)*. In extravascular haemolysis, plasma haemoglobin level is, therefore, barely raised.

Extravascular haemolysis is more common than the former.

Haemolytic anaemias are broadly classified into 2 main categories:

I. *Acquired haemolytic anaemias* caused by a variety of extrinsic environmental factors *(extracorpuscular)*.

II. *Hereditary haemolytic anaemias* are usually the result of intrinsic red cell defects *(intracorpuscular)*.

A simplified classification based on these mechanisms is given in Table 13.10.

Features of Haemolysis *(p. 385)*

General clinical features:

1. Presence of pallor of mucous membranes.
2. Positive family history in patients with congenital haemolytic anaemia.
3. Mild fluctuating jaundice due to unconjugated hyperbilirubinaemia.
4. Urine turns dark on standing due to excess of urobilinogen.
5. Splenomegaly is found in most chronic haemolytic anaemias.
6. Pigment gallstones are found in some cases.

Laboratory evaluation of haemolysis:

I. **Tests of increased red cell breakdown.**

1. *Serum bilirubin*—unconjugated (indirect) bilirubin is raised.
2. *Urine urobilinogen* is raised but there is no bilirubinuria.

TABLE 13.10: Classification of Haemolytic Anaemias.

I. ACQUIRED (EXTRACORPUSCULAR)

A. Antibody: Immunohaemolytic anaemias
  1. Autoimmune haemolytic anaemia (AIHA)
     i) Warm antibody AIHA
     ii) Cold antibody AIHA
  2. Drug-induced immunohaemolytic anaemia
  3. Isoimmune haemolytic anaemia

B. Mechanical trauma: Microangiopathic haemolytic anaemia

C. Direct toxic effects: Malaria, bacteria, infection and other agents

D. Acquired red cell membrane abnormalities: paroxysmal nocturnal haemoglobinuria (PNH)

E. Splenomegaly

II. HEREDITARY (INTRACORPUSCULAR)

A. Abnormalities of red cell membrane
  1. Hereditary spherocytosis
  2. Hereditary elliptocytosis (hereditary ovalocytosis)
  3. Hereditary stomatocytosis

B. Disorders of red cell interior
  1. *Red cell enzyme defects*
     i) Defects in the hexose monophosphate shunt: G6PD deficiency
     ii) Defects in the Embden-Meyerhof (or glycolytic) pathway: pyruvate kinase deficiency
  2. *Disorders of haemoglobin*
     i) Structurally abnormal haemoglobins (haemoglobinopathies): sickle syndromes, other haemoglobinopathies
     ii) Reduced globin chain synthesis: thalassaemias

---

3. *Faecal stercobilinogen* is raised.
4. *Serum haptoglobin* (α-globulin binding protein) is reduced or absent.
5. *Plasma lactic dehydrogenase* is raised.
6. *Evidences of intravascular haemolysis* in the form of haemoglobinaemia, haemoglobinuria, methaemoglobinaemia and haemosiderinuria.

II. Tests of increased red cell production.
1. *Reticulocyte count* reveals reticulocytosis.
2. *Routine blood film* shows macrocytosis, polychromasia and presence of normoblasts.
3. *Bone marrow* shows erythroid hyperplasia with usually raised iron stores.
4. *X-ray of bones* shows evidence of expansion of marrow space, especially in tubular bones and skull.

III. Tests of damage to red cells. These include the following:
1. *Routine blood film* shows a variety of abnormal morphological appearances of red cells (Table 13.11).
2. *Osmotic fragility* is increased.
3. *Autohaemolysis test* with or without addition of glucose.
4. *Coombs' antiglobulin test.*
5. *Electrophoresis* for abnormal haemoglobins.
6. *Estimation of HbA$_2$.*
7. *Estimation of HbF.*
8. *Tests for sickling.*
9. *Screening test for G6PD deficiency* and other enzymes (e.g. Heinz bodies test).

IV. Tests for shortened red cell life-span. A shortened red cell survival is best tested by ^{51}Cr labelling method.

TABLE 13.11: Red Cell Morphologic Features in Various Types of Haemolytic Anaemias.

	FEATURE	ETIOLOGY	TYPE OF HAEMOLYTIC ANAEMIA
1.	*Spherocytes*	Loss of spectrin from membrane	Hereditary spherocytosis AIHA
2.	*Target cells (Leptocytes)*	Increased ratio of surface area: volume	Thalassaemias Liver disease HbS disease HbC disease
3.	*Schistocytes*	Traumatic damage to red cell membrane	Microangiopathy
4.	*Sickle cells*	Polymerisation of HbS	Sickle syndromes
5.	*Acanthocytes (Spur cells)*	Abnormality in membrane lipids	Severe liver disease
6.	*Heinz bodies*	Precipitated Hb	Unstable Hb

I. ACQUIRED (EXTRACORPUSCULAR) HAEMOLYTIC ANAEMIAS *(p. 387)*

A. IMMUNOHAEMOLYTIC ANAEMIAS *(p. 387)*

Immunohaemolytic anaemias are a group of anaemias occurring due to antibody production by the body against its own red cells. Immune haemolysis in these cases may be induced by one of the following three types of antibodies:

1. *Autoimmune haemolytic anaemia (AIHA)* characterised by formation of autoantibodies against patient's own red cells. Depending upon the reactivity of autoantibody, AIHA is further divided into 2 types:

i) 'Warm' antibody AIHA in which the autoantibodies are reactive at body temperature (37°C).

ii) 'Cold' antibody AIHA in which the autoantibodies react better with patient's own red cells at 4°C.

2. *Drug-induced immunohaemolytic anaemia.*

3. *Isoimmune haemolytic anaemia* in which the antibodies are acquired by blood transfusions, pregnancies and haemolytic disease of the newborn.

An important diagnostic tool in all cases of immunohaemolytic anaemias is Coombs' antiglobulin test for detection of incomplete Rh-antibodies in saline directly (direct Coombs') or after addition of albumin (indirect Coombs').

'WARM' ANTIBODY AIHA *(p. 388)*

Warm antibodies reactive at body temperature and coating the red cells are generally IgG class antibodies and occasionally they are IgA. Red cells coated with IgG alongwith C3 on the surface further promote this red cell-leucocyte interaction, accounting for more severe haemolysis. The spleen is particularly efficient in trapping red cells coated with IgG antibodies. It is, thus, the major site of red cell destruction in warm antibody AIHA.

The disease may occur without any apparent cause (idiopathic) but about a quarter of patients develop this disorder as a complication of an underlying disease affecting the immune system, especially SLE, chronic lymphocytic leukaemia, lymphomas and certain drugs such as methyl DOPA, penicillin etc (Table 13.12).

CLINICAL FEATURES. The disease tends to have remissions and relapses. The usual clinical features are:

1. Chronic anaemia of varying severity with remissions and relapses.
2. Splenomegaly.
3. Occasionally hyperbilirubinaemia.

TABLE 13.12: Conditions Predisposing to Autoimmune Haemolytic Anaemia (AIHA).

A. *Warm antibody AIHA*
   1. Idiopathic (primary)
   2. Lymphomas-leukaemias e.g. non-Hodgkin's lymphoma, CLL, Hodgkin's disease
   3. Collagen vascular diseases e.g SLE
   4. Drugs e.g. methyl dopa, penicillin, quinidine group
   5. Post-viral

B. *Cold antibody AIHA*
   1. Cold agglutinin disease
   a) Acute: *Mycoplasma* infection, infectious mononucleosis
   b) Chronic: Idiopathic, lymphomas
   2. PCH (*Mycoplasma* infection, viral flu, measles, mumps, syphilis)

LABORATORY FINDINGS. These are as under:
1. Mild to moderate chronic anaemia.
2. Reticulocytosis.
3. Prominent spherocytosis in the peripheral blood film.
4. Positive direct Coombs' (antiglobulin) test for presence of warm antibodies on the red cell, best detected at 37°C.
5. A positive indirect Coombs' (antiglobulin) test at 37°C may indicate presence of large quantities of warm antibodies in the serum.
6. Unconjugated (indirect) hyperbilirubinaemia.
7. Co-existent immune thrombocytopenia alongwith occasional venous thrombosis may be present (termed Evans' syndrome).
8. In more severe cases, haemoglobinaemia and haemoglobinuria may be present.

'COLD' ANTIBODY AIHA (p. 388)

Antibodies which are reactive in the cold (4°C) may induce haemolysis under 2 conditions: cold agglutinin disease and paroxysmal cold haemoglobinuria.

1. Cold agglutinin disease. In cold agglutinin disease, the antibodies are IgM type which bind to the red cells best at 4°C. These cold antibodies are usually directed against the *I* antigen on the red cell surface. Agglutination of red blood cells by IgM cold agglutinins is most profound at very low temperature but upon warming to 37°C or above, disagglutination occurs quickly. Most cold agglutinins affect juvenile red blood cells.

   The etiology of cold antibody remains unknown. It is seen in the course of certain infections (e.g. *Mycoplasma* pneumonia, infectious mononucleosis) and in lymphomas.

2. Paroxysmal cold haemoglobinuria (PCH). In PCH, the cold antibody is an IgG antibody (Donath-Landsteiner antibody) which is directed against *P* blood group antigen and brings about complement-mediated haemolysis. Attacks of PCH are precipitated by exposure to cold. PCH is uncommon and may be seen in association with tertiary syphilis or as a complication of certain infections such as *Mycoplasma* pneumonia, flu, measles and mumps.

CLINICAL FEATURES. The clinical manifestations are due to haemolysis and not due to agglutination. These include:
1. Chronic anaemia worsened by exposure to cold.
2. Raynaud's phenomenon.
3. Cyanosis affecting the cold exposed regions such as tips of nose, ears, fingers and toes.
4. Haemoglobinaemia and haemoglobinuria occur on exposure to cold.

LABORATORY FINDINGS. The haematologic and biochemical findings are somewhat similar to those found in warm antibody AIHA except the thermal amplitude. These findings are: 1. Chronic anaemia. 2. Low reticulocyte count since young red cells are affected more. 3. Spherocytosis is less marked. 4. Positive direct Coombs' test for detection of C3 on the red cell surface but IgM responsible for C3 coating on red cells is not found. 5. The cold antibody titre is very high at 4°C and very low at 37°C (Donath-Landsteiner test).

Drug-induced Immunohaemolytic Anaemia *(p. 389)*

Drugs may cause immunohaemolytic anaemia by 3 different mechanisms:
1. α-methyl dopa type antibodies.
2. Penicillin-induced immunohaemolysis.
3. Innocent by stander immunohaemolysis.

Isoimmune Haemolytic Anaemia *(p. 389)*

Isoimmune haemolytic anaemias are caused by acquiring isoantibodies or alloantibodies by blood transfusions, pregnancies and in haemolytic disease of the newborn, discussed at the end of this chapter.

B. MICROANGIOPATHIC HAEMOLYTIC ANAEMIA *(p. 389)*

Microangiopathic haemolytic anaemia is caused by abnormalities in the microvasculature. It is generally due to mechanical trauma to the red cells in circulation and is characterised by red cell fragmentation (schistocytosis). There are 3 different ways by which microangiopathic haemolytic anaemia results:

1. EXTERNAL IMPACT. Direct external trauma to red blood cells, may cause haemolysis during various activities e.g. in prolonged marchers, joggers, karate players etc. These patients develop haemoglobinaemia, haemoglobinuria *(march haemoglobinuria).*

2. CARDIAC HAEMOLYSIS. A small proportion of patients who received prosthetic cardiac valves or artificial grafts develop haemolysis.

3. FIBRIN DEPOSIT IN MICROVASCULATURE. Deposition of fibrin in the microvasculature exposes the red cells to physical obstruction and eventual fragmentation of red cells and trapping of the platelets e.g.
i)   Abnormalities of the vessel wall e.g. in hypertension, eclampsia, disseminated cancers, transplant rejection, haemangioma etc.
ii) Thrombotic thrombocytopenic purpura.
iii) Haemolytic-uraemic syndrome.
iv) Disseminated intravascular coagulation (DIC)
v)   Vasculitis in collagen diseases.

C. HAEMOLYTIC ANAEMIA FROM DIRECT TOXIC EFFECTS *(p. 390)*

Haemolysis may result from direct toxic effects of certain agents. These include the following examples:
1. Malaria by direct parasitisation of red cells (black-water fever).
2. Bartonellosis by direct infection of red cells.
3. Septicaemia with Clostridium welchii.
4. Other microorganisms such as pneumococci, staphylococci and Escherichia coli.
5. Copper by direct haemolytic effect on red cells in Wilson's disease.
6. Lead poisoning
7. Snake and spider bites
8. Extensive burns.

D. PAROXYSMAL NOCTURNAL HAEMOGLOBINURIA (PNH) *(p. 390)*

PNH is a rare acquired disorder of red cell membrane in which there is chronic intravascular haemolysis due to undue sensitivity of red blood cells to complement due to defective synthesis of a red cell membrane protein. The defect affects all the cells of myeloid progenitor lineage (RBCs, WBCs, platelets).

PATHOGENESIS. PNH is considered as an acquired clonal disease of the cell membrane while normal clone also continues to proliferate. The defect in stem cells is a mutation affecting myeloid progenitor cells that normally is required for the biosynthesis of glycosyl phosphatidyl inositol (GPI) essential for anchoring of the cell. As a result of mutation, there is partial or complete deficiency of anchor protein. Out of about 20 such proteins described so far, the lack of two of the proteins—*decay accelerating factor (DAF, CD55)* and a *membrane inhibitor of reactive lysis (MIRL, CD59)*, makes the RBCs sensitive to the lytic effect of complement.

CLINICAL AND LABORATORY FINDINGS. These are as under:

i) Haemolytic anaemia. ii) Pancytopenia (mild granulocytopenia and thrombocytopenia frequent). iii) Intermittent clinical haemoglobinuria; acute haemolytic episodes occur at night identified by passage of brown urine in the morning. iv) Haemosiderinuria very common. v) Venous thrombosis common complication.

The presence of inordinate sensitivity of red blood cells, leucocytes and platelets to complement in PNH can be demonstrated *in vitro* by *Ham's test* using red cell lysis at acidic pH or by sucrose haemolysis test.

E.   HAEMOLYTIC ANAEMIA IN SPLENOMEGALY (*p. 390*)

Haemolytic anaemia is common in splenic enlargement from any cause. Normally, the spleen acts as a filter and traps the damaged red blood cells, destroys them and the splenic macrophages phagocytose the damaged red cells. A normal spleen poses no risk to normal red blood cells. But splenomegaly exaggerates the damaging effect to which the red cells are exposed. Besides haemolytic anaemia, splenomegaly is usually associated with pancytopenia.

II. HEREDITARY (INTRACORPUSCULAR)
    HAEMOLYTIC ANAEMIA (*p. 390*)

A. HEREDITARY ABNORMALITIES OF RED CELL MEMBRANE (*p. 390*)

Hereditary Spherocytosis (*p. 391*)

Hereditary spherocytosis is a common type of hereditary haemolytic anaemia of autosomal dominant inheritance in which the red cell membrane is abnormal.

PATHOGENESIS. The molecular abnormality in hereditary spherocytosis is a defect in proteins which anchor the lipid bilayer to the underlying cytoskeleton. These protein abnormalities are as under:

1. **Spectrin deficiency.** Almost all cases have deficiency in the structural protein of the red cell membrane, spectrin. Spectrin deficiency correlates with the severity of anaemia.

2. **Ankyrin abnormality.** About half the cases of hereditary spherocytosis have defect in ankyrin, protein that binds protein 3 and spectrin.

Inherited mutation in spectrin or ankyrin causes defect in anchoring of lipid bilayer cell membrane. Red cells with such unstable membrane but with normal volume, when released in circulation, lose their membrane further, till they can accommodate the given volume. This results in formation of spheroidal contour and smaller size of red blood cells, termed *microspherocytes*.

CLINICAL FEATURES. The major clinical features are:

1. *Anaemia* is usually mild to moderate. 2. *Splenomegaly* is a constant feature. 3. *Jaundice* occurs due to increased concentration of unconjugated (indirect) bilirubin. 4. *Pigment gallstones* are frequent.

LABORATORY FINDINGS. Salient laboratory findings are:

1. *Anaemia* of mild to moderate degree. 2. *Reticulocytosis,* usually 5-20%. 3. Blood film shows the characteristic *microspherocytes.* 4. MCV is usually normal or slightly decreased. 5. *Osmotic fragility is increased.* 6. *Autohaemolysis test* is similar to osmotic fragility test after incubation and shows increased spontaneous autohaemolysis. 7. *Direct Coombs' (antiglobulin) test* is negative.

Hereditary Elliptocytosis (Hereditary Ovalocytosis) *(p. 392)*

Hereditary elliptocytosis or hereditary ovalocytosis is another autosomal dominant disorder involving red cell membrane protein *spectrin.* Some patients have an inherited defect in erythrocyte membrane protein 4.1 that interconnects spectrin with actin in the cytoskeleton.

Hereditary Stomatocytosis *(p. 392)*

Stomatocytes are cup-shaped RBCs having one surface concave and the other side as convex. This causes a central slit-like or mouth-like appearance of red cells. The underlying defect is in membrane protein, *stomatin,* having autosomal dominant pattern of inheritance.

B.   HEREDITARY DISORDERS OF RED CELL INTERIOR *(p. 392)*

Inherited disorders involving the interior of the red blood cells are classified into 2 groups:

1.   Red cell enzyme defects: These cause defective red cell metabolism involving 2 pathways:

i)   *Defects in the hexose monophosphate shunt:* Common example is glucose-6-phosphate dehydrogenase (G6PD) deficiency.

ii)   *Defects in the Embden-Meyerhof (glycolytic) pathway:* Example is pyruvate kinase (PK) deficiency.

2.   Disorders of haemoglobin: These are divided into 2 subgroups:

i)   *Abnormal haemoglobins (haemoglobinopathies):* Examples are sickle syndromes and other haemoglobinopathies.

ii)   *Reduced globin chain synthesis:* Common examples are various types of thalassaemias.

G6PD DEFICIENCY (p. 393)

Among the defects in hexose monophosphate shunt, the most common is G6PD deficiency. It affects millions of people throughout the world. The G6PD gene is located on the X chromosome and its deficiency is, therefore, a sex (X)-linked trait affecting males, while the females are carriers and are asymptomatic. Several variants of G6PD have been described. The most common and significant clinical variant is A–(negative) type found in black males. Like the HbS gene, the A–type G6PD variant confers protection against malaria. Individuals with A–G6PD variant have shortened red cell life-span but without anaemia. However, these individuals develop haemolytic episodes on exposure to oxidant stress such as viral and bacterial infections, certain drugs, metabolic acidosis and on ingestion of fava beans (favism).

PATHOGENESIS. Individuals with inherited deficiency of G6PD, an enzyme required for hexose monophosphate shunt for glucose metabolism, fail to develop adequate levels of reduced glutathione in their red cells. This results in oxidation and precipitation of haemoglobin within the red cells forming Heinz bodies.

CLINICAL FEATURES. The clinical manifestations are those of an acute haemolytic anaemia within hours of exposure to oxidant stress. The haemolysis is, however, self-limiting even if the exposure to the oxidant is continued since it affects the older red cells only.

LABORATORY FINDINGS. These are as under:

1. During the period of acute haemolysis, there is rapid fall in haematocrit by 25-30%, features of intravascular haemolysis such as rise in plasma haemoglobin, haemoglobinuria, rise in unconjugated bilirubin and fall in plasma haptoglobin. Formation of Heinz bodies is visualised by means of supravital stains such as crystal violet, also called *Heinz body haemolytic anaemia.*

2. Between the crises, the affected patient generally has no anaemia. The red cell survival is, however, shortened.

PK DEFICIENCY *(p. 394)*

Pyruvate kinase (PK) deficiency is the only significant enzymopathy of the Embden-Meyerhof glycolytic pathway. The disorder is inherited as an autosomal recessive pattern.

LABORATORY FINDINGS. These are as under:
1. Normocytic and normochromic anaemia.
2. Reticulocytosis.
3. Blood film shows bizarre red cells.
4. Osmotic fragility is usually normal but after incubation it is increased.
5. Autohaemolysis is increased, but unlike hereditary spherocytosis, is not corrected by addition of glucose.
6. Direct specific enzyme assay on red cells is the only method of establishing the diagnosis.

ABNORMAL HAEMOGLOBINS (HAEMOGLOBINOPATHIES) *(p. 394)*

SICKLE SYNDROMES *(p. 394)*

The most important and widely prevalent type of haemoglobinopathy is due to the presence of sickle haemoglobin (HbS) in the red blood cells. The red cells with HbS develop 'sickling' when they are exposed to low oxygen tension. Sickle syndromes have the highest frequency in black race and in Central Africa where *falciparum* malaria is endemic. Patients with HbS are relatively protected against *falciparum* malaria. Sickle syndromes occur in 3 different forms:

Heterozygous State: Sickle Cell Trait *(p. 394)*

Sickle cell trait is a benign heterozygous state of HbS in which only one abnormal gene is inherited. Patients with AS develop no significant clinical problems except when they become severely hypoxic and may develop sickle cell crises.

LABORATORY FINDINGS. These patients have no anaemia and have normal appearance of red cells. But in hypoxic crisis, sickle cell crises develop. The diagnosis is made by 2 tests:
1. Demonstration of sickling. 2. Haemoglobin electrophoresis

Homozygous State: Sickle Cell Anaemia *(p. 395)*

Sickle cell anaemia (SS) is a homozygous state of HbS in the red cells in which an abnormal gene is inherited from each parent. SS is a severely malignant disorder associated with protean clinical manifestations and decreased life expectancy.

PATHOGENESIS. Following abnormalities are seen:

1. Basic molecular lesion: In HbS, basic genetic defect is the *single point mutation* in one amino acid out of 146 in haemoglobin molecule; there is *substitution of valine for glutamic acid* at the 6 residue position of the β-globin.

2. Mechanism of sickling: During deoxygenation, the red cells containing HbS change from biconcave disc shape to an elongated crescent-shaped or sickle-shaped cell. This process termed *sickling* occurs both within the intact red cells and *in vitro* in free solution.

3. Reversible-irreversible sickling: The oxygen-dependent sickling process is usually reversible.

4. Factors determining rate of sickling: These are:
i) Presence of non-HbS haemoglobins. ii) Intracellular concentration of HbS. iii) Total haemoglobin concentration. iv) Extent of deoxygenation. v) Acidosis and dehydration. vi) Increased concentration of 2, 3-BPG in the red cells.

CLINICAL FEATURES. The clinical manifestations of homozygous sickle cell disease are widespread. The symptoms begin to appear after 6th month of life when most of the HbF is replaced by HbS.

1. Anaemia. There is usually severe chronic haemolytic anaemia (primarily extravascular) with onset of aplastic crisis in between.

2. Vaso-occlusive phenomena. Patients of SS develop recurrent vaso-occlusive episodes throughout their lives due to obstruction to capillary blood flow by sickled red cells upon deoxygenation or dehydration.
i) *Microinfarcts* affecting particularly the abdomen, chest, back and joints and are the cause of recurrent painful crises in SS.
ii) *Macroinfarcts* involving most commonly the spleen (splenic sequestration, autosplenectomy), bone marrow (pains), bones (aseptic necrosis, osteomyelitis), lungs (pulmonary infections), kidneys (renal cortical necrosis), CNS (stroke), retina (damage) and skin (ulcers), and result in anatomic and functional damage to these organs.
    In addition to the features of anaemia and infarction, patients with SS have impaired growth and development and increased susceptibility to infection.

LABORATORY FINDINGS. These are as under:
1. Moderate to severe anaemia (haemoglobin concentration 6-9 g/dl).
2. The blood film shows sickle cells and target cells and features of splenic atrophy.
3. A positive sickling test.
4. Haemoglobin electrophoresis shows no normal HbA but shows predominance of HbS and 2-20% HbF.

Double Heterozygous States *(p. 396)*

Double heterozygous conditions involving combination of HbS with other haemoglobinopathies may occur. Most common among these are sickle-β-thalassaemia, sickle C disease (SC), and sickle D disease (SD). All these disorders behave like mild form of sickle cell disease.

Unstable-Hb Haemoglobinopathy *(p. 396)*

The unstable haemoglobins are those haemoglobin variants which undergo denaturation and precipitation within the red cells as Heinz bodies. These give rise to what is known as *congenital non-spherocytic haemolytic anaemia* or *congenital Heinz body haemolytic anaemia*. These disorders have either autosomal dominant inheritance or develop from spontaneous mutations.
    Over 100 unstable haemoglobins have been described. They are named according to the place where they are encountered.

THALASSAEMIA (p. 397)

The thalassaemias are a diverse group of hereditary disorders in which there is reduced rate of synthesis of one or more of the globin polypeptide chains.

Thus, thalassaemias, unlike haemoglobinopathies which are qualitative disorders of haemoglobin, are *quantitative abnormalities of polypeptide globin chain synthesis.*

Thalassaemias are genetically transmitted disorders. Normally, an individual inherits two β-globin genes located one each on two chromosomes 11, and two α-globin genes one each on two chromosomes 16, from each parent i.e. normal adult haemoglobin (HbA) is $\alpha_2 \beta_2$*. Depending upon whether the genetic defect or deletion lies in transmission of α- or β-globin chain genes, thalassaemias are classified into α- and β- thalassaemias.

A classification of various types of thalassaemias alongwith the clinical syndromes produced and salient laboratory findings are given in Table 13.13.

α-THALASSAEMIA *(p. 397)*

MOLECULAR PATHOGENESIS. α-thalassaemias are disorders in which there is defective synthesis of α-globin chains resulting in depressed production of haemoglobins that contain α-chains i.e. HbA, HbA_2 and HbF. The α-thalassaemias are most commonly due to deletion of one or more of the α-chain genes located on short arm of chromosome 16. Accordingly, α-thalassaemias are classified into 4 types:

1. Four α-gene deletion: Hb Bart's hydrops foetalis.
2. Three α-gene deletion: HbH disease.
3. Two α-gene deletion: α-thalassaemia trait.
4. One α-gene deletion: α-thalassaemia trait (carrier).

β-THALASSAEMIAS *(p. 399)*

MOLECULAR PATHOGENESIS. The β-thalassaemias are caused by decreased rate of β-chain synthesis resulting in reduced formation of HbA in the red cells. The molecular pathogenesis of the β-thalassaemias is more complex than that of α-thalassaemias. In contrast to α-thalassaemia, gene deletions rarely ever cause β-thalassaemia and is only seen in an entity called *hereditary persistence of foetal haemoglobin (HPFH)*. Instead, most of β-thalassaemias arise from different types of mutations of β–globin gene resulting from single base changes. The symbol β° is used to indicate the complete absence of synthesis while β⁺ denotes partial synthesis of the β-globin chains. Some of the important ones having effects on β-globin chain synthesis are as under.

i) Transcription defect. ii) Translation defect. iii) mRNA splicing defect.

Depending upon the extent of reduction in β-chain synthesis, there are 3 types of β-thalassaemia:

1. Homozygous form: β-Thalassaemia major. It is the most severe form of congenital haemolytic anaemia. It is further of 2 types:

i) β° *thalassaemia major* characterised by complete absence of β-chain synthesis.

ii) β⁺ *thalassaemia major* having incomplete suppression of β-chain synthesis.

2. β-Thalassaemia intermedia: It is β-thalassaemia of intermediate degree of severity that does not require regular blood transfusions. These cases are genetically heterozygous (β°/β or β⁺/β).

3. Heterozygous form: β-Thalassaemia minor (trait). It is a mild asymptomatic condition in which there is moderate suppression of β-chain synthesis.

---

*In a normal adult, distribution of haemoglobin is as under: HbA $(\alpha_2\beta_2)$ = 95-98%, HbA_2 $(\alpha_2\delta_2)$ (a minor variant of HbA) = 1.5-3.5%, HbF $(\alpha_2 \gamma_2)$ = less than 1%. But the level of HbF in children under 6 months is slightly higher.

TABLE 13.13: Classification of Thalassaemias.

TYPE	HB	HB-ELECTROPHORESIS	GENOTYPE	CLINICAL SYNDROME
α-Thalassaemias				
1. *Hydrops foetalis*	3-10 g/dl	Hb Barts (γ_4) (100%)	Deletion of four α-genes	Fatal *in utero* or in early infancy
2. *Hb-H disease*	2-12 g/dl	HbF (10%)	Deletion of three α-genes	Haemolytic anaemia
3. *α-Thalassaemia trait*	10-14 g/dl	Normal	Deletion of two α-genes	Microcytic hypochromic blood picture but no anaemia
β-Thalassaemias				
1. *β-Thalassaemia major*	< 5 g/dl	HbA (0-50%), HbF (50-98%)	$\beta^{thal}/\beta^{thal}$	Severe congenital haemolytic anaemia, requires blood transfusions
2. *β-Thalassaemia intermedia*	5-10 g/dl	Variable	Multiple mechanisms	Severe anaemia, but regular blood transfusions not required
3. *β-Thalassaemia minor*	10-12 g/dl	HbA_2 (4-9%) HbF (1-5%)	β^A/β^{thal}	Usually asymptomatic

Chapter Thirteen

Besides β-thalassaemia minor, a few uncommon globin chain combinations resulting in β-thalassaemia trait are as under:

i) *δβ-thalassaemia minor* in which there is total absence of both β and δ chain synthesis and is characterised by elevated HbF level but unlike β-thalassaemia minor there is normal or reduced HbA$_2$ level.

ii) *Hb Lepore syndrome* characterised by nonhomologous fusion of β- and δ-genes forming an abnormal haemoglobin called Hb Lepore (named after a family called Lepore). There is total absence of normal β-chain synthesis.

An individual may inherit one β-chain gene from each parent and produce heterozygous, homozygous, or double heterozygous states. Statistically, 25% of offsprings born to two heterozygotes (i.e. β-thalassaemia trait) will have the homozygous state i.e. β-thalassaemia major.

β-Thalassaemia Major (p. 400)

The β-thalassaemia major, also termed Mediterranean or Cooley's anaemia is the most common form of congenital haemolytic anaemia. More commonly, β-thalassaemia major is a homozygous state with either complete absence of β-chain synthesis (β° *thalassaemia major*) or only small amounts of β-chains are formed (β⁺ *thalassaemia major*).

CLINICAL FEATURES. 1. Anaemia starts appearing within the first 4-6 months of life. 2. Marked hepatosplenomegaly. 3. Expansion of bones. 4. Iron overload due to repeated blood transfusions.

LABORATORY FINDINGS. These are as under:

1. *Anaemia,* usually severe.

2. *Severe microcytic hypochromic red cell morphology,* marked anisopoikilo-cytosis, basophilic stippling, presence of many target cells, tear drop cells and normoblasts.

3. *Serum bilirubin* (unconjugated) is generally raised.

4. *Reticulocytosis* is generally present.

5. *MCV, MCH and MCHC* are significantly reduced.

6. *WBC count is* often raised with some shift to left of the neutrophil series.

7. *Platelet count* is usually normal.

8. *Decreased osmotic fragility.*

9. *Haemoglobin electrophoresis* shows presence of increased amounts of HbF, increased amount of HbA$_2$, and almost complete absence or presence of variable amounts of HbA.

10. *Bone marrow aspirate examination* shows normoblastic erythroid hyperplasia.

β-Thalassaemia Minor (p. 401)

The β-thalassaemia minor or β-thalassaemia trait, a heterozygous state, is a common entity characterised by moderate reduction in β-chain synthesis.

CLINICAL FEATURES. Clinically, the condition is usually asymptomatic and the diagnosis is generally made when the patient is being investigated for a mild chronic anaemia. The spleen may be palpable.

LABORATORY FINDINGS. These are as follows:

1. *Mild anaemia.*

2. *Blood film* shows mild anisopoikilocytosis, microcytosis and hypochromia, occasional target cells and basophilic stippling.

3. *Serum bilirubin* may be normal or slightly raised.

4. Mild *reticulocytosis* is often present.

5. *MCV, MCH and MCHC* may be slightly reduced.

6. *Decreased osmotic fragility.*

7. *Haemoglobin electrophoresis* is confirmatory for the diagnosis and shows about two-fold increase in HbA$_2$ and a slight elevation in HbF (2-3%).

Prevention of Thalassaemia *(p. 402)*

Finally, since thalassaemia is an inheritable disease, its prevention is possible by making an antenatal diagnosis. This is done by chorionic villous biopsy or cells obtained by amniocentesis and DNA studied by PCR amplification technique for presence of genetic mutations of thalassaemias.

APLASTIC ANAEMIA *(p. 402)*

Aplastic anaemia is defined as pancytopenia (i.e. simultaneous presence of anaemia, leucopenia and thrombocytopenia) resulting from aplasia of the bone marrow.

ETIOLOGY AND CLASSIFICATION. Based on the etiology, aplastic anaemia is classified into 2 main types: primary and secondary. The various causes that may give rise to both these types of aplastic anaemia are summarised in Table 13.14.

TABLE 13.14: Causes of Aplastic Anaemia.

A. PRIMARY APLASTIC ANAEMIA
1. *Fanconi's anaemia (congenital)*
2. *Immunologically-mediated (acquired)*

B. SECONDARY APLASTIC ANAEMIA
1. *Drugs*
i) Dose-related aplasia e.g. with antimetabolites (methotrexate), mitotic inhibitors (daunorubicin), alkylating agents (busulfan), nitrosourea, anthracyclines.
ii) Idiosyncratic aplasia e.g. with chloramphenicol, sulfa drugs, oxyphenbutazone, phenylbutazone, chlorpromazine, gold salts.
2. *Toxic chemicals* e.g. benzene derivatives, insecticides, arsenicals.
3. *Infections* e.g. infectious hepatitis, EB virus infection, AIDS, other viral illnesses.
4. Miscellaneous e.g. association with SLE and therapeutic X-rays.

CLINICAL FEATURES. 1. Anaemia and its symptoms like mild progressive weakness and fatigue. 2. Haemorrhage from various sites due to thrombocytopenia. 3. Infections of the mouth and throat. 4. The lymph nodes, liver and spleen are generally not enlarged.

LABORATORY FINDINGS. The diagnosis of aplastic anaemia is made after excluding other causes of pancytopenia (Table 13.15).

TABLE 13.15: Causes of Pancytopenia.

I. Aplastic anaemia (Table 13.14)
II. Pancytopenia with normal or increased marrow cellularity e.g.
1. Myelodysplastic syndromes
2. Hypersplenism
3. Megaloblastic anaemia
III. Paroxysmal nocturnal haemoglobinuria (page 390)
IV. Bone marrow infiltrations e.g.
1. Haematologic malignancies (leukaemias, lymphomas, myeloma)
2. Non-haematologic metastatic malignancies
3. Storage diseases
4. Osteopetrosis
5. Myelofibrosis

1. Anaemia. Haemoglobin levels are moderately reduced.

2. Leucopenia. The absolute granulocyte count is particularly low (below 1500/µl) with relative lymphocytosis.

3. Thrombocytopenia. Platelet count is always reduced.

4. Bone marrow aspiration. A bone marrow aspirate may yield a 'dry tap'. A trephine biopsy is generally essential for making the diagnosis which reveals patchy cellular areas in a hypocellular or aplastic marrow due to replacement by fat.

MYELOPHTHISIC ANAEMIA *(p. 404)*

Development of severe anaemia may result from infiltration of the marrow termed as myelophthisic anaemia. The causes for marrow infiltrations include:
- Haematologic malignancies (e.g. leukaemia, lymphoma, myeloma),
- Metastatic deposits from non-haematologic malignancies (e.g. cancer breast, stomach, prostate, lung, thyroid),
- Advanced tuberculosis,
- Primary lipid storage diseases (Gaucher's disease, Niemann-Pick's disease).
- Osteopetrosis and myelofibrosis may rarely cause myelophthisis.

The type of anaemia in myelophthisis is generally normocytic normochromic with some fragmented red cells, basophilic stippling and normoblasts in the peripheral blood. Thrombocytopenia is usually present but the leucocyte count is increased with slight shift-to-left of myeloid cells i.e. a picture of *leuco-erythroblastic reaction* consisting of immature myeloid cells and normoblasts is seen in the peripheral blood.

PURE RED CELL APLASIA *(p. 404)*

This is a rare syndrome involving a selective failure in the production of erythroid elements in the bone marrow but with normal granulopoiesis and megakaryocytopoiesis. Patients have normocytic normochromic anaemia with normal granulocyte and platelet count. Reticulocytes are markedly decreased or are absent.

Pure red cell aplasia exists in two forms:
- *Congenital red cell aplasia (Blackfan-Diamond syndrome)*
- *Acquired red cell aplasia* is seen in middle-aged adults in association with some other diseases, most commonly thymoma.

MYELODYSPLASTIC SYNDROMES *(p. 404)*

Myelodysplastic syndromes (MDS) or *preleukaemic syndromes* are a heterogeneous group of leukaemia-related conditions having abnormalities in development of different marrow elements in varying combinations. These conditions are, therefore, also termed as *dysmyelopoietic syndromes*. The various combinations of features include normocytic normochromic anaemia, presence of certain number of myeloblasts in the peripheral blood, neutropenia, thrombocytopenia and/or monocytosis.

The *FAB (French-American-British) classification* divides myelodysplastic syndromes into the following 5 groups (Table 13.16):

As per FAB classification, marrow may contain up to 30% myeloblasts in MDS and was considered as the dividing line for distinguishing cases of AML from MDS. However, as per recently described *WHO classification*, patients with blast count of 20-30% and labelled as RAEB-t in FAB classification have prognosis similar to patients with blast count above 30% (i.e. AML cases). Thus, as per WHO classification, marrow blast count for making the diagnosis of AML has been revised and brought down to 20%. Patients with FAB category of RAEB-t are currently considered and treated as cases of AML and the term RAEB-t stands excluded from MDS according to the WHO classification.

MDS is found more frequently in older people (above 50 years of age). The etiology remains unknown but an association with chemotherapy or radiation has been observed in some cases.

TABLE 13.16: French-American-British (FAB) Classification of Myelodysplastic Syndromes (MDS).

FINDINGS	RA	RARS	RAEB	CMML	RAEB-t
A. Incidence	28%	24%	23%	16%	9%
B. Peripheral Blood					
1. Haemoglobin	Low	Low	Low	Variable	Low
2. Myeloblasts	0-1%	0-1%	<5%	<5%	>5%
3. Monocytes	Rare	Rare	Rare	>1000/µl	Variable
C. Bone marrow					
1. Myeloblasts	<5%	<5%	5-20%	1-20%	20-30%
2. Ringed sideroblasts	±	>15%	±	±	±

Abbreviations: RA= refractory anaemia; RARS = refractory anaemia with ringed sideroblasts; RAEB = refractory anaemia with excess blasts; CMML= chronic myelomonocytic leukaemia; RAEB-t= refractory anaemia with excess blasts in transformation.

WHITE BLOOD CELLS *(p. 405)*

GRANULOPOIESIS *(p. 405)*

Site of Formation and Kinetics *(p. 405)*

All forms of granulocytes are produced in the bone marrow and are termed,'*myeloid series*'. These are: myeloblast (most primitive precursor), promyelocyte, myelocyte, metamyelocyte, band forms and segmented granulocyte (mature form). The myeloblast, promyelocyte and myelocyte form a '*proliferative or mitotic pool*', while the latter series i.e. metamyelocyte, band forms and segmented granulocytes make up a '*mature or post-mitotic pool*'. It takes about 12 days for formation of mature granulocytes from the myeloblast. Normally the bone marrow contains more myeloid cells than the erythroid cells in the ratio of 2:1 to 15:1 (average 3:1).

Myeloid Series *(p. 405)*

The development of myeloid cells from myeloblast takes place in the following sequence.

1. MYELOBLAST. The myeloblast is the earliest recognisable precursor of the granulocytes, normally comprising about 2% of the total marrow cells. The myeloblast varies considerably in size (10-18 µm in diameter), having a large round to oval nucleus nearly filling the cell, has fine nuclear chromatin and contains 2-5 well-defined pale nucleoli. The myeloblasts of acute myeloid leukaemia may, however, show the presence of rod-like cytoplasmic inclusions called *Auer's rods* which represent abnormal derivatives of primary azurophilic granules.

2. PROMYELOCYTE. The promyelocyte is slightly larger than the myeloblast (12-18 µm diameter). It possesses a round to oval nucleus, having fine nuclear chromatin which is slightly condensed around the nuclear membrane. The nucleoli are present but are less prominent and fewer than those in the myeloblast.

3. MYELOCYTE. The myelocyte is the stage in which specific or secondary granules appear in the cytoplasm, and accordingly, the cell can be identified at this stage as belonging to the neutrophilic, eosinophilic or basophilic myelocyte.

4. METAMYELOCYTE. The metamyelocyte stage is 10-18 µm in diameter and is characterised by a clearly indented or horseshoe-shaped nucleus without nucleoli. The nuclear chromatin is dense and clumped. The cytoplasm contains both primary and secondary granules.

Chapter Thirteen

5. BAND FORMS. Band form is juvenile granulocyte, 10-16 µm in diameter, characterised by further condensation of nuclear chromatin and transformation of nuclear shape into band configuration of uniform thickness.

Monocyte-Macrophage Series *(p. 407)*

1. MONOBLAST. The monoblast is the least mature of the recognisable cell of monocyte-macrophage series. It is very similar in appearance to myeloblasts except that it has ground-glass cytoplasm with irregular border and may show phagocytosis as indicated by the presence of engulfed red cells in the cytoplasm.

2. PROMONOCYTE. The promonocyte is a young monocyte, about 20 µm in diameter and possesses a large indented nucleus containing a nucleolus.

Lymphoid Series *(p. 407)*

1. LYMPHOBLAST. The lymphoblast is the earliest identifiable precursor of lymphoid cells and is a rapidly dividing cell. It is a large cell, 10-18 µm in diameter, containing a large round to oval nucleus having slightly clumped or stippled nuclear chromatin. The nuclear membrane is denser and the number of nucleoli is fewer (1-2) as compared with those in myeloblast (2-5). The cytoplasm is scanty, basophilic and non-granular.

The distinguishing morphologic features between the myeloblast and lymphoblast are summarised in Table 13.17.

TABLE 13.17: Morphologic Characteristics of the Blast Cells in Romanowsky Stains.

FEATURE	MYELOBLAST	LYMPHOBLAST
1. Size	10-18 µm	10-18 µm
2. Nucleus	Round or oval	Round or oval
3. Nuclear chromatin	Fine meshwork	Slightly clumped
4. Nuclear membrane	Very fine	Fairly dense
5. Nucleoli	2-5	1-2
6. Cytoplasm	Scanty, blue, agranular	Scanty, clear blue, agranular

2. PROLYMPHOCYTE. This stage is an intermediate stage between the lymphoblast and mature lymphocyte. These young lymphocytes are 9-18 µm in diameter, contain round to indented nucleus with slightly stippled or coarse chromatin and may have 0-1 nucleoli.

MATURE LEUCOCYTES IN HEALTH AND DISEASE *(p. 408)*

Normally, only mature leucocytes namely: polymorphs, lymphocytes, monocytes, eosinophils and basophils, are found in the peripheral blood. The normal range of total and differential leucocyte count (TLC and DLC) in health in adults and children is given in Table 13.18.

Polymorphs (Neutrophils) *(p. 408)*

MORPHOLOGY. A polymorphonuclear neutrophil (PMN), commonly called polymorph or neutrophil, is 12-15 µm in diameter. It consists of a characteristic dense nucleus, having 2-5 lobes and pale cytoplasm containing numerous fine violet-pink granules. These granules contain several enzymes and are of 2 types:

Primary or azurophilic granules are large and coarse and appear early at the promyelocyte stage. These granules contain the following:
i) Myeloperoxidase(MPO) used as marker for PMNs(CD13 marker). MPO is involved in formation of hydrogen peroxide which is an important oxygen free radical.

TABLE 13.18: Normal White Blood Cell Counts in Health.

	ABSOLUTE COUNT
TLC	
Adults	4,000–11,000/μl
Infants (Full term, at birth)	10,000–25,000/μl
Infants (1 year)	6,000–16,000/μl
Children (4–7 years)	5,000–15,000/μl
Children (8–12 years)	4,500–13,500/μl
DLC IN ADULTS	
Polymorphs (neutrophils) 40–75%	2,000–7,500/μl
Lymphocytes 20–50%	1,500–4,000/μl
Monocytes 2–10%	200–800/μl
Eosinophils 1–6%	40–400/μl
Basophils <l%	10–100/μl

ii) Hydrolases such as lysozymes, cathepsin, elastase and proteinase 3. MPO along with proteinase 3 is involved in ANCA-mediated vasculitis.

Secondary or specific granules are smaller and more numerous. These appear later at myelocyte stage, are MPO-negative.

The normal **functions** of neutrophils are as under:

1. *Chemotaxis.* 2. *Phagocytosis.* 3. *Killing.*

PATHOLOGIC VARIATIONS. These include variations in count, morphology and defective function.

Neutrophil leucocytosis. An increase in circulating neutrophils above 7,500/μl is the commonest type of leucocytosis and occurs most commonly as a response to acute bacterial infections. Some common causes of neutrophilia are as under:

1. *Acute infections, local or generalised,* especially by cocci but also by certain bacilli, fungi, spirochaetes, parasites and some viruses. For example: pneumonia, cholecystitis, salpingitis, meningitis, diphtheria, plague, peritonitis, appendicitis, actinomycosis, poliomyelitis, abscesses, furuncles, carbuncles, tonsillitis, otitis media, osteomyelitis etc.

2. *Other inflammations* e.g. tissue damage resulting from burns, operations, ischaemic necrosis (such as in MI), gout, collagen-vascular diseases, hypersensitivity reactions etc.

3. *Intoxication* e.g. uraemia, diabetic ketosis, eclampsia, poisonings by chemicals and drugs.

4. *Acute haemorrhage,* internal or external.

5. *Acute haemolysis.*

6. *Disseminated malignancies.*

7. *Myeloproliferative disorders* e.g. myeloid leukaemia, polycythaemia vera, myeloid metaplasia.

8. *Miscellaneous* e.g. following corticosteroid therapy, idiopathic neutrophilia.

Neutropenia. When the absolute neutrophil count falls below 2,500/μl, the patient is said to have neutropenia:

1. *Certain infections* e.g. typhoid, paratyphoid, brucellosis, influenza, measles, viral hepatitis, malaria, kala-azar etc.

2. *Overwhelming bacterial infections* especially in patients with poor resistance e.g. miliary tuberculosis, septicaemia.

3. *Drugs, chemicals and physical agents* which induce aplasia of the bone marrow cause neutropenia.

4. *Certain haematological and other diseases* e.g. pernicious anaemia, aplastic anaemia, cirrhosis of the liver with splenomegaly, SLE, Gaucher's disease.

5. *Cachexia and debility.*

6. *Anaphylactoid shock.*

VARIATIONS IN MORPHOLOGY

1. Granules. Heavy, dark staining, coarse toxic granules are characteristic of bacterial infections.

2. Vacuoles. In bacterial infections such as in septicaemia, cytoplasmic vacuolation may develop.

3. Döhle bodies. These are small, round or oval patches, 2-3 μm in size, in the cytoplasm. They are mostly seen in bacterial infections.

4. Nuclear abnormalities. These include: i) *Sex chromatin*, ii) A *'shift-to-left'*, iii) A *'shift-to-right'*, iv) *Pelger-Huët anomaly*.

DEFECTIVE FUNCTIONS. 1. Defective chemotaxis. 2. Defective phagocytosis. 3. Defective killing

Lymphocytes *(p. 410)*

MORPHOLOGY. Majority of lymphocytes in the peripheral blood are *small* (9-12 μm in diameter) but *large* lymphocytes (12-16 μm in diameter) are also found. Both small and large lymphocytes have round or slightly indented nucleus with coarsely-clumped chromatin and scanty basophilic cytoplasm. Plasma cells are derived from B lymphocytes under the influence of appropriate stimuli. The nucleus of plasma cell is eccentric and has cart-wheel pattern of clumped nuclear chromatin.

Functionally, there are 3 types of lymphocytes and possess distinct surface markers called clusters of differentiation (CD) which aid in identification of stage of their differentiation:

T lymphocytes i.e. thymus-dependent lymphocytes, which mature in the thymus and are also known as thymocytes. They are mainly involved in direct action on antigens and are therefore involved in *cell-mediated immune (CMI)* reaction mediated by its subsets such as cytotoxic (killer) T cells (CD3+), CD8+ T cells, and *delayed hypersensitivity reaction* by CD4+ T cells.

B lymphocytes i.e. bone marrow-dependent or bursa-equivalent lymphocytes as well as their derivatives, plasma cells, are the sources of specific immunoglobulin antibodies. They are, therefore, involved in *humoral immunity (HI) or circulating immune reactions*.

NK cells i.e. natural killer cells are those lymphocytes which morphologically have appearance of lymphocytes but do not possess functional features of T or B cells. As the name indicates they are identified with 'natural' or innate immunity and bring about direct 'killing' of microorganisms or lysis of foreign body.

PATHOLOGIC VARIATIONS. These include:

Lymphocytosis e.g.

1. *Certain acute infections* e.g. pertussis, infectious mononucleosis, viral hepatitis, infectious lymphocytosis.

2. *Certain chronic infections* e.g. brucellosis, tuberculosis, secondary syphilis.

3. *Haematopoietic disorders* e.g. lymphatic leukaemias, lymphosarcoma, heavy chain disease.

4. *Relative lymphocytosis* is found in viral exanthemas, convalescence from acute infections, thyrotoxicosis, conditions causing neutropenia.

Lymphopenia e.g.

1. Most acute infections. 2. Severe bone marrow failure. 3. Corticosteroid and immunosuppressive therapy. 4. Widespread irradiation.

Monocytes *(p. 411)*

MORPHOLOGY. The monocyte is the largest mature leucocyte in the peripheral blood measuring 12-20 μm in diameter. It possesses a large, central, oval, notched or indented or horseshoe-shaped nucleus which has characteristically fine reticulated chromatin network. The cytoplasm is abundant, pale blue and contains many fine granules and vacuoles.

The main **functions** of monocytes are: 1. Phagocytosis. 2. Antigen-presenting cells. 3. As mediator of inflammation.

PATHOLOGIC VARIATIONS. Some common causes of monocytosis are: 1. Certain bacterial infections. 2. Viral infections. 3. Protozoal and rickettsial infections e.g. malaria, typhus, trypanosomiasis, kala-azar. 4. Convalescence from acute infection. 5. Haematopoietic disorders e.g. monocytic leukaemia, lymphomas, myeloproliferative disorders, multiple myeloma, lipid storage disease. 6. Malignancies e.g. cancer of the ovary, stomach, breast. 7. Granulo-matous diseases e.g. sarcoidosis, inflammatory bowel disease. 8. Collagen-vascular diseases.

Eosinophils (p. 411)

MORPHOLOGY. Eosinophils are similar to segmented neutrophils in size (12-15 μm in diameter), and have coarse, deep red staining granules in the cytoplasm and have usually two nuclear lobes. Granules in eosinophils contain basic protein and stain more intensely for peroxidase than granules in the neutrophils. In addition, eosinophils also contain cell adhesion molecules, cytokines (IL-3, IL-5), and a protein that precipitates Charcot-Leyden crystals in lung tissues in asthmatic patients.

PATHOLOGIC VARIATIONS. These include:

Eosinophilia i.e. eosinophil count above 400/μl.
1. *Allergic disorders* e.g. bronchial asthma, urticaria, angioneurotic oedema, hay fever, drug hypersensitivity.
2. *Parasitic infestations* e.g. trichinosis, echinococcosis, intestinal parasitism.
3. *Skin diseases* e.g. pemphigus, dermatitis herpetiformis, erythema multiforme.
4. *Löeffler's syndrome.*
5. *Pulmonary infiltration with eosinophilia* (PIE) syndrome.
6. *Tropical eosinophilia.*
7. *Haematopoietic diseases* e.g. CML, polycythaemia vera, pernicious anaemia, Hodgkin's disease, following splenectomy.
8. *Malignant diseases* with metastases.
9. *Irradiation.*
10. *Miscellaneous disorders* e.g. polyarteritis nodosa, rheumatoid arthritis, sarcoidosis.

Eosinopenia. Adrenal steroids and ACTH induce eosinopenia in man.

Basophils (p. 411)

MORPHOLOGY. Basophils resemble the other mature granulocytes but are distinguished by coarse, intensely basophilic granules which usually fill the cytoplasm and often overlie and obscure the nucleus.

The granules of basophils contain heparin, histamine and 5-HT. In the tissues these cells become *mast cells.* Mast cells or basophils on degranulation are associated with histamine release.

PATHOLOGIC VARIATIONS. Basophilia is unusual and is found in the following conditions:
1. Chronic myeloid leukaemia. 2. Polycythaemia vera. 3. Myelosclerosis. 4. Myxoedema. 5. Ulcerative colitis. 6. Following splenectomy. 7. Hodgkin's disease. 8. Urticaria pigmentosa.

INFECTIOUS MONONUCLEOSIS (p. 412)

Infectious mononucleosis (IM) or glandular fever is a benign, self-limiting lymphoproliferative disease caused by Epstein-Barr virus (EBV), one of the herpesviruses. Infection may occur from childhood to old age but the classical acute infection is more common in teenagers and young adults. The infection is transmitted by person-to-person contact such as by kissing with transfer of virally-contaminated saliva. Groups of cases occur particularly in young people living together in boarding schools, colleges, camps and military institutions.

Pathogenesis *(p. 412)*

EBV, the etiologic agent for IM, is a B lymphotropic herpesvirus. The disease is characterised by fever, generalised lymphadenopathy, hepatosplenomegaly, sore throat, and appearance in blood of atypical 'mononucleosis cells'. The pathogenesis of these pathologic features is outlined below:

1. In a susceptible sero-negative host who lacks antibodies, the virus in the contaminated saliva *invades and replicates within epithelial cells* of the salivary gland and then enters B cells in the lymphoid tissues which possess receptors for EBV.

2. Viraemia and death of infected B cells causes an acute febrile illness and appearance of specific humoral antibodies. The appearance of antibodies marks the *disappearance of virus from the blood.*

3. *EBV-infected B cells undergo polyclonal activation and proliferation.* These cells perform two important roles which are the characteristic diagnostic features of IM:

i) They secrete *antibodies*—initially IgM but later IgG appears.
ii) They *activate T lymphocytes* of two types— CD8+ T lymphocytes and cytotoxic (suppressor) T cells.

4. The proliferation of these cells is responsible for *generalised lymphadenopathy and hepatosplenomegaly.*

5. The *sore throat* in IM may be caused by either necrosis of B cells or due to viral replication within the salivary epithelial cells.

Clinical Features *(p. 412)*

The incubation period of IM is 30-50 days in young adults, while children have shorter incubation period.

1. **During prodromal period (first 3-5 days),** the symptoms are mild such as malaise, myalgia, headache and fatigue.

2. **Frank clinical features (next 7-21 days),** commonly are fever, sore throat and bilateral cervical lymphadenopathy. Less commonly, splenomegaly (50% patients), hepatomegaly (10% cases), transient erythematous maculopapular eruption on the trunk and extremities, and neurologic manifestations are found.

Laboratory Findings *(p. 412)*

1. Blood picture. The peripheral blood shows a moderate rise in total white cell count (10,000-20,000/µl) with an absolute lymphocytosis. Essential to the diagnosis of IM is the presence of at least 10-12% *atypical T cells (or mononucleosis cells)* of the total lymphocytes in the peripheral blood. The mononucleosis cells are variable in appearance and are classed as Downey type I, II and III, of which Downey type I are found most frequently. These atypical T lymphocytes are usually of the size of large lymphocytes (12-16 µm diameter).

2. Serologic diagnosis

i) *Heterophile antibodies* against sheep red cells are found in the serum at high titer (Paul-Bunnell test) in 80-90% patients of IM, with a peak during the 2nd and 3rd week.

ii) *Specific antibody for EBV antigen.* The appearance of specific EBV antibody in the first 2-3 weeks can also be demonstrated.

iii) *EBV antigen.* If viral diagnostic facilities are available, EBV antigen can also be demonstrated.

3. Other laboratory findings. In addition, abnormalities of the liver function test may be found in some cases.

LEUKAEMOID REACTIONS *(p. 413)*

Leukaemoid reaction is defined as a reactive excessive leucocytosis in the peripheral blood resembling that of leukaemia in a subject who does not have leukaemia. In spite of confusing blood picture, the clinical features of leukaemia such as splenomegaly, lymphadenopathy and haemorrhages are usually absent and the features of underlying disorder causing the leukaemoid reaction are generally obvious.

Leukaemoid reaction may be myeloid or lymphoid; the former is much more common.

Myeloid Leukaemoid Reaction *(p. 414)*

The majority of leukaemoid reactions involve the granulocyte series. It may occur in association with a wide variety of diseases. These are as under:

1. *Infections* e.g. staphylococcal pneumonia, disseminated tuberculosis, meningitis, diphtheria, sepsis, endocarditis, plague, infected abortions etc.
2. *Intoxication* e.g. eclampsia, mercury poisoning, severe burns.
3. *Malignant diseases* e.g. multiple myeloma, myelofibrosis, Hodgkin's disease, bone metastases.
4. *Severe haemorrhage and severe haemolysis.*

LABORATORY FINDINGS. These are:

1. *Leucocytosis,* usually moderate, not exceeding 100,000/µl.
2. Proportion of *immature cells* mild to moderate, comprised by metamyelocytes, myelocytes (5-15%), and blasts fewer than 5% i.e. the blood picture simulates that of CML.
3. Infective cases may show *toxic granulation and Döhle bodies* in the cytoplasm of neutrophils.
4. *Neutrophil alkaline phosphatase (NAP) score* in the cytoplasm of mature neutrophils in leukaemoid reaction is characteristically high.
5. *Cytogenetic studies* may be helpful in exceptional cases which reveal negative Philadelphia chromosome in myeloid leukaemoid reaction but positive in cases of CML.
6. *Additional features* include anaemia, normal-to-raised platelet count, myeloid hyperplasia of the marrow and absence of infiltration by immature cells in organs and tissues.

Lymphoid Leukaemoid Reaction *(p. 414)*

Lymphoid leukaemoid reaction may be found in the following conditions:

1. *Infections* e.g. infectious mononucleosis, cytomegalovirus infection, pertussis (whooping cough), chickenpox, measles, infectious lymphocytosis, tuberculosis.
2. *Malignant diseases* may rarely produce lymphoid leukaemoid reaction.

LABORATORY FINDINGS. The blood picture is characterised by:

1. Leucocytosis not exceeding 100,000/µl.
2. The differential white cell count reveals mostly mature lymphocytes simulating the blood picture found in cases of CLL.

LEUKAEMIAS *(p. 414)*

The leukaemias are a group of disorders characterised by malignant transformation of blood-forming cells. The proliferation of leukaemic cells takes place primarily in the bone marrow, and in certain forms, in the lymphoid tissues. Ultimately, the abnormal cells appear in the peripheral blood raising the total white cell count to high level. In addition, features of bone marrow failure (e.g. anaemia, thrombocytopenia, neutropenia) and involvement of other organs (e.g. liver, spleen, lymph nodes, meninges, brain, skin etc) occur.

In general, leukaemias are classified on the basis of cell types predominantly involved, into *myeloid* and *lymphoid*, and on the basis of natural history of the disease, into *acute* and *chronic*. Thus, the main types are: *acute myeloblastic leukaemia* and *acute lymphoblastic leukaemia* (AML and ALL), and *chronic myeloid leukaemia* and *chronic lymphocytic leukaemia* (CML and CLL); *hairy cell leukaemia* (HCL) is an unusual variant of lymphoid neoplasia.

Etiology *(p. 414)*

The etiology of leukaemia is not known in most patients. However, a number of factors have been implicated.

1. GENETIC FACTORS. There is high concordance rate among identical twins if acute leukaemia develops in the first year of life. Families with excessive incidence of leukaemia have been identified.

2. ENVIRONMENTAL FACTORS. i) Ionising radiation. ii) Chemical carcinogens. iii) Certain drugs.

3. INFECTION. Induction of leukaemias in experimental animals by RNA viruses (retroviruses) has been studied for quite some time but more recently viral etiology of adult T cell leukaemia-lymphoma (ATLL) by a human retrovirus called human T cell leukaemia-lymphoma virus I (HTLV-I) and HTLV II for T cell variant of hairy cell leukaemia has been established.

Pathogenesis (Leukaemogenesis) *(p. 415)*

The leukaemia arises following *malignant transformation of a single clone of cells belonging to myeloid or lymphoid series, followed by proliferation of the transformed clone*. The evolution of leukaemia is multi-step process, and in many cases, acute leukaemia may develop after a pre-existing myelodysplastic or myeloproliferative disorder.

ACUTE LEUKAEMIAS *(p. 416)*

Acute leukaemias are characterised by predominance of undifferentiated leucocyte precursors or leukaemic blasts. Acute leukaemias may be derived from the myeloid stem cells called *acute myeloblastic leukaemia (AML)*, or from the lymphoid stem cells termed *acute lymphoblastic leukaemia (ALL)*.

Recently, more definite criteria for diagnosis and classification of acute leukaemias have been laid down by a group of French, American and British haematologists commonly called the *FAB classification*. According to this system, a leukaemia is acute if the bone marrow consists of more than 30% blasts. FAB classification divides AML into 8 subtypes (M0 to M7) and ALL into 3 subtypes (L1 to L3) as shown in Table 13.19. Another classification called *Revised European-American* classification of *Lymphoid* neoplasms (REAL classification) has been formulated and includes lymphoid leukaemias (acute and chronic) and non-Hodgkin's lymphomas since they represent the counterparts of neoplastic cells in the bone marrow and lymphoid tissue. More recently, WHO classification for AML has been proposed which takes into consideration cytogenetic and molecular abnormalities in different types.

Thus, the basis of these categorisation of leukaemias can be summed up as:

- *FAB classification* is based on *morphologic and cytochemical features.*
- *REAL classification* is based on *immunophenotypic features.*
- *WHO classification* is based on *cytogenetic and molecular features.*

TABLE 13:19: Revised FAB Classification of Acute Leukaemias.

FAB CLASS	PER CENT CASES	MORPHOLOGY	CYTOCHEMISTRY
ACUTE MYELOBLASTIC LEUKAEMIA (AML)			
M0: *Minimally differentiated AML*	2	Blasts lack definite cytologic and cytochemical features but have myeloid lineage antigens	Myeloperoxidase –
M1: *AML without maturation*	20	Myeloblasts predominate; few if any granules or Auer rods	Myeloperoxidase +
M2: *AML with maturation*	30	Myeloblasts with promyelocytes predominate; Auer rods may be present	Myeloperoxidase +++
M3: *Acute promyelocytic leukaemia*	5	Hypergranular promyelocytes; often with multiple Auer rods per cell	Myeloperoxidase +++
M4: *Acute myelomonocytic leukaemia (Naegeli type)*	30	Mature cells of both myeloid and monocytic series in peripheral blood; myeloid cells resemble M2	Myeloperoxidase ++ Non-specific esterase +
M5: *Acute monocytic leukaemia (Schilling type)*	10	Two subtypes: M5a shows poorly-differentiated monoblasts, M5b shows differentiated promonocytes and monocytes	Non-specific esterase ++
M6: *Acute erythroleukaemia (Di Guglielmo's syndrome)*	<5	Erythroblasts predominate (>50%); myeloblasts and promyelocytes also increased	Erythroblasts: PAS + Myeloblasts: myeloperoxidase +
M7: *Acute megakaryocytic leukaemia*	<5	Pleomorphic undifferentiated blasts predominate; react with antiplatelet antibodies	Platelet peroxidase +
ACUTE LYMPHOBLASTIC LEUKAEMIA (ALL)			
L1: *Childhood-ALL (B-ALL, and T-ALL)*	More common in children	Homogeneous small lymphoblasts; scanty cytoplasm, regular round nuclei, inconspicuous nucleoli	PAS ± Acid phosphatase ±
L2: *Adult-ALL (mostly T-ALL)*	More frequent in adults	Heterogeneous lymphoblasts; variable amount of cytoplasm, irregular or cleft nuclei, large nucleoli	PAS ± Acid phosphatase ±
L3: *Burkitt type-ALL (B-ALL)*	Uncommon	Large homogeneous lymphoblasts; round nuclei, prominent nucleoli, cytoplasmic vacuolation	PAS – Acid phosphatase –

Clinical Features (p. 416)

AML and ALL share many clinical features:

I. Due to Bone Marrow Failure

1. *Anaemia* producing pallor, lethargy, dyspnoea.

2. *Bleeding manifestations* due to thrombocytopenia.

3. *Infections* are quite common and include those of mouth, throat, skin, respiratory, perianal and other sites.

4. *Fever* is generally attributed to infections in acute leukaemia.

II. Due to Organ Infiltration

1. *Pain and tenderness of bones* (e.g. sternal tenderness) are due to bone infarcts or subperiosteal infiltrates by leukaemic cells.

2. *Lymphadenopathy* and enlargement of the *tonsils* are more common in ALL.

3. *Splenomegaly* of moderate grade is common, especially in ALL.

4. *Hepatomegaly* is frequently present due to leukaemic infiltration.

5. *Leukaemic infiltration of the kidney* may be present.

6. *Gum hypertrophy* due to leukaemic infiltration of the gingivae is a frequent finding in myelomonocytic (M4) and monocytic (M5) leukaemias.

7. *Chloroma or granulocytic sarcoma* is a localised tumour-forming mass occurring in the skin or orbit due to local infiltration of the tissues by leukaemic cells.

8. *Meningeal involvement* manifested by raised intracranial pressure, headache, nausea and vomiting, blurring of vision and diplopia are seen more frequently in ALL during haematologic remission.

9. *Other organ infiltrations* include testicular swelling in ALL and mediastinal compression in T cell type ALL.

Laboratory Findings (p. 417)

I. Blood picture

1. Anaemia. Anaemia is almost always present in acute leukaemias. It is generally severe, progressive and normochromic in type.

2. Thrombocytopenia. The platelet count is usually moderately to severely decreased (below 50,000/µl) but occasionally it may be normal.

3. White blood cells. The total WBC count ranges from subnormal-to-markedly elevated values. In 25% of patients, the total WBC count at presentation is reduced to 1,000-4,000 /µl. More often, however, there is progressive rise in white cell count which may exceed 100,000/µl in more advanced disease. The majority of leucocytes in the peripheral blood are blasts and there is often neutropenia due to marrow infiltration by leukaemic cells. Some patients present with pancytopenia and have a few blasts *(sub-leukaemic leukaemia)* or no blasts *(aleukaemic leukaemia)* in the blood.

II. Bone marrow examination

1. Cellularity. Typically, the marrow is hypercellular but sometimes a 'blood tap' or 'dry tap' occurs.

2. Leukaemic cells. The bone marrow is generally tightly packed with leukaemic blast cells. The essential criteria for diagnosis of acute leukaemia, as per FAB classification, is the presence of at least 30% blasts in the bone marrow. However, lately as per WHO classsification of leukaemias, these criteria have been revised upwards to 20% blasts in the marrow for labelling and treating a case as AML.

3. Erythropoiesis. Erythropoietic cells are reduced. Dyserythropoiesis, megaloblastic features and ring sideroblasts are commonly present.

4. Megakaryocytes. They are usually reduced or absent.

5. Cytogenetics. Chromosomal analysis of dividing leukaemic cells in the marrow shows karyotypic abnormalities in 75% of cases which may have a relationship to prognosis.

III. Cytochemistry

1. **Myeloperoxidase:** Positive in immature myeloid cells containing granules and Auer rods but negative in M0 myeloblasts.

2. **Sudan Black:** Positive in immature cells in AML.

3. **Periodic acid-Schiff (PAS):** Positive in immature lymphoid cells and in erythroleukaemia (M6).

4. **Non-specific esterase (NSE):** Positive in monocytic series (M4 and M5).

5. **Acid phosphatase:** Focal positivity in leukaemic blasts in ALL and diffuse reaction in monocytic cells (M4 and M5).

IV. Immunophenotyping.
AML cells express CD13 and CD33 antigens; M7 shows CD41 and CD42 positivity. Currently as per REAL-WHO classification for all lymphoid malignancies (lymphoid leukaemias and lymphomas), lymphoid leukaemias (both ALL and CLL) are subdivided on the basis of immunologic features by identification as regards their B or T cell origin. According to this classification, ALL is redivided into pre-B ALL, T cell ALL and B cell ALL with distinct cytogenetic and immunologic features (Table 13.20).

TABLE 13.20: WHO-REAL Classification of ALL on the Basis of Immunologic and Cytogenetic Features.

SUBTYPE	INCIDENCE	MARKERS	FAB SUBTYPE	CYTOGENETIC ABNORMALITIES
Pre-B ALL	75%	CD10+ (90%), TdT+	L1, L2	t(9;22) i.e. Philadelphia+ALL
B cell ALL	5%	CD10+ (50%), TdT-	L3	t(8;14) (Burkitt's leukaemia)
T cell ALL	20%	CD10+ (30%), TdT+	L1, L2	14q11

(TdT= terminal deoxynucleotidyl transferase)

V. Other Investigations. These include:

1. **Serum muramidase.** Serum levels of lysozyme (i.e. muramidase) are elevated in myelomonocytic (M4) and monocytic (M5) leukaemias.

2. **Serum uric acid.** Because of rapidly growing number of leukaemic cells, serum uric acid level is frequently increased.

The salient differences between the two main forms of acute leukaemia are summarised in Table 13.21.

CHRONIC LEUKAEMIAS (p. 420)

Chronic leukaemias are those haematologic malignancies in which the predominant leukaemic cells are initially well-differentiated and easily recognisable as regards their cell type. Chronic leukaemias are divided into 2 main types: chronic myeloid (granulocytic) leukaemia (CML or CGL), and chronic lymphocytic leukaemia (CLL).

CHRONIC MYELOID LEUKAEMIA (CML) (p. 420)

Chronic myeloid (myelogenous, granulocytic) leukaemia comprises about 20% of all leukaemias and its peak incidence is seen in 3rd and 4th decades of life. A distinctive variant of CML seen in children is called *juvenile CML*.

Clinical Features (p. 420)

1. Features of *anaemia* such as weakness, pallor, dyspnoea and tachycardia.

2. Symptoms due to *hypermetabolism* such as weight loss, lassitude, anorexia, night sweats.

TABLE 13.21: Contrasting Features of AML and ALL.

FEATURE	AML	ALL
1. *Common age*	Adults between 15-40 years; comprise 20% of childhood leukaemias	Children under 15 years; comprise 80% of childhood leukaemias
2. *Physical findings*	Splenomegaly + Hepatomegaly + Lymphadenopathy + Bony tenderness + Gum hypertrophy +	Splenomegaly ++ Hepatomegaly ++ Lymphadenopathy ++ Bony tenderness + Meningeal involvement +
3. *Laboratory findings*	Low-to-high TLC; predominance of myeloblasts and promyelocytes in blood and bone marrow; thrombocytopenia moderate to severe.	Low-to-high TLC, predominance of lymphoblasts in blood and bone marrow; thrombocytopenia moderate to severe.
4. *Cytochemical stains*	Myeloperoxidase +, Sudan black +, NSE + in M4 and M5, acid phosphatase (diffuse) + in M4 and M5	PAS +, acid phosphatase (focal) +
5. *Specific therapy*	Cytosine arabinoside, anthracyclines (daunorubicin, adriamycin) and 6-thioguanine	Vincristine, prednisolone, anthracyclines and L-asparaginase
6. *Response to therapy*	Remission rate low, duration of remission shorter	Remission rate high, duration of remission prolonged
7. *Median survival*	12-18 months	Children without CNS prophylaxis 33 months, with CNS prophylaxis 60 months; adults 12-18 months

3. *Splenomegaly* is almost always present and is frequently massive.

4. *Bleeding tendencies* such as easy bruising, epistaxis, menorrhagia and haematomas may occur.

5. Less *commonly,* features such as gout, visual disturbance, neurologic manifestations and priapism are present.

6. *Juvenile CML* is more often associated with lymph node enlargement than splenomegaly.

Laboratory Findings *(p. 421)*

I. Blood picture. The findings are as follows:

1. **Anaemia.** Anaemia is usually of moderate degree and is normocytic normochromic in type.

2. **White blood cells.** Characteristically, there is marked leucocytosis (approximately 200,000/µl or more at the time of presentation). The natural history of CML consists of 2 phases—chronic and blastic.

■ *The chronic phase of CML* begins as a myeloproliferative disorder and consists of excessive proliferation of myeloid cells of intermediate grade (i.e. myelocytes and metamyelocytes) and mature segmented neutrophils. Myeloblasts usually do not exceed 10% of cells in the peripheral blood and bone marrow.

■ *The blastic phase or blast crisis in CML* may be myeloid or lymphoid in origin. Myeloid blast crisis in CML is more common and resembles AML. However, unlike AML, Auer rods are never seen in myeloblasts of CML in blast crisis.

3. **Platelets.** The platelet count may be normal but is raised in about half the cases.

II. Bone marrow examination. These findings are:

1. Cellularity. Generally, there is hypercellularity.

2. Myeloid cells. The myeloid cells predominate in the bone marrow with increased myeloid-erythroid ratio.

3. Erythropoiesis. Erythropoiesis is normoblastic but there is reduction in erythropoietic cells.

4. Megakaryocytes. Megakaryocytes are conspicuous but are usually smaller in size than normal.

5. Cytogenetics. Cytogenetic studies on blood and bone marrow cells show the characteristic chromosomal abnormality called Philadelphia (Ph) chromosome formed by reciprocal translocation between part of long arm of chromosome 22 and part of long arm of chromosome 9{(t(9;22)} seen in 70-90% cases with CML.

III. Cytochemistry. The only significant finding on cytochemical stains is reduced scores of *neutrophil alkaline phosphatase (NAP)* which helps to distinguish CML from myeloid leukaemoid reaction in which case NAP scores are elevated.

CHRONIC LYMPHOCYTIC LEUKAEMIA (CLL) (p. 422)

Chronic lymphocytic leukaemia constitutes about 25% of all leukaemias and is predominantly a disease of the elderly (over 50 years of age) with a male preponderance (male-female ratio 2:1). Currently, CLL is considered as part of the common lymphoid malignancy of mature B cells termed CLL/SLL i.e. CLL for cases with peripheral blood involvement while SLL for those without blood spread.

Clinical Features (p. 422)

1. Features of *anaemia* such as gradually increasing weakness, fatigue and dyspnoea.
2. Enlargement of superficial *lymph nodes.*
3. *Splenomegaly* and *hepatomegaly* are usual.
4. *Haemorrhagic manifestations.*
5. *Infections,* particularly of respiratory tract.
6. *Less common* are: mediastinal pressure, tonsillar enlargement, disturbed vision, and bone and joint pains.

Laboratory Findings (p. 422)

I. Blood picture. The findings are:

1. Anaemia. Anaemia is usually mild to moderate and normocytic normochromic in type.

2. White blood cells. Typically, there is marked leucocytosis but less than that seen in CML (50,000-200,000/µl). Usually, more than 90% of leucocytes are mature small lymphocytes. Smear cells (degenerated forms) are present.

3. Platelets. The platelet count is normal or moderately reduced.

II. Bone marrow examination. These findings are:
1. Increased lymphocyte count (25-95%).
2. Reduced myeloid precursors.
3. Reduced erythroid precursors.

HAIRY CELL LEUKAEMIA (p. 423)

Hairy cell leukaemia (HCL), is an unusual and uncommon form of chronic leukaemia in which there is presence of abnormal mononuclear cells with hairy cytoplasmic projections in the bone marrow, peripheral blood and spleen. These cells are best recognised under phase contrast microscopy but may also be visible in routine blood smears. These leukaemic 'hairy cells' have characteristically positive cytochemical staining for *tartrate-resistant acid phosphatase*. The controversy on the origin of hairy cells whether these cells represent neoplastic T cells, B cells or monocytes, is settled with the molecular analysis of these cells which assigns them *B cell origin* expressing CD19, CD20 and CD22 antigen. In addition to B cell markers, hairy cells are also positive for CD11, CD25 and CD103.

Hairy cell leukaemia occurs in the older males. It is characterised clinically by the manifestations due to infiltration of reticuloendothelial organs (bone marrow, liver and spleen) and, hence, its previous name as *leukaemic reticuloendotheliosis*. Patients have susceptibility to infection with *M. avium intercellulare*. Laboratory diagnosis is made by the presence of pancytopenia due to marrow failure and splenic sequestration, and identification of characteristic hairy cells in blood and bone marrow which are positive for tartrate-resistant acid phosphatase (TRAP).

OTHER MYELOPROLIFERATIVE DISORDERS *(p. 423)*

Myeloproliferative disorders include 4 disorders: chronic myeloid leukaemia (CML), polycythaemia vera, myeloid metaplasia with myelosclerosis, and essential thrombocytosis (or primary/idiopathic thrombocythaemia).

POLYCYTHAEMIA VERA *(p. 423)*

Polycythaemia vera (PV) is characterised by increased production of all myeloid elements resulting in pancytosis, elevated haemoglobin concentration and splenomegaly. The term 'polycythaemia vera' or 'polycythaemia rubra vera' is used for *primary or idiopathic polycythaemia* only. *Secondary polycythaemia or erythrocytosis* may occur due to several causes e.g. high altitude, cardiovascular disease, pulmonary disease with alveolar hypoventilation, heavy smoking, inappropriate increase in erythropoietin (renal cell carcinoma, hydronephrosis, hepatocellular carcinoma, cerebellar haemangioblastoma, massive uterine leiomyoma).

In PV, unlike secondary polycythaemia, *the erythropoietin levels in serum and urine are reduced.*

CLINICAL FEATURES. PV is a disease of late middle life and is slightly more common in males. The disease generally runs a chronic but slowly progressive course. Clinical features are the result of hyperviscosity, hypervolaemia, hypermetabolism and decreased cerebral perfusion.
1. Headache, vertigo, tinnitus, visual alterations syncope or even coma.
2. Increased risk of thrombosis due to accelerated atherosclerosis.
3. Increased risk of haemorrhages due to increased blood volume and intrinsic platelet dysfunction.
4. Splenomegaly producing abdominal fullness.
5. Pruritus, especially after a bath.
6. Increased risk of urate stones and gout.

LABORATORY FINDINGS. These are as follows:
1. Raised haemoglobin concentration (above 17.5 g/dl in males and 15.5 g/dl in females).
2. Erythrocytosis (above 6 million/μl in males and 5.5 million/μl in females).
3. Haematocrit (PCV) above 55% in males and above 47% in females.
4. Mild to moderate leucocytosis (15,000-25,000/μl) with basophilia and raised neutrophil alkaline phosphatase scores.
5. Thrombocytosis with defective platelet function.

6. Bone marrow examination reveals erythroid hyperplasia or panhyperplasia.
7. Cytogenetic abnormalities such as trisomy are found in 10% cases of PV.

MYELOID METAPLASIA WITH MYELOFIBROSIS *(p. 424)*

Myeloid metaplasia with myelofibrosis, also called agnogenic (of unknown origin) myeloid metaplasia, primary myelofibrosis and myelosclerosis, is characterised by proliferation of neoplastic stem cells at multiple sites outside the bone marrow (i.e. extramedullary haematopoiesis), especially in the liver and spleen.

CLINICAL FEATURES. The disease begins in the late middle life and is gradual in onset.
1.   Anaemia with constitutional symptoms such as fatigue, weakness and anorexia.
2.   Massive splenomegaly producing abdominal discomfort, pain and dyspnoea.
3.   Hepatomegaly is present in half the cases.
4.   Petechial and other bleeding problems are found in about 20% cases.
5.   Less common findings are lymphadenopathy, jaundice, ascites, bone pain and hyperuricaemia.

LABORATORY FINDINGS. These are as follows:
1. *Mild anaemia* is usual except in cases where features of polycythaemia vera are coexistent.
2. *Leucocytosis* at the time of presentation but later there may be leucopenia.
3. *Thrombocytosis* initially but advanced cases show thrombocytopenia.
4. *Peripheral blood smear* shows bizarre red cell shapes, tear drop poikilocytes, basophilic stippling, nucleated red cells, immature leucocytes (i.e. leucoerythroblastic reaction), basophilia and giant platelet forms.
5. *Bone marrow aspiration* is generally unsuccessful and yields 'dry tap'. Examination of trephine biopsy shows focal areas of hypercellularity and increased reticulin network and variable amount of collagen.
6. *Extramedullary haematopoiesis* can be documented by liver biopsy or splenic aspiration.

ESSENTIAL THROMBOCYTOSIS *(p. 425)*

Essential thrombocytosis or primary (idiopathic) thrombocythaemia is another myeloproliferative disorder characterised by markedly elevated platelet count in the absence of any recognisable stimulus. *Secondary or reactive thrombocytosis,* on the other hand, occurs in response to known stimuli such as: chronic infection, haemorrhage, postoperative state, chronic iron deficiency, malignancy, rheumatoid arthritis and postsplenectomy.

CLINICAL FEATURES. The condition has an insidious onset and is more frequent in older people. Haemorrhagic and thrombotic events are common e.g.
1.   Arterial or venous thrombosis.
2.   Easy bruisability following minor trauma.
3.   Spontaneous bleeding.
4.   Transient ischaemic attack or frank stroke due to platelet aggregation in microvasculature of the CNS.

LABORATORY FINDINGS. These are as follows:
1.   Sustained elevation in platelet count (above 400,000 μl).
2.   Blood film shows many large platelets, megakaryocyte fragments and hypogranular forms.
3.   Consistently abnormal platelet functions, especially abnormality in platelet aggregation.
4.   Bone marrow examination reveals large number of hyperdiploid megakaryocytes and variable amount of increased fibrosis.

PLATELETS AND HAEMORRHAGIC DIATHESIS *(p. 425)*

THROMBOPOIESIS *(p. 425)*

Platelets are formed in the bone marrow by a process of fragmentation of the cytoplasm of megakaryocytes. Platelet production appears to be under the control of thrombopoietin, the nature and origin of which are not yet established. The stages in platelet production are: megakaryoblast, promegakaryocyte, megakaryocyte, and discoid platelets.

PLATELETS. Platelets are small (1-4 μm in diameter), discoid, non-nucleate structures containing red-purple granules. The normal platelet count ranges from 150,000-400,000/μl and its life-span is 7-10 days. Newly-formed platelets spend 24-36 hours in the spleen before being released into circulation but splenic stasis does not cause any injury to the platelets normally.

The main **function** of platelets is in haemostasis which includes two closely linked processes:

1. Primary haemostasis is the term used for platelet plug formation at the site of injury. It is an immediate phenomenon appearing within seconds of injury and is responsible for cessation of bleeding from microvasculature. Primary haemostasis involves three steps: platelet adhesion, platelet granule release and platelet aggregation which are regulated by changes in membrane phospholipids, and calcium.

2. Secondary haemostasis involves plasma coagulation system resulting in fibrin plug formation and takes several minutes for completion.

HAEMORRHAGIC DIATHESIS (BLEEDING DISORDERS) *(p. 426)*

Bleeding disorders or haemorrhagic diatheses are a group of disorders characterised by defective haemostasis with abnormal bleeding. The tendency to bleeding may be *spontaneous* in the form of small haemorrhages into the skin and mucous membranes (e.g. petechiae, purpura, ecchymoses), or there may be excessive external or internal bleeding *following trivial trauma* and surgical procedure (e.g. haematoma, haemarthrosis etc).

The causes of haemorrhagic diatheses may or may not be related to platelet abnormalities. These causes are broadly divided into the following 4 groups:

I. Haemorrhagic diathesis due to vascular abnormalities.

II. Haemorrhagic diathesis related to platelet abnormalities.

III. Disorders of coagulation factors.

IV. Combination of all these as occurs in disseminated intravascular coagulation (DIC).

INVESTIGATIONS OF HAEMOSTATIC FUNCTION *(p. 427)*

In general, the haemostatic mechanisms have 2 primary functions:

■ To promote *local haemostasis* at the site of injured blood vessel.

■ To ensure that the circulating blood remains in *fluid state* while in the vascular bed i.e. to prevent the occurrence of generalised thrombosis.

In order to perform these haemostatic functions, a delicate balance must exist among at least 5 components: (i) blood vessel wall; (ii) platelets; (iii) plasma coagulation factors; (iv) inhibitors; and (v) fibrinolytic system.

Anything that interferes with any of these components results in defective haemostasis with abnormal bleeding. In order to establish a definite diagnosis in any case suspected to have abnormal haemostatic functions, the following scheme is followed:

A. Comprehensive *clinical evaluation,* including the patient's history, family history and details of the site, frequency and character of haemostatic defect.

B. Series of *screening tests* for assessing the abnormalities in various components involved in maintaining haemostatic balance.

C. *Specific tests* to pinpoint the cause.

A brief review of general principles of tests used to investigate haemostatic abnormalities is summarised in Table 13.22.

TABLE 13.22: Screening Tests for Haemostasis (Coagulation Tests).

LABORATORY TEST	FACTOR/FUNCTION MEASURED	ASSOCIATED DISORDERS	
1. *Bleeding time*	Platelet function, vascular integrity	i)	Qualitative disorders of platelets
		ii)	von Willebrand's disease
		iii)	Quantitative disorders of platelets
		iv)	Acquired vascular disorders
2. *Platelet count*	Quantification of platelets	i)	Thrombocytopenia
		ii)	Thrombocytosis
3. *Prothrombin time*	Evaluation of extrinsic and common pathway (deficiency of factors I, II, V, VII, X)	i)	Oral anticoagulant therapy
		ii)	DIC
		iii)	Liver disease
4. *Partial thrombo-plastin time*	Evaluation of intrinsic and common pathway (deficiency of factors I, II, V, VIII, IX, X, XI, XII)	i)	Parenteral heparin therapy
		ii)	DIC
		iii)	Liver disease
5. *Thrombin time*	Evaluation of common pathway	i)	Afibrinogenaemia
		ii)	DIC
		iii)	Parenteral heparin therapy

HAEMORRHAGIC DIATHESES DUE TO VASCULAR DISORDERS (p. 430)

Vascular bleeding disorders, also called non-thrombocytopenic purpuras or vascular purpuras, are normally mild and characterised by petechiae, purpuras or ecchymoses confined to the skin and mucous membranes. The pathogenesis of bleeding is poorly understood since majority of the standard screening tests of haemostasis including the bleeding time, coagulation time, platelet count and platelet function, are usually normal. Vascular purpuras arise from damage to the capillary endothelium, abnormalities in the subendothelial matrix or extravascular connective tissue that supports the blood vessels, or from formation of abnormal blood vessels.

Vascular bleeding disorders may be *inherited* or *acquired*.

A. Inherited Vascular Bleeding Disorders (p. 430)

1. Hereditary haemorrhagic telangiectasia (Osler-Weber-Rendu disease). This is an uncommon inherited autosomal dominant disorder. The condition begins in childhood and is characterised by abnormally telangiectatic (dilated) capillaries. These telangiectasias develop particularly in the skin, mucous membranes and internal organs and are the source of frequent episodes of bleeding from nose and gastrointestinal tract.

2. Inherited disorders of connective tissue matrix. These include Marfan's syndome, Ehlers-Danlos syndrome and pseudoxanthoma elasticum, all of which have inherited defect in the connective tissue matrix and, thus, have fragile skin vessels and easy bruising.

B. Acquired Vascular Bleeding Disorders *(p. 430)*

1. Henoch-Schönlein purpura. Henoch-Schönlein or anaphylactoid purpura is a self-limited type of hypersensitivity vasculitis occurring in children and young adults. Circulating immune complexes are deposited in the vessel wall consisting of IgA, C3 and fibrin, and in some cases, properdin suggesting activation of alternate complement pathway as the trigger event.

2. Haemolytic-uraemic syndrome. Haemolytic-uraemic syndrome is a disease of infancy and early childhood in which there is bleeding tendency and varying degree of acute renal failure.

3. Simple easy bruising (Devil's pinches). Easy bruising of unknown cause is a common phenomenon in women of child-bearing age group.

4. Infection. Many infections cause vascular haemorrhages either by causing toxic damage to the endothelium or by DIC.

5. Drug reactions. Certain drugs form antibodies and produce hypersensitivity (or leucocytoclastic) vasculitis responsible for abnormal bleeding.

6. Steroid purpura. Long-term steroid therapy or Cushing's syndrome may be associated with vascular purpura due to defective vascular support.

7. Senile purpura. Atrophy of the supportive tissue of cutaneous blood vessels in old age may cause senile atrophy, especially in the dorsum of forearm and hand.

8. Scurvy. Deficiency of vitamin C causes defective collagen synthesis which causes skin bleeding as well as bleeding into muscles, and occasionally into the gastrointestinal and genitourinary tracts.

HAEMORRHAGIC DIATHESES DUE TO PLATELET DISORDERS *(p. 431)*

A. THROMBOCYTOPENIAS *(p. 431)*

Thrombocytopenia is defined as a reduction in the peripheral blood platelet count below the lower limit of normal i.e. below 150,000/μl. Thrombocytopenia is associated with abnormal bleeding that includes spontaneous skin purpura and mucosal haemorrhages as well as prolonged bleeding after trauma. However, spontaneous haemorrhagic tendency becomes clinically evident only after severe depletion of the platelet count to level of about 20,000/μl.

Thrombocytopenia may result from 4 main groups of causes: 1. Impaired platelet production. 2. Accelerated platelet destruction. 3. Splenic sequestration. 4. Dilutional loss.

A list of causes of thrombocytopenia is given in Table 13.23.

TABLE 13.23: Causes of Thrombocytopenia.

I.	**IMPAIRED PLATELET PRODUCTION**
	1. *Generalised bone marrow failure e.g.*
	Aplastic anaemia, leukaemia, myelofibrosis, megaloblastic anaemia, marrow infiltrations (carcinomas, lymphomas, multiple myeloma, storage diseases).
	2. *Selective suppression of platelet production e.g.*
	Drugs (quinine, quinidine, sulfonamides, PAS, rifampicin, anticancer drugs, thiazide diuretics), alcohol intake.
II.	**ACCELERATED PLATELET DESTRUCTION**
	1. *Immunologic thrombocytopenias e.g.*
	ITP (acute and chronic), neonatal and post-transfusion (isoimmune), drug-induced, secondary immune 'thrombocytopenia (post-infection, SLE, AIDS, CLL, lymphoma).
	2. *Increased consumption e.g.*
	DIC, TTP, giant haemangiomas, microangiopathic haemolytic anaemia.
III.	**SPLENIC SEQUESTRATION**
	Splenomegaly
IV.	**DILUTIONAL LOSS**
	Massive transfusion of old stored blood to bleeding patients.

IdiopathicThrombocytopenic Purpura (ITP) *(p. 431)*

Idiopathic thrombocytopenic purpura (ITP), also called immunologic thrombocytopenic purpura, is characterised by immunologic destruction of platelets and normal or increased megakaryocytes in the bone marrow.

PATHOGENESIS. On the basis of duration of illness, ITP is classified into acute and chronic forms, both of which have different pathogenesis.

Acute ITP. This is a self-limited disorder, seen most frequently in children following recovery from a viral illness (e.g. viral hepatitis, infectious mononucleosis, CMV infection) or an upper respiratory illness. The onset of acute ITP is sudden and thrombocytopenia is severe but recovery occurs within a few weeks to 6 months. The mechanism of acute ITP is by formation of *immune complexes* containing viral antigens, and by formation of *antibodies* against viral antigens which crossreact with platelets and lead to their immunologic destruction.

Chronic ITP. Chronic ITP occurs more commonly in adults, particularly in women of child-bearing age (20-40 years). The disorder develops insidiously and persists for several years. Though chronic ITP is idiopathic, similar immunologic thrombocytopenia may be seen in association with SLE, AIDS and autoimmune thyroiditis. The pathogenesis of chronic ITP is explained by formation of *anti-platelet autoantibodies,* usually by platelet-associated IgG humoral antibodies synthesised mainly in the spleen.

CLINICAL FEATURES. The clinical manifestation of ITP may develop abruptly as in cases of acute ITP, or the onset may be insidious as occurs in majority of cases of chronic ITP. The usual manifestations are petechial haemorrhages, easy bruising, and mucosal bleeding such as menorrhagia in women, nasal bleeding, bleeding from gums, melaena and haematuria.

LABORATORY FINDINGS. These are as under:

1. *Platelet count* is markedly reduced, usually in the range of 10,000-50,000/µl.

2. *Blood film* shows only occasional platelets which are often large in size.

3. *Bone marrow* shows increased number of megakaryocytes which have large non-lobulated single nuclei and may have reduced cytoplasmic granularity and presence of vacuoles.

4. With sensitive techniques, *anti-platelet IgG antibody* can be demonstrated on platelet surface or in the serum of patients.

5. *Platelet survival studies* reveal markedly reduced platelet life-span, sometimes less than one hour as against normal life-span of 7-10 days.

ThromboticThrombocytopenic Purpura (TTP) *(p. 433)*

Thrombotic thrombocytopenic purpura (TTP) is an uncommon but often fulminant and lethal disorder occurring in young adults. It is essentially characterised by triad of *thrombocytopenia, microangiopathic haemolytic anaemia and formation of hyaline fibrin microthrombi* within the microvasculature throughout the body. The intravascular microthrombi are composed predominantly of platelets and fibrin. The widespread presence of these platelet microthrombi is responsible for thrombocytopenia due to increased consumption of platelets, microangiopathic haemolytic anaemia and protean clinical manifestations involving different organs and tissues throughout the body.

PATHOGENESIS. Unlike DIC, a clinicopathologically related condition, activation of the clotting system is not the primary event in formation of microthrombi. TTP is initiated by endothelial injury followed by release of von Willebrand factor and other procoagulant material from endothelial cells, leading to the formation of microthrombi.

CLINICAL FEATURES. The clinical manifestations of TTP are due to microthrombi in the arterioles, capillaries and venules throughout the body. Besides features of thrombocytopenia and microangiopathic haemolytic anaemia, characteristic findings include fever, transient neurologic deficits and renal failure. The spleen may be palpable.

LABORATORY FINDINGS. These are as under:

1. Thrombocytopenia.

2. Microangiopathic haemolytic anaemia with negative Coombs' test.

3. Leucocytosis, sometimes with leukaemoid reaction.

4. Bone marrow examination reveals normal or slightly increased megakaryocytes accompanied with some myeloid hyperplasia.

5. Diagnosis is, however, established by examination of biopsy (e.g. from gingiva) which demonstrates typical microthrombi in arterioles, capillaries and venules, unassociated with any inflammatory changes in the vessel wall.

B. DISORDERS OF PLATELET FUNCTIONS *(p. 433)*

1. Hereditary Disorders *(p. 433)*

1. Defective platelet adhesion

i) *Bernard-Soulier syndrome* is an autosomal recessive disorder with inherited deficiency of a platelet membrane glycoprotein which is essential for adhesion of platelets to vessel wall.

ii) In *von Willebrand's disease,* there is defective platelet adhesion as well as deficiency of factor VIII .

2. Defective platelet aggregation. In *thrombasthenia (Glanzmann's disease),* there is failure of primary platelet aggregation with ADP or collagen due to inherited deficiency of two of platelet membrane glycoproteins.

3. Disorders of platelet release reaction. These disorders are characterised by normal initial aggregation of platelets with ADP or collagen but the subsequent release of ADP, prostaglandins and 5-HT is defective due to complex intrinsic deficiencies.

2. Acquired Disorders *(p. 433)*

1. Aspirin therapy. Prolonged use of aspirin leads to easy bruising and abnormal bleeding time.

2. Others. Several other acquired disorders are associated with various abnormalities in platelet functions at different levels. These include: uraemia, liver disease, multiple myeloma, Waldenström's macroglobulinaemia and various myeloproliferative disorders.

COAGULATION DISORDERS *(p. 434)*

A deficiency of each of the thirteen known plasma coagulation factors has been reported, which may be inherited or acquired. In general, these coagulation disorders are uncommon as compared with other bleeding disorders. Instead of spontaneous appearance of petechiae and purpuras, the plasma coagulation defects manifest more often in the form of large ecchymoses, haematomas and bleeding into muscles, joints, body cavities, GIT and urinary tract. For establishing the diagnosis, *screening tests for coagulation* (whole blood coagulation time, bleeding time, activated partial thromboplastin time and prothrombin time) are carried out, followed by *coagulation factor assays*.

Disorders of plasma coagulation factors may have hereditary or acquired origin.

Chapter Thirteen

Classic Haemophilia (Haemophilia A) *(p. 434)*

Classic haemophilia or haemophilia A is the second most common hereditary coagulation disorder next to von Willebrand's disease occurring due to deficiency or reduced activity of factor VIII (anti-haemophilic factor). The disorder is inherited as a sex-(X-) linked recessive trait and, therefore, manifests clinically in males, while females are usually the carriers. However, occasional women carriers of haemophilia may produce factor VIII levels far below 50% and become symptomatic carriers.

PATHOGENESIS. Haemophilia A is caused by quantitative reduction of factor VIII in 90% of cases, while 10% cases have normal or increased levels of factor VIII with reduced activity. Factor VIII is synthesised in hepatic parenchymal cells and regulates the activation of factor X in intrinsic coagulation pathway. Factor VIII circulates in blood complexed to another larger protein, von Willebrand's factor (vWF), which comprises 99% of the factor VIII-vWF complex. Normal haemostasis requires 25% factor VIII activity. Though occasional patients with 25% factor VIII level may develop bleeding, most symptomatic haemophilic patients have factor VIII levels below 5%.

CLINICAL FEATURES. Patients of haemophilia suffer from bleeding for hours or days after the injury. The clinical severity of the disease correlates well with plasma level of factor VIII activity. Haemophilic bleeding can involve any organ but occurs most commonly as recurrent painful haemarthroses and muscle haematomas, and sometimes as haematuria.

LABORATORY FINDINGS. These are as under:

1. Whole blood coagulation time is prolonged in severe cases only.

2. Prothrombin time is usually normal.

3. Activated partial thromboplastin time (APTT or PTTK) is typically prolonged.

4. Specific assay for factor VIII shows lowered activity.

Christmas Disease (Haemophilia B) *(p. 435)*

Inherited deficiency of factor IX (Christmas factor or plasma thromboplastin component) produces Christmas disease or haemophilia B. Haemophilia B is rarer than haemophilia A; its estimated incidence is 1 in 100,000 male births. The inheritance pattern and clinical features of factor IX deficiency are indistinguishable from those of classic haemophilia but accurate laboratory diagnosis is critical since haemophilia B requires treatment with different plasma fraction.

von Willebrand's Disease *(p. 435)*

von Willebrand's disease (vWD) is the most common hereditary coagulation disorder occurring due to qualitative or quantitative defect in von Willebrand's factor (vWF). Its incidence is estimated to be 1 in 1,000 individuals of either sex. The vWF comprises the larger fraction of factor VIII-vWF complex which circulates in the blood.

CLINICAL FEATURES. There are 3 major types of vWD:

Type I disease is the most common and is characterised by mild to moderate decrease in plasma vWF (50% activity).

Type II disease is much less common and is characterised by normal or near normal levels of vWF.

Type III disease is extremely rare and is the most severe form of the disease. These patients have no detectable vWF activity.

LABORATORY FINDINGS. 1. Prolonged bleeding time. 2. Normal platelet count. 3. Reduced plasma vWF concentration. 4. Defective platelet aggregation with ristocetin, an antibiotic. 5. Reduced factor. VIII activity.

Vitamin K Deficiency *(p. 436)*

Vitamin K is a fat-soluble vitamin which plays important role in haemostasis since it serves as a cofactor in the formation of 6 prothrombin complex proteins *(vitamin K-dependent coagulation factors)* synthesised in the liver: factor II, VII, IX, X, protein C and protein S. Vitamin K is obtained from green vegetables, absorbed in the small intestine and stored in the liver. Some quantity of vitamin K is endogenously synthesised by the bacteria in the colon.

■ **Neonatal vitamin K deficiency.** Deficiency of vitamin K in the newborn causes haemorrhagic disease of the newborn. Liver cell immaturity, lack of gut bacterial synthesis of the vitamin and low quantities in breast milk, all contribute to vitamin K deficiency in the newborn and may cause haemorrhage on 2nd to 4th day of life.

■ **Vitamin K deficiency in children and adult.** There are 3 major causes of vitamin K deficiency in childhood or adult life:
1. Inadequate dietary intake.
2. Intestinal malabsorption.
3. Loss of storage site due to hepatocellular disease.

Coagulation Disorders in Liver Disease *(p. 436)*

Since liver is the major site for synthesis and metabolism of coagulation factors, liver disease often leads to multiple haemostatic abnormalities. The liver also produces inhibitors of coagulation such as antithrombin III and protein C and S and plays a role in the clearance of activated factors and fibrinolytic enzymes.

The major causes of bleeding in liver diseases are as under:

I. Anatomic lesions. 1. Portal hypertension e.g. varices, splenomegaly with secondary thrombocytopenia. 2. Peptic ulceration. 3. Gastritis.

II. Hepatic dysfunctions, e.g. 1. Impaired hepatic synthesis of coagulation factors. 2. Impaired hepatic synthesis of coagulation inhibitors: protein C, protein S and antithrombin III. 3. Impaired absorption and metabolism of vitamin K. 4. Failure to clear activated coagulation factors causing DIC and systemic fibrinolysis.

III. Complications of therapy. These causes are: 1. Following massive transfusion leading to dilution of platelets and coagulation factors. 2. Infusion of activated coagulation proteins. 3. Following heparin therapy.

Fibrinolytic Defects *(p. 436)*

Normally, fibrinolysis consisting of plasminogen-plasmin and fibrin degradation products (FDPs) is an essential protective physiologic mechanism to limit the blood coagulation in the body. However, unchecked and excessive fibrinolysis may sometimes be the cause of bleeding. The causes of *primary pathologic fibrinolysis* leading to haemorrhagic defects are:
1. Deficiency of α_2-plasmin inhibitor following trauma or surgery.
2. Impaired clearance of tissue plasminogen activator e.g. in cirrhosis of liver.

DISSEMINATED INTRAVASCULAR COAGULATION (DIC) *(p. 436)*

Disseminated intravascular coagulation (DIC), also termed defibrination syndrome or consumption coagulopathy, is a complex thrombo-haemorrhagic disorder (intravascular coagulation and haemorrhage) occurring as a secondary complication in some systemic diseases.

ETIOLOGY. Although there are numerous conditions associated with DIC, most frequent causes are listed below:

1.   Massive tissue injury: in obstetrical syndromes (e.g. abruptio placentae, amniotic fluid embolism, retained dead foetus), massive trauma, metastatic malignancies, surgery.

2.   Infections: especially endotoxaemia, gram-negative and meningococcal septicaemia, certain viral infections, malaria, aspergillosis.

3.   Widespread endothelial damage: in aortic aneurysm, haemolytic-uraemic syndrome, severe burns, acute glomerulonephritis.

4.   Miscellaneous: snake bite, shock, acute intravascular haemolysis, heat stroke.

PATHOGENESIS. The sequence of events, in general, can be summarised as under.

1.   Activation of coagulation. The etiologic factors listed above initiate widespread activation of coagulation pathway by release of tissue factor.

2.   Thrombotic phase. Endothelial damage from the various thrombogenic stimuli causes generalised platelet aggregation and adhesion with resultant deposition of small thrombi and emboli throughout the microvasculature.

3.   Consumption phase. The early thrombotic phase is followed by a phase of consumption of coagulation factors and platelets.

4.   Secondary fibrinolysis. As a protective mechanism, fibrinolytic system is secondarily activated at the site of intravascular coagulation. Secondary fibrinolysis causes breakdown of fibrin resulting in formation of FDPs in the circulation.

CLINICAL FEATURES. There are 2 main features of DIC—*bleeding* as the most common manifestation, and *organ damage* due to ischaemia caused by the effect of widespread intravascular thrombosis such as in the kidney and brain.

LABORATORY FINDINGS. These are as follows:

1. The platelet count is low.
2. Blood film shows the features of microangiopathic haemolytic anaemia.
3. Prothrombin time, thrombin time and activated partial thromboplastin time, are all prolonged.
4. Plasma fibrinogen levels are reduced due to consumption in microvascular coagulation.
5. Fibrin degradation products (FDPs) are raised due to secondary fibrinolysis.

BLOOD GROUPS AND BLOOD TRANSFUSION *(p. 437)*

BLOOD GROUP ANTIGENS AND ANTIBODIES *(p. 437)*

The term *blood group* is applied to any well-defined system of red blood cell antigens which are inherited characteristics. Over 20 blood group systems having approximately 400 blood group antigens are currently recognised. The ABO and Rhesus (Rh) blood group systems are of major clinical significance.

ABO SYSTEM. This system consists of 3 major allelic genes: A,B and O, located on the long arm of chromosome 9. These genes control the synthesis of blood group antigens A and B. The serum of an individual contains naturally-occurring antibodies to A and/or B antigen, whichever antigen is lacking in the person's red cells (Table 13.24). In routine practice, the ABO type is determined

TABLE 13.24: The ABO Blood Groups.

BLOOD GROUP	ANTIGENS ON RED CELLS	NATURALLY-OCCURRING SERUM ANTIBODIES
AB	AB	None
A	A	Anti-B
B	B	Anti-A
O	O	Anti-A, Anti-B

by testing the red blood cells with anti-A and anti-B and by testing the serum against A, B and O red blood cells.

RHESUS SYSTEM. The Rhesus (Rh) blood group system was first discovered on human red cells by the use of antisera prepared by immunising rabbits with red cells from a Rhesus monkey.

D antigen is most strongly immunogenic and, therefore, clinically most important. In practice, Rh grouping is performed with anti-D antiserum. Individuals who are D-positive are referred to as *Rh-positive* and those who lack D antigen are termed *Rh-negative*.

BLOOD TRANSFUSION *(p. 439)*

A pre-transfusion compatibility testing is essential prior to any blood transfusion. The procedure consists of the following:

1. ABO and Rh(D) grouping of the patient *(recipient)*.
2. *Antibody screening* of the patient's serum to detect the presence of clinically significant antibodies.
3. Selecting the *donor* blood of the same ABO and Rh group.
4. *Cross-matching* the patient's serum against donor red cells to confirm donor-recipient compatibility.

Complications of Blood Transfusion *(p. 439)*

A carefully prepared and supervised blood transfusion is quite safe. However, in 5-6% of transfusions, untoward complications occur, some of which are minor while others are more serious and at times fatal.

Transfusion reactions are generally classified into 2 types: *immune* and *non-immune*.

I. Immunologic Transfusion Reactions. These are:

1. **Haemolytic transfusion reactions.** Haemolytic transfusion reaction may be *immediate* or *delayed*, *intravascular* or *extravascular*.

2. **Other allergic reactions.** Besides haemolytic transfusion reaction, others are: i) *Febrile reaction*. ii) *Anaphylactic shock*. iii) *Allergic reactions*. iv) *Graft-versus-host disease*.

II. Nonimmune Transfusion Reactions. These are:

1. **Circulatory overload.** Circulatory overload resulting in pulmonary congestion and acute heart failure is the most important and most common complication that may result in death following transfusion.

2. **Massive transfusion.** When the volume of stored blood transfused to bleeding patients exceeds their normal blood volume, it results in dilutional thrombocytopenia and dilution of coagulation factors.

3. **Transmission of infection.** Many diseases can be transmitted by transfusion of an infected blood. These include: hepatitis (HBV, HCV), CMV infection, syphilis, malaria, toxoplasmosis, infectious mononucleosis, brucellosis and AIDS (HIV infection).

4. Air embolism. Air embolism is unlikely to occur if the blood transfusion is carried out with plastic bags with negative pressure as is the usual practice now-a-days.

5. Thrombophlebitis. The complication of thrombophlebitis is more commonly associated with venesection for blood transfusion.

6. Transfusion haemosiderosis. Post-transfusion iron overload with deposition of iron in the tissues of the body occurs after repeated transfusions in the absence of any blood loss e.g. in thalassaemia major and in severe chronic refractory anaemias.

BLOOD COMPONENTS (p. 440)

Blood from donors is collected as whole blood in a suitable anticoagulant. Now-a-days it is a common practice to divide whole blood into components which include: packed RBCs, platelets, fresh-frozen plasma (FFP) and cryoprecipitate.

The procedure consists of initial centrifugation at low speed to separate whole blood into two parts: *packed RBCs* and *platelet-rich plasma (PRP)*. Subsequently, PRP is centrifuged at high speed to yield two parts: *random donor platelets* and *FFP*. *Cryoprecipitates* are obtained by thawing of FFP followed by centrifugation. *Apheresis* is the technique of direct collection of large excess of platelets from a single donor.

1. Packed RBCs. These are used to raise the oxygen-carrying capacity of blood and are used in normovolaemic patients of anaemia without cardiac disease.

2. Platelets. Transfusion of platelets is done in patients of thrombocytopenia who have haemorrhage.

3. Fresh frozen plasma. FFP contains plasma proteins and coagulation factors that includes albumin, protein C and S and antithrombin.

4. Cryoprecipitate. Cryoprecipitate is a source of insoluble plasma proteins, fibrinogen, factor VII and vWF.

HAEMOLYTIC DISEASE OF NEWBORN (p. 440)

Haemolytic disease of the newborn (HDN) results from the passage of IgG antibodies from the maternal circulation across the placenta into the circulation of the foetal red cells. Besides pregnancy, sensitisation of the mother may result from previous abortions and previous blood transfusion.

HDN can occur from incompatibility of ABO or Rh blood group system. ABO incompatibility is much more common but the HDN in such cases is usually mild, while Rh-D incompatibility results in more severe form of the HDN.

CLINICAL FEATURES. The HDN due to Rh-D incompatibility in its *severest form* may result in intrauterine death from *hydrops foetalis*. Moderate disease produces a baby born with severe anaemia and jaundice due to unconjugated hyperbilirubinaemia. When the level of unconjugated bilirubin exceeds 20 mg/dl, it may result in deposition of bile pigment in the basal ganglia of the CNS called *kernicterus* and result in permanent brain damage. *Mild disease*, however, causes only severe anaemia with or without jaundice.

LABORATORY FINDINGS. These are as under:

1. *Cord blood* shows variable degree of anaemia, reticulocytosis, elevated serum bilirubin and a positive direct Coombs' test if the cord blood is Rh-D positive.
2. Mother's blood is Rh-D negative with high plasma titre of anti-D.

■ SELF ASSESSMENT

1. **During foetal life, haematopoiesis commences in the bone marrow by:**
   A. 2nd to 3rd month
   B. 4th to 5th month
   C. 6th to 7th month
   D. 7th to 8th month

2. **Bone marrow trephine biopsy has advantage over aspiration since:**
   A. The former method is less time-consuming
   B. Romanowsky stains can be done in the former
   C. Architectural pattern of marrow is better in the former
   D. Cell morphology is better appreciated in the former

3. **Erythroid cells continue to proliferate upto the stage of:**
   A. Reticulocytes
   B. Late normoblasts
   C. Intermediate normoblasts
   D. Early normoblasts

4. **Weight of haemoglobin in RBC is:**
   A. 50%
   B. 70%
   C. 90%
   D. 99%

5. **Red cell membrane defects include the following *except:***
   A. Spherocytosis
   B. Ovalocytosis
   C. Leptocytosis
   D. Echinocytosis

6. **The following factors determine the release of oxygen from haemoglobin in tissue capillaries *except:***
   A. Nature of globin chains in Hb
   B. Bicarbonate ions in blood
   C. pH of blood
   D. Concentration of 2,3-BPG

7. **Absorption of iron is enhanced by the following *except:***
   A. Ascorbic acid
   B. Citric acid
   C. Tannates
   D. Sugars

8. **In iron deficiency anaemia, TIBC is:**
   A. Low
   B. Normal
   C. High
   D. Borderline

9. **Pappenheimer bodies are found in:**
   A. Sideroblasts
   B. Siderocytes
   C. Late normoblasts
   D. Intermediate normoblasts

10. **In anaemia of chronic disorders, serum ferritin is:**
    A. Normal
    B. Low
    C. Increased
    D. Absent

11. **Folate circulates in plasma as:**
    A. Methyl tetrahydrofolate
    B. Polyglutamate
    C. Monoglutamate
    D. Diglutamate

12. **Measurement of formiminoglutamic acid (FIGLU) for folate deficiency is done in:**
    A. Whole blood
    B. Serum
    C. Plasma
    D. Urine

13. **Pernicious anaemia causes pathologic changes in the anatomic region of stomach as under *except:***
    A. Antrum
    B. Body
    C. Body-fundic area
    D. Fundus

14. **In warm antibody autoimmune haemolytic anaemias, the antibody is commonly:**
    A. IgA
    B. IgG
    C. IgM
    D. IgD

15. **Cold agglutinin antibody in autoimmune haemolytic anaemia affects:**
    A. Mature erythrocytes
    B. Reticulocytes
    C. Siderocytes
    D. Late erythroblasts

16. **In paroxysmal nocturnal haemoglobinuria (PNH), the undue sensitivity of red cells to complement can be detected by:**
    A. Ham's test
    B. Heinz body test
    C. Direct Coombs' test
    D. Indirect Coombs' test

17. **In hereditary spherocytosis, the following membrane structure is deficient:**
    A. Band 3 protein
    B. Glycophorin
    C. Spectrin
    D. Glycolipid

18. **G6PD deficiency has the following genetic basis of inheritance:**
    A. Autosomal dominant
    B. Autosomal recessive
    C. Sex-linked trait
    D. Sex-linked homozygous

19. **The rate of sickling in sickle cell anaemia is directly correlated with the following factors *except:***
    A. Higher concentration of HbS
    B. Lower concentration of HbA
    C. Higher concentration of HbF
    D. Higher deoxygenation

20. **Molecular pathogenesis of α-thalassaemia involves:**
    A. Mutation in transcription promoter sequence
    B. Gene deletion
    C. Codon termination mutation
    D. mRNA splicing defect

21. **The pathognomonic abnormality in β-thalassaemia minor is:**
    A. Marked rise in HbA_2
    B. Marked rise in HbF
    C. Marked unconjugated hyperbilirubinaemia
    D. Marked anaemia

22. **In aplastic anaemia, there is generally:**
    A. Relative neutrophilia
    B. Relative lymphocytosis
    C. Microcytosis
    D. Reticulocyte count normal

23. **Among the various myelodysplastic syndromes, the following has worst prognosis:**
    A. Refractory anaemia with ringed sideroblasts (RARS)
    B. Refractory anaemia with excess of blasts (RAEB)
    C. Chronic myelomonocytic leukaemia (CMML)
    D. Refractory anaemia with excess of blasts in transformation (RAEBt)

24. **The following myeloid cells partake in mitosis *except:***
    A. Myelocytes
    B. Metamyelocytes
    C. Promyelocytes
    D. Myeloblast

25. **Basophils are increased in:**
    A. Bronchial asthma
    B. CML
    C. Angioneurotic oedema
    D. Corticosteroid therapy

26. **Heterophile antibody used to detect EBV infection in infectious mononucleosis is:**
    A. IgA
    B. IgD
    C. IgG
    D. IgM

27. **Atypical lymphoid cells (mononucleosis cells) in infectious mononucleosis are:**
    A. Monocytes
    B. CD8 + T lymphocytes
    C. Killer T cells
    D. B-lymphocytes

28. **Leucocyte alkaline phosphatase (LAP) scores are elevated in:**
    A. AML
    B. CML
    C. Myeloid metaplasia
    D. Myeloid leukaemoid reaction

29. **Radiation exposure is related to the following types of leukaemias *except:***
    A. AML
    B. CML
    C. ALL
    D. CLL

30. **Gum hypertrophy is a feature of the following FAB type of AML:**
    A. FAB type M1
    B. FAB type M2
    C. FAB type M3
    D. FAB type M4

31. **Myeloproliferative disorders include the following *except:***
    A. AML
    B. CML
    C. Polycythaemia vera
    D. Agnogenic myeloid metaplasia

32. **If a patient is on parenteral heparin therapy, the following test is used to monitor the administration:**
    A. Whole blood coagulation time
    B. Prothrombin time
    C. Thrombin time
    D. Activated partial thromboplastin time

33. **Chronic ITP is characterised by the following features *except:***
    A. Splenomegaly
    B. Reduced platelet lifespan
    C. Reduced number of megakaryocytes in the bone marrow
    D. Demonstration of anti-platelet IgG antibody

34. **For manifest bleeding haemophilia, the activity of factor VIII is generally:**
    A. More than 75%
    B. 50-75%
    C. 25-50%
    D. Below 25%

35. **Disseminated intravascular coagulation (DIC) is characterised by the following *except:***
    A. Thrombocytopenia
    B. Microangiopathic haemolytic anaemia
    C. Presence of FDPs in the blood
    D. Normal prothrombin time

36. **Naturally-occurring antibodies in the serum of a non-transfused person are:**
    A. IgA
    B. IgD
    C. IgG
    D. IgM

37. **Prussian blue staining for iron is positive in the following *except:***
    A. Pappenheimer bodies
    B. Howell-Jolly bodies
    C. Ferritin
    D. Haemochromatosis

38. **The major molecular abnormality in PNH is the deficiency of following protein:**
    A. Ankyrin
    B. Spectrin
    C. Decay-accelerating factor
    D. Stomatin

KEY

1 = B	2 = C	3 = C	4 = C
5 = C	6 = B	7 = C	8 = C
9 = B	10 = C	11 = A	12 = D
13 = A	14 = B	15 = B	16 = A
17 = C	18 = C	19 = C	20 = B
21 = A	22 = B	23 = D	24 = B
25 = B	26 = D	27 = C	28 = D
29 = D	30 = D	31 = A	32 = D
33 = C	34 = D	35 = D	36 = D
37 = B	38 = C		

14

The Lymphoid System

The lymphoid system tissues consisting of peripheral lymphoid organs (lymph nodes, spleen, mucosa-associated lymphoid tissue—MALT, pharyngeal lymphoid tissue) and thymus are closely interlinked with the function of the bone marrow.

LYMPH NODES (p. 442)

NORMAL STRUCTURE (p. 442)

The inner structure of the lymph node is divided into a peripheral cortex and central medulla. The *cortex* consists of several rounded aggregates of lymphocytes called *lymphoid follicles*. The follicle has a pale-staining germinal centre surrounded by small dark-staining lymphocytes called the mantle zone. The deeper region of the cortex or *paracortex* is the zone between the peripheral cortex and the inner medulla. The capsule and the structure within the lymph node are connected by supportive delicate reticulin framework.

Functionally, the lymph node is divided into T and B lymphocyte zones:

■ *B-cell zone* lies in the follicles in the cortex, the mantle zone and the interfollicular space, while *plasma cells* are also present in the interfollicular zone.

■ *T-cell zone* is predominantly present in the medulla.

There are two main functions of the lymph node—to mount immune response in the body, and to perform the function of active phagocytosis for particulate material. Besides T and B-cells, the follicular centre has *dendritic histiocytes* and antigen presenting *Langerhans' histiocytes* (formerly together called tingible body macrophages due to engulfment of particulate material) and *endothelial cells*. The follicular centre is a very active zone where lymphocytes from peripheral blood continuously enter and leave, interact with macrophage-histiocytes and endothelial cells and undergo maturation and transformation. Lymphocytes and endothelial cells have surface molecules which interact and serve as 'addresses' so that endothelial cells can direct the lymphocytes; these molecules are appropriately termed as *addressins* or *homing receptors*.

REACTIVE LYMPHADENITIS (p. 443)

Lymph nodes undergo reactive changes in response to a wide variety of stimuli which include microbial infections, drugs, environmental pollutants, tissue injury, immune-complexes and neoplasia. However, the most common causes of lymph node enlargement are inflammatory and immune reactions, aside from primary malignant neoplasms and metastatic tumour deposits.

Acute Nonspecific Lymphadenitis (p. 443)

All kinds of acute inflammations may cause acute nonspecific lymphadenitis in the nodes draining the area of inflamed tissue. Most common causes are microbiologic infections or their breakdown products, and foreign bodies in the wound or into the circulation etc. Most frequently involved lymph nodes are: *cervical* (due to infections in the oral cavity), *axillary* (due to infection in the arm), *inguinal* (due to infection in the lower extremities), and *mesenteric* (due to acute appendicitis, acute enteritis etc).

G/A The affected lymph nodes are enlarged 2-3 times their normal size and may show abscess formation if the involvement is extensive.

M/E The sinusoids are congested, widely dilated and oedematous and contain numerous neutrophils. The lymphoid follicles are prominent with presence of many mitoses and phagocytosis. In more severe cases, necrosis may occur and neutrophil abscesses may form.

Chronic Nonspecific Lymphadenitis *(p. 444)*

Chronic nonspecific lymphadenitis, commonly called *reactive lymphoid hyperplasia,* is a common form of inflammatory reaction of draining lymph nodes as a response to antigenic stimuli such as repeated attacks of acute lymphadenitis and lymph from malignant tumours.

G/A The affected lymph nodes are usually enlarged, firm and non-tender.

M/E The features of 3 patterns of reactive lymphoid hyperplasia are as under:

1. **Follicular hyperplasia** is the most frequent pattern, particularly encountered in children. Besides nonspecific stimulation, a few specific causes are: rheumatoid arthritis, toxoplasmosis, syphilis and AIDS.

i)   Enlargement and prominence of the germinal centres of lymphoid follicles (proliferation of B-cell areas).

ii)   Parafollicular and medullary regions are more cellular.

iii) There is hyperplasia of mononuclear phagocytic cells lining the lymphatic sinuses in the lymph node.

■ *Angiofollicular lymphoid hyperplasia* or *Castleman's disease* is a clinicopathologic variant of follicular hyperplasia. Two histologic forms are distinguished:

i)   *Hyaline-vascular type* is more common (90% cases) and is characterised by the presence of hyalinised arterioles in small lymphoid follicles and proliferation of vessels in the interfollicular area.

ii)   *Plasma cell form* is less common and is characterised by plasma cell hyperplasia and vascular proliferation in the interfollicular region.

2. **Paracortical lymphoid hyperplasia** is due to hyperplasia of T-cell-dependent area of the lymph node. Amongst the important causes are immunologic reactions caused by drugs (e.g. dilantin), vaccination, viruses (e.g. infectious mononucleosis) and autoimmune disorders. Its histologic features are:

i)   Expansion of the paracortex (T-cell area) with increased number of T-cell transformed immunoblasts.

ii)   Encroachment by the enlarged paracortex on the lymphoid follicles.

iii) Hyperplasia of the mononuclear phagocytic cells in the lymphatic sinuses. Variants of paracortical lymphoid hyperplasia are:

■ *Angioimmunoblastic lymphadenopathy* is characterised by diffuse hyperplasia of immunoblasts rather than paracortical hyperplasia only, and there is proliferation of blood vessels.

■ *Dermatopathic lymphadenopathy* occurs in lymph node draining an area of skin lesion.

3. **Sinus histiocytosis or sinus hyperplasia** is a very common type found in regional lymph nodes draining inflammatory lesions, or as an immune reaction of the host to a draining malignant tumour or its products. The hallmark of histologic diagnosis is the expansion of the sinuses by proliferating large histiocytes containing phagocytosed material.

■ *Sinus histiocytosis with massive lymphadenopathy* is characterised by marked enlargement of lymph nodes, especially of the neck, in young adolescents.

HIV-related Lymphadenopathy *(p. 445)*

The presence of enlarged lymph nodes of more than 1 cm diameter at two or more extra-inguinal sites for more than 3 months without any other obvious cause is frequently the earliest symptom of primary HIV infection.

M/E 1. *In the early stage* marked follicular hyperplasia is the dominant finding.

2 *In the intermediate stage,* there is a combination of follicular hyperplasia and follicular involution.

3. *In the last stage,* there is decrease in the lymph node size indicative of prognostic marker of disease progression.

MALIGNANT LYMPHOMAS *(p. 445)*

Lymphomas are malignant tumours of lymphoreticular origin i.e. from lymphocytes and histiocytes and their precursor cells. However, two distinct clinicopathologic groups are routinely distinguished:

I. *Hodgkin's lymphoma* or *Hodgkin's disease (HD)* characterised by pathognomonic presence of Reed-Sternberg cells. This group comprises about 25% of all cases of malignant lymphomas.

II. *Non-Hodgkin's lymphomas (NHL)* are more common and comprise the rest of cases.

HODGKIN'S DISEASE *(p. 445)*

Hodgkin's disease (HD) primarily arises within the lymph nodes and involves the extranodal sites secondarily. The incidence of the disease has bimodal peaks—one in young adults between the age of 15 and 35 years and the other peak after 5th decade of life. The HD is more prevalent in young adult males than females. The classical diagnostic feature is the presence of *Reed-Sternberg (RS) cell (or Dorothy-Reed-Sternberg cell).*

Etiopathogenesis *(p. 445)*

The nature and origin of RS cells, which are the real neoplastic cells in HD, have been a matter of considerable debate. One main reason for this difficulty in their characterisation is that in HD, unlike most other malignancies, the number of neoplastic cells (i.e. RS cells) is very small (less than 5%) which are interspersed in the predominant reactive cells. The following possible hypotheses are suggested:

1. EBV. Recently, on the basis of molecular studies, genome of EBV has been identified in majority of cases of mixed cellularity type and some cases of nodular sclerosis HD.

2. Genetic etiology. HD is 99 times more common in identical twin of an affected case compared with general population.

3. Cytokines. Presence of reactive inflammatory cells in the HD is due to secretion of cytokines from the RS cells e.g. IL-5 (growth factor for eosinophils), IL-13 (for autocrine stimulation of RS cells) and transforming growth factor-β (for fibrogenesis).

Classification *(p. 445)*

The diagnosis of HD requires accurate microscopic diagnosis by biopsy, usually from lymph node, and occasionally from other tissues. Unlike NHL, there is only one universally accepted classification of HD i.e. *Rye classification* adopted since 1966:

1) Lymphocyte-predominance type, 2) Nodular-sclerosis type, 3) Mixed-cellularity type, 4) Lymphocyte-depletion type.

More recently , however, according to the new WHO classification of all malignancies of lymphoid tissues (Harris et al, 1999) which takes into account clinical, morphologic, immunologic and genetic information, HD has been divided into 2 main groups:

I. Nodular lymphocyte-predominant HD (a new type).

II. Classic HD (includes all the 4 above subtypes in the Rye classification).

The salient features of the 4 conventional histologic subtypes of HD are summarised in Table 14.1.

TABLE 14.1: Modified Rye Classification of Hodgkin's Disease.

HISTOLOGIC SUBTYPE	INCIDENCE	MAIN PATHOLOGY	RS CELLS	PROGNOSIS
I. CLASSIC HD				
Lymphocyte-predominance	5%	Proliferating lymphocytes, a few histiocytes	Few, classic and polyploid type, CD15–, CD80–, CD20+	Excellent
Nodular sclerosis	70%	Lymphoid nodules, collagen bands	Frequent, lacunar type, CD15+, CD30+	Very good
Mixed cellularity	22%	Mixed infiltrate	Numerous, classic type, CD15+, CD30+	Good
Lymphocyte-depletion Diffuse fibrotic and reticular variants)	1%	Scanty lympho-cytes, atypical histiocytes, fibrosis	Numerous, pleomorphic type, CD15+, CD30+	Poor
II. NODULAR LYMPHOCYTE-PREDOMINANT HD				
	2%	Proliferation of small lympho-cytes, nodular pattern of growth	Sparse number of RS cells, CD45+, EMA+, CD15–, CD30–	Chronic relapsing, may transform into large B cell NHL

Reed-Sternberg Cell *(p. 446)*

The diagnosis of Hodgkin's disease rests on identification of RS cells, though uncommonly similar cells can occur in infectious mononucleosis and other forms of lymphomas. Therefore, additional cellular and architectural features of the biopsy must be given due consideration for making the histologic diagnosis.

There are several morphologic variants of RS cells which characterise different histologic subtypes of HD:

1. **Classic RS cell** is a large cell which has characteristically a bilobed nucleus appearing as mirror image of each other but occasionally the nucleus may be multilobed. Each lobe of the nucleus contains a prominent, eosinophilic, inclusion-like nucleolus with a clear halo around it, giving an owl-eye appearance. The cytoplasm of cell is abundant and amphophilic.

2. **Lacunar type RS cell** is smaller and in addition to above features has a pericellular space or lacuna in which it lies. It is characteristically found in nodular sclerosis variety of HD.

3. **Polyploid type (or popcorn or lymphocytic-histiocytic i.e. L and H) RS cells** are seen in lymphocyte predominance type of HD.

4. Pleomorphic RS cells are a feature of lymphocyte depletion type. These cells have pleomorphic and atypical nuclei.

Immunophenotyping of RS cells reveals monoclonal lymphoid cell origin of RS cell from B-cells in most subtypes of Hodgkin's disease. RS cells in all types of Hodgkin's diseases, except in lymphocyte predominance type, express immunoreactivity for CD15 and CD30. RS cells in lymphocyte predominance type, however, are negative for both CD15 and CD30, but positive for CD20.

G/A The affected lymph nodes initially remain discrete but later are matted together. The sectioned surface is homogeneous and fishflesh-like in *lymphocyte predominance type,* nodular due to scarring in *nodular sclerosis type,* and abundance of necrosis in *mixed cellularity* and *lymphocyte depletion types.*

M/E The criteria for diagnosis of histologic subtypes are as under:

I. Classic HD

As per WHO classification, classic group of HD includes 4 types of HD of older Rye classification:

1. Lymphocyte-predominance type. The lymphocyte-predominance type of HD is characterised by proliferation of small lymphocytes admixed with a varying number of histiocytes forming nodular or diffuse pattern.

i)   *Nodular form* is characterised by replacement of nodal architecture by numerous large neoplastic nodules.

ii)   *Diffuse form* does not have discernible nodules but instead there is diffuse proliferation of cells.

However, currently nodular form of lymphocyte predominent HD has been categorised separately due to its distinct immunophenotyping features and prognosis.

For making the diagnosis, definite demonstration of RS cells is essential which are few in number, requiring a thorough search. In addition to typical RS cells, *polyploid variant* having polyploid, and twisted nucleus (popcorn-like) may be found in some cases.

2.   Nodular-sclerosis type. Nodular sclerosis is the most frequent type of HD, seen more commonly in women than in men. It is characterised by two essential features:

i)   *Bands of collagen:* Variable amount of fibrous tissue is characteristically present in the involved lymph nodes.

ii)   *Lacunar type RS cells:* Characteristic lacunar type of RS cells with distinctive pericellular halo are present.

In addition to these 2 characteristics, the nodules between the fibrous septa consist predominantly of lymphocytes and macrophages, sometimes with foci of necrosis.

3.   Mixed-cellularity type. This form of HD generally replaces the entire affected lymph nodes by heterogeneous mixture of various types of apparently normal cells. These include proliferating lymphocytes, histiocytes, eosinophils, neutrophils and plasma cells. Some amount of fibrosis and focal areas of necrosis are generally present. Typical RS cells are frequent.

4.   Lymphocyte-depletion type. In this type of HD, the lymph node is depleted of lymphocytes. There are two variants of lymphocyte-depletion HD:

i)   *Diffuse fibrotic variant* is hypocellular and the entire lymph node is replaced by diffuse fibrosis, appearing as homogeneous, fibrillar hyaline material. The area of hyalinosis contains some lymphocytes, atypical histiocytes (Hodgkin cells), and numerous typical and atypical (pleomorphic) RS cells.

ii)   *Reticular variant* is much more cellular and consists of large number of atypical pleomorphic histiocytes, scanty lymphocytes and a few typical RS cells.

II. Nodular Lymphocyte-predominant HD

This is a newly described entity which is distinct from the classic HD described above. This type was previously included in lymphocyte predominant type of HD. Its peculiarities are as under:

i) These cases of HD have a nodular growth pattern (similar to nodular sclerosis type).

ii) Like lymphocyte-predominant pattern of classic type, there is predominance of small lymphocyte with sparse number of RS cells.

iii) These cases of HD have distinctive immunophenotyping: CD45 positive, epithelial membrane (EMA) positive but negative for the usual markers for RS cells (CD15 and CD30 negative).

iv) Though generally it has a chronic relapsing course, but some cases of this type of HD may transform in to large B-cell NHL.

Clinical Features *(p. 448)*

Hodgkin's disease is particularly frequent among young and middle-aged adults. All histologic subtypes of HD, except the nodular sclerosis variety, are more common in males.

1. Most commonly, patients present with painless, movable and firm *lymphadenopathy*. The cervical and mediastinal lymph nodes are involved most frequently. Other lymph node groups like axillary, inguinal and abdominal are involved sometimes.

2. Approximately half the patients develop *splenomegaly* during the course of the disease. *Liver enlargement* too may occur.

3. *Constitutional symptoms* (type B symptoms) are present in 25-40% of patients. The most common is low-grade fever with night sweats and weight loss.

Other Laboratory Findings *(p. 448)*

Haematologic abnormalities:

1. A moderate, normocytic and normochromic *anaemia* is often present.

2. *Serum iron and TIBC* are low but marrow iron stores are normal or increased.

3. *Marrow infiltration* by the disease may produce marrow failure with leucoerythroblastic reaction.

4. *Routine blood counts* reveal moderate leukaemoid reaction. Cases with pruritus frequently show peripheral eosinophilia.

5. *Platelet count* is normal or increased.

6. *ESR* is invariably elevated.

Immunologic abnormalities:

1. There is progressive fall in immunocompetent T-cells with *defective cellular immunity*. There is reversal of CD4: CD8 ratio and anergy to routine skin tests.

2. *Humoral antibody production* is normal in untreated patients until late in the disease.

Staging *(p. 449)*

Following biopsy and histopathologic classification of HD, the extent of involvement of the disease (i.e. staging) is studied so as to select the proper treatment and assess the prognosis. *The Ann Arbor staging classification* takes into account both clinical and pathologic stage of the disease.

The suffix *A* or *B* are added to the above stages depending upon whether the three constitutional symptoms (fever, night sweats and unexplained weight loss exceeding 10% of normal) are absent (A) or present (B). The suffix *E* or *S* are used for extranodal involvement and splenomegaly respectively (Table 14.2).

TABLE 14.2: Ann Arbor Staging Classification of Hodgkin's Disease.

Stage I	I	Involvement of a single lymph node region.
(A or B)	I$_E$	Involvement of a single extra-lymphatic organ or site.
Stage II	II	Involvement of two or more lymph node regions on the same
(A or B)		side of the diaphragm.
	II$_E$	(or) with localised contiguous involvement of an extranodal organ or site.
Stage III	III	Involvement of lymph node regions on both sides of the
(A or B)		diaphragm.
	III$_E$	(or) with localised contiguous involvement of an extranodal organ or site.
	III$_S$	(or) with involvement of spleen.
	III$_{ES}$	(or) both features of III$_E$ and III$_S$.
Stage IV	IV	Multiple or disseminated involvement of one or
(A or B)		more extra-lymphatic organs or tissues with or without lymphatic involvement.

A = asymptomatic; B = presence of constitutional symptoms;
E = extranodal involvement; S = splenomegaly

Prognosis *(p. 449)*

With use of aggressive radiotherapy and chemotherapy, the outlook for Hodgkin's disease has improved significantly.

■ With appropriate treatment, the overall 5 years survival rate for *stage I and II A* is as high as about 100%, while the advanced stage of the disease may have upto 50% 5-year survival rate.

■ Patients with *lymphocyte-predominance type* of HD tend to have localised form of the disease and have excellent prognosis.

■ The *nodular sclerosis* variety too has very good prognosis but those patients with larger mediastinal mass respond poorly to both chemotherapy and radiotherapy.

■ The *mixed cellularity type* occupies intermediate clinical position between the lymphocyte predominance and the lymphocyte-depletion type, but patients with disseminated disease and systemic manifestations do poorly.

■ The *lymphocyte-depletion type* is usually disseminated at the time of diagnosis and is associated with constitutional symptoms. These patients usually have the most aggressive form of the disease.

NON-HODGKIN'S LYMPHOMAS *(p. 449)*

Non-Hodgkin's lymphomas (NHL) are the malignant neoplasms of the immune system of the body and are more common than Hodgkin's lymphoma. The biologic and clinical behaviour of NHL are quite distinct from HD and thus the two are quite different diseases. NHL is most frequent in young adults (20-40 years). Its incidence is showing an upward trend due to increasing incidence of AIDS.

Majority of NHL arise in lymph nodes (65%) while the remaining 35% take origin in extranodal lymphoid tissues.

Etiopathogenesis *(p. 450)*

Malignant lymphomas are considered as the clonal proliferation of immune cells. About 65% of NHL are of B-lymphocyte origin, 35% of T-lymphocytes, and less than 2% are histiocytic derivatives. The following etiologic factors have been shown to have strong association with the development of NHL.

1. Infections. *i) Viral infections:* Epstein-Barr virus (EBV) in endemic variety of Burkitt's lymphoma and post-transplant lymphoma, human-T-cell leukaemia virus type I (HTLV-I) in adult T-cell lymphoma-leukaemia, HIV in diffuse large B-cell lymphoma and Burkitt's lymphoma, hepatitis C virus in lymphoplasmacytic lymphoma, and human herpes virus 8 (HHV-8) in primary effusion lymphoma. *ii) Bacteria.* Helicobacter pylori in MALT lymphoma of the stomach.

2. Immunodeficiency diseases. Various inherited and acquired immunodeficiency diseases including AIDS and iatrogenic immunosuppression induced by chemotherapy or radiation, are associated with subsequent development of lymphomatous transformation.

3. Autoimmune disease association. A few autoimmune diseases such as Sjögren's syndrome, nontropical sprue, rheumatoid arthritis and SLE are associated with higher incidence of NHL.

4. Chemical and drug exposure. Long-term exposure to drugs such as phenytoin, radiation, prior chemotherapy and agriculture chemicals have all been associated with development of NHL. Patients treated for HD can develop NHL.

A number of cytogenetic abnormalities have been detected in cases of NHL, most important of which are chromosomal translocations involving antigen receptor genes, immunoglobulin genes, or overexpression of *BCL*-2 protein.

Classification *(p. 450)*

Unlike Hodgkin's disease in which Rye classification is the only universally accepted classification since 1966 with some modifications, the pathologic classification of NHL has been difficult for both pathologists and clinicians. Several classifications have been described at different times adding further confusion. The widely used classification systems of NHL (in chronologic order) are: *Rappaport* (1966), *Lukes-Collins* (1974), *Working Formulations for clinical usage* (1982), REAL (1994), and WHO classification (1999). These classifications are given in Table 14.3.

WORKING FORMULATIONS FOR CLINICAL USAGE. This classification proposed in 1982 by a panel of experts from National Cancer Institute of the US incorporates the best features of all previous classification systems, and as the name implies, has strong clinical relevance. Based on the natural history of disease and long-term survival studies, working Formulations divides all NHLs into 3 prognostic groups:

- *Low-grade NHL:* 5-year survival 50-70%;
- *Intermediate-grade NHL:* 5-year survival 35-45%; and
- *High-grade NHL:* 5-year survival 25-35%.

In this classification, no attempt is made to determine whether the tumour cells are B-cells, T-cells or macrophages.

REAL CLASSIFICATION. International Lymphoma Study Group in 1994 has proposed another classification called *revised European-American* classification of *lymphoid* neoplasms abbreviated as REAL classification. This classification is based on the hypothesis that all forms of lymphoid malignancies (NHLs as well as lymphoblastic leukaemias) represent malignant counterparts of normal population of immune cells (B-cells, T-cells and histiocytes) present in the lymph node and bone marrow. It is believed that lymphoid malignancies arise due to arrest at the various differentiation stages of B and T-cells since tumours of histiocytic origin are quite uncommon. Accordingly, it is considered essential to understand and correlate the differentiation stages of B and T-cells with various lymphoid malignancies. REAL classification divides all lymphoid malignancies into two broad groups, each having further subtypes (Table 14.3):

TABLE 14.3: Classification of NHL.

RAPPAPORT CLASSIFICATION (1966)

A) Nodular NHL
1. Lymphocytic, well-differentiated
2. Lymphocytic, poorly-differentiated
3. Lymphocytic and histiocytic, mixed

B) Diffuse NHL
1. Lymphocytic, well-differentiated
2. Lymphocytic, poorly-differentiated
3. Lymphocytic and histiocytic, mixed
4. Histiocytic
5. Lymphoblastic
6. Diffuse undifferentiated, Burkitt's and non-Burkitt's

LUKES-COLLINS CLASSIFICATION (1974)

A) B-cell NHL
1. Small lymphocytic
2. Plasmacytoid lymphocytic
3. Follicular centre cell (small cleaved and large cleaved, small non-cleaved and large non-cleaved)
4. Immunoblastic

B) T-cell NHL
1. Small lymphocytic
2. Convoluted lymphocytic
3. Cerebriform lymphocytic
4. Immunoblastic

C) Histiocytic NHL

D) Undefined (U) NHL

WORKING FORMULATIONS FOR CLINICAL USAGE (1982)

I. Low-grade
A) Small lymphocytic
B) Follicular, predominantly small cleaved cell
C) Follicular, mixed small and large cleaved cell

II. Intermediate-grade
D) Follicular, predominantly large cell
E) Diffuse, small cleaved cell
F) Diffuse, mixed small and large cell
G) Diffuse, large, cell

III. High-grade
H) Large cell, immunoblastic
I) Lymphoblastic
J) Small non-cleaved cell (Burkitt's)

IV. Miscellaneous
1. Adult T-cell leukaemia/lymphoma
2. Cutaneous T-cell lymphoma
3. Histiocytic (Histiocytic medullary reticulosis)

REAL CLASSIFICATION (1994)

I. Leukaemias and lymphomas of B-cell origin (Pan-B CD19,20 positive)

A) Indolent B-cell malignancies
i) Chronic lymphocytic leukaemia/small lymphocytic lymphoma
ii) Hairy cell leukaemia
iii) Follicular lymphomas (grade I small cleaved, grade II mixed small and large)
iv) Lymphoplasmacytoid lymphoma/Waldenström's macroglobulinaemia
v) Marginal zone lymphoma (lymphoma of mucosa associated lymphoid tissue (MALT), splenic lymphoma)

B) Aggressive B-cell malignancies
i) Diffuse large cell lymphoma
ii) Follicular large cell lymphoma (grade III)

Contd...

Table 14.3 (contd...)

        iii)   Mantle cell lymphoma
        iv)   Burkitt's lymphoma
        v)   Plasmacytoma/myeloma

II.   **Leukaemias and lymphomas of T-cell origin**
      (CD2,7 positive)
      a)   **Indolent T-cell malignancies**
          i)   T-CLL, T-prolymphocytic leukaemia
          ii)   Cutaneous T-cell lymphoma (Sézary's syndrome mycosis fungoides)
      b)   **Aggressive T-cell malignancies**
          i)   Peripheral T-cell NHL
          ii)   Angioimmunoblastic T-cell lymphoma
          iii) Intestinal T-cell lymphoma
          iv) Adult T-ALL

WHO CLASSIFICATION (1999)

I. B-cell neoplasms

Precursor B-cell malignancies:

Precursor B lymphoblastic leukaemia/lymphoma (precursor B-cell ALL)

Mature (Peripheral) B-cell malignancies:

1.   B-cell CLL/SLL (chronic lymphocytic leukaemia/small lymphocytic lymphoma)
2.   Plasma cell myeloma/plasmacytoma (page 459)
3.   Extranodal marginal zone B-cell lymphoma, MALT type
4.   Mantle cell lymphoma
5.   Follicular lymphoma
6.   Diffuse large B-cell lymphoma
7.   Burkitt's lymphoma/Burkitt cell leukaemia
8.   Other B-cell malignancies:
     i)   B-cell prolymphocytic leukaemia
     ii)   Hairy cell leukaemia
     iii) Splenic marginal zone B-cell lymphoma
     iv) Lymphoplasmacytic lymphoma
     v)   Nodal marginal zone lymphoma (Monocytoid B-cell lymphoma)

II. T-cell neoplasms

Precursor T-cell malignancies:

Precursor T lymphoblastic lymphoma/leukaemia (Precursor T-cell ALL)

Mature (Peripheral) T-cell malignancies:

1.   Mycosis fungoides/Sézary syndrome
2.   Adult T-cell lymphoma/leukaemia (HTLV-I +)
3.   Anaplastic large T/null cell lymphoma, primary systemic type
4.   Peripheral T-cell lymphoma, not otherwise specified
     i)   Angioimmunoblastic T-cell lymphoma
     ii)   Extranodal NK/T-cell lymphoma, nasal type
     iii) Enteropathy-type T-cell lymphoma
     iv) Hepatosplenic T-cell lymphoma
5.   Other T-cell malignanies:
     i)   T-cell prolymphocytic leukaemia
     ii)   T-cell granular lymphocytic leukaemia
     iii) Aggressive NK cell leukaemia

■ *Leukaemias and lymphomas of B-cell origin:* B-cell derivation comprises 80% cases of lymphoid leukaemias and 90% cases of NHLs. All these tumours express Pan-B (CD19) antigen besides other markers.

■ *Leukaemias and lymphomas of T-cell origin:* T-cell malignancies comprise the remainder 20% cases of lymphoid leukaemia and 10% cases of NHLs. T-cell malignancies reflect the stages of T-cell ontogeny. The most widely expressed T-cell antigens are CD3 and CD7.

WHO CLASSIFICATION. In 1999, the same group of workers (Harris et al) who described REAL classification revised their classification under the aegis of WHO. Although this classification has many similarities with REAL classification as regards identification of B and T cell types, WHO classification has more classes. Besides, it takes into consideration clinicopathologic and immunologic profile of all lymphoid malignancies, and has a better clinical and therapeutic relevance.

G/A The affected group of lymph nodes are enlarged in majority of cases of NHL. Any lymph node group may be involved but most commonly affected are the cervical, supraclavicular and axillary groups. Less commonly at the time of diagnosis, there may be enlargement of lymphoid tissue elsewhere such as in the tonsils, spleen, stomach, bone etc. Initially, the lymph nodes are discrete and separate from one another but later the lymph nodes form a large matted mass due to infiltration into the surrounding connective tissue.

M/E

I. B-CELL NEOPLASMS
PRECURSOR B-CELL MALIGNANCIES

Precursor B-cell lymphocytic leukaemia-lymphoma *(Diffuse lymphoblastic; Convoluted T-cell lymphoma; Lymphoblastic lymphoma).* This is the most common form of ALL in children; rarely presentation may be in the form of lymphoma in children or adults. The diagnosis is made by bone marrow biopsy which shows malignant cells of precursor B cell origin as demonstrated by immunophenotyping (CD10, 19, 20, 22, HLA-DR and TdT positive) and characteristic cytogenetic abnormalities, most often t(9;22) i.e. Philadelphia positive-ALL.

MATURE (PERIPHERAL) B-CELL MALIGNANCIES

1. B-cell CLL/SLL (Chronic lymphocytic leukaemia—small lymphocytic lymphoma). *(Diffuse, well-differentiated lymphocytic; B-small lymphocytic and plasmacytoid lymphoma; Small lymphocytic lymphoma).* As the name implies, this subtype may present as leukaemia or lymphoma. As lymphoid leukaemia, this is the most common form, while as NHL it constitutes about 4% of all NHLs. The diagnosis of B-cell CLL is made by circulating lymphocytosis in excess of 4,000/μl with typical smudge or basket cells in the peripheral blood due to damaged nuclei of malignant lymphocytes. These cells are of monoclonal B-cell origin having immunologic features of mantle zone B-cells (typically positive for CD5; other markers are CD19, 20, 22 and for HLA-DR) and cytogenetic abnormalities (most commonly trisomy 12). Cases with lymphadenopathy at presentation show replacement of the lymph node by diffuse proliferation of well-differentiated, mature, small and uniform lymphocytes without any cytologic atypia or significant mitoses and having features of immunophenotype as for B-cell CLL.

Some cases of SLL may transform into more aggressive diffuse large B-cell lymphoma, or may be associated with occurrence of an IgM monoclonal gammopathy called Waldenström's macroglobulinaemia.

2. Extranodal marginal zone B-cell lymphoma of MALT type. This type comprises about 8% of all NHLs. In the previous classification, it was included under SLL, but currently it is categorised separately for 2 reasons: etiologic association with *H. pylori* infection and occurrence at extranodal sites. Most frequent is gastric lymphoma of MALT type with its characteristic etiologic association with *H. pylori*; other extranodal sites for this subtype of NHL are intestine, orbit, lung, thyroid, salivary glands and CNS. Morphologically, it is characterised by diffuse infiltration by monoclonal small B lymphocytes which are negative for CD5.

3. Mantle cell lymphoma. This subtype of NHL comprises about 6% of all NHLs. It was earlier included in SLL but has been identified as a separate subtype recently due to characteristic chromosomal translocation, t(11;14) and overexpression of *BCL-1* and surface immunoglobulins IgM and IgD protein. However, both SLL and mantle cell NHL are positive for CD5 antigen.

4. Follicular lymphoma *(Nodular, poorly-differentiated lymphocytic; Follicular centre cell, small/large cleaved lymphoma; Follicular, predominantly small/large cleaved cell lymphoma).* Follicular lymphomas comprise approximately 22% of all NHLs. Morphologically, as the name suggests, this form of follicular lymphoma is characterised by follicular or nodular pattern of growth. The nuclei of tumour cells may vary from predominantly small cleaved (or indented) to predominantly large cleaved variety. The former is more common, has infrequent mitoses and the rate of growth slow (low grade), while the patients with large cell lymphoma have high proliferation and progress rapidly (high grade).

5. Diffuse large B-cell lymphoma *(Diffuse poorly-differentiated lymphocytic/ Diffuse histiocytic; Follicular centre cell, large, cleaved/non-cleaved diffuse lymphoma).* Diffuse large B-cell lymphoma is the most common comprising about 35% of all NHLs. This variety is the diffuse counterpart of follicular large cleaved cell lymphoma i.e. it is composed of large cleaved cells spread in a diffuse pattern. Immunophenotypic markers for pan-B cells (CD19, CD20) are positive, besides overexpression of surface immunoglobulins (IgM, IgG and light chains) and of *BCL-2* protein.

6. Burkitt's lymphoma/leukaemia *(Diffuse undifferentiated Burkitt's and Non-Burkitt's; Follicular centre cell, small non-cleaved cell lymphoma; Small non-cleaved cell lymphoma).* Burkitt's lymphoma/leukaemia is an uncommon tumour in adults but comprises about 30% of childhood NHLs. Burkitt's leukaemia corresponds to L3 ALL of FAB grouping and is uncommon. Three subgroups of Burkitt's lymphoma are recognised: *African endemic, sporadic and immunodeficiency-associated*, but histologically all three are similar. The tumour cells are intermediate in size, non-cleaved, and homogeneous in size and shape. The nuclei are round to oval and contain 2-5 nucleoli. The cytoplasm is basophilic and contains lipid vacuolation. The tumour cells have a very high mitotic rate, and therefore high cell death. This feature accounts for presence of numerous macrophages in the background of this tumour containing phagocytosed tumour debris giving it a 'starry sky' appearance.

Immunophenotypically, the tumour cells are positive for CD19 and CD10 and surface immunoglobulin IgM. Typical cytogenetic abnormalities in the tumour cells are t(8;22) involving *MYC* gene on chromosome 8, with overexpression of MYC protein having transforming activity.

7. Other B-cell malignancies. A few other types are:

i) B-cell prolymphocytic leukaemia is involvement of blood and bone marrow by large B lymphocytes having prominent nucleoli.

ii) Hairy cell leukaemia is a rare B-cell malignancy characterised by presence of hairy cells in the blood and bone marrow and splenomegaly.

iii) Splenic marginal zone lymphoma is another uncommon B-cell neoplasm in which the splenic white pulp is infiltrated by small monoclonal B lymphocytes.

iv) Lymphoplasmacytic lymphoma is tissue manifestation of Waldenström's macroglobulinaemia. Etiologic association of this form of lymphoma with hepatitis C virus infection has also been proposed.

v) Nodal marginal zone lymphoma (monocytoid B-cell lymphoma) is another uncommon subtype of aggressive NHL.

II. T-CELL NEOPLASMS
PRECURSOR T-CELL MALIGNANCIES

Precursor T-cell lymphoblastic leukaemia/lymphoma. As the name implies, these cases may present as ALL or as lymphoma. Like precursor B-cell NHL, this subtype is also more common in children under 4 years of age. Since the precursor T-cells differentiate in the thymus, this tumour often presents as mediastinal mass and pleural effusion and progresses rapidly to develop leukaemia in the blood and bone marrow. Morphologically, precursor B and T-cell ALL/lymphoma are indistinguishable. However, immunophenotype of T-cell subtype is positive for CD2, CD7 and TdT.

MATURE (PERIPHERAL) T-CELL MALIGNANCIES

1. Mycosis fungoides/Sézary syndrome. Mycosis fungoides is a slowly evolving cutaneous T-cell lymphoma occurring in middle aged adult males. The condition is often preceded by eczema or dermatitis for several years (*premycotic stage*). This is followed by infiltration by CD4+T-cells in the epidermis and dermis as a plaque (*plaque stage*) and eventually as *tumour stage*. The disease may spread to viscera and to peripheral blood as a leukaemia characterised by Sézary cells having cerebriform nuclei termed as Sézary syndrome.

2. Adult T-cell lymphoma/leukaemia (ATLL). This is an uncommon T-cell malignancy but has gained much prominence due to association with retrovirus, human T-cell lymphotropic virus-I (HTLV-I). The infection is acquired by blood transfusion, breast milk, sexual route or transplacentally. The involved lymph nodes have proliferation of CD4 positive large atypical T-cells with indented nuclei, called 'flower cells', most prominent in the paracortical zone. The blood also shows large pleomorphic T-cell leukaemia.

3. Anaplastic large T/Null cell lymphoma. This relatively newer entity is the T-cell counterpart of diffuse large B-cell lymphoma and was previously included under malignant histiocytosis or diagnosed as anaplastic carcinoma. There is diffuse infiltration of lymph nodes by anaplastic T-cells/null cells positive for CD30 (Ki 1).

4. Peripheral T-cell lymphomas. This group includes a variety of aggressive T-cell lymphomas which are morphologically heterogeneous but have common immunotypic features of mature T-cells (CD4+, CD8+, or both). These are more common in young adults and often have bone marrow involvement at presentation. The subtypes of peripheral T-cell lymphomas include the following syndromes:

i) Angioimmunoblastic T-cell lymphoma is relatively more common subtype, comprising about 20% of all T-cell NHLs.

ii) Extranodal T/NK cell lymphoma of nasal type is involvement of upper airways by the monoclonal T-cells.

iii) Enteropathy type T-cell lymphoma is a rare aggressive lymphoma seen in association with untreated cases of gluten-sensitive enteropathy.

iv) Hepatosplenic T-cell lymphoma, unlike other lymphomas which occur as tumour masses, is characterised by sinusoidal infiltration of the liver, spleen and bone marrow by monoclonal T-cells.

Clinical Features *(p. 457)*

1) Superficial lymphadenopathy, 2) Constitutional symptoms, 3) Oropharyngeal involvement 4) Abdominal disease, 5) Other organs. Involvement of the skin or brain occurs in certain subtypes of NHL.

Other Laboratory Findings *(p. 458)*

Haematologic abnormalities:

1. Anaemia of normocytic normochromic type.

2. Advanced disease with marrow infiltration may show neutropenia, thrombocytopenia and leucoerythroblastic reaction.

Chapter Fourteen

3. Lymphosarcoma cell leukaemia (leukaemic conversion of NHL) occurs in some patients.

4. Marrow involvement by NHL is seen in 20% of cases.

5. Hyperuricaemia and hypercalcaemia occur late in the disease.

Immunologic abnormalities:

Immunologic studies reveal that majority of NHLs are of B lymphocyte origin. There may be associated monoclonal excess of immunoglobulins, usually IgG or IgM. Plasmacytoid lymphoma may produce excess of a heavy chain or a light chain.

Staging *(p. 458)*

The Ann Arbor staging system developed for Hodgkin's disease is used for staging NHL too. This staging system depends upon the number and location of nodal and extranodal sites involved, and presence or absence of constitutional (B) symptoms.

Prognosis *(p. 458)*

Low-grade lymphomas usually progress slowly and local radiotherapy brings about remission lasting for upto 10 years in 75% cases. More extensive disease is treated with combination chemotherapy and local radiotherapy. Patients with histiocytic lymphoma and T-cell leukaemia/lymphoma have an extremely poor prognosis.

The salient features to distinguish Hodgkin's disease and non-Hodgkin's lymphoma are summarised in Table 14.4.

TABLE 14.4: Contrasting Features of Hodgkin's Disease and Non-Hodgkin's Lymphoma.

	FEATURE	HODGKIN'S	NON-HODGKIN'S
1.	*Cell derivation*	B-cell mostly	90% B 10% T
2.	*Nodal involvement*	Localised, may spread to contiguous nodes	Disseminated nodal spread
3.	*Extranodal spread*	Uncommon	Common
4.	*Bone marrow involvement*	Uncommon	Common
5.	*Constitutional symptoms*	Common	Uncommon
6.	*Chromosomal defects*	Aneuploidy	Translocations, deletions
7.	*Spill-over*	Never	May spread to blood
8.	*Prognosis*	Better (75-85% cure)	Bad (30-40% cure)

LYMPH NODE METASTATIC TUMOURS *(p. 458)*

The regional lymph nodes draining the site of a primary malignant tumour are commonly enlarged. This enlargement may be due to benign *reactive hyperplasia* or *metastatic tumour deposits.*

1. **Benign reactive hyperplasia,** is due to immunologic reaction by the lymph node in response to tumour-associated antigens.

2. **Metastatic deposits** in regional lymph nodes occurs most commonly from carcinomas and malignant melanoma. Sarcomas generally disseminate

by the haematogenous route but uncommonly may metastasise to the regional lymph nodes. Metastatic tumour cells from the primary malignant tumour are drained via lymphatics into the subcapsular sinuses initially but subsequently the lymph node stroma is also invaded.

PLASMA CELL DISORDERS (p. 459)

The plasma cell disorders are characterised by abnormal proliferation of immunoglobulin-producing cells and result in accumulation of monoclonal immunoglobulin in serum and urine. The group as a whole is known by various synonyms such as *plasma cell dyscrasias, paraproteinaemias, dysproteinaemias and monoclonal gammopathies*. The group comprises the following four disease entities:

1) Multiple myeloma, 2) Waldenström's macroglobulinaemia, 3) Heavy chain disease, 4) Primary amyloidosis.

The feature common to all plasma cell disorders is the neoplastic proliferation of cells derived from B-lymphocyte lineage.

MULTIPLE MYELOMA (p. 459)

Multiple myeloma is a multifocal malignant proliferation of plasma cells derived from a single clone of cells (i.e. monoclonal). The tumour, its products (M component), and the host response result in the most important and most common syndrome in the group of plasma cell disorders that produces osseous as well as extraosseous manifestations. Multiple myeloma primarily affects the elderly (peak incidence in 5th-6th decades) and increases in incidence with age. It is rare under the age of 40 and is slightly more common in males.

Etiopathogenesis (p. 459)

Myeloma is a monoclonal proliferation of B-cells. The etiology of myeloma remains unknown. However, following factors have been implicated:
1) Radiation exposure, 2) Those exposed to petroleum products, 3) Farmers, wood workers, leather workers are more prone.

As regards its pathogenesis, following concepts have been proposed:

1. Genetic abnormalities. i) Translocation t(11;14)(q13;q32) is the most common.
ii) Overexpression of *MYC* or *RAS* genes in some cases.
iii) Mutation in p53 (TP53) and *RB* gene in some cases.

2. Role of growth factor. Interleukin (IL)-6 has been found to play role in B-cell proliferation in myeloma. Infection of the marrow macrophages with human herpes virus 8 with resultant release of viral IL-6 may be responsible for stimulation of neoplastic process in myeloma.

MORPHOLOGY Myeloma affects principally the bone marrow though in the course of the disease other organs are also involved.

I. OSSEOUS (BONE MARROW) LESIONS. In more than 95% of cases, multiple myeloma begins in the bone marrow. In the majority of cases, the disease involves multiple bones. By the time the diagnosis is made, most of the bone marrow is involved. Most commonly affected bones are those with red marrow i.e. skull, spine, ribs and pelvis, but later long bones of the limbs are also involved. Radiographically, these lesions appear as punched out, rounded, 1-2 cm sized defects in the affected bone.

G/A The normal bone marrow is replaced by soft, gelatinous, reddish-grey tumours. The affected bone usually shows focal or diffuse osteoporosis.

M/E The diagnosis of multiple myeloma can be usually established by examining bone marrow aspiration from an area of bony rarefaction.

i)   **Cellularity:** There is usually hypercellularity of the bone marrow.

ii)   **Myeloma cells:** Myeloma cells constitute 15-30% of the marrow cellularity. These cells may form clumps or sheets, or may be scattered among the normal haematopoietic cells. Myeloma cells may vary in size from small, differentiated cells resembling normal plasma cells to large, immature and undifferentiated cells. Binucleate and multinucleate cells are sometimes present. The nucleus of myeloma cell is commonly eccentric similar to plasma cells but usually lacks the cart-wheel chromatin pattern seen in classical plasma cells. Nucleoli are frequently present.

In addition to multiple myeloma, *plasmacytosis* in the bone marrow can occur in some other disorders. These are: aplastic anaemia, rheumatoid arthritis, SLE, cirrhosis of liver, metastatic cancer and chronic inflammation. However, in all these conditions the plasma cells are mature and they do not exceed 10% of the total marrow cells.

II.   EXTRAOSSEOUS LESIONS. Some of the commonly involved sites are as under:

1.   Blood. Approximately 50% of patients with multiple myeloma have a few atypical plasma cells in the blood. Other changes in the blood in myeloma are the presence of anaemia (usually normocytic normochromic type), marked red cell rouleaux formation due to hyperviscosity of blood, and an elevated ESR.

2.   Myeloma kidney. Renal involvement in myeloma called myeloma nephrosis occurs in many cases. The main mechanism of myeloma kidney is by filtration of light chain proteins (Bence Jones proteins) which are precipitated in the distal convoluted tubules in combination with Tamm-Horsfall proteins as tubular casts.

3.   Myeloma neuropathy. Infiltration of the nerve trunk roots by tumour cells produces nonspecific polyneuropathy.

4.   Systemic amyloidosis. Systemic primary generalised amyloidosis (AL amyloid) may occur in 10% cases of multiple myeloma and involve multiple organs and systems.

5.   Liver, spleen involvement. Involvement of the liver and spleen by myeloma cells sufficient to cause hepatomegaly, and splenomegaly occurs in a small percentage of cases.

Clinical Features *(p. 461)*

The clinical manifestations of myeloma result from the effects of infiltration of the bones and other organs by neoplastic plasma cells and from immunoglobulin synthesis. The principal clinical features are as under :

1.   *Bone pain* is the most common symptom. The pain usually involves the back and ribs. Pathological fractures may occur causing persistent localised pain.

2.   *Susceptibility to infections* is the next most common clinical feature. Particularly common are bacterial infections such as pneumonias and pyelonephritis.

3.   *Renal failure* occurs in about 25% of patients, while renal pathology occurs in 50% of cases.

4.   *Anaemia* occurs in majority of patients of myeloma.

5.   *Bleeding tendencies* may appear in some patients due to thrombocytopenia, deranged platelet function and interaction of the M component with coagulation factors.

6.   *Neurologic symptoms* occur in a minority of patients.

7.   *Hyperviscosity syndrome* owing to hyperglobulinaemia may produce headache, fatigue, visual disturbances and haemorrhages.

8. *Biochemical abnormalities* include:

i) hypercalcaemia;

ii) hyperuricaemia from necrosis of tumour mass and from uraemia related to renal failure; and

iii) along with other globulins, there is increased β-2 microglobulins in urine and serum.

Diagnosis *(p. 461)*

The diagnosis of myeloma is made by classic *triad* of features:

1) marrow plasmacytosis of more than 10%; 2) radiologic evidence of lytic bony lesions; and 3) demonstration of serum and/or urine M component.

There is rise in the total serum protein concentration due to *paraprotein-aemia*. Paraproteins are abnormal immunoglobulins or their parts circulating in plasma and excreted in urine. The most common paraprotein is *IgG* seen in two-third cases of myeloma, *IgA* in one-third, and rarely there may be *IgM* or *IgD* paraproteins, or various combinations.

About two-third cases of myeloma excrete Bence Jones (light chain) proteins in the urine, consisting of either kappa or lambda light chains, alongwith presence of Bence Jones paraproteins in the serum.

The median survival is 2 years after the diagnosis is made. The terminal phase is marked by the development of pancytopenia, severe anaemia and sepsis.

WALDENSTRÖM'S MACROGLOBULINAEMIA *(p. 462)*

Waldenström's macroglobulinaemia is an uncommon malignant proliferation of monoclonal B lymphocytes which secrete IgM paraproteins called macroglobulins as they have high molecular weight. The condition is more common in men over 50 years of age and behaves clinically like a slowly progressive lymphoma.

HEAVY CHAIN DISEASES *(p. 463)*

Heavy chain diseases are rare malignant proliferations of B-cells accompanied by monoclonal excess of one of the heavy chains. Depending upon the type of excessive heavy chain, three types—γ, α and μ, of heavy chain diseases are distinguished.

LANGERHANS' CELL HISTIOCYTOSIS *(p. 463)*

Langerhans' cell histiocytosis is a group of malignant proliferations of histiocytes and macrophages. Earlier, this group was referred to as histiocytosis-X and included three conditions: eosinophilic granuloma, Hand-Schüller-Christian disease and Letterer-Siwe syndrome. Now, it is known that:

■ *firstly*, histiocytosis-X are not proliferations of unknown origin (X-for unknown) but proliferating cells are in fact Langerhans' cells of marrow origin. Langerhans' cells are normally present mainly in the epidermis but also in some other organs; and

■ *secondly*, the three conditions included under histiocytosis-X are actually different expression of the same basic disorder. This has been made possible by demonstration of common antigens on these cells (positive for S-100 protein, CD1, CD 74 and HLA-DR) as well as by ultrastructural features of Langerhans' cell or Birbeck granules in the cytoplasm.

Eosinophilic Granuloma *(p. 463)*

Unifocal eosinophilic granuloma is more common (60%) than the multifocal variety which is often a component of Hand-Schüller-Christian disease. Most of the patients are children and young adults, predominantly males. The condition commonly presents as a solitary osteolytic lesion in the femur, skull, vertebrae, ribs and pelvis. The diagnosis requires biopsy of the lytic bone lesion.

M/E The lesion consists largely of closely-packed aggregates of macrophages admixed with variable number of eosinophils. The macrophages contain droplets of fat or a few granules of brown pigment indicative of phagocytic activity. A few multinucleate macrophages may also be seen. The cytoplasm of a few macrophages may contain rod-shaped inclusions called *histiocytosis-X bodies.*

Hand-Schüller-Christian Disease *(p. 464)*

A triad of features consisting of *multifocal bony defects, diabetes insipidus* and *exophthalmos* is termed Hand-Schüller-Christian disease. The disease develops in children under 5 years of age. The multifocal lytic bony lesions may develop at any site.

M/E The lesions are indistinguishable from those of unifocal eosinophilic granuloma.

Letterer-Siwe Disease *(p. 464)*

Letterer-Siwe disease is an acute clinical syndrome of unknown etiology occurring in infants and children under three years of age. The disease is characterised by hepatosplenomegaly, lymphadenopathy, thrombocytopenia, anaemia and leucopenia. There is generalised hyperplasia of tissue macrophages in various organs.

M/E The involved organs contain aggregates of macrophages which are pleomorphic and show nuclear atypia. The cytoplasm of these cells contains vacuoles and rod-shaped *histiocytosis-X bodies.*

SPLEEN *(p. 464)*

NORMAL STRUCTURE *(p. 464)*

The spleen is the largest lymphoid organ of the body. Under normal conditions, the average weight of the spleen is about 150 gm in the adult. From the capsule extend connective tissue *trabeculae* into the pulp of the organ and serve as supportive network. Blood enters the spleen by the splenic artery which divides into branches that penetrate the spleen via trabeculae. From the trabeculae arise small branches called *central arterioles.*

M/E The red pulp consists of a network of thin-walled venous sinuses and adjacent blood spaces. The blood spaces contain blood cells, lymphocytes and macrophages and appear to be arranged in cords called *splenic cords* or *cords of Billroth.* The white pulp is made up of lymphocytes surrounding an eccentrically placed arteriole. The periarteriolar lymphocytes are mainly T-cells, while at other places the lymphocytes have a germinal centre composed principally of B-cells surrounded by densely packed lymphocytes.

The spleen is a lymphoreticular organ that performs at least the following four *functions:*

1. it is an organ of the immune system where B and T lymphocytes multiply and help in *immune responses.*

2. active role in *sequestering* and removing normal and abnormal blood cells.

3. plays a role in *regulating portal blood flow.*

4. the spleen may become the site of *extramedullary haematopoiesis.*

SPLENOMEGALY (p. 465)

Enlargement of the spleen termed splenomegaly, occurs in a wide variety of disorders which increase the cellularity and vascularity of the organ. Many of the causes are exaggerated forms of normal splenic function. Based on mechanisms, an abbreviated list of causes of splenomegaly is given in Table 14.5. Most of these conditions have been discussed elsewhere.

TABLE 14.5: Causes of Splenomegaly.

I. **INFECTIONS**
 1. Malaria
 2. Leishmaniasis
 3. Typhoid
 4. Infectious mononucleosis
 5. Bacterial septicaemia
 6. Bacterial endocarditis
 7. Tuberculosis
 8. Syphilis
 9. Viral hepatitis
 10. AIDS

II. **DISORDERS OF IMMUNOREGULATION**
 1. Rheumatoid arthritis
 2. SLE
 3. Immune haemolytic anaemia
 4. Immune thrombocytopenias
 5. Immune neutropenias

III. **ALTERED SPLENIC BLOOD FLOW**
 1. Cirrhosis of liver
 2. Portal vein obstruction
 3. Splenic vein obstruction
 4. Congestive heart failure

IV. **LYMPHO-HAEMATOGENOUS MALIGNANCIES**
 1. Hodgkin's disease
 2. Non-Hodgkin's lymphomas
 3. Multiple myeloma
 4. Leukaemias
 5. Myeloproliferative disorders (e.g. CML, polycythaemia vera, myeloid metaplasia with myelofibrosis)

V. **DISEASES WITH ABNORMAL ERYTHROCYTES**
 1. Thalassaemias
 2. Spherocytosis
 3. Sickle cell disease
 4. Ovalocytosis

VI. **STORAGE DISEASES**
 1. Gaucher's disease
 2. Niemann-Pick's disease

VII. **MISCELLANEOUS**
 1. Amyloidosis
 2. Primary and metastatic splenic tumours
 3. Idiopathic splenomegaly

The **degree of splenomegaly** varies with the disease entity:

■ *Mild enlargement (upto 5 cm)* occurs in CVC of spleen in CHF, acute malaria, typhoid fever, bacterial endocarditis, SLE, rheumatoid arthritis and thalassaemia minor.

■ *Moderate enlargement (upto umbilicus)* occurs in hepatitis, cirrhosis, lymphomas, infectious mononucleosis, haemolytic anaemia, splenic abscesses and amyloidosis.

■ *Massive enlargement (below umbilicus)* occurs in CML, myeloid metaplasia with myelofibrosis, storage diseases, thalassaemia major, chronic malaria, leishmaniasis and portal vein obstruction.

Mild to moderate splenomegaly is usually symptomless, while a massively enlarged spleen may cause dragging sensation in the left hypochondrium. Spleen becomes palpable only when it is enlarged.

G/A An enlarged spleen is heavy and firm. The capsule is tense and thickened. The sectioned surface of the organ is firm with prominent trabeculae.

M/E There is dilatation of sinusoids with prominence of splenic cords. The white pulp is atrophic while the trabeculae are thickened. Long-standing congestion may produce haemorrhages and *Gamna-Gandy bodies* resulting in *fibrocongestive splenomegaly,* also called *Banti's spleen.*

HYPERSPLENISM *(p. 466)*

The term hypersplenism is used for conditions which cause excessive removal of erythrocytes, granulocytes or platelets from the circulation. The mechanism for excessive removal could be due to increased sequestration of cells in the spleen by altered splenic blood flow or by production of antibodies against respective blood cells. The criteria for hypersplenism are as under:

1. Splenomegaly.
2. Splenic destruction of one or more of the cell types in the peripheral blood causing anaemia, leucopenia, thrombocytopenia, or pancytopenia.
3. Bone marrow cellularity is normal or hyperplastic.
4. Splenectomy is followed by improvement in the severity of blood cytopenia.

EFFECTS OF SPLENECTOMY *(p. 466)*

Splenectomy in a normal individual is followed by significant haematologic alterations. Induction of similar haematologic effects is made use in the treatment of certain pathologic conditions.

1. Red cells: There is appearance of target cells in the blood film. Howell-Jolly bodies are present in the red cells as they are no longer cleared by the spleen. Osmotic fragility test shows increased resistance to haemolysis. There may be appearance of normoblasts.

2. White cells: There is leucocytosis reaching its peak in 1-2 days after splenectomy. There is shift-to-left of the myeloid cells with appearance of some myelocytes.

3. Platelets: Within hours after splenectomy, there is rise in platelet count upto 3-4 times normal.

SPLENIC RUPTURE *(p. 466)*

The most common cause of splenic rupture or laceration is blunt trauma. The trauma may be direct or indirect. Non-traumatic or spontaneous rupture occurs in an enlarged spleen but almost never in a normal spleen. In acute infections, the spleen can enlarge rapidly to 2 to 3 times its normal size causing acute splenic enlargement termed *acute splenic tumour* e.g. in pneumonias, septicaemia, acute endocarditis etc.

Rupture of spleen is an acute surgical emergency due to rapid blood loss and haemoperitoneum. Sometimes fragments of splenic tissue are autotransplanted within the peritoneal cavity and grow into tiny spleens there *(splenosis).*

TUMOURS *(p. 466)*

■ **Primary tumours** of the spleen are extremely rare. The only notable benign tumours are haemangiomas and lymphangioma, while examples of primary malignant neoplasms are Hodgkin's disease and non-Hodgkin's lymphomas.

■ **Secondary tumours** occur late in the course of disease and represent haematogenous dissemination of the malignant tumour. Splenic metastases appear as multiple nodules. The most frequent primary sites include: lung, breast, prostate, colon and stomach.

THYMUS *(p. 467)*

NORMAL STRUCTURE *(p. 467)*

The thymus gland is a complex lymphoreticular organ lying buried within the mediastinum. At birth, the gland weighs 10-35 gm and grows in size upto puberty, following which there is progressive involution in the elderly. In the adult, thymus weighs 5-10 gm.

The histologic structure of the lobule shows *outer cortex* and *inner medulla*. Both cortex and medulla contain two types of cells:

■ **The epithelial cells** are similar throughout the thymus gland. These cells have elongated cytoplasmic processes forming network in which thymocytes and macrophages are found. *Hassall's corpuscles* are distinctive structures within the medulla composed of onion skin-like concentrically arranged epithelial cells having central area of keratinisation.

■ **Thymocytes** are predominantly present in the cortex. These cells include immature T lymphocytes in the cortex and mature T lymphocytes in the medulla.

The main **function** of the thymus is in the cell-mediated immunity by T-cells and by secretion of thymic hormones such as *thymopoietin* and *thymosin-*α_1.

THYMIC HYPOPLASIA AND AGENESIS *(p. 467)*

Thymic hypoplasia and agenesis are acquired and congenital disorders respectively in which the gland is either unusually small or absent. These conditions are various types of hereditary (primary) immunodeficiency diseases such as DiGeorge's syndrome, severe combined immunodeficiency and reticular dysgenesis.

THYMIC HYPERPLASIA *(p. 467)*

Enlargement of the thymus or failure to involute produces thymic hyperplasia. Hyperplasia is usually associated with appearance of lymphoid follicles in the medulla of the thymus and is called *thymic follicular hyperplasia*. Most common cause of follicular hyperplasia of the thymus is myasthenia gravis.

THYMOMA *(p. 467)*

Most common primary tumour present in the anterosuperior mediastinum is thymoma. Although thymus is a lymphoepithelial organ, the term thymoma is used for the tumour of epithelial origin. Most of the patients are adults.

G/A The tumour is spherical, measuring 5-10 cm in diameter with an average weight of 150 gm. Sectioned surface is soft, yellowish, lobulated and may be either homogeneous or contain cysts due to the presence of haemorrhage and necrosis.

M/E The tumour has a thick fibrous capsule from which extend collagenous septa into the tumour dividing it into lobules. The tumour consists of neoplastic epithelial cells and variable number of non-neoplastic lymphocytes. Thymoma may be of following types:

Benign thymoma is more common. It consists of epithelial cells which are similar to the epithelial cells in the medulla of thymus and hence also called as medullary thymoma.

Malignant thymoma is less common and is further of 2 types:

Type 1 is cytologically benign looking but aggressive and invades the mediastinal structures locally.

Type 2 is also called thymic carcinoma and has cytologic features of cancer.

Thymomas are known for their association with paraneoplastic syndrome. These include: myasthenia gravis (most common), hypogammaglobulinaemia, erythroid hypoplasia (pure red cell aplasia), peripheral T cell leukaemia, multiple myeloma.

■ SELF ASSESSMENT

1. **The following type of reactive lymphadenitis in the draining lymph nodes of some cancers renders better prognosis due to good host immune response:**
   A. Follicular hyperplasia
   B. Sinus histiocytosis
   C. Paracortical hyperplasia
   D. Immunoblastic lymphadenopathy

2. **Reed-Sternberg cells are generally believed to be of:**
   A. T cell origin
   B. B cell origin
   C. Follicular reticulum cells
   D. Macrophages

3. **Lacunar type of RS cells are a feature of following type of Hodgkin's disease:**
   A. Lymphocyte-predominance
   B. Nodular sclerosis
   C. Mixed cellularity
   D. Lymphocyte-depletion

4. **RS cells of all types of Hodgkin's disease are positive for CD15 and CD30 markers *except* in:**
   A. Lymphocyte predominance
   B. Nodular sclerosis
   C. Mixed cellularity
   D. Lymphocyte-depletion

5. **The following classification systems have been used for classifying non-Hodgkin's lymphoma *except:***
   A. Rappaport classification
   B. Rye classification
   C. Working formulation
   D. R.E.A.L. classification

6. **The following type of non-Hodgkin's lymphoma more commonly produces CLL-like picture after spill over into peripheral blood:**
   A. Small lymphocytic lymphoma
   B. Follicular, small cleaved cell lymphoma
   C. Follicular, mixed small and large cleaved cell lymphoma
   D. Follicular, predominantly large cell lymphoma

7. **The most common type of non-Hodgkin's lymphomas are:**
   A. B cell type
   B. T cell type
   C. Null cell type
   D. Histiocytic type

8. **Most common type of paraproteinaemia is:**
   A. IgA
   B. IgD
   C. IgG
   D. IgM

9. **M-band is seen in multiple myeloma on electrophoresis in the region of:**
   A. Alpha-1 (α1) globulin
   B. Alpha-2 (α2) globulin
   C. Beta (β) globulin
   D. Gamma (γ) globulin

10. **Langerhans' cell histiocytosis includes the following entities** *except:*
   - A. Eosinophilic granuloma
   - B. Hand-Schüller-Christian disease
   - C. Histiocytic lymphoma
   - D. Letterer-Siwe disease

11. **Massive enlargement of spleen (below umbilicus) may occur generally from the following causes** *except:*
   - A. Chronic myeloid leukaemia
   - B. CVC spleen
   - C. Thalassaemia major
   - D. Chronic malaria

12. **Hypersplenism is characterised by the following features** *except:*
   - A. Pancytopenia
   - B. Hypocellular bone marrow
   - C. Splenomegaly
   - D. Splenectomy improves the blood cytopenia

13. **Acute splenic tumour means:**
   - A. Rapidly developing primary splenic lymphoma
   - B. Rapidly developing metastatic carcinoma
   - C. Splenic enlargement due to systemic acute infection
   - D. Splenic enlargement due to infiltration by leukaemia

14. **The following virus is strongly implicated in the etiology of Hodgkin's disease:**
   - A. HPV
   - B. HSV
   - C. EBV
   - D. HCV

15. **RS cells in lymphocyte predominance type of Hodgkin's disease are positive for following marker:**
   - A. CD 15
   - B. CD 20
   - C. CD 30
   - D. CD 45

KEY

1 = B	2 = B	3 = B	4 = A
5 = B	6 = A	7 = A	8 = C
9 = D	10 = C	11 = B	12 = B
13 = C	14 = C	15 = B	

Chapter Fourteen

15

The Respiratory System

LUNGS (p. 468)

ANATOMY. The normal *adult right lung* weighs 375 to 550 gm (average 450 gm) and is divided by two fissures into three lobes—the upper, middle and lower lobes. The weight of the normal *adult left lung* is 325 to 450 gm (average 400 gm) and has one fissure dividing it into two lobes—the upper and the lower lobes, while the middle lobe is represented by the lingula.

The right main bronchus is more vertical so that aspirated foreign material tends to pass down to the right lung rather than to the left. The trachea, major bronchi and their branchings possess cartilage, smooth muscle and mucous glands in their walls, while the bronchioles have smooth muscle but lack cartilage as well as the mucous glands. Between the tracheal bifurcation and the smallest bronchi, about 8 divisions take place. The *bronchioles* so formed further undergo 3 to 4 divisions leading to the *terminal bronchioles* which are less than 2 mm in diameter. The part of the lung tissue distal to a terminal bronchiole is called an *acinus*. A cluster of about 5 acini supplied by terminal bronchioles and enclosed by visible fibrous septa is termed as the *pulmonary lobule*. An **acinus** consists of 3 parts:

1. Several (usually 3 to 5 generations) *respiratory bronchioles* originate from a terminal bronchiole.
2. Each respiratory bronchiole divides into several *alveolar ducts*.
3. Each alveolar duct opens into many *alveolar sacs (alveoli)* which are blind ends of the respiratory passages.

The lungs have double blood supply—oxygenated blood from the bronchial arteries and venous blood from the pulmonary arteries, and there is mixing of the blood to some extent.

HISTOLOGY. The bronchi and their subdivisions upto bronchioles are lined by pseudostratified columnar ciliated epithelial cells, also called *respiratory epithelium*. These cells are admixed with mucus-secreting goblet cells which decrease in number as the bronchioles are approached.

The **alveolar walls or alveolar septa** are the sites of exchange between the blood and air and have the following microscopic features:

1. The *capillary endothelium* lines the anastomotic capillaries in the alveolar walls.
2. The capillary endothelium and the alveolar lining epithelial cells are separated by the *capillary basement membrane and some interstitial tissue*.
3. The *alveolar epithelium* consists of 2 types of cells: *type I* or *membranous pneumocytes* are the most numerous covering about 95% of alveolar surface, and *type II* or *granular pneumocytes* project into the alveoli and are covered by microvilli.
4. The *alveolar macrophages* belonging to mononuclear-phagocyte system are present either free in the alveolar spaces or are attached to the alveolar cells.
5. The *pores of Kohn* are the sites of alveolar connections between the adjacent alveoli and allow the passage of bacteria and exudate.

PAEDIATRIC LUNG DISEASE (p. 470)

CONGENITAL CYSTS (p. 470)

Developmental defects involving deficiency of bronchial or bronchiolar cartilage, elastic tissue and muscle result in congenital cystic disease of lungs. A single large cyst of this type occupying almost a lobe is called *pneumatocele*. Multiple small cysts are more common and give sponge-like appearance to the lung. The cysts are thin-walled and dilated and generally lined by flattened ciliated epithelium.

BRONCHOPULMONARY SEQUESTRATION *(p. 470)*

Sequestration is the presence of lobes or segments of lung tissue which are not connected to the airway system.

■ **Intralobar sequestration** is the sequestered bronchopulmonary mass within the pleural covering of the affected lung.

■ **Extralobar sequestration** is the sequestered mass of lung tissue lying outside the pleural investing layer such as in the base of left lung or below the diaphragm.

NEONATAL RESPIRATORY DISTRESS SYNDROME (HYALINE MEMBRANE DISEASE) *(p. 470)*

Neonatal respiratory distress syndrome (RDS) or hyaline membrane disease (HMD) characterised by formation of pulmonary hyaline membrane is the most common and serious form of disease of the newborn infants. The condition begins with dyspnoea a few hours after birth with tachypnoea, hypoxia and cyanosis and in severe cases death occurs in a few hours. The mortality rate is high (20 to 30%) and is still higher in babies under 1 kg of body weight.

ETIOLOGY. The following clinical settings are commonly associated with neonatal RDS:
1. Preterm infants. 2. Infants born to diabetic mothers. 3. Delivery by caesarean section. 4. Infants born to mothers with previous premature infants. 5. Excessive sedation of the mother causing depression in respiration of the infant. 6. Birth asphyxia from various causes. 7. Male preponderance (1.5 to 2 times) over female babies.

Besides all these factors causing respiratory distress, a number of cases of neonatal RDS remain idiopathic.

PATHOGENESIS. *Entry of air into alveoli is essential for formation of HMD i.e. dead born infants do not develop HMD.* The basic defect in neonatal RDS is a deficiency of pulmonary surfactant, normally synthesised by type II alveolar cells.

The sequence of events is schematically illustrated in Fig. 15.1.

G/A The lungs are normal in size and reddish purple in colour. They are solid and airless so that they sink in water.

M/E 1. The presence of collapsed alveoli (atelectasis) alternating with dilated alveoli.
2. Formation of characteristic eosinophilic hyaline membranes lining the respiratory bronchioles, alveolar ducts and the proximal alveoli. The membrane is largely composed of fibrin admixed with cell debris derived from necrotic alveolar cells.
3. Vascular congestion, focal haemorrhages and dilatation of septal lymphatics.
4. Absence of inflammatory reaction.

BRONCHOPULMONARY DYSPLASIA *(p. 471)*

Bronchopulmonary dysplasia occurs as a complication in infants treated for neonatal RDS with oxygen and assisted ventilation.

M/E There is organisation of hyaline membranes resulting in fibrous thickening of the alveolar walls, bronchiolitis, peribronchial fibrosis, and development of emphysema.

Chapter Fifteen

NEONATAL HYPOXIA

↓ Alveolar surfactant

↑ Alveolar surface tension

Atelectasis

Hypoventilation

Pulmonary hypoperfusion

Ischaemic damage
(Capillary endothelium
and alveolar cells)

Exudation of plasma proteins

Fibrinogen

Fibrin

HYALINE MEMBRANE

Fig. 15.1: Schematic representation of sequence of events leading to the formation of hyaline membrane in neonatal respiratory distress syndrome.

ATELECTASIS AND COLLAPSE *(p. 471)*

ATELECTASIS. Stillborn infants have total atelectasis, while the newborn infants with weak respiratory action develop incomplete expansion of the lungs and clinical atelectasis. The common causes are prematurity, cerebral birth injury, CNS malformations and intrauterine hypoxia.

G/A The lungs are small, dark blue, fleshy and non-crepitant.

M/E The alveolar spaces in the affected area are small with thick interalveolar septa. The alveolar spaces contain proteinaceous fluid with a few epithelial squames and meconium.

COLLAPSE. Pulmonary collapse or secondary atelectasis in children and adults may occur from various causes:

1. **Compressive collapse.** Pressure from outside causes compressive collapse e.g. by massive pleural effusion, haemothorax, pneumothorax, intrathoracic tumour, high diaphragm and spinal deformities.

2. **Obstructive/absorptive collapse.** Obstruction of a bronchus or many bronchioles causes absorption of oxygen in the affected alveoli followed by collapse e.g. by viscid mucus secretions in bronchial asthma, chronic bronchitis, bronchiectasis, bronchial tumours and aspiration of foreign bodies.

3. **Contraction collapse.** This type occurs due to localised fibrosis in lung causing contraction followed by collapse.

BRONCHIOLITIS AND BRONCHIOLITIS OBLITERANS *(p. 472)*

Bronchiolitis and bronchiolitis obliterans are the inflammatory conditions affecting the small airways occurring predominantly in older paediatric age group and in quite elderly persons. A number of etiologic factors have been stated to cause this condition. These include viral infection (frequently adenovirus and respiratory syncytial virus), bacterial infection, fungal infection, inhalation of toxic gases (e.g. in silo-fillers' disease) and aspiration of gastric contents.

M/E The lumina of affected bronchioles are narrow and occluded by fibrous plugs. The bronchiolar walls are inflamed and are infiltrated by lymphocytes and plasma cells.

SUDDEN INFANT DEATH SYNDROME *(p. 472)*

Sudden infant death syndrome or crib death is an uncommon condition seen mainly in the western countries. It affects infants in the age group of 2 to 6 months. The condition is seen in premature babies born to mothers who have been smokers and indulged in drug abuse.

ADULT RESPIRATORY DISTRESS SYNDROME (ARDS) *(p. 472)*

Adult respiratory distress syndrome (ARDS) is known by various synonyms such as shock-lung syndrome, diffuse alveolar damage (DAD), acute alveolar injury, traumatic wet lungs and post-traumatic respiratory insufficiency. ARDS is a syndrome caused by diffuse alveolar capillary damage and clinically characterised by sudden and severe respiratory distress, tachypnoea, tachycardia, cyanosis and severe hypoxaemia that fails to respond to oxygen therapy and assisted ventilation unlike neonatal RDS described above.

ETIOLOGY. Diffuse alveolar damage in ARDS may occur from a number of causes: 1. Shock due to sepsis, trauma, burns 2. Diffuse pulmonary infections, chiefly viral pneumonia 3. Pancreatitis 4. Oxygen toxicity 5. Inhalation of toxins and irritants e.g. smoke, war gases, nitrogen dioxide, metal fumes etc. 6. Narcotic overdose 7. Drugs e.g. salicylates, colchicine 8. Aspiration pneumonitis 9. Fat embolism 10. Radiation.

PATHOGENESIS. The basic initiating event in the pathogenesis of ARDS is diffuse damage to the alveolocapillary wall by one of the injurious factors listed above.

The mechanism of acute injury depends upon the *imbalance between pro-inflammatory and anti-inflammatory cytokines.*

1. Activated pulmonay macrophages release *proinflammatory cytokines* such as interleukin (IL) 8, IL1, and tumour necrosis factor (TNF), while macrophage inhibitory factor (MIF) helps to sustain inflammation in the alveoli.

2. Besides the role of cytokines in acute injury, a few *fibrogenic cytokines* such as transforming growth factor- α (TGF-α) and platelet-derived growth factor (PDGF) play a role in repair process by stimulation of proliferation of fibroblast and collagen.

As a result of lining of the alveoli with hyaline membranes, there is loss of surfactant causing collapse with pulmonary oedema called 'stiff lung'. There is an attempt at regeneration of alveolar cells by proliferation of type II alveolar cells. A stiff lung of ARDS may undergo complete recovery, or may undergo organisation by proliferation of interstitial cells leading to interstitial fibrosis or even death.

G/A The lungs are characteristically stiff, congested and heavy.

M/E 1. Interstitial and intra-alveolar oedema.
2. Necrosis of alveolar epithelial cells with formation of hyaline membranes.
3. Congestion and intra-alveolar haemorrhages.
4. Changes of bronchopneumonia.
5. In organising stage, there may be interstitial fibrosis and regenerating flat alveolar epithelial cells lining the denuded alveoli.

PULMONARY HYPERTENSION *(p. 474)*

Normally, the blood pressure in the pulmonary arterial circulation is much lower than the systemic blood pressure; it does not exceed 30/15 mmHg even during exercise (normally, blood pressure in the pulmonary veins is between 3 and 8 mmHg). Pulmonary hypertension is defined as a systolic blood pressure in the pulmonary arterial circulation above 30 mmHg. Pulmonary hypertension is broadly classified into 2 groups:

Primary (Idiopathic) Pulmonary Hypertension *(p.474)*

Primary or idiopathic pulmonary hypertension is an uncommon condition of unknown cause. The diagnosis can be established only after a thorough search for the usual causes of secondary pulmonary hypertension. The patients are usually young females between the age of 20 and 40 years, or children around 5 years of age.

ETIOPATHOGENESIS. Though the etiology of primary pulmonary hypertension is unknown, a number of etiologic factors have been suggested to explain its pathogenesis:
1. A neurohumoral vasoconstrictor mechanism
2. Unrecognised thromboemboli or amniotic fluid emboli during pregnancy
3. There is a suggestion that primary pulmonary hypertension may be a form of collagen vascular disease.
4. Pulmonary veno-occlusive disease characterised by fibrous obliteration of small pulmonary veins.
5. Ingestion of substances like 'bush tea', oral contraceptives and appetite depressant agents like aminorex.
6. Familial occurrence.

Secondary Pulmonary Hypertension *(p. 474)*

When pulmonary hypertension occurs secondary to a recognised lesion in the heart or lungs, it is termed as secondary pulmonary hypertension. It is the more common type and may be encountered at any age, but more frequently over the age of 50 years.

ETIOPATHOGENESIS. Based on the underlying mechanism, causes of secondary pulmonary hypertension are divided into the following 3 groups:

A. Passive pulmonary hypertension. This is the commonest and is produced by diseases raising pressure in the pulmonary veins e.g. 1. Mitral stenosis. 2. Chronic left ventricular failure.

B. Hyperkinetic (Reactive) pulmonary hypertension. In this group are included causes in which the blood enters the pulmonary arteries in greater volume or at a higher pressure e.g. 1. Patent ductus arteriosus. 2. Atrial or ventricular septal defects.

C. Vaso-occlusive pulmonary hypertension. All such conditions which produce progressive diminution of the vascular bed in the lungs are included in this group. Vaso-occlusive causes may be further sub-divided into 3 types:

1. *Obstructive type,* e.g. i) Multiple emboli or thrombi. ii) Sickle cell disease iii) Schistosomiasis.

2. *Obliterative type,* e.g. i) Chronic emphysema. ii) Chronic bronchitis. iii) Bronchiectasis. iv) Pulmonary tuberculosis. v) Pneumoconiosis.

3. *Vasoconstrictive type,* e.g. i) In residents at high altitude. ii) Pathologic obesity (Pickwickian disease). iii) Upper airway disease such as tonsillar hypertrophy. iv) Neuromuscular diseases such as poliomyelitis. v) Severe kyphoscoliosis.

MORPHOLOGY. Irrespective of the type of pulmonary hypertension (primary or secondary), chronic cases invariably lead to cor pulmonale. The pathologic changes are confined to the right side of the heart and pulmonary arterial tree in the lungs. There is hypertrophy of the right ventricle and dilatation of the right atrium. The vascular changes are similar in primary and secondary types and involve the entire arterial tree from the main pulmonary arteries down to the arterioles:

1. **Arterioles and small pulmonary arteries:** i) Medial hypertrophy. ii) Thickening and reduplication of elastic laminae. iii) Plexiform pulmonary arteriopathy.

2. **Medium-sized pulmonary arteries:** i) Medial hypertrophy. ii) Concentric intimal thickening. iii) Adventitial fibrosis. iv) Thickening and reduplication of elastic laminae.

3. **Large pulmonary arteries:** i) Atheromatous deposits.

PNEUMONIAS *(p. 475)*

Pneumonia is defined as acute inflammation of the lung parenchyma distal to the terminal bronchioles which consist of the respiratory bronchiole, alveolar ducts, alveolar sacs and alveoli. The terms 'pneumonia' and 'pneumonitis' are often used synonymously for inflammation of the lungs, while 'consolidation' (meaning solidification) is the term used for macroscopic and radiologic appearance of the lungs in pneumonia.

PATHOGENESIS. The microorganisms gain entry into the lungs by one of the following four routes:

1. Inhalation of the microbes. 2. Aspiration of organisms. 3. Haematogenous spread from a distant focus. 4. Direct spread from an adjoining site of infection.

Failure of defense mechanisms and presence of certain predisposing factors result in pneumonias. These conditions are as under:

1. Altered consciousness. 2. Depressed cough and glottic reflexes. 3. Impaired mucociliary transport. 4. Impaired alveolar macrophage function. 5. Endobronchial obstruction. 6. Leucocyte dysfunctions.

CLASSIFICATION. On the basis of the anatomic part of the lung parenchyma involved, pneumonias are traditionally classified into 3 main types:

1. Lobar pneumonia. 2. Bronchopneumonia (or Lobular pneumonia). 3. Interstitial pneumonia.

A. BACTERIAL PNEUMONIA *(p. 476)*

Bacterial infection of the lung parenchyma is the most common cause of pneumonia or consolidation of one or both the lungs. Two types of acute bacterial pneumonias are distinguished—lobar pneumonia and broncho-(lobular-) pneumonia, each with distinct etiologic agent and morphologic changes.

1. Lobar Pneumonia *(p. 476)*

Lobar pneumonia is an acute bacterial infection of a part of a lobe, the entire lobe, or even two lobes of one or both the lungs.

ETIOLOGY. Following types are described:

1. **Pneumococcal pneumonia.** More than 90% of all lobar pneumonias are caused by *Streptococcus pneumoniae*, a lancet-shaped diplococcus. Out of various types, type 3-*S. pneumoniae* causes particularly virulent form of lobar pneumonia.

2. **Staphylococcal pneumonia.** *Staphylococcus aureus* causes pneumonia by haematogenous spread of infection.

3. **Streptococcal pneumonia.** β-haemolytic streptococci may rarely cause pneumonia such as in children after measles or influenza.

4. **Pneumonia by gram-negative aerobic bacteria.** Less common causes of lobar pneumonia are gram-negative bacteria like *Haemophilus influenzae*,

Klebsiella pneumoniae (Friedlander's bacillus), Pseudomonas, Proteus and *Escherichia coli.*

MORPHOLOGY. Laennec's original description divides lobar pneumonia into 4 sequential pathologic phases:

1. STAGE OF CONGESTION: INITIAL PHASE The initial phase represents the early acute inflammatory response to bacterial infection and lasts for 1 to 2 days.

G/A The affected lobe is enlarged, heavy, dark red and congested. Cut surface exudes blood-stained frothy fluid.

M/E i) Dilatation and congestion of the capillaries in the alveolar walls.

ii) Pale eosinophilic oedema fluid in the air spaces.

iii) A few red cells and neutrophils in the intra-alveolar fluid.

iv) Numerous bacteria demonstrated in the alveolar fluid by Gram's staining.

2. RED HEPATISATION: EARLY CONSOLIDATION This phase lasts for 2 to 4 days. The term hepatisation in pneumonia refers to liver-like consistency of the affected lobe on cut section.

G/A The affected lobe is red, firm and consolidated. The cut surface of the involved lobe is airless, red-pink, dry, granular and has liver-like consistency.

M/E i) The oedema fluid of the preceding stage is replaced by strands of fibrin.

ii) There is marked cellular exudate of neutrophils and extravasation of red cells.

iii) Many neutrophils show ingested bacteria.

iv) The alveolar septa are less prominent than in the first stage due to cellular exudation.

3. GREY HEPATISATION: LATE CONSOLIDATION This phase lasts for 4 to 8 days.

G/A The affected lobe is firm and heavy. The cut surface is dry, granular and grey in appearance with liver-like consistency. The change in colour from red to grey begins at the hilum and spreads towards the periphery. Fibrinous pleurisy is prominent.

M/E i) The fibrin strands are dense and more numerous.

ii) The cellular exudate of neutrophils is reduced due to disintegration of many inflammatory cells. The red cells are also fewer. The macrophages begin to appear in the exudate.

iii) The cellular exudate is often separated from the septal walls by a thin clear space.

iv) The organisms are less numerous and appear as degenerated forms.

4. RESOLUTION: This stage begins by 8th to 9th day if no chemotherapy is administered and is completed in 1 to 3 weeks. However, antibiotic therapy induces resolution on about 3rd day.

G/A The previously solid fibrinous constituent is liquefied by enzymatic action, eventually restoring the normal aeration in the affected lobe. The process of softening begins centrally and spreads to the periphery. The cut surface is grey-red or dirty brown and frothy, yellow, creamy fluid can be expressed on pressing.

M/E i) Macrophages are the predominant cells in the alveolar spaces, while neutrophils diminish in number. Many of the macrophages contain engulfed neutrophils and debris.

ii) Granular and fragmented strands of fibrin in the alveolar spaces are seen due to progressive enzymatic digestion.

iii) Alveolar capillaries are engorged.

iv) There is progressive removal of fluid content as well as cellular exudate from the air spaces.

COMPLICATIONS. Since the advent of antibiotics, serious complications of lobar pneumonia are uncommon. However, they may develop in neglected cases and in patients with impaired immunologic defenses. These are as under:

1. Organisation. In about 3% of cases, resolution of the exudate does not occur but instead it is organised. There is ingrowth of fibroblasts from the alveolar septa resulting in fibrosed, tough, airless leathery lung tissue.

2. Pleural effusion. About 5% of treated cases of lobar pneumonia develop inflammation of the pleura with effusion.

3. Empyema. Less than 1% of treated cases of lobar pneumonia develop encysted pus in the pleural cavity termed empyema.

4. Lung abscess. A rare complication of lobar pneumonia is formation of lung abscess.

5. Metastatic infection. Occasionally, infection in the lungs and pleural cavity in lobar pneumonia may extend into the pericardium and the heart causing purulent pericarditis, bacterial endocarditis and myocarditis.

CLINICAL FEATURES. The major symptoms are: shaking chills, fever, malaise with pleuritic chest pain, dyspnoea and cough with expectoration which may be mucoid, purulent or even bloody. The common physical findings are fever, tachycardia, and tachypnoea, and sometimes cyanosis if the patient is severely hypoxaemic. There is generally a marked neutrophilic leucocytosis. Blood cultures are positive in about 30% of cases. Chest radiograph may reveal consolidation.

II. Bronchopneumonia (Lobular Pneumonia) *(p. 479)*

Bronchopneumonia or lobular pneumonia is infection of the terminal bronchioles that extends into the surrounding alveoli resulting in patchy consolidation of the lung. The condition is particularly frequent at extremes of life (i.e. in infancy and old age), as a terminal event in chronic debilitating diseases and as a secondary infection following viral respiratory infections such as influenza, measles etc.

ETIOLOGY. The common organisms responsible for bronchopneumonia are staphylococci, streptococci, pneumococci, *Klebsiella pneumoniae*, *Haemophilus influenzae*, and gram-negative bacilli like *Pseudomonas* and coliform bacteria.

G/A Bronchopneumonia is identified by patchy areas of red or grey consolidation affecting one or more lobes, frequently found bilaterally and more often involving the lower zones of the lungs due to gravitation of the secretions. On cut surface, these patchy consolidated lesions are dry, granular, firm, red or grey in colour, 3 to 4 cm in diameter, slightly elevated over the surface and are often centred around a bronchiole. These patchy areas are best picked up by passing the fingertips on the cut surface.

M/E i) Acute bronchiolitis. ii) Suppurative exudate, consisting chiefly of neutrophils, in the peribronchiolar alveoli. iii) Thickening of the alveolar septa by congested capillaries and leucocytic infiltration. iv) Less involved alveoli contain oedema fluid.

COMPLICATIONS. The complications of lobar pneumonia may occur in bronchopneumonia as well. However, complete resolution of bronchopneumonia is uncommon. There is generally some degree of destruction of the bronchioles resulting in foci of bronchiolar fibrosis that may eventually cause bronchiectasis.

CLINICAL FEATURES. The patients of bronchopneumonia are generally infants or elderly individuals. There may be history of preceding bed-ridden

Chapter Fifteen

illness, chronic debility, aspiration of gastric contents or upper respiratory infection.

The salient features of the two main types of bacterial pneumonias are contrasted in Table 15.1.

TABLE 15.1: Contrasting Features of Lobal Pneumonia and Bronchopneumonia.

	FEATURE	LOBAR PNEUMONIA	BRONCHOPNEUMONIA
1.	*Definition*	Acute bacterial infection of a part of a lobe of one or both lungs, or the entire lobe/s	Acute bacterial infection of the terminal bronchioles extending in to adjoining alveoli
2.	*Age group*	More common in adults	Commoner at exteremes of age–infants and old age
3.	*Predisposing factors*	More often affects healthy individuals	Preexisting diseases e.g. chronic debility, terminal illness, flu, measles
4.	*Common etiologic agents*	Pneumococci, *Klebsiella pneuminae*, staphylococci, streptococci	Staphylococci, streptococci, Pseudomonas, *Haemophilus influenzae*
5.	*Pathologic features*	Typical case passes through stages of congestion (1-2 days), early (2-4 days) and late consolidation (4-8 days), followed by resolution (1-3 weeks)	Patchy consolidation with central granularity, alveolar exudation, thickened septa
6.	*Investigations*	Neutrophilic leucocytosis, positive blood culture, X-ray shows consolidation	Neutrophilic leucocytosis, positive blood culture, X-ray shows mottled focal opacities
7	*Prognosis*	Better response to treatment, resolution common, prognosis good	Response to treatment variable, organisation may occur, prognosis poor
8.	*Complications*	Less common; pleural effusion, empyema, lung abscess, organisation	Brochiectasis may occur; other complications same as for lobar pneumoina

B. VIRAL AND MYCOPLASMAL PNEUMONIA (PRIMARY ATYPICAL PNEUMONIA) *(p. 480)*

Viral and mycoplasmal pneumonia is characterised by patchy inflammatory changes, largely confined to interstitial tissue of the lungs, without any alveolar exudate. Other terms used for these respiratory tract infections are *interstitial pneumonitis*, reflecting the interstitial location of the inflammation, and *primary atypical pneumonia*, atypicality being the absence of alveolar exudate commonly present in other pneumonias. Interstitial pneumonitis may occur in all ages.

ETIOLOGY. Interstitial pneumonitis is caused by a wide variety of agents, the most common being *respiratory syncytial virus* (RSV). Others are *Mycoplasma pneumoniae* and many viruses such as influenza and parainfluenza viruses, adenoviruses, rhinoviruses, coxsackieviruses and cytomegaloviruses (CMV).

G/A Depending upon the severity of infection, the involvement may be patchy to massive and widespread consolidation of one or both the lungs. The lungs are heavy, congested and subcrepitant. Sectioned surface of the lung exudes small amount of frothy or bloody fluid.

M/E i) **Interstitial inflammation:** There is thickening of alveolar walls due to congestion, oedema and mononuclear inflammatory infiltrate comprised by lymphocytes, macrophages and some plasma cells.

ii) Necrotising bronchiolitis: This is characterised by foci of necrosis of the bronchiolar epithelium, inspissated secretions in the lumina and mononuclear infiltrate in the walls and lumina.

iii) Reactive changes: The lining epithelial cells of the bronchioles and alveoli proliferate in the presence of virus and may form multinucleate giant cells and syncytia in the bronchiolar and alveolar walls.

vi) Alveolar changes: In severe cases, the alveolar lumina may contain oedema fluid, fibrin, scanty inflammatory exudate and coating of alveolar walls by pink, hyaline membrane similar to the one seen in respiratory distress syndrome.

COMPLICATIONS. The major complication of interstitial pneumonitis is superimposed bacterial infection and its complications. Most cases of interstitial pneumonitis recover completely.

CLINICAL FEATURES. Majority of cases of interstitial pneumonitis initially have upper respiratory symptoms with fever, headache and muscle-aches. A few days later appears dry, hacking, non-productive cough with retrosternal burning due to tracheitis and bronchitis. Chest radiograph may show patchy or diffuse consolidation.

C. OTHER TYPES OF PNEUMONIAS *(p. 481)*

1. *Pneumocystis carinii* Pneumonia *(p. 481)*

Pneumocystis carinii, a protozoon widespread in the environment, causes pneumonia by inhalation of the organisms as an opportunistic infection in neonates and immunosuppressed people. Almost 100% cases of AIDS develop opportunistic infection, most commonly *Pneumocystis carinii* pneumonia.

II. *Legionella* Pneumonia *(p. 482)*

Legionella pneumonia or legionnaire's disease is an epidemic illness caused by gram-negative bacilli, *Legionella pneumophila* that thrives in aquatic environment. It was first recognised following investigation into high mortality among those attending American Legion Convention in Philadelphia in July 1976. The epidemic occurs in summer months by spread of organisms through contaminated drinking water or in air-conditioning cooling towers. Impaired host defenses in the form of immunodeficiency, corticosteroid therapy, old age and cigarette smoking play important roles.

III. Aspiration (Inhalation) Pneumonia *(p. 482)*

Aspiration or inhalation pneumonia results from inhaling different agents into the lungs. These substances include food, gastric contents, foreign body and infected material from oral cavity. A number of factors predispose to inhalation pneumonia which include: unconsciousness, drunkenness, neurological disorders affecting swallowing, drowning, necrotic oropharyngeal tumours, in premature infants and congenital tracheo-oesophageal fistula.

1. Aspiration of small amount of **sterile foreign matter** such as acidic gastric contents produce *chemical pneumonitis*. It is characterised by haemorrhagic pulmonary oedema with presence of particles in the bronchioles.

2. **Non-sterile aspirate** causes widespread *bronchopneumonia* with multiple areas of necrosis and suppuration.

IV. Hypostatic Pneumonia *(p. 483)*

Hypostatic pneumonia is the term used for collection of oedema fluid and secretions in the dependent parts of the lungs in severely debilitated, bed-ridden patients. The accumulated fluid in the basal zone and posterior part of lungs gets infected by bacteria from the upper respiratory tract and sets in bacterial pneumonia.

V. Lipid Pneumonia *(p. 483)*

Another variety of noninfective pneumonia is lipid pneumonia. It is of 2 types:

1. Exogenous lipid pneumonia. This is caused by aspiration of a variety of oily materials. These are: inhalation of oily nasal drops, regurgitation of oily medicines from stomach (e.g. liquid paraffin), administration of oily vitamin preparation to reluctant children or to debilitated old patients.

2. Endogenous lipid pneumonia. Endogenous origin of lipids causing pneumonic consolidation is more common. The sources of origin are tissue breakdown following obstruction to airways e.g. obstruction by bronchogenic cancer, tuberculosis and bronchiectasis.

LUNG ABSCESS *(p. 483)*

Lung abscess is a localised area of necrosis of lung tissue with suppuration. It is of 2 types:

■ *Primary lung abscess* that develops in an otherwise normal lung. The commonest cause is aspiration of infected material.

■ *Secondary lung abscess* that develops as a complication of some other disease of the lung or from another site.

ETIOPATHOGENESIS. The microorganisms commonly isolated from the lungs in lung abscess are streptococci, staphylococci and various gram-negative organisms. These are introduced into the lungs from one of the following mechanisms:

1. Aspiration of infected foreign material. 2. Preceding bacterial infection. 3. Bronchial obstruction. 4. Septic embolism. 5. Miscellaneous (i) Infection in pulmonary infarcts. (ii) Amoebic abscesses. (iii) Trauma to the lungs. (iv) Direct extension from a suppurative focus.

G/A Abscesses may be of variable size from a few millimeters to large cavities, 5 to 6 cm in diameter. The cavity often contains exudate. An acute lung abscess is initially surrounded by acute pneumonia and has poorly-defined ragged wall. With passage of time, the abscess becomes chronic and develops fibrous wall.

M/E The characteristic feature is the destruction of lung parenchyma with suppurative exudate in the lung cavity. The cavity is initially surrounded by acute inflammation in the wall but later there is replacement by exudate of lymphocytes, plasma cells and macrophages. In more chronic cases, there is considerable fibroblastic proliferation forming a fibrocollagenic wall.

FUNGAL INFECTIONS OF LUNG *(p. 484)*

Fungal infections of the lung are more common than tuberculosis in the United States of America. These infections in healthy individuals are rarely serious but in immunosuppressed individuals may prove fatal. Some of the common examples of fungal infections of the lung are: 1. Histoplasmosis. 2. Coccidio-idomycosis. 3. Cryptococcosis. 4. Blastomycosis. 5. Aspergillosis. 6. Mucor-mycosis. 7. Candidiasis.

CHRONIC OBSTRUCTIVE PULMONARY DISEASE *(p. 485)*

Chronic obstructive pulmonary disease (COPD) or chronic obstructive airways disease (COAD) are commonly used clinical terms for a group of pathological conditions in which there is chronic, partial or complete, obstruction to the airflow at any level from trachea to the smallest airways resulting in functional disability of the lungs. The following 4 entities are included in COPD:

I) Chronic bronchitis II) Emphysema III) Bronchial asthma IV) Bronchiectasis.

I. CHRONIC BRONCHITIS (p. 485)

Chronic bronchitis is a common condition defined clinically as persistent cough with expectoration on most days for at least three months of the year for two or more consecutive years. The cough is caused by oversecretion of mucus. The condition is more common in middle-aged males than females; approximately 20% of adult men and 5% of adult women have chronic bronchitis, but only a minority of them develop serious disabling COPD or cor pulmonale.

ETIOPATHOGENESIS. The two most important etiologic factors responsible for majority of cases of chronic bronchitis are: cigarette smoking and atmospheric pollution. Other contributory factors are occupation, infection, familial and genetic factors.

G/A The bronchial wall is thickened, hyperaemic and oedematous. Lumina of the bronchi and bronchioles may contain mucus plugs and purulent exudate.

M/E Just as there is clinical definition, there is histologic definition of chronic bronchitis by increased Reid index. *Reid index* is the ratio between thickness of the submucosal mucous glands (i.e. hypertrophy and hyperplasia) in the cartilage-containing large airways to that of the total bronchial wall. The bronchial epithelium may show squamous metaplasia and dysplasia. There is little chronic inflammatory cell infiltrate. The non-cartilage containing small airways show goblet cell hyperplasia and intraluminal and peribronchial fibrosis.

II. EMPHYSEMA (p. 486)

The WHO has defined pulmonary emphysema as combination of permanent dilatation of air spaces distal to the terminal bronchioles and the destruction of the walls of dilated air spaces. *Thus, emphysema is defined morphologically, while chronic bronchitis is defined clinically.*

CLASSIFICATION. By strictly adhering to the WHO definition of pulmonary emphysema, it is classified, according to the portion of the acinus involved, into 5 types: while a number of other conditions to which the term 'emphysema' is losely applied are, in fact, examples of 'overinflation' (Table 15.2).

TABLE 15.2: Classification of 'True Emphysema' and 'Overinflation'.

A. TRUE EMPHYSEMA

1. Centriacinar (centrilobular) emphysema
2. Panacinar (panlobular) emphysema
3. Paraseptal (distal acinar) emphysema
4. Irregular (para-cicatricial) emphysema
5. Mixed (unclassified) emphysema

B. OVERINFLATION

1. Compensatory overinflation (compensatory emphysema)
2. Senile hyperinflation (aging lung, senile emphysema)
3. Obstructive overinflation (infantile lobar emphysema)
4. Unilateral translucent lung (unilateral emphysema)
5. Interstitial emphysema (surgical emphysema)

ETIOPATHOGENESIS. The commonest form of COPD is the combination of chronic bronchitis and pulmonary emphysema. Chronic bronchitis, however, does not always lead to emphysema nor all cases of emphysema have changes of chronic bronchitis. The association of the two conditions is principally linked to the common etiologic factors; most importantly, *tobacco smoke* and *air pollutants*. Other less significant contributory factors are occupational exposure, infection and somewhat poorly-understood familial and genetic influences. The few conditions are contrasted in Table 15.3.

TABLE 15.3: Contrasting Salient Features of 'Predominant Bronchitis' and 'Predominant Emphysema'.

	FEATURE	PREDOMINANT BRONCHITIS	PREDOMINANT EMPHYSEMA
1.	*Age at diagnosis*	About 50 years	About 60 years
2.	*Underlying pathology*	Hypertrophy of mucus-producing cells	Inflammatory narrowing of bronchioles and destruction of septal walls
3.	*Dyspnoea*	Late, mild	Early, severe
4.	*Cough*	Before dyspnoea starts	After dyspnoea starts
5.	*Sputum*	Copious, purulent	Scanty, mucoid, less frequent
6.	*Bronchial infections*	More frequent	Less frequent
7.	*Respiratory insufficiency*	Repeated	Terminal
8.	*Cyanosis*	Common ('blue-bloaters')	Rare ('pink-puffers')
9.	*Lung capacity*	Normal	Increased (barrel-chest)
10.	*Blood gas values*	↓ pO_2, ↓ pCO_2, no compensatory hyperventilation	pO_2 and pCO_2 usually within normal limits due to compensatory hyperventilation
11.	*Cor pulmonale*	Frequent	Rare and terminal
12.	*Chest X-ray*	Large heart, prominent vessels	Small heart, hyperinflated lungs

However, the pathogenesis of the most significant event in emphysema, the *destruction of the alveolar walls*, is not linked to bronchial changes but is closely related to deficiency of serum alpha-1-antitrypsin (α1-protease inhibitor) commonly termed *protease-antiprotease hypothesis* detailed below.

Protease-antiprotease hypothesis. Alpha-1-antitrypsin (α-1-AT), also called α1-protease inhibitor (α-1-Pi), is a glycoprotein that forms the normal constituent of the α1-globulin fraction of the plasma proteins on serum electrophoresis. The single gene locus that codes for α-1-AT is located on the long arm of chromosome 15. It is normally synthesised in the liver and is distributed in the circulating blood, tissue fluids and macrophages. The normal function of α1-AT is to inhibit proteases and hence its name α1-protease inhibitor. The proteases (mainly elastases) are derived from neutrophils. Neutrophil elastase has the capability of digesting lung parenchyma but is inhibited from doing so by anti-elastase effect of α1-AT.

There are several known alleles of α1-AT which have an autosomal codominant inheritance pattern and are classified as normal (*PiMM*), deficient (*PiZZ*), null type (*Pi null null*) having no detectable level, and dysfunctional (*PiSS*) type having about half the normal level.

■ The most common abnormal phenotype in classic α1-AT deficiency is *homozygous state PiZZ* resulting from a single amino acid substitution Glu → Lys which causes spontaneous polymerisation of α1-AT and inhibits its release from the liver.

■ Clinically significant deficiency is also associated with *homozygous Pi null null* and heterozygous *Pi nullZ*.

■ The *heterozygote pattern* of *PiMZ* has intermediate levels which is not sufficient to produce clinical deficiency, but heterozygote individuals who smoke heavily have higher risk of developing emphysema.

The α1-AT deficiency develops in adults and causes pulmonary emphysema in smokers as well as in non-smokers, though the smokers become symptomatic about 15 years earlier than non-smokers.

The mechanism of alveolar wall destruction in emphysema by elastolytic action is based on the imbalance between proteases (chiefly *elastase)* and anti-proteases (chiefly *anti-elastase):*

■ By decreased anti-elastase activity i.e. deficiency of α-1 antitrypsin.

■ By increased activity of elastase i.e. increased neutrophilic infiltration in the lungs causing excessive elaboration of neutrophil elastase.

G/A The lungs are voluminous, pale with little blood. The edges of the lungs are rounded. Mild cases show dilatation of air spaces visible with hand lens. Advanced cases show subpleural bullae and blebs bulging outwards from the surface of the lungs with rib markings between them. The *bullae* are air-filled cyst-like or bubble-like structures, larger than 1 cm in diameter. They are formed by the rupture of adjacent air spaces while *blebs* are the result of rupture of alveoli directly into the subpleural interstitial tissue.

M/E Depending upon the type of emphysema, there is dilatation of air spaces and destruction of septal walls of part of acinus involved i.e. respiratory bronchioles, alveolar ducts and alveolar sacs. Changes of bronchitis may be present. Bullae and blebs when present show fibrosis and chronic inflammation of the walls.

CLINICAL FEATURES. Cases of 'predominant emphysema' develop clinical features after about one-third of the pulmonary parenchyma is damaged which occurs most severely in panacinar emphysema. The age at the time of diagnosis is often a decade later (about 60 years) than the age for predominant bronchitis (about 50 years).

A. Morphology of Individual Types of Emphysema *(p. 488)*

1. CENTRIACINAR (CENTRILOBULAR) EMPHYSEMA. It is characterised by initial involvement of respiratory bronchioles i.e. the central or proximal part of the acinus. This is the type of emphysema that usually coexists with chronic bronchitis and occurs predominantly in smokers and in coal miners' pneumoconiosis.

2. PANACINAR (PANLOBULAR) EMPHYSEMA. Panacinar or panlobular emphysema is the other common type. In this type, all portions of the acinus are affected but not of the entire lung. Panacinar emphysema is most often associated with α1-antitrypsin deficiency in middle-aged smokers and is the one that produces the most characteristic anatomical changes in the lung in emphysema.

3. PARASEPTAL (DISTAL ACINAR) EMPHYSEMA. This type of emphysema involves distal part of acinus while the proximal part is normal. Paraseptal or distal acinar emphysema is localised along the pleura and along the perilobular septa. The involvement is seen adjacent to the areas of fibrosis and atelectasis and involves upper part of lungs more severely than the lower. This form of emphysema is seldom associated with COPD but is the common cause of spontaneous pneumothorax in young adults.

4. IRREGULAR (PARA-CICATRICIAL) EMPHYSEMA. This is the most common form of emphysema, seen surrounding scars from any cause. The involvement is irregular as regards the portion of acinus involved as well as within the lung as a whole.

5. MIXED (UNCLASSIFIED) EMPHYSEMA. Quite often, the same lung may show more than one type of emphysema. It is usually due to more severe involvement resulting in loss of clearcut distinction between one type of emphysema and the other.

B. Morphology of Types of Overinflation *(p. 490)*

A group of lung conditions of heterogeneous etiology characterised by overinflation of the parts of acini but without significant destruction of the walls are sometimes loosely termed emphysema.

1. COMPENSATORY OVERINFLATION (COMPENSATORY EMPHYSEMA). When part of a lung or a lobe of lung is surgically removed, the residual lung parenchyma undergoes compensatory hyperinflation so as to fill the pleural cavity.

2. SENILE HYPERINFLATION (AGING LUNG, SENILE EMPHYSEMA). In old people, the lungs become voluminous due to loss of elastic tissue, thinning and atrophy of the alveolar ducts and alveoli. The alveoli are thin-walled and distended throughout the lungs but there is no significant destruction of the septal walls.

3. OBSTRUCTIVE OVERINFLATION (INFANTILE LOBAR EMPHYSEMA). Partial obstruction to the bronchial tree such as by a tumour or a foreign body causes overinflation of the region supplied by obstructed bronchus.

4. UNILATERAL TRANSLUCENT LUNG (UNILATERAL EMPHYSEMA). This is a form of overinflation in which one lung or one of its lobes or segments of a lobe are radiolucent. The condition occurs in adults and there is generally a history of serious pulmonary infection in childhood, probably bronchiolitis obliterans.

5. INTERSTITIAL EMPHYSEMA (SURGICAL EMPHYSEMA). The entry of air into the connective tissue framework of the lung is called interstitial or surgical emphysema. The usual sources of entry of air into stroma of the lung are rupture of alveoli or of larger airways. The causes are as under:

i) Violent coughing with bronchiolar obstruction e.g. in children with whooping cough, bronchitis, in patients with obstruction to the airways by foreign bodies, blood clots and exposure to irritant gases.

ii) Rupture of the oesophagus, trauma to the lung, or major bronchus and trachea.

iii) Entry of air through surgical incision.

iv) Fractured rib puncturing the lung parenchyma.

v) Sudden change in atmospheric pressure e.g. in decompression sickness.

The condition may affect patients of all ages. On rupture of alveoli, the leaked air enters the fibrous connective tissue of the alveolar walls from where it extends into the fibrous septa of the lung, into the mediastinum, the pleura, and even the subcutaneous tissues. Escape of air into the pleural cavity may cause pneumothorax.

III. BRONCHIAL ASTHMA *(p. 491)*

Asthma is a disease of airways that is characterised by increased responsiveness of the tracheobronchial tree to a variety of stimuli resulting in widespread spasmodic narrowing of the air passages which may be relieved spontaneously or by therapy. Asthma is an episodic disease manifested clinically by paroxysms of dyspnoea, cough and wheezing. However, a severe and unremitting form of the disease termed *status asthmaticus* may prove fatal.

Bronchial asthma is common and prevalent worldwide; in the United States about 4% of population is reported to suffer from this disease. It occurs at all ages but nearly 50% of cases develop it before the age of 10 years. In adults, both sexes are affected equally but in children there is 2:1 male-female ratio.

ETIOPATHOGENESIS AND TYPES. Based on the stimuli initiating bronchial asthma, two broad etiologic types are traditionally described: *extrinsic (allergic,* *atopic)* and *intrinsic (idiosyncratic, non-atopic) asthma.* A third type is a *mixed pattern* in which the features do not fit clearly into either of the two main types. The contrasting features of the two main types are summed up in Table 15.4.

TABLE 15.4: Contrasting Features of the Two Major Types of Asthma.

	FEATURE	EXTRINSIC ASTHMA	INTRINSIC ASTHMA
1.	*Age at onset*	In childhood	In adult
2.	*Personal/family history*	Commonly present	Absent
3.	*Preceding allergic illness (atopy)*	Present *(e.g.* rhinitis, urticaria, eczema)	Absent
4.	*Allergens*	Present (dust, pollens, danders etc)	None
5.	*Drug hypersensitivity*	None	Present (usually to aspirin)
6.	*Serum IgE levels*	Elevated	Normal
7.	*Associated chronic bronchitis, nasal polyps*	Absent	Present
8.	*Emphysema*	Unusual	Common

G/A The lungs are overdistended due to over-inflation.

M/E 1. The mucus plugs contain normal or degenerated respiratory epithelium forming twisted strips called *Curschmann's spirals.*
2. The sputum usually contains numerous eosinophils and diamond-shaped crystals derived from eosinophils called *Charcot-Leyden crystals.*
3. The bronchial wall shows thickened basement membrane of the bronchial epithelium, submucosal oedema and inflammatory exudate. There is hypertrophy of submucosal glands as well as of the bronchial smooth muscle.
4. Changes of bronchitis and emphysema may supervene, especially in intrinsic asthma.

IV. BRONCHIECTASIS (p. 493)

Bronchiectasis is defined as abnormal and irreversible dilatation of the bronchi and bronchioles (greater than 2 mm in diameter) developing secondary to inflammatory weakening of the bronchial walls. The most characteristic clinical manifestation of bronchiectasis is persistent cough with expectoration of copious amounts of foul-smelling, purulent sputum.

ETIOPATHOGENESIS. The origin of inflammatory destructive process of bronchial walls is nearly always a result of two basic mechanisms:
■ *Endobronchial obstruction* by foreign body, neoplastic growth or enlarged lymph nodes causes resorption of air distal to the obstruction with consequent atelectasis and retention of secretions.
■ *Infection* may be secondary to local obstruction and impaired systemic defense mechanism promoting bacterial growth, or infection may be a primary event.
    These 2 mechanisms—endobronchial obstruction and infection, are seen in a number of clinical settings.

1. Hereditary and congenital factors e.g. (i) Congenital bronchiectasis (ii) Cystic fibrosis (iii) Hereditary immune deficiency diseases (iv) Immotile cilia syndrome (v) Atopic bronchial asthma.

2. Obstruction. Post-obstructive bronchiectasis, unlike the congenital-hereditary forms, is of the localised variety, usually confined to one part of the bronchial system. The causes of endobronchial obstruction include foreign bodies, endobronchial tumours, compression by enlarged hilar lymph nodes and post-inflammatory scarring (e.g. in healed tuberculosis) all of which favour the development of post-obstructive bronchiectasis.

3. As secondary complication. *Necrotising pneumonias* such as in staphylococcal suppurative pneumonia and *tuberculosis* may develop bronchiectasis as a complication.

G/A The lungs may be involved diffusely or segmentally. Bilateral involvement of lower lobes occurs most frequently. More vertical air passages of left lower lobe are more often involved than the right. The pleura is usually fibrotic and thickened with adhesions to the chest wall. The dilated airways, depending upon their gross or bronchographic appearance, have been subclassified into the following different types: (i) Cylindrical (ii) Fusiform (iii) Saccular (iv) Varicose.

Cut surface of the affected lobes, generally the lower zones, shows characteristic honey-combed appearance.

M/E i) The bronchial epithelium may be normal, ulcerated or may show squamous metaplasia.

ii) The bronchial wall shows infiltration by acute and chronic inflammatory cells and destruction of normal muscle and elastic tissue with replacement by fibrosis.

iii) The intervening lung parenchyma shows fibrosis, while the surrounding lung tissue shows changes of interstitial pneumonia.

iv) The pleura in the affected area is adherent.

CLINICAL FEATURES. The clinical manifestations of bronchiectasis typically consist of chronic cough with foul-smelling sputum production, haemoptysis and recurrent pneumonia. Sinusitis is a common accompaniment of diffuse bronchiectasis. Development of clubbing of the fingers, metastatic abscesses (often to the brain), amyloidosis and cor pulmonale are late complications occurring in cases uncontrolled for years.

CHRONIC RESTRICTIVE PULMONARY DISEASE *(p. 494)*

The second large group of diffuse lung disease is 'chronic restrictive pulmonary disease' characterised by reduced expansion of lung parenchyma with decreased total lung capacity.

Restrictive lung disease includes 2 types of conditions:

A. Restriction due to chest wall disorder. These causes are: 1. Kyphoscoliosis 2. Poliomyelitis 3. Severe obesity 4. Pleural diseases.

B. Restriction due to interstitial and infiltrative diseases. These are diseases characterised by non-infectious involvement of the interstitial connective tissue of lung parenchyma. The conditions included in this group are as under:

I) Pneumoconiosis. II) Immunologic lung diseases. III) Collagen-vascular diseases. IV) Idiopathic pulmonary fibrosis. V) Sarcoidosis (Chapter 6).

The **pathogenesis** of the interstitial lung disease is explained by inflammatory reaction causing initial alveolitis in response to various stimuli. In alveolitis, there is accumulation of lymphocytes, macrophages, neutrophils and eosinophils, all of which result in inflammatory destruction of the pulmonary parenchyma followed by fibrosis. Eventually, there is widespread destruction of alveolar capillary walls resulting in end-stage lung or 'honeycomb lung'.

The *major clinical manifestations* of restrictive lung diseases are dyspnoea, tachypnoea and cyanosis, but no wheezing so characteristic of COPD.

I. PNEUMOCONIOSES *(p. 495)*

Pneumoconiosis is the term used for lung diseases caused by inhalation of dust, mostly at work. These diseases are, therefore, also called 'dust diseases' or 'occupational lung diseases'.

The type of lung disease varies according to the nature of inhaled dust. Some dusts are inert and cause no reaction and no damage at all, while others cause immunologic damage and predispose to tuberculosis or to neoplasia. The factors which determine the extent of damage caused by inhaled dusts are:

1. size and shape of the particles;
2. their solubility and physico-chemical composition;
3. the amount of dust retained in the lungs;
4. the additional effect of other irritants such as tobacco smoke; and
5. host factors such as efficiency of clearance mechanism and immune status of the host.

In general, most of the inhaled dust particles larger than 5 μm reach the terminal airways where they are ingested by alveolar macrophages. Most of these too are eliminated by expectoration but the remaining accumulate in alveolar tissue. Of particular interest are the particles smaller than 1 μm which are deposited in the alveoli most efficiently. The tissue response to inhaled dust may be one of the following three types:

■ *Fibrous nodules* e.g. in coal-workers' pneumoconiosis and silicosis.
■ *Interstitial fibrosis* e.g. in asbestosis.
■ *Hypersensitivity reaction* e.g. in berylliosis.

Coal-Workers' Pneumoconiosis *(p. 496)*

This is the commonest form of pneumoconiosis and is defined as the lung disease resulting from inhalation of coal dust particles, especially in coal miners engaged in handling soft bituminous coal for a number of years, often 20 to 30 years. It exists in 2 forms—a milder form of the disease called *simple coal workers' pneumoconiosis* and an advanced form termed *progressive massive fibrosis* (complicated coal-miners' pneumoconiosis).

PATHOGENESIS. Pathogenetically, it appears that anthracosis, simple coal-workers' pneumoconiosis and progressive massive fibrosis are different stages in the evolution of fully-developed coal-workers' pneumoconiosis. However, progressive massive fibrosis develops in a small proportion of cases (2-8%) of simple coal-workers' pneumoconiosis. A number of predisposing factors have been implicated in this transformation:

1. Older age of the miners. 2. Severity of coal dust burden engulfed by macrophages. 3. Prolonged exposure (20 to 30 years) to coal dust. 4. Concomitant tuberculosis. 5. Additional role of silica dust.

Activation of alveolar macrophage plays the most significant role in the pathogenesis of progressive massive fibrosis by release of various mediators.

SIMPLE COAL-WORKERS' PNEUMOCONIOSIS. G/A The lung parenchyma shows small, black focal lesions, measuring less than 5 mm in diameter and evenly distributed throughout the lung but have a tendency to be more numerous in the upper lobes. These are termed *coal macules,* and if palpable are called *nodules.* The air spaces around coal macules are dilated with little destruction of alveolar walls. Similar blackish pigmentations are found on the pleural surface and in the regional lymph nodes.

M/E 1. Coal macules are composed of aggregates of dust-laden macrophages. These are present in the alveoli and in the bronchiolar and alveolar walls.
2. There is some increase in the network of reticulin and collagen in the coal macules.
3. Respiratory bronchioles and alveoli surrounding the macules are distended without significant destruction of the alveolar walls.

PROGRESSIVE MASSIVE FIBROSIS. G/A Besides the coal macules and nodules of simple pneumoconiosis, there are larger, hard, black scattered areas measuring more than 2 cm in diameter and sometimes massive. They are usually bilateral and located more often in the upper parts of the lungs posteriorly. Sometimes, these masses break down centrally due to ischaemic necrosis or due to tuberculosis forming cavities filled with black semifluid resembling India ink.

M/E 1. The fibrous lesions are composed almost entirely of dense collagen and carbon pigment.

2. The wall of respiratory bronchioles and pulmonary vessels included in the massive scars are thickened and their lumina obliterated.

3. There is scanty inflammatory infiltrate of lymphocytes and plasma cells.

4. The alveoli surrounding the scars are markedly dilated.

RHEUMATOID PNEUMOCONIOSIS (CAPLAN'S SYNDROME). The development or rheumatoid arthritis in a few cases of coal-workers' pneumoconiosis, silicosis or absestosis is termed rheumatoid pneumoconiosis or Caplan's syndrome.

G/A The lungs have rounded, firm nodules with central necrosis, cavitation or calcification.

M/E The lung lesions are modified rheumatoid nodules with central zone of dust-laden fibrinoid necrosis enclosed by palisading fibroblasts and mono-nuclear cells.

CLINICAL FEATURES. Simple coal-workers' pneumoconiosis is the mild form of disease characterised by chronic cough with black expectoration. The radiological findings of nodularities in the lungs appear after working for several years in coal mines. Progressive massive fibrosis is, however, a serious disabling condition manifested by progressive dyspnoea and chronic cough with jet-black sputum. Tuberculosis and rheumatoid arthritis are more common in coal miners than the general population. Coal workers have increased risk of developing carcinomas of the stomach, probably due to swallowing of coal dust containing carcinogens. But bronchogenic carcinoma does not appear to be more common in coal-miners than in other groups.

Silicosis *(p. 499)*

Historically, silicosis used to be called knife grinders' lung. Silicosis is caused by prolonged inhalation of silicon dioxide, commonly called silica. Silica constitutes about one-fourth of earth's crust. Therefore, a number of occupations engaged in silceous rocks or sand and products manufactured from them are at increased risk. These include miners (e.g. of granite, sandstone, slate, coal, gold, tin and copper), quarry workers, tunnellers, sandblasters, grinders, ceramic workers, foundry workers and those involved in the manufacture of abrasives containing silica. Peculiar to India are the occupational exposure to pencil, slate and agate grinding industry carrying high risk of silicosis (agate = sort of very hard stone containing silica).

PATHOGENESIS. Silicosis appears after prolonged exposure to silica dust, often a few decades. Besides, it depends upon a number of other factors such as total dose, duration of exposure, the type of silica inhaled and individual host factors. The following sequence of events has been proposed:

1. Silica particles between 0.5 to 5μm size on reaching the alveoli are taken by the macrophages which undergo necrosis. New macrophages engulf the debris and thus a repetitive cycle of *phagocytosis and necrosis* is set up.

2. Some silica-laden macrophages are carried to the respiratory bronchioles, alveoli and in the interstitial tissue. The *cellular aggregates* containing silica become associated with lymphocytes, plasma cells, mast cells and fibroblasts.

3. Silica dust is *fibrogenic*. Crystalline form, particularly quartz, is more fibrogenic than non-crystalline form of silica.

4. As noted above, silica is *cytotoxic* and kills the macrophages which engulf it. The released silica dust activates viable macrophages leading to secretion of macrophage-derived growth factors.

5. Simultaneously, there is *activation of T and B lymphocytes*. This results in increased serum levels of immunoglobulins (IgG and IgM), antinuclear antibodies, rheumatoid factor.

G/A The chronic silicotic lung is studded with well-circumscribed, hard, fibrotic nodules, 1 to 5 mm in diameters. They are scattered throughout the lung parenchyma but are initially more often located in the upper zones of the lungs.

M/E 1. The silicotic nodules are located in the region of respiratory bronchioles, adjacent alveoli, pulmonary arteries, in the pleura and the regional lymph nodes.

2. The *silicotic nodules* consist of central hyalinised material with scanty cellularity and some amount of dust.

3. The collagenous nodules have cleft-like spaces between the lamellae of collagen which when examined polariscopically may demonstrate numerous birefringent particles of silica.

4. The severe and progressive form of the disease may result in coalescence of adjacent nodules and cause complicated silicosis similar to progressive massive fibrosis of coal-workers' pneumoconiosis.

5. The intervening lung parenchyma may show hyperinflation or emphysema.

6. Cavitation when present may be due to ischaemic necrosis in the nodules, or may reveal changes of tuberculosis or rheumatoid pneumoconiosis (Caplan's syndrome).

Asbestos Disease *(p. 500)*

Asbestos as a mineral is known to mankind for more than 4000 years but its harmful effects have come to light during the last few decades. In general, if *coal is lot of dust and little fibrosis, asbestos is little dust and lot of fibrosis.* Prolonged exposure for a number of years to asbestos dust produces three types of severe diseases: *asbestosis of lungs, pleural disease and tumours.* In nature, asbestos exists as long thin fibrils which are fire-resistant and can be spun into yarns and fabrics suitable for thermal and electrical insulation and has many applications in industries.

There are two major geometric forms of asbestos:

■ *Serpentine* consisting of curly and flexible fibres. It includes the most common chemical form *chrysotile* (white asbestos) comprising more than 90% of commercially used asbestos.

■ *Amphibole* consists of straight, stiff and rigid fibres. It includes the less common chemical forms *crocidolite* (blue asbestos), *amosite* (brown asbestos), *tremolite, anthophyllite* and *actinolyte.* However, the group of amphibole, though less common, is more important since it is associated with induction of malignant pleural tumours, particularly in association with crocidolite.

PATHOGENESIS. How asbestos causes all these lesions is not clearly understood but the following mechanisms have been suggested.

1. The inhaled asbestos fibres are *phagocytosed by alveolar macrophages* from where they reach the interstitium.

2. The asbestos-laden macrophages release *chemo-attractants* for neutrophils and for more macrophages.

3. Asbestos fibres are coated with glycoprotein and endogenous haemosiderin to produce characteristic beaded or dumbbell-shaped *asbestos bodies.*

4. All types of asbestos are *fibrogenic* and result in interstitial fibrosis.

5. A few *immunological abnormalities* such as antinuclear antibodies and rheumatoid factor have been found in cases of asbestosis.

6. Asbestos fibres are *carcinogenic*, the most carcinogenic being crocidolite. There is high incidence of bronchogenic carcinoma in asbestosis.

A. ASBESTOSIS. The gross pulmonary fibrosis caused by asbestos exposure and histologic demonstration of asbestos bodies on asbestos fibres is termed asbestosis.

G/A The affected lungs are small and firm with cartilage-like thickening of the pleura. The sectioned surface shows variable degree of pulmonary fibrosis, especially in the subpleural areas and in the bases of lungs.

M/E 1. There is non-specific interstitial fibrosis.

2. There is presence of characteristic *asbestos bodies* in the involved areas.

3. There may be changes of emphysema.

4. The involvement of hilar lymph nodes in asbestosis is not as significant as in silicosis.

B. PLEURAL DISEASE. Pleural disease in asbestos exposure may produce one of the following 3 types of lesions:

1. Pleural Effusion. It develops in about 5% of asbestos workers and is usually serious type.

2. Visceral pleural fibrosis. Quite often, asbestosis is associated with dense fibrous thickening of the visceral pleura encasing the lung.

3. Pleural plaques. Fibrocalcific pleural plaques are the most common lesions associated with asbestos exposure.

G/A The lesions appear as circumscribed, flat, small (upto 1 cm in diameter), firm or hard, bilateral nodules.

M/E They consist of hyalinised collagenous tissue which may be calcified so that they are visible on chest X-ray.

C. TUMOURS. Asbestos exposure predisposes to a number of cancers.

1. Bronchogenic carcinoma is the most common malignancy in asbestos workers. Its incidence is 5 times higher in non-smoker asbestos workers than the non-smoker general population and 10 times higher in smoker asbestos workers than the other smokers.

2. Malignant mesothelioma is an uncommon tumour but association with asbestos exposure is present in 30 to 80% of cases with mesothelioma.

CLINICAL FEATURES. Asbestosis is a slow and insidious illness. The patient may remain asymptomatic for a number of years in spite of radiological evidence of calcific pleural plaques and parenchymatous changes. However, onset of interstitial fibrosis brings about dyspnoea with dry or productive cough.

Berylliosis *(p. 502)*

Berylliosis is caused by heavy exposure to dust or fumes of metallic beryllium or its salts. Beryllium was used in the past in fluorescent tubes and light bulbs but currently it is principally used in nuclear and aerospace industries and in the manufacture of electrical and electronic equipments. Two forms of pulmonary berylliosis are recognised:

ACUTE BERYLLIOSIS. Acute berylliosis occurs in individuals who are unusually sensitive to it and are heavily exposed to it for 2 to 4 weeks.

CHRONIC BERYLLIOSIS. Chronic berylliosis develops in individuals who are sensitised to it for a number of years, often after a delay of 20 or more years. The disease is a cell-mediated hypersensitivity reaction in which the metal beryllium acts as a hapten. The condition is characterised by development of non-caseating epithelioid granulomas like those of sarcoidosis.

II. IMMUNOLOGIC LUNG DISEASE *(p. 502)*

Hypersensitivity (Allergic) Pneumonitis *(p. 502)*

Hypersensitivity pneumonitis are a group of immunologically-mediated interstitial lung diseases occurring in workers inhaling a variety of organic (biologic) antigenic materials. The condition may have an *acute* onset due to isolated exposure or may be *chronic* due to repeated low-dose exposure.

ETIOPATHOGENESIS. A list of important organic (biologic) dusts which may be inhaled to produce hypersensitivity pneumonitis. The immunologic mechanisms underlying hypersensitivity pneumonitis from any of these causes appear to be either type III immune-complex disease or type IV delayed-hypersensitivity reaction.

1. Farmers' lung. 2. Bagassosis. 3. Byssinosis. 4. Bird-breeders' (Bird-fanciers') lung. 5. Mushroom-workers' lung. 6. Malt-workers' lung. 7. Maple-bark disease. 8. Silo-fillers' disease

Pulmonary Eosinophilia *(p. 503)*

Pulmonary eosinophilia, eosinophilic pneumonias or pulmonary infiltration with eosinophilia (PIE) syndrome are a group of immunologically-mediated lung diseases characterised by combination of 2 features:

■ Infiltration of the lungs in chest radiographs; and
■ Elevated eosinophil count in the peripheral blood.

ETIOPATHOGENESIS. PIE syndrome has a number of diverse causes and pathogenesis:

1. Löeffler's syndrome is characterised by eosinophilia in the blood and typical wandering radiologic shadows.

2. Tropical pulmonary eosinophilia is caused by the passage of larvae of worms through the lungs e.g. in filariasis, ascariasis.

3. Secondary chronic pulmonary eosinophilia occurs secondary to adverse drug reactions; infection with fungi, bacteria, and helminths.

4. Idiopathic chronic eosinophilic pneumonia is characterised by prominent focal areas of consolidation of the lung.

5. Hypereosinophilic syndrome is occurrence of eosinophilia of over 1500/μl for more than 6 months without any identifiable cause and without eosinophilic infiltrates in the lungs and other organs.

Goodpasture's Syndrome *(p. 503)*

Goodpasture's syndrome is combination of necrotising haemorrhagic interstitial pneumonitis and rapidly progressive glomerulonephritis.

ETIOPATHOGENESIS. The condition results from immunologic damage produced by anti-basement membrane antibodies formed against antigens common to the glomerular and pulmonary basement membranes. The trigger for initiation of this autoimmune response is not clear; it could be virus infection, exposure to hydrocarbons and smoking.

G/A The lungs are heavy with red-brown areas of consolidation.

M/E In acute stage, there are focal areas of haemorrhages in the alveoli and focal necrosis in the alveolar walls.

In more chronic cases, there is organisation of the haemorrhage leading to interstitial fibrosis and filling of alveoli with haemosiderin-laden macrophages.

Pulmonary Alveolar Proteinosis *(p. 504)*

Pulmonary alveolar proteinosis is a rare chronic disease in which the distal airspaces of the lungs are filled with granular, PAS-positive, eosinophilic material with abundant lipid in it. The condition can occur at any age from infancy to old age.

III. COLLAGEN-VASCULAR DISEASE (p. 504)

A number of collagen diseases may result in chronic interstitial fibrosis and destruction of blood vessels.

1. **Scleroderma (Progressive Systemic Sclerosis).** The lungs are involved in 80% cases of scleroderma. Interstitial pulmonary fibrosis is the most common form of pulmonary involvement.

2. **Rheumatoid Arthritis.** Pulmonary involvement in rheumatoid arthritis may result in pleural effusion, interstitial pneumonitis, necrobiotic nodules and rheumatoid pneumoconiosis (Caplan's syndrome).

3. **Systemic Lupus Erythematosus.** Patients with systemic lupus erythematosus (SLE) commonly develop some form of lung disease during the course.

4. **Sjögren's Syndrome.** Patients with Sjögren's syndrome often have rheumatoid arthritis and associated pulmonary changes.

5. **Dermatomyositis and Polymyositis.** Interstitial pneumonitis and interstitial fibrosis commonly accompany dermatomyositis and polymyositis.

6. **Wegener's Granulomatosis.** Wegener's granulomatosis is an inflammatory lesion having 4 components—granulomas of the upper respiratory tract, granulomas of the lungs, systemic vasculitis and focal necrotising glomerulonephritis. *Localised or limited form* of the disease occurs in the lungs without involvement of other organs.

IV. IDIOPATHIC PULMONARY FIBROSIS (p. 505)

Diffuse interstitial fibrosis can occur as a result of a number of pathologic entities such as pneumoconiosis, hypersensitivity pneumonitis and collagen-vascular disease. However, in half the cases of diffuse interstitial fibrosis, no apparent cause or underlying disease is identifiable.

PATHOGENESIS. The pathogenesis of idiopathic pulmonary fibrosis is unknown and the condition is diagnosed by excluding all known causes of interstitial fibrosis. However, evidences point toward immunologic mechanism:
1. High levels of autoantibodies such as rheumatoid factor and antinuclear antibodies.
2. Elevated titres of circulating immune complexes.
3. Immunofluorescent demonstration of the deposits of immunoglobulins and complement on the alveolar walls in biopsy specimens.

MORPHOLOGY. **G/A** The lungs are firm, heavier with reduced volume. Honey-combing (i.e. enlarged, thick-walled air spaces) develops in parts of lung, particularly in the subpleural region.

M/E **In early stage,** there is widening of the alveolar septa by oedema and cellular infiltrate by mononuclear inflammatory cells. The alveolar lining cells may show hyperplasia at places and are flattened at other places. There is often formation of hyaline membranes.

   In advanced stage, there is organisation of the alveolar exudate and replacement fibrosis in the alveoli as well as in the interstitial septal wall with variable amount of inflammation.

TUMOURS OF LUNGS (p. 505)

A number of benign and malignant tumours occur in the lungs but the primary lung cancer, commonly termed bronchogenic carcinoma, is the most common (95% of all primary lung tumours). The lung is also the commonest site for metastasis from carcinomas and sarcomas. A histologic classification of various benign and malignant tumours of lungs is given in Table 15.5.

BRONCHOGENIC CARCINOMA (p. 505)

Though the term bronchogenic carcinoma is commonly used for cancer of the lungs, it includes carcinomas having bronchial as well as bronchiolar origin.

TABLE 15.5: Histological Classification of Lung Tumours.

I. **EPITHELIAL TUMOURS**

  A. **Benign**
    1. Papilloma
    2. Adenoma

  B. **Dysplasia and carcinoma in situ**

  C. **Malignant**
    Bronchogenic carcinoma
    1. Squamous cell (epidermoid) carcinoma
    2. Small cell carcinoma
      i) Oat cell carcinoma
      ii) Intermediate cell carcinoma
      iii) Combined oat cell carcinoma
    3. Adenocarcinoma
      i) Acinar adenocarcinoma
      ii) Papillary adenocarcinoma
      iii) Bronchiolo-alveolar carcinoma
      iv) Solid carcinoma with mucus formation
    4. Large cell carcinoma
    5. Adenosquamous carcinoma

    Other carcinomas
    1. Pulmonary neuroendocrine tumour (carcinoid tumour)
    2. Bronchial gland carcinomas
      i) Adenoid cystic carcinoma
      ii) Mucoepidermoid carcinoma

II. **SOFT TISSUE TUMOURS**

  (Fibroma, fibrosarcoma; leiomyoma, leiomyosarcoma; lipoma, chondroma, haemangioma, lymphangioma, granular cell myoblastoma)

III. **PLEURAL TUMOURS**
  A. **Benign mesothelioma**
  B. **Malignant mesothelioma**

IV. **MISCELLANEOUS TUMOURS**
    1. Carcinosarcoma
    2. Pulmonary blastoma
    3. Malignant melanoma
    4. Malignant lymphoma

V. **SECONDARY TUMOURS**

VI. **TUMOUR-LIKE LESIONS**
    1. Hamartomas
    2. Eosinophilic granuloma
    3. Inflammatory pseudotumours

INCIDENCE. Bronchogenic carcinoma is the most common primary malignant tumour in men in industrialised nations and accounts for nearly one-third of all cancer deaths in both sexes.

ETIOPATHOGENESIS. The high incidence of lung cancer is associated with a number of etiologic factors.

1. Smoking. The most important factor for rise in the incidence of bronchogenic carcinoma is tobacco smoking. About 80% of lung cancer occurs in active smokers.

i) Total dose: There is a direct statistical correlation between death rate from lung cancer and the total amount of cigarettes smoked e.g.

■ An average regular smoker has 10 times greater risk of developing lung cancer than a non-smoker.

■ The risk of smokers of more than 2 packs (40 cigarettes) per day for 20 years is 20 times greater.

■ Cessation of smoking by a regular smoker results in gradual decline in the chances of developing lung cancer. After 10 years of abstinence from smoking, the risk is not greater than in a non-smoker.

■ Pipe and cigar smokers, though have higher risk than non-smokers but are at lesser risk than cigarette smokers.

ii) Histologic alterations: The association of tobacco smoking is strongest for squamous cell carcinoma and small cell carcinoma of the lung. More than 90% of smokers have epithelial changes in the respiratory tract in the form of squamous metaplasia, dysplasia or carcinoma *in situ*.

iii) Mechanism: How tobacco smoking causes lung cancer is not quite clear.
■ Analysis of the tar from cigarette smoke has revealed a number of known carcinogens (e.g. polycyclic aromatic hydrocarbons, nitrosamines) and tumour promoters (e.g. phenol derivatives).
■ In experimental animal studies, it has been possible to induce cancer by skin painting experiments with smoke-tar.

2. Atmospheric pollution. There is increased risk of developing bronchogenic carcinoma in nonsmokers living in industrialised and smoky cities than in the less polluted rural areas.

3. Occupational causes. There are number of well-established occupational causes of lung cancer. These include workers exposed to asbestos, radiation of all types, bis-ethers, nickel, beryllium, arsenic, metallic iron and iron-oxide.

4. Dietary factors. Susceptibility to respiratory cancers is increased in vitamin A deficiency. Smokers with low vitamin A intake have a greater risk of lung cancer than those with vitamin A-rich diet. The incidence of lung cancer is inversely related to socioeconomic level reflecting their dietary pattern.

5. Genetic factors. The risk of developing lung cancer in the relatives of lung cancer patients is two and half times greater than that in the general population.

6. Chronic scarring. Peripheral adenocarcinomas occur more frequently in areas of chronic scarring caused by chronic inflammatory changes, old tuberculosis, asbestosis, chronic interstitial fibrosis, old infarcts and in scleroderma.

G/A Two types are recognised:

1. Hilar type: Most commonly, the lung cancer arises in the main bronchus or one of its segmental branches in the hilar parts of the lung, more often on the right side. The tumour begins as a small roughened area on the bronchial mucosa at the bifurcation. As the tumour enlarges, it thickens the bronchial mucosa producing nodular or ulcerated surface. As the nodules coalesce, the carcinoma grows into a friable spherical mass, 1 to 5 cm in diameter, narrowing and occluding the lumen. The cut surface of the tumour is yellowish-white with foci of necrosis and haemorrhages which may produce cavitary lesions (Table 15.6 sums up a list of common conditions having *pulmonary cavitary lesions* or 'honey-comb lung' during the course of different lung diseases).

2. Peripheral type: A small proportion of lung cancers, chiefly adenocarcinomas including bronchioloalveolar carcinomas, originate from a small peripheral bronchiole but the exact site of origin may not be discernible. The tumour may be a single nodule or multiple nodules in the periphery of the lung producing pneumonia-like consolidation of a large part of the lung. The cut surface of the tumour is greyish and mucoid.

M/E As per the World Health Organisation recommendations (see Table 15.5), bronchogenic carcinoma is divided into 5 main histologic types: squamous cell or epidermoid carcinoma (35-50%), small cell carcinoma (20-25%), adenocarcinoma (15-35%), large cell carcinoma (10-15%), and combined squamous cell carcinoma and adenocarcinoma (adenosquamous carcinoma,

TABLE 15.6: Conditions Producing Pulmonary Cavities (Honey-Comb Lung).

A. INFECTIONS

  1. Pulmonary tuberculosis
  2. Primary lung abscess (e.g. due to aspiration)
  3. Secondary lung abscess (e.g. preceding pneumonia, pyaemia, sepsis)
  4. Bronchiectasis
  5. Fungal infections (e.g. aspergillosis, mucormycosis)
  6. Actinomycosis
  7. Nocardiosis

B. NON-INFECTIOUS CAUSES

  1. Pneumoconiosis (e.g. simple coal-workers' pneumoconiosis, silicosis asbestosis)
  2. Bronchogenic carcinoma
  3. Metastatic lung tumours
  4. Wegener's granulomatosis
  5. Pulmonary infarction
  6. Congenital cysts
  7. Idiopathic pulmonary fibrosis

1-3%). However, for therapeutic purposes, bronchogenic carcinoma can be classified into three groups:
1. Small cell carcinoma (20-25%)
2. Non-small cell carcinomas (70-75%) (includes squamous cell carcinoma, adenocarcinoma, and large cell carcinoma)
3. Combined/mixed patterns (5-10%).

The distinction between small cell and non-small cell carcinomas is important because the two not only differ in morphology, but there are major differences in immunophenotyping and response to treatment (Table 15.7):

M/E Following features are observed:

1. Squamous cell (epidermoid) carcinoma: This is the most common type of bronchogenic carcinoma found more commonly in men, particularly with history of tobacco smoking. These tumours usually arise in a large bronchus and are prone to massive necrosis and cavitation. The tumour is diagnosed microscopically by identification of either intercellular bridges or keratinisation. The tumour may show varying histologic grades of differentiation such as well-differentiated, moderately-differentiated and poorly-differentiated. Occasionally, a variant of squamous cell carcinoma, *spindle cell carcinoma,* having biphasic pattern of growth due to the presence of a component of squamous cell carcinoma and the other sarcoma-like spindle cell component, is found.

2. Small cell carcinoma: Small cell carcinomas are frequently hilar or central in location, have strong relationship to cigarette smoking and are highly malignant tumours. They are most often associated with ectopic hormone production because of the presence of neurosecretory granules in majority of tumour cells which are similar to those found in argentaffin or Kulchitsky cells normally found in bronchial epithelium. By immunohistochemistry, these tumour cells are positive for neuroendocrine markers: chromogranin, neuron-specific enolase (NSE) and synaptophysin. Small cell carcinomas have 3 subtypes:

i) *Oat cell carcinoma* is composed of uniform, small cells, larger than lymphocytes with dense, round or oval nuclei having diffuse chromatin, inconspicuous nucleoli and very sparse cytoplasm (*oat* = a form of grain). These cells are organised into cords, aggregates and ribbons or around small blood vessels forming pseudorosettes.

ii) *Small cell carcinoma, intermediate cell type* is composed of cells slightly larger than those of oat cell carcinoma and have similar nuclear characteristics but have more abundant cytoplasm. These cells are organised into lobules.

TABLE 15.7: Comparison of Features of Small Cell and Non-small Cell Carcinoma of the Lung.

	FEATURE	SMALL CELL CARCINOMA	NON-SMALL CELL CARCINOMA
1.	**Etiologic relationship**	Strongly related to tobacco smoking	Smoking implicated, other factors: pollution, chronic scars, asbestos exposure
2.	**Morphology**		
	i) Pattern	Diffuse sheets	Squamous or glandular pattern
	ii) Nuclei	Hyperchromatic, fine chromatin	Pleomorphic, coarse chromatin
	iii) Nucleoli	Indistinct	Prominent
	iv) Cytoplasm	Scanty	Abundant
3.	**Neuroendocrine markers** (e.g. dense-core granules on EM, chromogranin, synaptophysin, neuron-specific enolase, CD56, CD57)	Present	Absent
4.	**Epithelial markers** (e.g. epithelial membrane antigen, carcinoembryonic antigen, cytokeratin)	Present	Present
5.	**Mucin**	Absent	Present in adenocarcinoma
6.	**HLA, β2 micro-globulin**	Absent to low	Present
7.	**Peptide hormone production**	Gastrin, ACTH, ADH, calcitonin	Parathormone
8.	**Genetic abnormalities**	3p allele loss, *RB* and *TP* 53 mutations	3p allele loss, *p16/CDKN2A* and *RAS* mutations
9.	**Treatment type**	Radiotherapy and/or chemotherapy	Surgical resection possible, limited response to radiotherapy and/or chemotherapy
10.	**Prognosis**	Poor	Better

iii) *Combined oat cell carcinoma* is a tumour in which there is a definite component of oat cell carcinoma with squamous cell and/or adenocarcinoma.

3. Adenocarcinoma: Adenocarcinoma, also called *peripheral carcinoma* due to its location and *scar carcinoma* due to its association with areas of chronic scarring, is the most common bronchogenic carcinoma in women and is slow-growing. Adenocarcinoma is further subclassified into 4 types:

i) *Acinar adenocarcinoma* which has predominance of glandular structure and often occurs in the larger bronchi.

ii) *Papillary adenocarcinoma* which has a pronounced papillary configuration and is frequently peripherally located in the lungs and is found in relation to pulmonary scars (scar carcinoma).

iii) *Bronchiolo-alveolar carcinoma* is characterised by cuboidal to tall columnar and mucus-secreting epithelial cells growing along the existing alveoli and forming numerous papillary structures.

4. Large cell carcinoma: These are undifferentiated carcinomas which lack the specific features by which they could be assigned into squamous cell carcinoma or adenocarcinoma. Large cell carcinomas are more common in men, have strong association with cigarette smoking and are highly malignant tumours. The tumour cells have large nuclei, prominent nucleoli, abundant cytoplasm and well-defined cell borders.

5. Adenosquamous carcinoma: These are a small proportion of peripheral scar carcinomas having clear evidence of both keratinisation and glandular differentiation.

SPREAD. Bronchogenic carcinoma can invade the adjoining structures directly, or may spread by lymphatic and haematogenous routes.

1. Direct spread. The tumour extends directly by invading through the wall of the bronchus and destroys and replaces the peribronchial lung tissue. As it grows further, it spreads to the opposite bronchus and lung, into the pleural cavity, the pericardium and the myocardium and along the great vessels of the heart causing their constriction.

2. Lymphatic spread. Initially, hilar lymph nodes are affected. Later, lymphatic metastases occur to the other groups leading to spread to mediastinal, cervical, supraclavicular and para-aortic lymph nodes.

3. Haematogenous spread. Distant metastases via blood stream are widespread and early. The sites affected, in descending order of involvement, are: the liver, adrenals, bones, pancreas, brain, opposite lung, kidneys and thyroid.

CLINICAL FEATURES. These are quite variable.

1. Local symptoms. Most common local complaints are cough, chest pain, dyspnoea and haemoptysis. A list of various causes of haemoptysis is given in Table 15.8.

TABLE 15.8: Causes of Haemoptysis.

A. INFLAMMATORY

1. Bronchitis
2. Bronchiectasis
3. Tuberculosis
4. Lung abscess
5. Pneumonias

B. NEOPLASTIC

1. Primary and metastatic lung cancer
2. Bronchial adenoma

C. OTHERS

1. Pulmonary thromboembolism
2. Left ventricular failure
3. Mitral stenosis
4. Trauma
5. Foreign bodies
6. Primary pulmonary hypertension
7. Haemorrhagic diathesis

2. Bronchial obstructive symptoms. Occlusion of a bronchus may result in bronchopneumonia, lung abscess and bronchiectasis in the lung tissue distal to the site of obstruction and cause their attendant symptoms like fever, productive cough, pleural effusion and weight loss.

3. Symptoms due to metastases. Distant spread may produce varying features and sometimes these are the first manifestation of lung cancer. These include: superior vena caval syndrome, painful bony lesions, paralysis of recurrent nerve and other neurologic manifestations resulting from brain metastases.

4. Paraneoplastic syndromes. A number of paraneoplastic syndromes are associated with lung cancer.

i) Ectopic hormone production: a) ACTH, producing Cushing's syndrome. b) ADH, inducing hyponatraemia. c) Parathormone, causing hypercalcaemia.

d) Calcitonin, producing hypocalcaemia. e) Gonadotropins, causing gynaecomastia. f) Serotonin, associated with carcinoid syndrome.

ii) Other systemic manifestations:

a) *Neuromuscular* e.g. polymyositis, myopathy, peripheral neuropathy and subacute cerebellar degeneration.

b) *Skeletal* e.g. clubbing and hypertrophic osteoarthropathy.

c) *Cutaneous* e.g. acanthosis nigricans and dermatomypathy.

d) *Cardiovascular* e.g. migratory thrombophlebitis (Trousseau's syndrome), nonbacterial thrombotic endocarditis.

e) *Haematologic* e.g. abnormalities in coagulation and leukaemoid reaction.

STAGING AND PROGNOSIS. The widely accepted clinical staging of lung cancer is according to the TNM classification, combining features of primary *T*umours, *N*odal involvement and distant *M*etastases. TNM staging divides all lung cancers into the following 4 stages:

Occult: Malignant cells in the broncho-pulmonary secretions but no evidence of primary tumour or metastasis.

Stage I: Tumour less than 3 cm, with or without ipsilateral nodal involvement, no distant metastasis.

Stage II: Tumour larger than 3 cm, with ipsilateral hilar lymph node involvement, no distant metastasis.

Stage III: Tumour of any size, involving adjacent structures, involving contralateral lymph nodes or distant metastasis.

In general, tumour size larger than 5 cm has worse prognosis. Symptomatic patients, particularly with systemic symptoms, fare far badly than the non-symptomatic patients. The overall prognosis of bronchogenic carcinoma is dismal; 5-year survival rate with surgery combined with radiotherapy or chemotherapy is about 9%. Adenocarcinoma and squamous cell carcinoma which are localised, are resectable and have a slightly better prognosis. *Small cell carcinoma has the worst prognosis* since surgical treatment is ineffective though the tumour is sensitive to radiotherapy and chemotherapy.

NEUROENDOCRINE TUMOURS (BRONCHIAL CARCINOID) *(p. 512)*

Bronchial carcinoids are tumours of low grade malignancy arising from neuroendocrine (Kulchitsky) cells of bronchial mucosa in common with cell of origin for small cell carcinomas described above. Formerly, they used to be classified as 'bronchial adenomas' but now it is known that these tumours are locally invasive and have the capacity to metastasise.

G/A Bronchial carcinoids most commonly arise from a major bronchus and project into the bronchial lumen as a spherical polypoid mass, 3-4 cm in diameter. Less commonly, the tumour may grow into the bronchial wall and produce collar-button like lesion. The overlying bronchial mucosa is usually intact. Cut surface of the tumour is yellow-tan in colour.

M/E The tumour is composed of uniform cuboidal cells forming aggregates, trabeculae or ribbons separated by fine fibrous septa. The tumour cells have abundant, finely granular cytoplasm and oval central nuclei with clumped nuclear chromatin.

CLINICAL FEATURES. Most of the symptoms in bronchial carcinoids occur as a result of bronchial obstruction such as cough, haemoptysis, atelectasis and secondary infection. About 5-10% of bronchial carcinoids metastasise to the liver and these cases are capable of producing carcinoid syndrome.

HAMARTOMA *(p. 512)*

Hamartoma is a tumour-like lesion composed of an abnormal admixture of pulmonary tissue components and is discovered incidentally as a coin-lesion in the chest-X-ray.

■ **Chondromatous hamartoma** is more common and usually asymptomatic. It forms a solitary, spherical mass, 2-5 cm in diameter, usually at the periphery of the lung.

■ **Leiomyomatous hamartoma** has a prominent smooth muscle component and bronchiolar structures.

METASTATIC LUNG TUMOURS *(p. 513)*

Secondary tumours of the lungs are more common than the primary pulmonary tumours. Metastases from carcinomas as well as sarcomas arising from anywhere in the body may spread to the lung by haematogenous or lymphatic routes, or by direct extension. Blood-borne metastases are the most common since emboli of tumour cells from any malignant tumour entering the systemic venous circulation are likely to be lodged in the lungs. Metastases are most common in the peripheral part of the lung forming single or multiple, discrete nodular lesions which appear radiologically as *'cannon-ball secondaries'.* Less frequently, the metastatic growth is confined to peribronchiolar and perivascular locations which is due to spread via lymphatics.

Most common sources of metastases in the lungs are: carcinomas of the bowel, breast, thyroid, kidney, pancreas, lung (ipsilateral or contralateral) and liver. Other tumours which frequently metastasise to the lungs are osteogenic sarcoma, neuroblastoma, Wilms' tumour, melanoma, lymphomas and leukaemias.

PLEURA *(p. 513)*

NORMAL STRUCTURE *(p. 513)*

Visceral pleura covers the lungs and extends into the fissures while the parietal pleura limits the mediastinum and covers the dome of the diaphragm and inner aspect of the chest wall. The two layers between them enclose pleural cavity which contains less than 15 ml of clear serous fluid.

INFLAMMATIONS *(p. 513)*

Inflammatory involvement of the pleura is commonly termed *pleuritis or pleurisy*. Depending upon the character of resultant exudate, it can be divided into following:

1. SEROUS, FIBRINOUS AND SEROFIBRINOUS PLEURITIS. Acute inflammation of the pleural sac (acute pleuritis) can result in serous, serofibrinous and fibrinous exudate. Most of the causes of such pleuritis are infective in origin, particularly within the lungs, such as tuberculosis, pneumonias, pulmonary infarcts, lung abscess and bronchiectasis. Other causes include a few collagen diseases (e.g. rheumatoid arthritis and disseminated lupus erythematosus).

2. SUPPURATIVE PLEURITIS (EMPYEMA THORACIS). Bacterial or mycotic infection of the pleural cavity that converts a serofibrinous effusion into purulent exudate is termed suppurative pleuritis or empyema thoracis. The most common cause is direct spread of pyogenic infection from the lung.

In empyema, the exudate is yellow-green, creamy pus that accumulates in large volumes. In time, tough fibrocollagenic adhesions develop which obliterate the cavity.

3. HAEMORRHAGIC PLEURITIS. Haemorrhagic pleuritis differs from haemothorax in having inflammatory cells or exfoliated tumour cells in the exudate. The causes of haemorrhagic pleuritis are metastatic involvement of the pleura, bleeding disorders and rickettsial diseases.

NON-INFLAMMATORY PLEURAL EFFUSIONS *(p. 513)*

1. HYDROTHORAX. Hydrothorax is non-inflammatory accumulation of serous fluid within the pleural cavities. Hydrothorax may be unilateral or bilateral depending upon the underlying cause. Occasionally, an effusion is limited to part of a pleural cavity by preexisting pleural adhesions.

The most common cause of hydrothorax, often bilateral, is congestive heart failure. Other causes are renal failure, cirrhosis of liver, Meig's syndrome pulmonary oedema and primary and secondary tumours of the lungs.

The non-inflammatory serous effusion in hydrothorax is clear and straw-coloured and has the characteristics of transudate with a specific gravity of under 1.012, protein content below 1 gm/dl and little cellular content.

If the fluid collection in pleural cavity is less than 300 ml (normal is less than 15 ml), no signs or symptoms are produced and may be apparent in chest X-ray in standing posture as obliterated costodiaphragmatic angle.

2. HAEMOTHORAX. Accumulation of pure blood in the pleural cavity is termed as haemothorax. The most common causes of haemothorax are trauma to the chest wall or to the thoracic viscera and rupture of aortic aneurysm. It is important to remove the blood from the pleural cavity as early as possible.

3. CHYLOTHORAX. Chylothorax is an uncommon condition in which there is accumulation of milky fluid of lymphatic origin into the pleural cavity. Chylothorax results most commonly from rupture of the thoracic duct by trauma or obstruction of the thoracic duct such as by malignant tumours, most often malignant lymphomas.

PNEUMOTHORAX *(p. 514)*

An accumulation of air in the pleural cavity is called pneumothorax. It may occur in one of the three circumstances:

i) Spontaneous pneumothorax occurs due to spontaneous rupture of alveoli in any form of pulmonary disease. Most commonly, spontaneous pneumothorax occurs in association with emphysema, asthma and tuberculosis. Other causes include chronic bronchitis in an old patient, bronchiectasis, pulmonary infarction and bronchial cancer.

ii) Traumatic pneumothorax is caused by trauma to the chest wall or lungs, ruptured oesophagus or stomach, and surgical operations of the thorax.

iii) Therapeutic (artificial) pneumothorax used to be employed formerly in the treatment of chronic pulmonary tuberculosis in which air was introduced into the pleural sac so as to collapse the lung and limit its respiratory movements.

TUMOURS OF PLEURA *(p. 514)*

Pleural tumours may be primary or secondary. Secondary tumours in the pleura are more common. The only important primary tumour of pleura is mesothelioma.

MESOTHELIOMA *(p. 514)*

Mesothelioma is an uncommon tumour arising from mesothelial lining of serous cavities, most often in pleural cavity, and rarely in peritoneal cavity and pericardial sac. Mesotheliomas are of 2 types—*benign (solitary) and malignant (diffuse)*. The biologic behaviour of pleural mesotheliomas is usually predicted by their gross appearance.

Benign (Solitary) Mesothelioma *(p. 514)*

Benign or solitary mesothelioma is also called as pleural fibroma. *Asbestos exposure plays no role in etiology of benign mesothelioma.*

G/A It consists of a solitary, circumscribed, small, firm mass, generally less than 3 cm in diameter. Cut surface shows whorls of dense fibrous tissue.

M/E The tumour is predominantly composed of whorls of collagen fibres and reticulin with interspersed fibroblasts. Rarely, mesothelial-lined clefts are seen in the tumour.

Malignant (Diffuse) Mesothelioma *(p. 515)*

Malignant or diffuse mesothelioma is rare. It is a highly malignant tumour associated with high mortality. The tumour is significant in view of its *recognised association with occupational exposure to asbsestos* (particularly crocidolite) for a number of years, usually 20 to 40 years. About 90% of malignant mesotheliomas are asbestos-related.

G/A The tumour is characteristically diffuse, forming a thick, white, fleshy coating over the parietal and visceral surfaces.

M/E Malignant mesothelioma may have the following patterns:

i) Epithelial pattern resembles an adenocarcinoma, consisting of tubular and tubulo-papillary formations. The tumour cells are usually well-differentiated, cuboidal, flattened or columnar cells.

ii) Sarcomatoid pattern consists of spindle cell sarcoma resembling fibrosarcoma. The tumour cells are arranged in a storiform pattern with abundant collagen between them.

iii) Biphasic pattern shows mixed growth having epithelial as well as sarcomatoid pattern. Usually, there are slit-like or gland-like spaces lined by neoplastic mesothelial cells separated by proliferating spindle-shaped tumour cells.

Asbestos bodies are found in the lungs of most patients with malignant mesothelioma of any histologic type.

SECONDARY PLEURAL TUMOURS *(p. 516)*

Metastatic malignancies in the pleura are more common than the primary tumours and appear as small nodules scattered over the lung surface. The most frequent primary malignant tumours metastasising to the pleura are of the lung and breast through lymphatics, and ovarian cancers via haematogenous route.

■ **SELF ASSESSMENT**

---

1. **Source of pulmonary surfactant is:**
   A. Alveolar macrophages
   B. Type I pneumocytes
   C. Type II pneumocytes
   D. Capillary basement membrane

2. **The basic defect in neonatal hyaline membrane disease is:**
   A. Shock due to sepsis
   B. Deficient production of surfactant
   C. Inhalation of toxins
   D. Aspiration pneumonitis

3. **Adult respiratory distress syndrome occurs from the following causes *except:***
   A. Pancreatitis
   B. Oxygen toxicity
   C. Deficiency of surfactant
   D. Diffuse pulmonary infections

4. **Primary atelectasis is defined as:**
   A. Incomplete expansion of a previously unexpanded lung
   B. Reduction in size of a previously expanded lung due to compression
   C. Reduction in size of a lung due to obstruction
   D. Reduction in lung size due to contraction

Chapter Fifteen

5. **Pulmonary hypertension is defined as systolic blood pressure in the pulmonary arterial circulation above the following cut off figure:**
   A. 120 mmHg
   B. 90 mmHg
   C. 60 mmHg
   D. 30 mmHg

6. **Bronchopneumonia is grossly characterised by:**
   A. Diffuse consolidation of a lobe or lobes of one or both lungs
   B. Diffuse consolidation of a lobe of one lung
   C. Diffuse consolidation of a lobe of both lungs
   D. Patchy consolidation of a lobe or lobes of one or both lungs

7. **The most common causative organism for lobar pneumonia is:**
   A. Staphylococci
   B. Streptococci
   C. Pneumococci
   D. Haemophilus

8. **Viral pneumonias are characterised by the following features** *except:*
   A. Presence of interstitial inflammation
   B. Presence of alveolar exudate
   C. Necrotising bronchiolitis
   D. Multinucleate giant cells in the bronchiolar wall

9. **The organism in *Pneumocystis carinii* pneumonia is:**
   A. Mycoplasma
   B. Fungus
   C. Protozoa
   D. Chlamydia

10. **Lung abscess secondary to aspiration pneumonia develops more often in:**
    A. Lower lobe of right lung
    B. Lower lobe of left lung
    C. Upper lobe of either lung
    D. Middle lobe of right lung

11. **Reid index used as a criteria of quantitation in chronic bronchitis is the ratio of thickness of:**
    A. Bronchial mucosa to that of bronchial wall
    B. Submucosal glands to that of bronchial wall
    C. Bronchial cartilage to that of bronchial wall
    D. Inflammatory infiltrate to that of bronchial wall

12. **The most fibrogenic dust in pneumoconiosis is:**
    A. Coal
    B. Asbestos
    C. Silica
    D. Beryllium

13. **Classic α-1 antitrypsin deficiency in emphysema has the following phenotype of protease inhibitor:**
    A. PiMM
    B. PiZZ
    C. PiMZ
    D. PiMO

14. **The extent of damage to pulmonary parenchyma is severest in the following type of emphysema:**
    A. Centriacinar
    B. Panacinar
    C. Distal acinar
    D. Irregular

15. **Emphysema associated most often with α_1 antitrypsin deficiency is:**
    A. Panacinar
    B. Centriacinar
    C. Distal acinar
    D. Irregular

16. **Serum IgE levels are elevated in:**
    A. Intrinsic bronchial asthma
    B. Extrinsic bronchial asthma
    C. Predominant chronic bronchitis
    D. Predominant emphysema

17. **Bronchiectasis commonly develops in the following microanatomic zone of bronchial tree:**
    A. Acini beyond respiratory bronchioles
    B. Acini beyond terminal bronchioles
    C. Terminal bronchioles less than 2 mm diameter
    D. Bronchioles more than 2 mm diameter

18. **Restrictive lung disease is characterised by the following features** *except:*
    A. Dyspnoea
    B. Tachypnoea
    C. Cyanosis
    D. Wheezing

19. Inhaled dust particles of the following size are generally eliminated by expectoration:
    A. Smaller than 1 µm
    B. 1-3 µm
    C. 3-5 µm
    D. Larger than 5 µm

20. Bronchogenic carcinoma has increased incidence in the following pneumoconiosis:
    A. Coal workers' pneumoconiosis
    B. Silicosis
    C. Asbestosis
    D. Berylliosis

21. Silicosis occurs in following occupational exposure *except:*
    A. Ceramic workers
    B. Foundry workers
    C. Textile workers
    D. Construction workers

22. Out of various forms of asbestos, the following type is implicated in etiology of malignant pleural tumour:
    A. Chrysotite
    B. Crocidolite
    C. Amosite
    D. Anthophyllite

23. Caplan's syndrome may develop in the following types of pneumoconiosis *except:*
    A. Coal-workers' pneumoconiosis
    B. Asbestosis
    C. Berylliosis
    D. Silicosis

24. Non-caseating sarcoid-like epithelioid cell granulomas are seen in:
    A. Silicosis
    B. Asbestosis
    C. Coal-workers' pneumoconiosis
    D. Chronic berylliosis

25. The following histologic types of bronchogenic carcinoma have strong association with cigarette smoking *except:*
    A. Squamous cell carcinoma
    B. Small cell carcinoma
    C. Large cell carcinoma
    D. Adenocarcinoma

26. The following type of bronchogenic carcinoma has worst prognosis:
    A. Squamous cell carcinoma
    B. Small cell carcinoma
    C. Large cell carcinoma
    D. Adenocarcinoma

27. Bronchial carcinoid arises from:
    A. Columnar ciliated epithelium
    B. Goblet cells
    C. Kulchitsky cells
    D. Alveolar lining cells

28. The following tumour does not have association with occupational exposure to asbestosis:
    A. Benign mesothelioma
    B. Malignant mesothelioma
    C. Bronchogenic carcinoma
    D. Laryngeal carcinoma

29. Macrophage-derived fibrogenic cytokine is:
    A. IL-1
    B. IL-8
    C. TNF
    D. TGF α

30. The most important mutation in small cell carcinoma is in the following gene:
    A. *RB* gene
    B. *MYC* gene
    C. *CDK* gene
    D. *RAS* gene

KEY

1 = C	2 = B	3 = C	4 = A
5 = D	6 = D	7 = C	8 = B
9 = C	10 = A	11 = B	12 = C
13 = B	14 = B	15 = A	16 = B
17 = D	18 = D	19 = D	20 = C
21 = C	22 = B	23 = C	24 = D
25 = D	26 = B	27 = C	28 = A
29 = D	30 = A		

Chapter Fifteen

16

The Eye, ENT and Neck

EYE (p.517)

NORMAL STRUCTURE (p.517)

The *globe of the eye* is composed of 3 layers: the cornea-sclera, choroid-iris, and retina.

The **cornea** consists of stratified epithelium which may be regarded as continuation of the conjunctiva over the cornea.

The **sclera** is composed of dense fibrous tissue which is thickest at the back of the eyeball.

The **choroid** is the vascular membrane in contact with the sclera. The choroid becomes thickened anteriorly forming ciliary body, ciliary processes and contains ciliary muscle.

The **iris** is the continuation of the choroid which extends in front of the lens. It is similar in structure to the choroid but contains pigment cells.

The **uveal tract** consists of 3 parts—the choroid and ciliary body posteriorly, and the iris anteriorly.

The **retina** is part of the central nervous system and corresponds in extent to the choroid which it lines internally. The retina is composed of a number of layers of cells and their synapses.

The **lens** is the biconvex mass of laminated transparent tissue with elastic capsule.

The **anterior chamber** is the space filled with the aqueous humour, and is bounded by the cornea in front and the iris behind, with anterior surface of the lens exposed in the pupil.

The **posterior chamber** containing aqueous humour is the triangular space between the back of the iris, the anterior surface of the lens and ciliary body forming its apex at the pupillary margin.

The **vitreous chamber** is the large space behind the lens containing gelatinous material, the vitreous humour.

CONGENITAL LESIONS (p.518)

RETROLENTAL FIBROPLASIA (RETINOPATHY OF PREMATURITY). This is a developmental disorder occurring in premature infants who have been given oxygen-therapy at birth. The basic defect lies in the developmental prematurity of the retinal blood vessels which are extremely sensitive to high dose of oxygen-therapy.

RETINITIS PIGMENTOSA. Retinitis pigmentosa is a group of systemic and ocular diseases of unknown etiology, characterised by degeneration of the retinal pigment epithelium.

INFLAMMATORY CONDITIONS (p.518)

Inflammatory conditions of the eye are designated according to the tissue affected. 'Uveitis' is the commonly used term for the ocular inflammation of the uveal tract which is the most vascular tissue of the eye.

STYE (HORDEOLUM). Stye or 'external hordeolum' is an acute suppurative inflammation of the sebaceous glands of Zeis, the apocrine glands of Moll and the eyelash follicles.

CHALAZION. Chalazion is the chronic inflammatory process involving the meibomian glands. It occurs as a result of obstruction to the drainage of secretions. The inflammatory process begins with destruction of meibomian glands and duct and subsequently involves tarsal plate.

ENDOPHTHALMITIS. Endophthalmitis is an acute suppurative intraocular inflammation which may be of exogenous or endogenous origin. The exogenous agents may be bacteria, viruses or fungi introduced into the eye during an accidental or surgical perforating wound. The endogenous agents include opportunistic infections which may cause endophthalmitis via haematogenous route.

CONJUNCTIVITIS AND KERATOCONJUNCTIVITIS. Conjunctiva and cornea are constantly exposed to various types of physical, chemical, microbial (bacteria, fungi, viruses) and allergic agents and hence prone to develop acute, subacute and chronic inflammations. In the acute stage, there is corneal oedema and infiltration by inflammatory cells, affecting the transparency of the cornea. In the more chronic form of inflammation, there is proliferation of small blood vessels in the normally avascular cornea and infiltration by lymphocytes and plasma cells (pannus formation).

TRACHOMA AND INCLUSION CONJUNCTIVITIS. Both these conditions are caused by *Chlamydia* or TRIC agents. Trachoma is caused by *C. trachomatis* while inclusion conjunctivitis is caused by *C. oculogenitalis*. Trachoma is widely prevalent in the underdeveloped and developing countries of the world and is responsible for blindness on a large scale. The end-result is extensive corneal and conjunctival cicatrisation accounting for blindness in trachoma.

GRANULOMATOUS UVEITIS. A number of chronic granulomatous conditions may cause granulomatous uveitis. These include bacteria (e.g. tuberculosis, leprosy, syphilis), viruses (e.g. CMV disease, herpes zoster), fungi (e.g. aspergillosis, blastomycosis, phycomycosis, histoplasmosis), and certain parasites (e.g. toxoplasmosis, onchocerciasis).

SYMPATHETIC OPHTHALMIA (SYMPATHETIC UVEITIS). This is an uncommon condition in which there is bilateral diffuse granulomatous uveitis following penetrating injury to one eye. The condition probably results from an autosensitivity reaction to injured uveal tissue.

VASCULAR LESIONS *(p. 519)*

DIABETIC RETINOPATHY. Diabetic retinopathy is an important cause of blindness. It is related to the degree and duration of glycaemic control. The condition develops in more than 60% of diabetics 15 years or so after the onset of disease, and in about 2% of diabetics causes blindness. Other ocular complications of diabetes include glaucoma, cataract and corneal disease. Most cases of diabetic retinopathy occur over the age of 50 years. The risk is greater in type 1 diabetes mellitus (IDDM) than in type 2 diabetes mellitus, although in clinical practice there are more patients of diabetic retinopathy due to type 2 diabetes mellitus because of its higher prevalence.

M/E Two types of changes are described in diabetic retinopathy:

1. *Background (non-proliferative) retinopathy:*
i) Basement membrane shows varying thickness
ii) Degeneration of pericytes
iii) Capillary microaneurysms
iv) 'Waxy exudates' accumulate in the vicinity of microaneurysms
v) 'Dot and blot haemorrhages' in the deeper layers of retina
vi) Soft 'cotton-wool spots' appear on the retina which are microinfarcts of nerve fibre layers.

2. *Proliferative retinopathy (retinitis proliferans):*
i) Neovascularisation of the retina at the optic disc

ii) Friability of newly-formed blood vessels

iii) Proliferation of astrocytes and fibrous tissue

iv) Fibrovascular and gliotic tissue contracts to cause retinal detachment and blindness.

HYPERTENSIVE RETINOPATHY. In hypertensive retinopathy, the retinal arterioles are reduced in their diameter leading to retinal ischaemia. In acute severe hypertension as happens at the onset of malignant hypertension and in toxaemia of pregnancy, the vascular changes are in the form of spasms, while in chronic hypertension the changes are diffuse in the form of onion-skin thickening of the arteriolar walls with narrowing of the lumina. Features of hypertensive retinopathy include the following:

i) Variable degree of arteriolar narrowing due to arteriolosclerosis.

ii) 'Flame-shaped' haemorrhages in the retinal nerve fibre layer.

iii) Macular star i.e. exudates radiating from the centre of macula.

iv) Cotton-wool spots i.e. fluffy white bodies in the superficial layer of retina.

v) Microaneurysms.

vi) Arteriovenous nicking i.e. kinking of veins at sites where sclerotic arterioles cross veins.

vii) Hard exudates due to leakage of lipid and fluid into macula.

RETINAL INFARCTS. Infarcts of the retina may result from thrombosis or embolism in central artery of the retina, causing ischaemic necrosis of the inner two-third of the retina while occlusion of the posterior ciliary arteries causes ischaemia of the inner photoreceptor layer only. The usual causes of thrombosis and embolism are atherosclerosis, hypertension and diabetes.

MISCELLANEOUS CONDITIONS (p. 520)

PINGUECULA AND PTERYGIUM. Pinguecula is a degenerative condition of the collagen of the bulbar conjunctiva. Clinically, the condition appears as raised yellowish lesions on the interpalpebral bulbar conjunctiva of both eyes in middle-aged and elderly patients.

Pterygium is a lesion closely related to pinguecula but differs from the latter by being located at the limbus and often involves the cornea.

SENILE MACULAR DEGENERATION. Age-related degeneration of the macular region of the retina is an important cause of bilateral central visual loss in the elderly people.

RETINAL DETACHMENT. Retinal detachment is the separation of the neurosensory retina from the retinal pigment epithelium. Normally, the rods and cones of the photoreceptor layer are interdigitated with projections of the retinal pigment epithelium, but the two can separate readily in many disease processes.

PHTHISIS BULBI. Phthisis bulbi is the end-stage of advanced degeneration and disorganisation of the entire eyeball in which the intraocular pressure is decreased and the eyeball shrinks. The causes of such end-stage blind eye are trauma, glaucoma and intraocular inflammations.

CATARACT. The cataract is the opacification of the normally crystalline lens. The various causes of cataract are: senility, congenital (e.g. rubella, galacto-saemia), traumatic (e.g. penetrating injury, electrical injury) and metabolic (e.g. diabetes). The most common is, however, idiopathic senile cataract.

GLAUCOMA. Glaucoma is a group of ocular disorders that have in common increased intraocular pressure. Glaucoma is one of the leading causes of blindness because of the ocular tissue damage produced by raised intraocular pressure. In almost all cases, glaucoma occurs due to impaired outflow of aqueous humour, though there is a theoretical possibility of increased production of aqueous by the ciliary body causing glaucoma. The obstruction to the aqueous flow may occur as a result of developmental malformations (**congenital glaucoma**); or due to complications of some other diseases such as uveitis, trauma, intraocular haemorrhage and tumours (**secondary glaucoma**); or may be **primary glaucoma** which is typically bilateral and is the most common type.

PAPILLOEDEMA. Papilloedema is oedema of the optic disc resulting from increased intracranial pressure. This is due to anatomic continuation of the subarachnoid space of the brain around the optic nerve so that raised intracranial pressure is passed onto the optic disc area. In *acute papilloedema*, there is oedema, congestion and haemorrhage at the optic disc. In *chronic papilloedema*, there is degeneration of nerve fibres, gliosis and optic atrophy.

SJÖGREN'S SYNDROME. Sjögren's syndrome is characterised by triad of keratoconjunctivitis sicca, xerostomia (sicca syndrome) and rheumatoid arthritis.

MIKULICZ'S SYNDROME. This is characterised by inflammatory enlargement of lacrimal and salivary glands. The condition may occur with Sjögren's syndrome, or with some diseases like sarcoidosis, leukaemia, lymphoma and macroglobulinaemia.

TUMOURS AND TUMOUR-LIKE LESIONS *(p. 522)*

The eye and its adnexal structures are the site of a variety of benign and malignant tumours as well as tumour-like lesions.

Inflammatory Pseudotumours *(p. 522)*

These are a group of inflammatory enlargements, especially in the orbit, which clinically look like tumours but surgical exploration and pathologic examination fail to reveal any evidence of neoplasm.

G/A These lesions are circumscribed and sometimes have fibrous capsule.

M/E Many of the lesions can be placed in well-established categories such as tuberculous, syphilitic, mycotic, parasitic, foreign-body granuloma etc, while others show non-specific histologic appearance having abundant fibrous tissue, lymphoid follicles and inflammatory infiltrate with prominence of eosinophils.

Sebaceous Carcinoma *(p. 522)*

This is the most frequent tumour of the eyelid next only to basal cell carcinoma, although it is very rare tumour elsewhere in the body. It arises either from the meibomian glands in the tarsus or from Zeis' glands of eyelash follicles. The tumour is seen more commonly in the upper eyelid (basal cell carcinoma is seen more frequently in the lower eyelid).

G/A The tumour appears as a localised or diffuse swelling of the tarsus, or may be in the form of ulcerated or papillomatous tumour at the lid margin.

M/E The tumour may show well-differentiated lobules of tumour cells with sebaceous differentiation, or may be poorly-differentiated tumour requiring confirmation by fat stains.

Uveal Malignant Melanoma *(p. 522)*

Malignant melanomas arising from neural crest-derived pigment epithelium of the uvea is the most common primary ocular malignancy in the white adults in North America and Europe.

G/A The malignant melanoma appears as a pigmented mass, most commonly in the posterior choroid, and less often in the ciliary body and iris. The mass projects into the vitreous cavity with retina covering it.

M/E Age-old classification of Callender (1931) which has prognostic significance is still followed with some modifications:

1. *Spindle A melanoma* is composed of uniform, spindle-shaped cells containing spindled nuclei. Nucleoli are indistinct and mitotic figures are rare.

2. *Spindle B melanoma* is composed of larger and plump spindle-shaped cells with ovoid nuclei. Nucleoli are conspicuous and a few mitotic figures are present.

3. *Epithelioid melanoma* consists of larger, irregular and pleomorphic cells with larger nuclei and abundant acidophilic cytoplasm. These tumours are the most malignant of the uveal melanomas and have poor prognosis (35% 10-year survival).

4. *Mixed cell type melanomas* have features of spindle cell type as well as of epithelioid cell type. These are more common tumours and carry an intermediate prognosis (45% 10-year survival).

In general, uveal malignant melanomas are usually slow-growing, late metastasising and have a better prognosis than malignant melanoma of the skin.

Retinoblastoma *(p. 523)*

This is the most common malignant ocular tumour in children. It may be present at birth or recognised in early childhood before the age of 4 years. Retinoblastoma has some peculiar features. About 60% cases of retinoblastoma are sporadic and the remaining 40% are familial. Familial tumours are often multiple and multifocal and transmitted as an autosomal dominant trait by retinoblastoma susceptibility gene *(RB)* located on chromosome 13. Such individuals have a higher incidence of bilateral tumours and have increased risk of developing second primary tumour, particularly osteogenic sarcoma.

G/A The tumour characteristically appears as a white mass within the retina which may be partly solid and partly necrotic. The tumour may be *endophytic* when it protrudes into the vitreous, or *exophytic* when it grows between the retina and the pigment epithelium.

M/E As the name implies, the tumour is composed of undifferentiated retinal cells with tendency towards formation of photo-receptor elements. In the better differentiated area, the tumour cells are characteristically arranged in rosettes. The rosettes may be of 2 types—*Flexner-Wintersteiner rosettes* characterised by small tumour cells arranged around a lumen with their nuclei away from the lumen, and *Homer-Wright rosettes* having radial arrangement of tumour cells around the central neurofibrillar structure.

Salient features of retinoblastoma are contrasted with those of uveal melanoma in Table 16.1.

TABLE 16.1: Uveal Malignant Melanoma *versus* Retinoblastoma.

	FEATURE	MELANOMA	RETINOBLASTOMA
1.	*Inheritance*	Rare	About 40% cases
2.	*Age*	>50 years	Birth to 4 years
3.	*Race*	Common in Caucasians, uncommon in blacks	No predisposition
4.	*Location*	Most commonly choroid	Retina
5.	*Bilaterality*	Rare	Common (30%)
6.	*Cell of origin*	Melanocytes	Retinal neurons
7.	*Colour of tumour*	Grey black	Creamy
8.	*Spread*	Haematogenous common, rarely via optic nerve	Common via both haematogenous and optic nerve

MetastaticTumours *(p. 523)*

Ocular metastatic tumours are quite common, choroid being the preferential site for metastasis. Common primary tumours that metastasise in the eye are cancers of the breast in women and lung in men. Involvement of the eye by leukaemia and malignant lymphoma is present in some cases.

EAR *(p. 524)*

NORMAL STRUCTURE *(p. 524)*

The ear is divided into 3 parts:

The **external ear** comprises the auricle or pinna composed of cartilage, the external cartilaginous meatus and the external bony meatus.

The **middle ear** consists of 3 parts—the uppermost portion is the *attic,* the middle portion is *mesotympanum,* and the lowermost portion is the *hypotympanum.*

The **inner ear** or labyrinth consists of bony capsule embedded in the petrous bone and contains the membranous labyrinth.

INFLAMMATORY LESIONS *(p. 525)*

OTITIS MEDIA. This is the term used for inflammatory involvement of the middle ear. It may be acute or chronic. The usual source of infection is via the eustachian tube and the common causative organisms are *Streptococcus pneumoniae, Haemophilus influenzae* and β-*Streptococcus haemolyticus.* Otitis media may be suppurative, serous or mucoid. Acute suppurative otitis media (SOM) clinically presents as tense and hyperaemic tympanic membrane alongwith pain and tenderness and sometimes mastoiditis as well. Chronic SOM manifests clinically as draining ear with perforated tympanic membrane and partially impaired hearing.

RELAPSING POLYCHONDRITIS. This is an uncommon autoimmune disease characterised by complete loss of glycosaminoglycans resulting in destruction of cartilage of the ear, nose, eustachian tube, larynx and lower respiratory tract.

CHONDRODERMATITIS NODULARIS CHRONICA HELICIS. This condition involves the external ear superficially and presents as a 'painful nodule of the ear'. The skin in this location is in direct contact with the cartilage without protective subcutaneous layer.

MISCELLANEOUS CONDITIONS *(p. 525)*

CAULIFLOWER EAR. This is an acquired deformity of the external ear due to degeneration of cartilage as a result of repeated trauma as occurs in boxers and wrestlers.

OTOSCLEROSIS. This is a dystrophic disease of labyrinth of the temporal bone. The footplate of stapes first undergoes fibrous replacement and is subsequently replaced by sclerotic bone.

TUMOURS AND TUMOUR-LIKE LESIONS *(p. 525)*

Tumours and tumour-like conditions are relatively more common in the external than the middle and inner ear.

AURAL (OTIC) POLYPS. Aural or otic polyps are tumour-like lesions arising from the middle ear as a complication of the chronic otitis media and project into the external auditory canal.

CERUMEN-GLAND TUMOURS. Tumours arising from cerumen-secreting apocrine sweat glands of the external auditory canal are cerumen-gland adenomas or cerumen-gland adenocarcinomas and are counter-parts of sweat gland tumours.

CHOLESTEATOMA (KERATOMA). This is a post-inflammatory 'pseudo-tumour' found in the middle ear or mastoid air cells. There is invariable history of acute or chronic otitis media. A marginal perforation is generally present through which the squamous epithelium enters the middle ear and results in exfoliation of squamous and formation of the keratin.

JUGULAR PARAGANGLIOMA (GLOMUS JUGULARE TUMOUR, NON-CHROMAFFIN PARAGANGLIOMA). Tumours originating from parasympathetic ganglia are called 'paraganglioma' and are named according to the location of the tissue of origin. The one arising from glomus jugulare bodies of the middle ear (jugulotympanic bodies) is called jugular paraganglioma or chemodectoma or non-chromaffin paraganglioma and is the most common benign tumour of the middle ear. Histologically similar tumours are seen in the carotid bodies and vagus.

ACOUSTIC NEUROMA (ACOUSTIC SCHWANNOMA). This is a tumour of Schwann cells of 8th cranial nerve. It is usually located in the internal auditory canal and cerebellopontine angle. It is a benign tumour similar to ·other schwannomas but by virtue of its location and large size, may produce compression of the important neighbouring tissues.

NOSE AND PARANASAL SINUSES *(p. 526)*

NORMAL STRUCTURE *(p. 526)*

The external nose and the septum are composed of bone and cartilage. On the lateral wall of the nasal cavity, there is a system of 3 ridges on each side known as conchae or turbinates—the inferior, middle and superior.

INFLAMMATORY CONDITIONS *(p. 526)*

ACUTE RHINITIS (COMMON COLD). Acute rhinitis or common cold is the common inflammatory disorder of the nasal cavities that may extend into the nasal sinuses. It begins with rhinorrhoea, nasal obstruction and sneezing.

ALLERGIC RHINITIS (HAY FEVER). Allergic rhinitis occurs due to sensitivity to allergens such as pollens. It is an IgE-mediated immune response consisting of an early acute response due to degranulation of mast cells, and a delayed prolonged response in which there is infiltration by leucocytes.

SINUSITIS. Acute sinusitis is generally a complication of acute or allergic rhinitis and rarely secondary to dental sepsis. The ostia are occluded due to inflammation and oedema and the sinuses are full. *'Mucocele'* is filling up of the sinus with mucus while *'empyema'* of the sinus occurs due to collection of pus.

NASAL POLYPS. Nasal polyps are pedunculated grape-like masses of tissue. They are the end-result of prolonged chronic inflammation causing polypoid thickening of the mucosa. They may be *allergic* or *inflammatory*. They are commonly bilateral and the middle turbinate is the common site. *Antrochoanal polyps* originate from the mucosa of the maxillary sinus and appear in the nasal cavity. Morphologically, nasal and antro-choanal polyps are identical.·

G/A They are gelatinous masses with smooth and shining surface.

M/E They are composed of loose oedematous connective tissue containing some mucous glands and varying number of inflammatory cells like lymphocytes, plasma cells and eosinophils. The polyps are covered by respiratory epithelium which may show squamous metaplasia.

RHINOSPORIDIOSIS. Rhinosporidiosis is caused by a fungus, *Rhinosporidium seeberi*. Typically it occurs in a nasal polyp but may be found in other locations like nasopharynx, larynx and conjunctiva. The disease is common in India and Sri Lanka.

M/E Besides the structure of inflammatory or allergic polyp, large number of organisms of the size of erythrocytes with chitinous wall are seen in the thick-walled *sporangia*. Each sporangium may contain a few thousand spores. On rupture of a sporangium, the spores are discharged into the submucosa or on to the surface of the mucosa.

RHINOSCLEROMA. This is a chronic destructive inflammatory lesion of the nose and upper respiratory airways caused by diplobacilli, *Klebsiella rhinoscleromatis*. The condition is endemic in parts of Africa, America, South Asia and Eastern Europe.

M/E There is extensive infiltration by foamy histiocytes containing the organisms (Mikulicz cells) and other chronic inflammatory cells like lymphocytes and plasma cells.

GRANULOMAS. Many granulomatous inflammations may involve the nose:

1. **Tuberculosis or lupus** of the nose is uncommon and occurs secondary to pulmonary tuberculosis and usually produces ulcerative lesions on the anterior part of the septum of the nose.

2. **Leprosy** begins as a nodule that may ulcerate and perforate the septum.

3. **Syphilis** may involve the nose in congenital form causing destruction of the septum, or in acquired tertiary syphilis in the form of gummas perforating the septum.

4. **Aspergillosis** may involve the paranasal sinuses where the septate hyphae grow to form a mass called *aspergilloma*.

5. **Mucormycosis** is an opportunistic infection caused by *Mucorales* which are non-septate hyphae and invade the nerves and blood vessels.

6. **Wegener's granulomatosis** is a form of necrotising vasculitis with granuloma formation affecting the upper respiratory tract, lungs and kidneys.

7. **Lethal midline granuloma or polymorphic reticulosis** is a rare and lethal lesion of the upper respiratory tract that causes extensive destruction of cartilage and necrosis of tissues and does not respond to antibiotic treatment. Besides the necrosis, lymphoid infiltrates of pleomorphic and atypical cells admixed with small lymphocytes, plasma cells and macrophages are seen. Currently, the condition is considered to be a T cell lymphoma.

TUMOURS *(p. 528)*

Benign Tumours *(p. 528)*

1. **CAPILLARY HAEMANGIOMA.** Capillary haemangioma of the septum of nose is a common benign lesion. If the surface is ulcerated and the lesion contains inflammatory cell infiltrate, it resembles inflammatory granulation tissue and is called *'haemangioma of granulation tissue type'* or *'granuloma pyogenicum'*.

2. **PAPILLOMAS.** Papillomas may occur in the nasal vestibule, nasal cavity and paranasal sinuses. They are mainly of 2 types—*fungiform papilloma* with exophytic growth, and *inverted papilloma* with everted growth.

Malignant Tumours *(p. 528)*

1. OLFACTORY NEUROBLASTOMA OR ESTHESIONEUROBLASTOMA.

It occurs over the olfactory mucosa as a polypoid mass that may invade the paranasal sinuses or skull. It is a highly malignant small cell tumour of neural crest origin that may, at times, be indistinguishable from other small cell malignancies like rhabdomyosarcoma, undifferentiated carcinoma, lymphoma or Ewing's sarcoma.

2. CARCINOMAS. Majority of carcinomas of the nasal cavity and paranasal sinuses are squamous cell carcinomas. They are seen more commonly in the elderly with history of heavy smoking and severe chronic sinusitis, in nickel refinery workers and in wood workers.

PHARYNX *(p. 528)*

NORMAL STRUCTURE *(p. 528)*

The pharynx has 3 parts—the nasopharynx, oropharynx (pharynx proper) and the laryngopharynx. The whole of pharynx is lined by stratified squamous epithelium.

INFLAMMATORY CONDITIONS *(p. 528)*

LUDWIG'S ANGINA. This is a severe, acute streptococcal cellulitis involving the neck, tongue and back of the throat. The condition often proves fatal due to glottic oedema, asphyxia and severe toxaemia.

VINCENT'S ANGINA. Vincent's angina is a painful condition of the throat characterised by local ulceration of the tonsils, mouth and pharynx. The causative organism is *Vincent's bacillus.*

DIPHTHERIA. Diphtheria is an acute communicable disease caused by *Corynebacterium diphtheriae.* It usually occurs in children and results in the formation of a yellowish-grey *pseudomembrane* in the mucosa of nasopharynx, oropharynx, tonsils, larynx and trachea. *C. diphtheriae* elaborates an exotoxin that causes necrosis of the epithelium which is associated with abundant fibrinopurulent exudate resulting in the formation of pseudomembrane. Absorption of the exotoxin in the blood may lead to more distant injurious effects such as myocardial necrosis, polyneuritis, parenchymal necrosis of the liver, kidney and adrenals.

TONSILLITIS. Tonsillitis caused by staphylococci or streptococci may be acute or chronic. *Acute tonsillitis* is characterised by enlargement, redness and inflammation. Acute tonsillitis may progress to acute follicular tonsillitis in which crypts are filled with debris and pus giving it follicular appearance. *Chronic tonsillitis* is caused by repeated attacks of acute tonsillitis in which case the tonsils are small and fibrosed.

PERITONSILLAR ABSCESS (QUINSY). Peritonsillar abscess or quinsy occurs as a complication of acute tonsillitis. The causative organisms are staphylococci or streptococci which are associated with infection of the tonsils. The patient complains of acute pain in the throat, trismus, difficulty in speech and inability to swallow.

RETROPHARYNGEAL ABSCESS. Formation of abscess in the soft tissue between the posterior wall of the pharynx and the vertebral column is called retropharyngeal abscess. It occurs due to infection of the retropharyngeal lymph nodes.

TUMOURS *(p. 529)*

NASOPHARYNGEAL ANGIOFIBROMA. This is a peculiar tumour that occurs exclusively in adolescent males (10-20 years of age) suggesting the role of testosterone hormone in its production. Though a benign tumour of the nasopharynx, it may grow into paranasal sinuses, cheek and orbit but does not metastasise.

M/E The tumour is composed of 2 components as the name suggests—numerous small endothelium-lined vascular spaces and the stromal cells which are myofibroblasts.

NASOPHARYNGEAL CARCINOMA. Nasopharyngeal carcinoma is a common cancer in South-East Asia, especially prevalent in people of Chinese descent under 45 years of age. Genetic susceptibility and role of Epstein-Barr virus are considered important factors in its etiology. In fact, EBV-genome is found virtually in all cases of nasopharyngeal carcinoma unlike Burkitt's lymphoma, another EBV-associated tumour.

M/E Non-keratinising and keratinising squamous cell carcinomas are identical in morphology to typical tumours in other locations. The undifferentiated carcinoma, also called as transitional cell carcinoma, is characterised by masses and cords of cells which are polygonal to spindled and have large vesicular nuclei. A variant of undifferentiated carcinoma is *'lymphoepithelioma'* in which undifferentiated carcinoma is infiltrated by abundant non-neoplastic mature lymphocytes.

MALIGNANT LYMPHOMA. The lymphoid tissue of the nasopharynx and tonsils may be the site for development of malignant lymphomas which resemble similar tumours elsewhere in the body.

LARYNX *(p. 529)*

NORMAL STRUCTURE *(p. 529)*

The larynx is composed of cartilages which are bound together by ligaments and muscles and is covered by mucous membrane. The cartilages of the larynx are of 2 types—unpaired and paired.

The larynx as well as trachea are lined by respiratory epithelium, except over the true vocal cords and the epiglottis, which are lined by stratified squamous epithelium.

INFLAMMATORY CONDITIONS *(p. 529)*

ACUTE LARYNGITIS. This may occur as a part of the upper or lower respiratory tract infection. Atmospheric pollutants like cigarette smoke, exhaust fumes, industrial and domestic smoke etc predispose the larynx to acute bacterial and viral infections.

CHRONIC LARYNGITIS. Chronic laryngitis may occur from repeated attacks of acute inflammation, excessive smoking, chronic alcoholism or vocal abuse. The surface is granular due to swollen mucous glands. There may be extensive squamous metaplasia.

TUBERCULOUS LARYNGITIS. Tuberculous laryngitis occurs secondary to pulmonary tuberculosis.

ACUTE OEDEMA OF THE LARYNX. This hazardous condition is an acute inflammatory condition, causing swelling of the larynx that may lead to airway obstruction and death by suffocation.

TUMOURS *(p. 530)*

Both benign and malignant tumours occur in the larynx. The common examples of benign tumours are papillomas and polyps, while laryngeal carcinoma is an important example amongst malignant tumours.

LARYNGEAL PAPILLOMAS. These tumours are found more frequently in children between 1 and 6 years of age and are often multiple, while the adults have usually a single lesion. Multiple juvenile papillomas may undergo spontaneous regression at puberty. *Papova* group of viruses (human papilloma virus, HPV) have been implicated in the etiology of papillomas of the larynx.

G/A The lesions appear as warty growths on the true vocal cords.

M/E Papillomas are composed of finger-like papillae, each papilla contains fibrovascular core covered by stratified squamous epithelium.

LARYNGEAL POLYPS. Laryngeal polyps are seen mainly in adults and are found more often in heavy smokers and in individuals subjected to vocal abuse.

G/A It is a small lesion, less than 1 cm in diameter, rounded, smooth.

M/E The nodules have prominent oedema with sparse fibrous tissue and numerous irregular and dilated vascular channels.

LARYNGEAL CARCINOMA. Cancer of the larynx in 99% of cases is squamous cell carcinoma. Rarely, adenocarcinoma and sarcoma are encountered. Squamous carcinoma of the larynx occurs in males beyond 4th decade of life. Important etiologic factor is heavy smoking of cigarettes, cigar or pipe; other factors include excessive alcohol consumption, radiation and asbestos exposure.

1. *Glottic* is the most common location, found in the region of true vocal cords and anterior and posterior commissures.

2. *Supraglottic* involving ventricles and arytenoids.

3. *Subglottic* in the walls of subglottis.

4. *Marginal zone* between the tip of epiglottis and ary-epiglottic folds.

5. *Laryngo-(hypo-) pharynx* in the pyriform fossa, postcricoid fossa and posterior pharyngeal wall.

G/A The glottic carcinoma is the most common form and appears as a small, pearly white, plaque-like thickening.

M/E Keratinising and non-keratinising squamous carcinomas of varying grades are found. Two special varieties of squamous carcinoma in the larynx are: *verrucous carcinoma* which is a well-differentiated squamous carcinoma, and *spindle cell carcinoma* which has elongated tumour cells resembling sarcoma (pseudosarcoma).

Cervical lymph node metastasis of laryngeal carcinoma are found in a good proportion of cases at the time of diagnosis.

NECK *(p. 530)*

NORMAL STRUCTURE *(p. 530)*

The neck is the region from where important structures like oesophagus, trachea, carotid arteries, great veins and nerve trunks pass down. Besides, the neck has structures such as carotid body, sympathetic ganglia, larynx, thyroid, parathyroids and lymph nodes.

I. Medial (Midline) Cervical Cysts *(p. 531)*

1. THYROGLOSSAL CYST. Thyroglossal cyst arises from the vestiges of thyroglossal duct that connects the foramen caecum at the base of the tongue with the normally located thyroid gland. The cyst is located in the midline, generally at the level of hyoid bone, and rarely at the base of the tongue.

M/E The cyst is lined by respiratory and/or stratified squamous epithelium.

2. MIDLINE DERMOID CYST. Dermoid cyst located in the midline of the neck occurs due to sequestration of dermal cells along the lines of closure of embryonic clefts. The cyst contains paste-like pultaceous material.

M/E It is lined by epidermis and may contain skin adnexal structures.

II. Lateral Cervical Cysts *(p. 531)*

1. BRANCHIAL (LYMPHOEPITHELIAL) CYST. Branchial or lymphoepithelial cyst arises from incomplete closure of 2nd or 3rd branchial clefts. The cyst is generally located anterior to the sternocleidomastoid muscle near the angle of the mandible.

M/E The cyst is lined by stratified squamous or respiratory epithelium, covering subepithelial lymphoid tissue aggregates or follicles with germinal centres.

2. PARATHYROID CYST. Parathyroid cyst is a lateral cyst of the neck usually located deep to the sternocleidomastoid muscle at the angle of the mandible.

ME Parathyroid cyst is lined by flattened cuboidal to low columnar epithelium and the cyst wall may contain any type of parathyroid cells.

3. CERVICAL THYMIC CYST. Cervical thymic cyst originates from cystic degeneration of Hassall's corpuscles.

M/E The cyst is lined by stratified squamous epithelium and the cyst wall may contain thymic structures.

4. CYSTIC HYGROMA. Cystic hygroma is a lateral swelling at the root of the neck, usually located behind the sternocleidomastoid muscle. It may be present congenitally or may manifest in the first 2 years of life. It is usually multilocular and may extend into the mediastinum and pectoral region.

M/E Cystic hygroma is a diffuse lymphangioma containing large cavernous spaces lined by endothelium and containing lymph fluid.

I. Primary Tumours *(p. 531)*

1. CAROTID BODY TUMOUR (CHEMODECTOMA, CAROTID BODY PARAGANGLIOMA). Carotid body tumour arises in the carotid bodies which are situated at the bifurcation of the common carotid arteries. Carotid bodies are normally part of the chemoreceptor system and the cells of this system are sensitive to changes in the pH and arterial oxygen tension and are also the storage site for catecholamines.

2. TORTICOLLIS (FIBROMATOSIS COLLI, WRY NECK). This is a deformity in which the head is bent to one side while the chin points to the other side. The deformity may occur as congenital torticollis or may be an acquired form. The *acquired form* may occur secondary to fracture dislocation of the cervical spine, Pott's disease of the cervical spine, scoliosis, spasm of the muscles of neck, exposure to chill causing myositis, and contracture following burns or wound healing.

3. MALIGNANT LYMPHOMAS. Various forms of non-Hodgkin's lymphomas and Hodgkin's disease occur in the cervical lymph nodes.

II. Secondary Tumours *(p. 532)*

Cervical lymph nodes are common site for metastases of a large number of carcinomas. These include: squamous cell carcinoma of the lips, mouth, tongue, larynx and oesophagus; transitional cell carcinoma of the pharynx and nasopharynx; thoracic and abdominal cancers such as of stomach, lungs, ovaries, uterus and testis.

Chapter Sixteen

■ **SELF ASSESSMENT**

1. **Chalazion is chronic inflammatory process involving:**
   A. Sebaceous gland of Zeis
   B. Apocrine gland of Moll
   C. Meibomian glands
   D. Eyelash follicle
2. **Proliferative retinopathy consists of the following lesions *except:***
   A. Capillary microaneurysms
   B. Neovascularisation of the retina at optic disc
   C. Vitreous haemorrhages
   D. Proliferation of astrocytes and fibrous tissue around blood vessels

3. **Hypertensive retinopathy has the following features** *except:*
   A. Flame-shaped haemorrhages in retinal nerve layer
   B. Arteriolosclerosis
   C. Vitreous haemorrhages
   D. Microaneurysm

4. **Mikulicz's syndrome is inflammatory enlargement of lacrimal and salivary glands which may occur with following conditions** *except:*
   A. Sjögren's syndrome   B. Sarcoidosis
   C. Tuberculosis   D. Lymphoma

5. **Sebaceous carcinoma occurs most commonly at:**
   A. Axilla   B. Groin
   C. Upper eyelid   D. Lower eyelid

6. **Following histologic type of uveal malignant melanoma has the worst prognosis:**
   A. Spindle A   B. Spindle B
   C. Epithelioid   D. Mixed

7. **The most common ocular metastatic tumour is from the following primary cancer:**
   A. Melanoma   B. Breast
   C. Epidermoid   D. Neuroblastoma

8. **Aural polyps are generally of the following type:**
   A. Allergic   B. Inflammatory
   C. Fungal   D. Neoplastic

9. **Cholesteatoma of the mastoid is categorised as a lesion of the following type:**
   A. Benign tumour   B. Malignant tumour
   C. Hamartoma   D. Inflammatory pseudotumour

10. **Rhinoscleroma of the nose is a lesion of the following type:**
    A. Benign tumour   B. Malignant tumour
    C. Hamartoma   D. Bacterial

11. **Wegener's granulomatosis generally produces lesions in the following tissues** *except:*
    A. Nose   B. Ears
    C. Lungs   D. Kidneys

12. **Nasopharyngeal angiofibroma has the following features** *except:*
    A. It is endemic in people of South-East Asia
    B. It occurs exclusively in adolescent males
    C. It is a benign nasopharyngeal tumour
    D. Testosterone hormone plays a role in its etiology

13. **Nasopharyngeal carcinoma has the following features** *except:*
    A. It is common cancer in South-East Asia
    B. It occurs in males exclusively
    C. EB virus plays a role in its etiology
    D. The prognosis is usually fatal

14. **Subaceous carcinoma is commonest tumour in the following location:**
    A. Upper eyelid   B. Lower eyelid
    C. External auditory canal   D. Lip

15. **Lateral cervical cysts of the neck include the following examples** *except:*
    A. Branchial cyst   B. Thyroglossal cyst
    C. Cervical thymic cyst   D. Parathyroid cyst

KEY

1 = C	2 = A	3 = C	4 = C
5 = C	6 = C	7 = B	8 = B
9 = D	10 = D	11 = B	12 = A
13 = B	14 = A	15 = B	

17

The Oral Cavity and Salivary Glands

ORAL SOFT TISSUES *(p. 533)*

NORMAL STRUCTURE *(p. 533)*

The mucous membrane of the mouth consists of squamous epithelium covering vascularised connective tissue. The epithelium is keratinised over the hard palate, lips and gingiva, while elsewhere it is non-keratinised. Mucous glands (minor salivary glands) are scattered throughout the oral mucosa.

DEVELOPMENTAL ANOMALIES *(p. 533)*

1. FACIAL CLEFTS. *Cleft upper lip (harelip) and cleft palate,* alone or in combination, are the commonest developmental anomalies of the face.

2. FORDYCE'S GRANULES. Fordyce's granules are symmetric, small, light yellow macular spots on the lips and buccal mucosa and represent collections of sebaceous glands.

3. LEUKOEDEMA. This is an asymptomatic condition occurring in children and is characterised by symmetric, grey-white areas on the buccal mucosa.

4. DEVELOPMENTAL DEFECTS OF THE TONGUE. These are:

i) Macroglossia is the enlargement of the tongue, usually due to lymphangioma or haemangioma, and sometimes due to amyloid tumour.

ii) Microglossia and aglossia are rare congenital anomalies representing small-sized and absence of tongue respectively.

iii) Fissured tongue (scrotal, furrowed or grooved tongue) is a genetically-determined condition characterised by numerous small furrows or grooves on the dorsum of the tongue.

iv) Bifid tongue is a rare condition occurring due to failure of the two lateral halves of the tongue to fuse in the midline.

v) Tongue tie occurs when the lingual fraenum is quite short, or when the fraenum is attached near the tongue tip.

vi) Hairy tongue is not a true developmental defect, but is mentioned here alongwith other similar conditions.

MUCOCUTANEOUS LESIONS *(p. 534)*

1. LICHEN PLANUS. Characteristically, oral lichen planus appears as interlacing network of whitening or keratosis on the buccal mucosa.

2. VESICULAR LESIONS. These are similar to skin lesions.

i) Pemphigus vulgaris. Vesicular oral lesions appear invariably in all cases at some time in the course of pemphigus vulgaris.

ii) Pemphigoid. Vesicles or bullae appear on oral mucosa as well as on conjunctiva in pemphigoid and are seen more often in older women.

iii) Erythema multiforme. Subepithelial vesicles may occur on the skin as well as mucosae.

iv) Stevens-Johnson syndrome is a rather fatal and severe form of erythema multiforme involving oral and other mucous membranes occurring following ingestion of sulfa drugs.

v) Epidermolysis bullosa is a hereditary condition having subepidermal bullae on the skin as well as has oral lesions.

INFLAMMATORY DISEASES *(p. 534)*

1. STOMATITIS. Inflammation of the mucous membrane of the mouth is called stomatitis. It can occur in the course of many different diseases.

i) Aphthous ulcers (Canker sores) is the commonest form of oral ulceration. The etiology is unknown but may be precipitated by emotional factors, stress, allergy, hormonal imbalance, nutritional deficiencies, gastrointestinal disturbances, trauma etc.

ii) Herpetic stomatitis is an acute disease occurring in infants and young children. It is the most common manifestation of primary infection with herpes simplex virus. The lesions are in the form of vesicles around the lips.

iii) Necrotising stomatitis (Noma or Cancrum oris) occurs more commonly in poorly-nourished children like in kwashiorkor; infectious diseases such as measles; immunodeficiencies and emotional stress.

iv) Mycotic infections. The common ones are:
- *Cervicofacial actinomycosis* is the commonest form of the disease developing at the angle of the mandible.
- *Candidiasis (moniliasis or thrush)* is caused by *Candida albicans* which is a commensal in the mouth. It appears as an opportunistic infection in immunocompromised host.

2. GLOSSITIS. Acute glossitis characterised by swollen papillae occurs in eruptions of measles and scarlet fever. In **chronic glossitis**, the tongue is raw and red without swollen papillae and is seen in malnutrition such as in pellagra, ariboflavinosis and niacin deficiency.

3. SYPHILITIC LESIONS. Oral lesions may occur in primary, secondary, tertiary and congenital syphilis.
i) Extragenital chancre of *primary syphilis* occurs most commonly on the lips.
ii) Secondary syphilis shows maculopapular eruptions and mucous patches in the mouth.
iii) In the *tertiary syphilis*, gummas or diffuse fibrosis may be seen on the hard palate and tongue.
iv) Oral lesions of the *congenital syphilis* are fissures at the angles of mouth and characteristic peg-shaped notched Hutchinson's incisors.

4. TUBERCULOUS LESIONS. Involvement of the mouth in tuberculosis is rare.

5. HIV INFECTION. HIV infection of low grade as well as full-blown acquired immunodeficiency syndrome (AIDS) are associated with oral manifestations such as opportunistic infections, malignancy, hairy leukoplakia and others.

PIGMENTARY LESIONS *(p. 535)*

Oral and labial melanotic pigmentation may be observed in certain systemic and metabolic disorders such as Addison's disease, Albright syndrome, Peutz-Jeghers syndrome and haemochromatosis. All types of pigmented naevi as well as malignant melanoma can also occur in oral cavity.

TUMOURS AND TUMOUR-LIKE LESIONS *(p. 535)*

A. TUMOUR-LIKE LESIONS *(p. 535)*

A number of proliferative lesions arising from the oral tissues are tumour-like masses which clinically may resemble neoplasms.

1. FIBROUS GROWTHS. Fibrous growths of the oral soft tissues are very common. These are not true tumours (unlike intraoral fibroma and papilloma), but are instead inflammatory or irritative in origin. A few common varieties are as under:

(i) Fibroepithelial polyps, (ii) Fibrous epulis, and (iii) Denture hyperplasia.

2. PYOGENIC GRANULOMA. This is an elevated, bright red swelling of variable size occurring on the lips, tongue, buccal mucosa and gingiva. It is a vasoproliferative inflammatory lesion. *Pregnancy tumour* is a variant of pyogenic granuloma.

3. MUCOCELE. Also called mucous cyst, it is a cystic dilatation of the mucous glands of the oral mucosa.

4. RANULA. It is a large mucocele located on the floor of the mouth. The cyst is lined by true epithelial lining.

5. DERMOID CYST. This tumour-like mass in the floor of the mouth represents a developmental malformation. The cyst is lined by stratified squamous epithelium. The cyst wall contains sebaceous glands, sweat glands, hair follicles and other mature tissues.

B. BENIGN TUMOURS *(p. 536)*

1. SQUAMOUS PAPILLOMA. Papilloma can occur anywhere in the mouth and has the usual papillary or finger-like projections.

2. HAEMANGIOMA. Haemangioma can occur anywhere in the mouth; when it occurs on tongue it may cause macroglossia. It is most commonly capillary type, although cavernous and mixed types may also occur.

3. LYMPHANGIOMA. Lymphangioma may develop most commonly on the tongue producing macroglossia; on the lips producing macrocheilia, and on the cheek. *Cystic hygroma* is a special variety of lymphangioma occurring in children on the lateral side of neck.

4. FIBROMA. The true fibroma of mouth is relatively uncommon benign tumour and is more often a tumour-like lesion (discussed above).

5. FIBROMATOSIS GINGIVAE. This is a fibrous overgrowth of unknown etiology involving the entire gingiva. Sometimes the fibrous overgrowth is so much that the teeth are covered by fibrous tissue.

6. TUMOURS OF MINOR SALIVARY GLANDS. Minor salivary glands present in the oral cavity may sometimes be the site of origin of salivary tumours similar to those seen in the major salivary glands. Pleomorphic adenoma is a common example.

7. GRANULAR CELL MYOBLASTOMA. This is an unusual oral benign tumour, seen more often in the tongue.

C. ORAL LEUKOPLAKIA (WHITE LESIONS) *(p. 536)*

DEFINITION. Leukoplakia *(white plaque)* may be clinically defined as a white patch or plaque on the oral mucosa, exceeding 5 mm in diameter, which cannot be rubbed off nor can be classified into any other diagnosable disease. However, from the pathologist's point of view, the term 'leukoplakia' is reserved for epithelial thickening which may range from completely benign to atypical and to premalignant cellular changes.

INCIDENCE. It occurs more frequently in males than females. The lesions may be of variable size and appearance. The sites of predilection, in descending order of frequency, are: cheek mucosa, angles of mouth, alveolar mucosa, tongue, lip, hard and soft palate, and floor of the mouth. In about 4-6% cases of leukoplakia, carcinomatous change is reported.

ETIOLOGY. The etiological factors are similar to those suggested for carcinoma of the oral mucosa. *It has the strongest association with the use of tobacco in various forms* e.g. in heavy smokers (especially in pipe and cigar smokers) and improves when smoking is discontinued, and in those who chew tobacco as in paan, paan masaala, zarda, gutka etc. The condition is also known by other names such as *smokers keratosis* and *stomatitis nicotina*. Other etiological factors implicated are chronic friction such as with ill-fitting dentures or jagged teeth, and local irritants like excessive consumption of alcohol and very hot and spicy foods and beverages.

G/A The lesions of leukoplakia may appear white, whitish-yellow, or red-velvety of more than 5 mm diameter and variable in appearance.

M/E Leukoplakia is of 2 types:

1. Hyperkeratotic type. This is characterised by an orderly and regular hyperplasia of squamous epithelium with hyperkeratosis on the surface.

2. Dysplastic type. When the changes such as irregular stratification of the epithelium, focal areas of increased and abnormal mitotic figures, hyperchromatism, pleomorphism, loss of polarity and individual cell keratinisation are present, the lesion is considered as epithelial dysplasia. If the epithelial dysplasia is extensive so as to involve the entire thickness of the epithelium, the lesion is called carcinoma *in situ* which may progress to invasive carcinoma.

Squamous Cell (Epidermoid) Carcinoma *(p. 537)*

Oral cancer is a disease with very poor prognosis because it is not recognised and treated when small and early.

INCIDENCE. Squamous cell (epidermoid) carcinoma comprises 90% of all oral malignant tumours and 5% of all human malignancies. The peak incidence in the UK and the USA is from 55 to 75 years of age, whereas in India it is from 40 to 45 years of age. Oral cancer is a very frequent malignancy in India, Sri Lanka and some Eastern countries, probably related to habits of betel-nut chewing and reversed smoking. These sites, in descending order of frequency, are: the lips (more commonly lower), tongue, anterior floor of mouth, buccal mucosa in the region of alveolar lingual sulcus, and palate.

ETIOLOGY. A number of etiological factors have been implicated:

Strong association:

i) Tobacco smoking and tobacco chewing causing leukoplakia is the most important factor as discussed above.

ii) Chronic alcohol consumption.

iii) Human papilloma virus infection, particularly HPV 16, 18 and 33 types.

Weak association:

i) Chronic irritation from ill-fitting denture or jagged teeth.

ii) Submucosal fibrosis as seen in Indians consuming excess of chillies.

iii) Poor orodental hygiene.

iv) Nutritional deficiencies.

v) Exposure to sunlight (in relation to lip cancer).

vi) Exposure to radiation.

vii) Plummer-Vinson syndrome, characterised by atrophy of the upper alimentary tract.

G/A Squamous cell carcinoma of oral cavity may have the following types:

i) *Ulcerative type*—is the most frequent type and is characterised by indurated ulcer and firm everted or rolled edges.

ii) *Papillary or verrucous type*—is soft and wartlike growth.

iii) *Nodular type*—appears as a firm, slow growing submucosal nodule.

iv) *Scirrhous type*—is characterised by infiltration into deeper structures.

All these types may appear on a background of leukoplakia or erythroplasia of the oral mucosa. Enlarged cervical lymph nodes may sometimes be present.

M/E Squamous cell carcinoma ranges from well-differentiated keratinising carcinoma to highly-undifferentiated neoplasm. Changes of epithelial dysplasia are often present in the surrounding areas of the lesion.

Carcinoma of the lip has a more favourable prognosis due to visible and easily accessible location and less frequent metastasis to the regional lymph nodes. *Verrucous carcinoma,* on the other hand, is composed of very well-differentiated squamous epithelium with minimal atypia and hence has very good prognosis.

TEETH AND PERIODONTAL TISSUES *(p. 539)*

NORMAL STRUCTURE *(p. 539)*

The teeth are normally composed of 3 calcified tissues, namely: enamel, dentine and cementum; and the pulp composed of connective tissue. The teeth are surrounded by the portion of oral mucosa called the gingiva or gum.

Enamel is the outer covering of teeth composed almost entirely of inorganic material (as in bone) which can be demonstrated in ground sections only as it is lost in decalcified section.

Dentine lies under the enamel and comprises most of the tooth substance. It is composed of organic material in the form of collagen fibrils as well as inorganic material in the form of calcium phosphates as in bone.

Cementum is the portion of tooth which covers the dentine at the root of tooth and is the site where periodontal ligament is attached.

Dental pulp is inner to dentine and occupies the pulp cavity and root canal. It consists of connective tissue, blood vessels and nerves.

DENTAL CARIES *(p. 539)*

Dental caries is the most common disease of dental tissues, causing destruction of the calcified tissues of the teeth.

ETIOPATHOGENESIS. Dental caries is essentially a disease of modern society, associated with diet containing high proportion of refined carbohydrates. Enamel is largely composed of inorganic material which virtually disintegrates. Dentine contains organic material also which is left after decalcification. Bacteria present in the oral cavity cause proteolysis of the remaining organic material of dentine so that the process of destruction is complete.

Caries occurs chiefly in the areas of pits and fissures, mainly of the molars and premolars, where food retention occurs, and in the cervical part of the tooth.

G/A The earliest change is the appearance of a small, chalky-white spot on the enamel which subsequently enlarges and often becomes yellow or brown and breaks down to form carious cavity.

M/E Inflammation (pulpitis) and necrosis of pulp take place. There is evidence of reaction of the tooth to the carious process in the form of *secondary dentine,* which is a layer of odontoblasts laid down under the original dentine.

SEQUELAE OF CARIES. Common sequelae are as under:

1. **Pulpitis.** Pulpitis may be acute or chronic.

■ *Acute pulpitis* is accompanied by severe pain which may be continuous, throbbing or dull, and is accentuated by heat or cold. It is often accompanied by mild fever and leucocytosis.

■ *Chronic pulpitis* occurs when pulp is exposed widely. It is often not associated with pain. Chronically inflamed pulp tissue may protrude through the cavity forming polyp of the pulp.

2. Apical granuloma. Pulpitis may lead to spread of infection through the apical foramen into the tissues surrounding the root of the tooth.

3. Apical abscess. An apical granuloma or acute pulpitis may develop into apical abscess. Acute abscess is very painful, while pus in chronic abscess may escape through root canal and cause further complications like osteomyelitis, cellulitis, cerebral abscess.

PERIODONTAL DISEASE *(p. 540)*

Chronic inflammation and degeneration of the supporting tissues of teeth resulting in teeth loss is a common condition.

The inflammatory periodontal disease affects adults more commonly. Pregnancy, puberty and use of drugs like dilantin are also associated with periodontal disease more often. The disease begins as *chronic marginal gingivitis,* secondary to bacterial plaques around the teeth such as due to calculus (tartar) on the tooth surface.

M/E Chronic marginal gingivitis is characterised by heavy chronic inflammatory cell infiltrate, destruction of collagen, and epithelial hyperplasia so as to line the pocket. Untreated chronic marginal gingivitis slowly progresses to *chronic periodontitis* or *pyorrhoea.*

EPITHELIAL CYSTS OF JAW *(p. 541)*

Radicular Cyst *(p. 541)*

Radicular cyst, also called as apical, periodontal or simply dental cyst, is the most common cyst originating from the dental tissues. It arises consequent to inflammation following destruction of dental pulp such as in dental caries, pulpitis, and apical granuloma. Most often, radicular cyst is observed at the apex of an erupted tooth and sometimes contains thick pultaceous material.

M/E The radicular cyst is lined by nonkeratinised squamous epithelium. Epithelial rete processes may penetrate the underlying connective tissues. Radicular cyst of maxilla may be lined by respiratory epithelium. The cyst wall is fibrous and contains chronic inflammatory cells (lymphocytes, plasma cells with Russell bodies and macrophages), hyaline bodies and deposits of cholesterol crystals which may be associated with foreign body giant cells.

DENTIGEROUS (FOLLICULAR) CYST *(p. 541)*

Dentigerous cyst arises from enamel of an unerupted tooth. The mandibular third molars and the maxillary canines are most often involved. Dentigerous cysts are less common than radicular cysts and occur more commonly in children and young individuals.

M/E Dentigerous cyst is composed of a thin fibrous tissue wall lined by stratified squamous epithelium. Thus, the cyst may resemble radicular cyst, except that chronic inflammatory changes so characteristic of radicular cyst, are usually absent in dentigerous cyst.

ODONTOGENIC TUMOURS *(p. 542)*

Odontogenic tumours are a group of uncommon lesions of jaw derived from the odontogenic apparatus. These tumours are usually benign but some have malignant counterparts.

Ameloblastoma *(p. 542)*

Ameloblastoma is the most common benign but locally invasive epithelial odontogenic tumour. It is commonest in the 3rd to 5th decades of life.

Preferential sites are the mandible in the molar-ramus area and the maxilla. The tumour originates from dental epithelium of the enamel itself or its epithelial residues. Sometimes, the tumour may arise from the epithelial lining of a dentigerous cyst or from basal layer of oral mucosa. Radiologically, typical picture is of a multilocular destruction of bone.

G/A The tumour is greyish-white, usually solid, sometimes cystic, replacing and expanding the affected bone.

M/E Ameloblastoma can show different patterns:

i) Follicular pattern is the most common. The tumour consists of follicles of variable size and shape and separated from each other by fibrous tissue. The structure of follicles is similar to that of enamel organ consisting of central area of stellate cells resembling stellate reticulum.

ii) Plexiform pattern is the next common pattern after follicular pattern. The tumour epithelium is seen to form irregular plexiform masses or network of strands.

iii) Acanthomatous pattern is squamous metaplasia within the islands of tumour cells.

iv) Basal cell pattern of ameloblastoma is similar to basal cell carcinoma of the skin.

v) Granular cell pattern is characterised by appearance of acidophilic granularity in the cytoplasm of tumour cells.

Odontogenic Adenomatoid Tumour (Adeno-ameloblastoma) *(p. 543)*

This is a benign tumour seen more frequently in females in their 2nd decade of life. The tumour is commonly associated with an unerupted tooth and thus closely resembles dentigerous cyst radiologically.

M/E The lesion has extensive cyst formations. The wall of cyst contains scanty fibrous connective tissue in which are present characteristic tubule-like structures composed of epithelial cells and hence the name 'adenomatoid' (gland-like).

Odontogenic Carcinoma *(p. 544)*

i)   *Malignant ameloblastoma* is the term used for the uncommon metastasising ameloblastoma.

ii) *Ameloblastic carcinoma* is the term employed for the ameloblastic tumour having cytologic features of malignancy in the primary tumour.

iii) *Primary intraosseous carcinoma* may develop within the jaw from the rests of odontogenic epithelium.

iv) Rarely, carcinomas may arise from the odontogenic epithelium lining the *odontogenic cysts.*

SALIVARY GLANDS *(p. 544)*

NORMAL STRUCTURE *(p. 544)*

There are two main groups of salivary glands—major and minor. The major salivary glands are the three paired glands: parotid, submandibular and sublingual. The minor salivary glands are numerous and widely distributed in the mucosa of oral cavity.

M/E The salivary glands are tubuloalveolar glands and may contain mucous cells, serous cells, or both. The parotid gland is purely serous. The submandibular gland is mixed type but is predominantly serous, whereas the sublingual gland is predominantly mucous type.

SALIVARY FLOW DISTURBANCES *(p. 544)*

SIALORRHOEA (PTYALISM). Increased flow of saliva is termed sialorrhoea or ptyalism. It occurs commonly due to: stomatitis, teething, mentally retarded state, schizophrenia, neurological disturbances, increased gastric secretion and sialosis (i.e. uniform, symmetric, painless hypertrophy of salivary glands).

XEROSTOMIA. Decreased salivary flow is termed xerostomia. It is associated with the following conditions: Sjögren's syndrome, sarcoidosis, mumps parotitis, Mikulicz's syndrome, megaloblastic anaemia, dehydration, drug intake (e.g. antihistamines, antihypertensives, antidepressants).

SIALADENITIS *(p. 544)*

Inflammation of salivary glands, sialadenitis, may be acute or chronic, the latter being more common. It can occur due to the following causes:

1. Viral infections. The most common inflammatory lesion of the salivary glands particularly of the parotid glands, is mumps occurring in children of school-age. It is characterised by triad of pathological involvement—*epidemic parotitis (mumps), orchitis-oophoritis, and pancreatitis.* Involvement of testis and pancreas may lead to their atrophy.

2. Bacterial and mycotic infections. Bacterial infections may cause acute sialadenitis more often. Sometimes there are recurrent attacks of acute parotitis when parotitis becomes chronic.

i) *Acute sialadenitis.* The causes are: a) Acute infectious fevers. b) Acute postoperative parotitis (ascent of microorganisms up to the parotid duct from the mouth). c) General debility. d) Old age. e) Dehydration.

ii) *Chronic sialadenitis.* It may result from the following:

a) Recurrent obstructive type. Recurrent obstruction due to calculi (sialolithiasis), stricture, surgery, injury etc may cause repeated attacks of acute sialadenitis by ascending infection and then chronicity.

b) Recurrent non-obstructive type. Recurrent mild ascending infection of the parotid gland may occur due to non-obstructive causes which reduce salivary secretion like due to intake of drugs causing hyposalivation (e.g. antihistamines, antihypertensives, antidepressants), effect of irradiation and congenital malformations of the duct system.

c) Chronic inflammatory diseases. Tuberculosis, actinomycosis and other mycoses may rarely occur in the salivary glands.

3. Autoimmune disease. Two such conditions are:

i) *Sjögren's syndrome* characterised by triad of dry eyes (keratoconjunctivitis sicca), dry mouth (xerostomia) and rheumatoid arthritis.

ii) *Mikulicz's syndrome* is the combination of inflammatory enlargement of salivary and lacrimal glands with xerostomia.

G/A Irrespective of the underlying etiology of sialadenitis, there is swelling of the affected salivary gland, usually restricted by the fibrous capsule.

M/E Acute viral sialadenitis in mumps shows swelling and cytoplasmic vacuolation of the acinar epithelial cells and degenerative changes in the ductal epithelium. *Chronic and recurrent sialadenitis* is characterised by increased lymphoid tissue in the interstitium, progressive loss of secretory tissue and replacement by fibrosis.

TUMOURS OF SALIVARY GLANDS *(p. 545)*

The major as well as minor salivary glands can give rise to a variety of benign and malignant tumours (Table 17.1). The major glands, particularly the parotid

TABLE 17.1: Classification of Salivary Gland Tumours.

A. BENIGN

1. Adenomas

   i) Pleomorphic adenoma (Mixed tumour) (65-80%)

   ii) Monomorphic adenoma

      (a) Warthin's tumour (Papillary cystadenoma lymphomatosum, Adenolymphoma) (5-10%)

      (b) Oxyphil adenoma (Oncocytomas) (< 1%)

      (c) Other types (Myoepithelioma, Basal cell adenoma, Clear cell adenoma) (uncommon)

2. Mesenchymal tumours (rare)

B. MALIGNANT

1. Mucoepidermoid carcinoma (5-10%)
2. Malignant mixed tumour

   i) Carcinoma in pleomorphic adenoma (2%)

   ii) Carcinosarcoma (rare)

   iii) Metastasising mixed salivary tumour (rare)

3. Adenoid cystic carcinoma (cylindroma) (3-10%)
4. Acinic cell carcinoma (2-3%)
5. Adenocarcinoma (l-3%)
6. Epidermoid carcinoma (l-3%)
7. Undifferentiated carcinoma (<I%)
8. Miscellaneous (rare)

glands (85%), are the most common sites. Majority of the parotid gland tumour (65-85%) are benign, while in the other major and minor salivary glands 35-50% of the tumours are malignant.

Pleomorphic Adenoma (Mixed Salivary Tumour) *(p. 546)*

This is the most common tumour of major (60-75%) and minor (50%) salivary glands. Pleomorphic adenoma is the commonest tumour in the parotid gland and occurs less often in other major and minor salivary glands. The tumour is commoner in women and is seen more frequently in 3rd to 5th decades of life. The tumour is solitary, smooth-surfaced but sometimes nodular, painless and slow-growing.

G/A Pleomorphic adenoma is a circumscribed, pseudoencapsulated, rounded, at times multilobulated, firm mass, 2-5 cm in diameter, with bosselated surface. The cut surface is grey-white and bluish, variegated, semitranslucent, usually solid but occasionally may show small cystic spaces.

M/E The pleomorphic adenoma is characterised by pleomorphic or 'mixed' appearance in which there are epithelial elements present in a matrix of mucoid, myxoid and chondroid tissue:

■ **The epithelial component** may form various patterns like ducts, acini, tubules, sheets and strands of cells of ductal or myoepithelial origin. The ductal cells are cuboidal or columnar, and the underlying myoepithelial cells may be polygonal or spindle-shaped resembling smooth muscle cells.

■ **The mesenchymal elements** are present as loose connective tissue and as myxoid, mucoid and chondroid matrix, which simulates cartilage *(pseudocartilage)* but is actually connective tissue mucin.

PROGNOSIS. Pleomorphic adenoma is notorious for recurrences, sometimes after many years. The main factors responsible for the tendency to recur are incomplete surgical removal due to proximity to the facial nerve, multiple foci of tumour, pseudoencapsulation, and implantation in the surgical field.

Monomorphic Adenomas *(p. 546)*

a) WARTHIN'S TUMOUR (PAPILLARY CYSTADENOMA LYMPHO-MATOSUM, ADENOLYMPHOMA). It is a benign tumour of the parotid gland comprising about 8% of all parotid neoplasms, seen more commonly in men from 4th to 7th decades of life. Rarely, it may arise in the submandibular gland or in minor salivary glands.

G/A The tumour is encapsulated, round or oval with smooth surface. The cut surface shows characteristic slit-like or cystic spaces, containing milky fluid and having papillary projections.

M/E The tumour shows 2 components:
■ **The epithelial parenchyma** is composed of glandular and cystic structures having papillary arrangement and lined by characteristic eosinophilic epithelium.
■ **The lymphoid stroma** is present under the epithelium in the form of prominent lymphoid tissue, often with germinal centres.

b) OXYPHIL ADENOMA (ONCOCYTOMA). It is a benign slow-growing tumour of the major salivary glands. The tumour consists of parallel sheets, acini or tubules of large cells with glandular eosinophilic cytoplasm (oncocytes).

c) OTHER TYPES OF MONOMORPHIC ADENOMAS. Uncommon ones are:
i) Myoepithelioma is an adenoma composed exclusively of myoepithelial cells which may be arranged in tubular, alveolar or trabecular pattern.
ii) Basal cell adenoma is characterised by the type and arrangement of cells resembling basal cell carcinoma of the skin.
iii) Clear cell adenoma has spindle-shaped or polyhedral cells with clear cytoplasm.

Mucoepidermoid Carcinoma *(p. 548)*

The status of 'mucoepidermoid tumour' as an intermediate grade tumour in the previous classification has undergone upgradation to full-fledged mucoepidermoid carcinoma now having the following peculiar features:
■ It is the most *common malignant* salivary gland tumour (both in the major and minor glands).
■ The *parotid gland* amongst the major salivary glands and the minor salivary glands in the *palate* are the most common sites.
■ The common age group affected is 30-60 years but it is also the most common malignant salivary gland tumour affecting *children and adolescents*.
■ It is the most common example of *radiation-induced* malignant tumour, especially therapeutic radiation.

G/A The tumour is usually circumscribed but not encapsulated. It varies in size from 1 to 4 cm.

M/E The tumour is classified into low, intermediate and high grade depending upon the degree of differentiation and tumour invasiveness. The tumour is composed of combination of epidermoid cells and mucus-secreting cells (as the name implies) as also cells with intermediate differentiation between these two cell types and clear cells.

Malignant Mixed Tumour *(p. 548)*

Malignant mixed tumour comprises three distinct clinicopathologic entities:
■ Carcinoma arising in benign mixed salivary gland tumour (carcinoma *ex* pleomorphic adenoma);
■ Carcinosarcoma; and
■ Metastasising mixed salivary tumour.
    Carcinoma *ex* pleomorphic adenoma is more common while the other two are rare tumours. Approximately 2 to 5% of pleomorphic adenomas reveal areas of frank malignancy.

G/A The tumour is poorly-circumscribed with irregular infiltrating margin.

M/E Besides the typical appearance of pleomorphic adenoma, malignant areas show cytologic features of carcinoma such as anaplasia, nuclear hyperchromatism, large nucleolisation, mitoses and evidence of invasive growth.

Adenoid Cystic Carcinoma (Cylindroma) (p. 548)

This is a highly malignant tumour due to its typical infiltrative nature, especially along the nerve sheaths. Adenoid cystic carcinoma is histologically characterised by cribriform appearance i.e. the epithelial tumour cells of duct-lining and myoepithelial cells are arranged in duct-like structures or masses of cells, having typical fenestrations or cyst-like spaces and hence the name 'adenoid cystic'.

Acinic Cell Carcinoma (p. 548)

This is a rare tumour composed of acinic cells resembling serous cells of normal salivary gland. These cells are arranged in sheets or acini and have characteristic basophilic granular cytoplasm. The degree of atypia may vary from a benign cytologic appearance to cellular features of malignancy.

Adenocarcinoma (p. 549)

Adenocarcinoma of the salivary gland does not differ from adenocarcinoma elsewhere in the body. It may have some variants such as mucoid adeno-carcinoma, clear-cell adenocarcinoma and papillary cystadenocarcinoma.

Epidermoid Carcinoma (p. 549)

This rare tumour has features of squamous cell carcinoma with keratin formation and has intercellular bridges.

Undifferentiated Carcinoma (p. 549)

This highly malignant tumour consists of anaplastic epithelial cells which are too poorly differentiated to be placed in any other known category.

Miscellaneous Malignant Tumours (p. 549)

Some rare malignant tumour of epithelial and mesenchymal origin are melanoma, sebaceous carcinoma, undifferentiated carcinoma, lymphoma, fibrosarcoma and leiomyosarcoma and are similar in morphology to such tumours elsewhere in the body.

Chapter Seventeen

■ SELF ASSESSMENT

1. **The following tissues are lined by keratinised stratified squa-mous epithelium *except:***
   A. Hard palate
   B. Soft palate
   C. Lips
   D. Gingiva
2. **Fordyce's granules are composed of the following:**
   A. Sebaceous glands
   B. Sweat glands
   C. Fibrous tissue
   D. Epithelial hyperplasia
3. **Patients of AIDS have the following type of oral leukoplakia:**
   A. Speckled
   B. Nodular
   C. Hairy
   D. Wrinkled
4. **The most common gross pattern of carcinoma of oral cavity is:**
   A. Papillary
   B. Nodular
   C. Ulcerative
   D. Scirrhous

5. **The following type of dental cyst is more often associated with development of ameloblastoma:**
   A. Radicular cyst
   B. Dentigerous cyst
   C. Primordial cyst
   D. Gingival cyst

6. **Majority of salivary gland tumours originate from:**
   A. Acini
   B. Ducts
   C. Mesenchyme
   D. Combination of various tissues

7. **The pseudocartilage or matrix in mixed salivary tumour is a product of:**
   A. Connective tissue mucin
   B. Ductal epithelial cell origin
   C. Myoepithelial cell origin
   D. Combination of all mucins

8. **Most common malignant salivary gland tumour is:**
   A. Malignant mixed tumour
   B. Mucoepidermoid carcinoma
   C. Adenoid cyst carcinoma
   D. Adenocarcinoma

9. **The most common malignant salivary gland tumour in children is:**
   A. Acinic cell tumour
   B. Adenoid cystic carcinoma
   C. Mucoepidermoid carcinoma
   D. Adenocarcinoma

10. **Malignant salivary gland tumour that commonly spreads along the nerves is:**
    A. Malignant mixed salivary tumour
    B. Mucoepidermoid carcinoma
    C. Acinic cell carcinoma
    D. Adenoid cystic carcinoma

KEY

1 = B	2 = A	3 = C	4 = C
5 = B	6 = B	7 = C	8 = B
9 = C	10 = D		

18

The Gastrointestinal Tract

OESOPHAGUS *(p. 550)*

NORMAL STRUCTURE *(p. 550)*

The oesophagus is a muscular tube extending from the pharynx to the stomach. In an adult, this distance measures 25 cm. However, from the clinical point of view, the distance from the incisor teeth to the gastro-oesophageal junction is about 40 cm.

M/E The wall of the oesophagus consists of following layers.

■ The **mucosa** is composed of non-keratinising stratified squamous epithelium overlying lamina propria. At the lower end of the oesophagus, there is sudden change from stratified squamous epithelium to mucin-secreting columnar epithelium for a distance of 0.5 to 1.5 cm; this is called the *junctional mucosa.*

■ The **submucosa** consists of loose connective tissue with sprinkling of lymphocytes, plasma cells, and occasional eosinophil and mast cell.

■ The **muscularis propria** is composed of 2 layers of smooth muscle—an inner circular coat and an outer longitudinal coat.

■ The **adventitia/serosa** is the outer covering of oesophagus. Serosa is present in intra-abdominal part of oesophagus only.

ANOMALIES AND DYSFUNCTIONS *(p. 551)*

Oesophageal Atresia and Tracheo-oesophageal Fistula *(p. 551)*

In about 85% of cases, congenital atresia of the oesophagus is associated with tracheo-oesophageal fistula, usually at the level of tracheal bifurcation. Morphologically, the condition is recognised by cord-like non-canalised segment of oesophagus having blind pouch at both ends.

Achalasia (Cardiospasm) *(p. 551)*

Achalasia of the oesophagus is a neuromuscular dysfunction due to which the cardiac sphincter fails to relax during swallowing and results in progressive dysphagia and dilatation of the oesophagus *(mega-oesophagus).*

ETIOLOGY. The exact etiology is not known. It may be congenital. Emotional stress has been believed to contribute to the onset of the disease. Chagas' disease, an epidemic parasitosis with *Trypansoma cruzi* has also been found to be associated with alterations of Auerbach's plexus.

G/A There is dilatation above the short contracted terminal segment of the oesophagus. Muscularis propria of the wall may be of normal thickness, hypertrophied as a result of obstruction, or thinned out due to dilatation.

Hiatus Hernia *(p. 551)*

Hiatus hernia is the herniation or protrusion of the stomach through the oesophageal hiatus of the diaphragm. Oesophageal hiatal hernia is the cause of diaphragmatic hernia in 98% of cases. In symptomatic cases, especially the elderly women, the clinical features are heartburn (retrosternal burning sensation) and regurgitation of gastric juice into the mouth.

ETIOLOGY. The basic defect is the failure of the muscle fibres of the diaphragm that form the margin of the oesophageal hiatus. This occurs due to shortening of the oesophagus which may be congenital or acquired.

i) **Congenitally short oesophagus** may be the cause of hiatus hernia in a small proportion of cases.

ii) More commonly, it is **acquired** due to secondary factors which cause fibrous scarring of the oesophagus e.g. a) Degeneration of muscle due to aging. b) Increased intra-abdominal pressure such as in pregnancy, abdominal tumours etc. c) Recurrent oesophageal regurgitation and spasm causing inflammation and fibrosis. d) Increase in fatty tissue in obese people.

G/A Three patterns are observed:

i) **Sliding or oesophago-gastric hernia** is the most common, occurring in 85% of cases. The herniated part of the stomach appears as supra-diaphragmatic bell due to sliding up on both sides of the oesophagus.

ii) **Rolling or para-oesophageal hernia** is seen in 10% of cases. This is a true hernia in which cardiac end of the stomach rolls up para-oesophageally, producing an intrathoracic sac.

iii) **Mixed or transitional hernia** constitutes the remaining 5% cases in which there is combination of sliding and rolling hiatus hernia.

Oesophageal Diverticula *(p. 552)*

Diverticula are the outpouchings of oesophageal wall at the point of weakness. They may be congenital or acquired.

Congenital diverticula occur either at the upper end of the oesophagus or at the bifurcation of trachea.

Acquired diverticula may be of 2 types:

a) Pulsion (Zenker's) type—is seen in the region of hypopharynx and occurs due to oesophageal obstruction such as due to chronic oesophagitis, carcinoma etc.

b) Traction type—occurs in the lower third of oesophagus from contraction of fibrous tissue such as from pleural adhesions, scar tissue of healed tuberculous lesions in the hilum, silicosis etc.

Complications of diverticula include obstruction, infection, perforation, haemorrhage and carcinoma.

Oesophageal Webs and Rings *(p. 552)*

WEBS. Those located in the upper oesophagus, seen more commonly in adult women, and associated with dysphagia, iron deficiency anaemia and chronic atrophic glossitis (Plummer-Vinson syndrome) are called 'webs'.

RINGS. Those located in the lower oesophagus, not associated with iron-deficiency anaemia, nor occurring in women alone, are referred to as 'Schatzki's rings'.

HAEMATEMESIS OF OESOPHAGEAL ORIGIN *(p. 552)*

1. **OESOPHAGEAL VARICES.** Oesophageal varices are tortuous, dilated and engorged oesophageal veins, seen along the longitudinal axis of oesophagus. They occur as a result of elevated pressure in the portal venous system, most commonly in cirrhosis of the liver. Less common causes are: portal vein thrombosis, hepatic vein thrombosis (Budd-Chiari syndrome) and pylephlebitis.

2. **MALLORY-WEISS SYNDROME.** In this condition, there is lacerations of mucosa at the gastro-oesophageal junction following minor trauma such as by vomiting, retching or vigorous coughing.

3. RUPTURE OF THE OESOPHAGUS. Rupture of the oesophagus may occur following trauma, during oesophagoscopy, indirect injury (e.g. due to sudden acceleration and deceleration of the body) and spontaneous rupture.

4. OTHER CAUSES. i) Bursting of aortic aneurysm. ii) Vascular erosion by malignant growth. iii) Hiatus hernia. iv) Oesophageal cancer. v) Purpuras. vi) Haemophilia.

INFLAMMATORY LESIONS *(p. 553)*

Reflux (Peptic) Oesophagitis *(p. 553)*

Reflux of the gastric juice is the commonest cause of oesophagitis.

PATHOGENESIS. Gastro-oesophageal reflux, to an extent, may occur in normal healthy individuals after meals and in early pregnancy. However, in some clinical conditions, the gastro-oesophageal reflux is excessive, resulting in inflammation of the lower oesophagus. These conditions are as under:

i) Sliding hiatus hernia, ii) chronic gastric and duodenal ulcers, iii) nasogastric intubation, iv) persistent vomiting, v) surgical vagotomy, vi) neuropathy in alcoholics, diabetics, and vii) oesophago-gastrostomy.

Endoscopically, the demarcation between normal squamous and columnar epithelium at the junctional mucosa is lost. In advanced cases, there are features of chronic disease such as nodularity, strictures, ulcerations and erosions.

M/E The reflux changes in the distal oesophagus include basal cell hyperplasia and deep elongation of the papillae touching close to the surface epithelium.

Barrett's Oesophagus *(p. 553)*

This is a condition in which, following reflux oesophagitis, stratified squamous epithelium of the lower oesophagus is replaced by columnar epithelium (columnar metaplasia). Barrett's oesophagus is a premalignant condition evolving sequentially from Barrett's epithelium → dysplasia → carcinoma *in situ* → invasive adenocarcinoma.

Endoscopically, the affected area is red and velvety. Hiatus hernia and peptic ulcer at squamo-columnar junction (Barrett's ulcer) are frequently associated.

M/E The most common finding is the replacement of squamous epithelium by metaplastic columnar cells. Barrett's oesophagus may be composed of

- intestinal epithelium;
- fundic gastric glands; or
- cardiac mucous glands.

Other cells present in the glands may be Paneth cells, goblet cells, chief cells, parietal cells, mucus-secreting cells and endocrine cells.

Dysplastic changes of the columnar epithelium or glands may be present. Long-standing cases of Barrett's oesophagus have 5-8% risk of developing adenocarcinoma of the oesophagus.

Infective Oesophagitis *(p. 554)*

A number of opportunistic infections in immunosuppressed individuals can cause oesophagitis e.g. i) Candida (Monilial) oesophagitis. ii) Herpes simplex (Herpetic oesophagitis). iii) Cytomegalovirus. iv) Tuberculosis.

CARCINOMA OF OESOPHAGUS *(p. 554)*

Carcinoma of the oesophagus is diagnosed late, after symptomatic oesophageal obstruction (dysphagia) has developed and the tumour has transgressed the anatomical limits of the organ.

Chapter Eighteen

ETIOLOGY. A number of conditions and factors have been implicated:

1. Diet and personal habits: i) Heavy smoking ii) Alcohol consumption iii) Intake of foods contaminated with fungus iv) Nutritional deficiency of vitamins and trace elements

2. Oesophageal disorders: i) Oesophagitis (especially Barrett's oesophagus in adenocarcinoma) ii) Achalasia iii) Hiatus hernia iv) Diverticula v) Plummer-Vinson syndrome.

3. Other factors: i) Race ii) Family history iii) Genetic factors.

At molecular level, abnormality of *TP53* (earlier known as p53) tumour suppressor gene has been found associated with a number of above risk factors, notably with consumption of tobacco and alcohol, and in cases having proven Barrett's oesophagus.

Carcinoma of the oesophagus is mainly of 2 types—squamous cell (epidermoid) and adenocarcinoma.

SQUAMOUS CELL (EPIDERMOID) CARCINOMA. Squamous cell or epidermoid carcinoma comprises 90% of primary oesophageal cancers. It is exceeded in incidence by carcinoma colon, rectum and stomach amongst all the gastrointestinal cancers. Half of the squamous cell carcinomas of oesophagus occur in the middle third, followed by lower third, and the upper third of oesophagus in that order of frequency.

G/A 3 types are recognised:

i) *Polypoid fungating type*—is the most common form.

ii) *Ulcerating type*—It looks grossly like a necrotic ulcer with everted edges.

iii) *Diffuse infiltrating type*—appears as an annular, stenosing narrowing of the lumen.

M/E Majority of the squamous cell carcinomas of the oesophagus are well-differentiated or moderately-differentiated.

ADENOCARCINOMA. Adenocarcinoma of the oesophagus constitutes less than 10% of primary oesophageal cancer. It occurs predominantly in men in their 4th to 5th decades. The common locations are lower and middle third of the oesophagus. These tumours have a strong and definite association with Barrett's oesophagus in which there are foci of gastric or intestinal type of epithelium.

G/A Oesophageal adenocarcinoma appears as nodular, elevated mass in the lower oesophagus.

M/E Adenocarcinoma of the oesophagus can have 3 patterns: i) Intestinal type ii) Adenosquamous type iii) Adenoid cystic type.

SPREAD. The oesophageal cancer spreads locally as well as to distant sites.

i) Local spread. This is the most important mode of spread and is of great importance for surgical treatment. The local spread may occur in the transverse as well as longitudinal direction.

ii) Lymphatic spread. Submucosal lymphatic permeation may lead to multiple satellite nodules away from the main tumour.

iii) Haematogenous spread. Blood-borne metastases from the oesophageal cancer are rare, probably because the death occurs early due to invasion of important structures.

STOMACH *(p. 556)*

NORMAL STRUCTURE *(p. 556)*

The stomach is 'gland with cavity', extending from its junction with lower end of the oesophagus (cardia) to its junction with the duodenum (pylorus). The *lesser curvature* is inner concavity on the right, while the *greater curvature* is the outer convexity on the left side of the stomach.

The stomach has 5 anatomical regions:

1. Cardia is the oesophago-gastric junction and lacks the sphincter.

2. Fundus is the portion above the horizontal line drawn across the oesophago-gastric junction.

3. Body is the middle portion of the stomach between the fundus and the pyloric antrum.

4. Pyloric antrum is the distal third of the stomach.

5. Pylorus is the junction of distal end of the stomach with the duodenum. It has powerful sphincter muscle.

Gastric canal is the relatively fixed portion of the pyloric antrum and the adjoining lesser curvature; it is the site for numerous pathological changes such as gastritis, peptic ulcer and gastric carcinoma.

M/E The wall of the stomach consists of 4 layers:

1. Serosa is derived from the peritoneum which is deficient in the region of lesser and greater curvatures.

2. Muscularis consists of 3 layers of smooth muscle fibres—the outer longitudinal, the middle circular and the inner oblique.

3. Submucosa is a layer of loose fibroconnective tissue binding the mucosa to the muscularis loosely.

4. Mucosa consists of 2 layers—superficial and deep.

i)   *THE SUPERFICIAL LAYER* consists of a single layer of surface epithelium composed of regular, mucin-secreting, tall columnar cells with basal nuclei.

■   *Cardiac mucosa* is the transition zone between the oesophageal squamous mucosa and the oxyntic mucosa of the fundus and body.

■   *Oxyntic mucosa* lines both gastric fundus and body.

■   *Antral mucosa* lines the pyloric antrum.

ii)   *THE DEEP LAYER* consists of glands that open into the bottom of the crypts. Depending upon the structure, these glands are of 3 types:

a)   *Glands of the cardia* are simple tubular or compound tubulo-racemose, lined by mucin secreting cells.

b)   *Glands of the body-fundus* are long, tubular and tightly packed which may be coiled or dilated. There are 4 types of cells present in the glands of body-fundic mucosa:

■   *Parietal (Oxyntic) cells*—are the most numerous and line the superficial (upper) part of the glands.

■   *Chief (Peptic) cells*—are the dominant cells in the deeper (lower) parts of the glands.

■   *Mucin-secreting neck cells*—are small and fewer.

■   *Endocrine (Kulchitsky or Enterochromaffin) cells*—are widely distributed in the mucosa of all parts of the alimentary tract.

c)   *Glands of the pylorus* are much longer than the body-fundic glands. These are simple tubular glands which are often coiled.

The secretory products of the gastric mucosa are the *gastric juice* and the *intrinsic factor*, required for absorption of vitamin B_{12}.

GASTRIC ANALYSIS *(p. 558)*

In various diseases of the stomach, the laboratory tests to measure gastric secretions (consisting of gastric acid, pepsin, mucus and intrinsic factor) and serum gastrin are of particular significance (Table 18.1).

PYLORIC STENOSIS *(p. 559)*

Hypertrophy and narrowing of the pyloric lumen occurs predominantly in male children as a congenital defect *(infantile pyloric stenosis)*. The *adult form* is rarely seen.

TABLE 18.1: Gastric Analysis.

A. TESTS FOR GASTRIC SECRETIONS

1. ***Tests for gastric acid secretions***
   - i) Histamine stimulation
   - ii) Histalog stimulation
   - iii) Pentagastrin (peptavlon) stimulation
   - iv) Insulin meal (Hollander test)
   - v) Tubeless analysis
2. ***Tests for pepsin***
   Pepsin inhibitors
3. ***Tests for mucus***
   Protein content of mucus
4. ***Tests for intrinsic factor***

B. TESTS FOR GASTRIN

1. ***Serum gastrin***
2. ***Gastrin provocation tests***
   - i) Secretin test
   - ii) Calcium infusion test

ETIOLOGY. The exact cause of *congenital (infantile)* pyloric stenosis is not known but it appears to have familial clustering and recessive genetic origin.

G/A and M/E There is hypertrophy as well as hyperplasia of the circular layer of muscularis in the pyloric sphincter accompanied by mild degree of fibrosis.

CLINICAL FEATURES 1. Vomiting, 2. visible peristalsis, 3. palpable lump, 4. constipation, and 5. loss of weight.

BEZOARS (p. 560)

Bezoars are foreign bodies in the stomach, usually in patients with mental illness who chew these substances. Some of the common bezoars are:

- *Trichobezoars* composed of a ball of hair.
- *Phytobezoars* composed of vegetable fibres, seeds or fruit skin.
- *Trichophytobezoars* combining both hair and vegetable matter.

GASTRITIS (p. 560)

The term 'gastritis' is commonly employed for any clinical condition with upper abdominal discomfort like indigestion or dyspepsia in which the specific clinical signs and radiological abnormalities are absent. The condition is of great importance due to its relationship with peptic ulcer and gastric cancer. Broadly speaking, gastritis may be of 2 types—acute and chronic.

Acute Gastritis (p. 560)

Acute gastritis is a transient acute inflammatory involvement of the stomach, mainly mucosa.

ETIOPATHOGENESIS. A variety of etiologic agents have been implicated:

1. Diet and personal habits: Highly spiced food, excessive alcohol consumption, malnutrition, heavy smoking.

2. Infections: *Bacterial infections* e.g. *Helicobacter pylori,* diphtheria, salmonellosis, pneumonia, staphylococcal food poisoning. *Viral infections* e.g. viral hepatitis, influenza, infectious mononucleosis.

3. Drugs: Intake of drugs like non-steroidal anti-inflammatory drugs (NSAIDs), aspirin.

4. Chemical and physical agents: Intake of corrosive chemicals, gastric irradiation, and freezing.

5. Severe stress: Emotional factors, extensive burns, trauma, and surgery.

G/A The gastric mucosa is oedematous with abundant mucus and haemorrhagic spots.

M/E Depending upon the stage, there is variable amount of oedema and infiltration by neutrophils in the lamina propria. In acute haemorrhagic and erosive gastritis, the mucosa is sloughed off and there are haemorrhages on the surface.

Chronic Gastritis (p. 561)

Chronic gastritis is the commonest histological change observed in biopsies from the stomach.

ETIOPATHOGENESIS. All the causative factors of acute gastritis described above may result in chronic gastritis too. Recurrent attacks of acute gastritis may result in chronic gastritis. Some additional causes are as under:
1. *Reflux of duodenal contents into the stomach,* 2. infection with *H. pylori* is strongly implicated, 3. *associated disease of the stomach and duodenum,* such as gastric or duodenal ulcer, gastric carcinoma, 4. *chronic hypochromic anaemia,* and 5. *immunological factors* such as autoantibodies to gastric parietal cells in atrophic gastritis and autoantibodies against intrinsic factor.

CLASSIFICATION. Based on the type of mucosa affected (i.e. cardiac, body, pyloric, antral or transitional), a clinicopathologic classification has been proposed (Table 18.2).

TABLE 18.2: Classification of Gastritis.

A. ACUTE GASTRITIS

1. Acute *H. pylori* gastritis
2. Other acute infective gastritis (bacteria, viruses, fungi, parasites)
3. Acute non-infective gastritis

B. CHRONIC GASTRITIS

1. Type A (autoimmune)	:	Body-fundic predominant
2. Type B (*H. pylori*-related) gastritis	:	Antral-predominant
3. Type AB (environmental)	:	Antral-body gastritis
4. Chemical (reflux) gastritis	:	Antral-body predominant
5. Uncommon forms of gastritis		

1. Type A Gastritis (Autoimmune gastritis). Type A gastritis involves mainly the body-fundic mucosa. It is also called autoimmune gastritis due to the presence of circulating antibodies and is sometimes associated with other autoimmune diseases such as Hashimoto's thyroiditis and Addison's disease. Due to depletion of gastric acid-producing mucosal area, there is hypo- or achlorhydria, and hyperplasia of gastrin-producing G cells in the antrum resulting in hypergastrinaemia.

2. Type B Gastritis (*H. pylori*-related). Type B gastritis mainly involves the region of antral mucosa and is more common. It is also called hypersecretory gastritis due to excessive secretion of acid, commonly due to infection with *H. pylori*. These patients may have associated peptic ulcer.

3. Type AB Gastritis (Environmental gastritis, Chronic atrophic gastritis). Type AB gastritis affects the mucosal region of A as well as B types (body-fundic and antral mucosa). This is the most common type of gastritis in all age groups. It is also called environmental gastritis because a number of as yet unidentified environmental factors have been implicated in its etiopathogenesis.

G/A The gastric mucosa may be normal, atrophied, or oedematous.

M/E Based on: i) the extent of inflammatory changes in the mucosa (i.e. superficial or deep); ii) the activity of inflammation (i.e. quiescent or active; acute or chronic); and iii) the presence of and type of metaplasia (i.e. intestinal or pseudo-pyloric), a simple classification has been proposed as given below.

However, *Sydney system* of recording of histologic changes in gastritis is more acceptable since it takes into account following multiple parameters:

i) *Etiology* (*H. pylori*, autoimmune, NSAIDs, infections).

ii) *Location* (pangastritis, predominant antral, predominant body-fundic).

iii) *Morphology* (depth of inflammation—superficial or deep, severity of inflammation, type of inflammation, atrophy, metaplasia).

iv) *Some special features* (e.g. granulomas, eosinophilic gastritis, erosions, necrosis, haemorrhages).

1. CHRONIC SUPERFICIAL GASTRITIS. As the name suggests there is inflammatory infiltrate consisting of plasma cells and lymphocytes in the superficial layer of the gastric mucosa, *but there are no histological changes in the deep layer of mucosa containing gastric glands*. Chronic superficial gastritis may resolve completely or may progress to chronic gastric atrophy.

H. pylori, a spiral-shaped bacteria, is found in almost all active cases of chronic superficial gastritis and about 65% of quiescent cases. The organism is identified on the epithelial layer on the luminal surface and does not invade the mucosa. It is not seen on areas with intestinal metaplasia.

Although most patients of chronic superficial gastritis due to *H. pylori* remain asymptomatic, they may develop chronic atrophic gastritis, gastric atrophy, peptic ulcer disease and malignant transformation (Fig. 18.1).

Fig. 18.1: Consequences of long-term *H. pylori* gastritis.

2. CHRONIC ATROPHIC GASTRITIS. In this stage, *there is inflammatory cell infiltrate in the deeper layer of the mucosa and atrophy of the epithelial elements including destruction of the glands*. Two types of metaplasia are commonly associated with atrophic gastritis:

i) Intestinal metaplasia. It is more common and involves antral mucosa more frequently. Characteristic histologic feature is the presence of intestinal type mucus-goblet cells; Paneth cells and endocrine cells may also be present.

ii) **Pseudopyloric metaplasia.** It involves the body glands which are replaced by proliferated mucous neck cells, conforming in appearance to normal pyloric glands. Its significance is not known.

3. **GASTRIC ATROPHY.** There is thinning of the gastric mucosa with loss of glands but no inflammation.

4. **CHRONIC HYPERTROPHIC GASTRITIS (MÉNÉTRIER'S DISEASE).** This is an uncommon condition characterised pathologically by enormous thickening of gastric rugal folds resembling cerebral convolutions, affecting mainly the region of fundic-body mucosa and characteristically sparing antral mucosa.

M/E The gastric pits are elongated and are tortuous. The mucosa is markedly thickened and parts of muscularis mucosae may extend into the thickened folds.

5. **UNCOMMON FORMS OF CHRONIC GASTRITIS.** These include:

i) **Gastric candidiasis.** Infection with *Candida albicans* may occur as an opportunistic infection in immunosuppressed and debilitated individuals.

ii) **Eosinophilic gastritis.** This condition is characterised by diffuse thickening of the pyloric antrum due to oedema and extensive infiltration by eosinophils and probably has an allergic basis.

iii) **Chronic follicular gastritis.** This is a variant of chronic atrophic gastritis in which numerous lymphoid follicles are present in the mucosa and submucosa of the stomach.

iv) **Haemorrhagic (Erosive) gastritis.** In this condition, there are superficial erosions and mucosal haemorrhages, usually following severe haematemesis.

v) **Granulomatous gastritis.** Rarely, granulomas may be present in the gastric mucosa such as in tuberculosis, sarcoidosis, Crohn's disease.

PEPTIC ULCERS *(p. 563)*

Peptic ulcers are the areas of degeneration and necrosis of gastrointestinal mucosa exposed to acid-peptic secretions. Though they can occur at any level of the alimentary tract that is exposed to hydrochloric acid and pepsin, they occur most commonly (98-99%) in either the duodenum or the stomach in the ratio of 4:1.

Acute Peptic (Stress) Ulcers *(p. 563)*

Acute peptic ulcers or stress ulcers are multiple, small mucosal erosions, seen most commonly in the stomach but occasionally involving the duodenum.

ETIOLOGY. These ulcers occur following severe stress. The causes are:
i) *Psychological stress*
ii) *Physiological stress* e.g. shock, severe trauma, septicaemia, extensive burns (Curling's ulcers in the posterior aspect of the first part of the duodenum), intracranial lesions (Cushing's ulcers developing from hyperacidity following excessive vagal stimulation), drug intake (e.g. aspirin, steroids, butazolidine, indomethacin), local irritants (e.g. alcohol, smoking, coffee etc.).

PATHOGENESIS. It is not clear how the mucosal erosions occur in stress ulcers because actual hypersecretion of gastric acid is demonstrable in only Cushing's ulcers occurring from intracranial conditions such as due to brain trauma, intracranial surgery and brain tumours. In all other etiologic factors, gastric acid secretion is normal or below normal. In these conditions, the possible hypotheses for genesis of stress ulcers are as follows:
1. Ischaemic hypoxic injury to the mucosal cells.
2. Depletion of the gastric mucus 'barrier' rendering the mucosa susceptible to attack by acid-peptic secretions.

G/A Acute stress ulcers are multiple (more than three ulcers in 75% of cases). They are more common anywhere in the stomach, followed in decreasing frequency by occurrence in the first part of duodenum.

M/E The stress ulcers are shallow and do not invade the muscular layer. The margins and base may show some inflammatory reaction depending upon the duration of the ulcers.

Chronic Peptic Ulcers (Gastric and Duodenal Ulcers) *(p. 564)*

If not specified, chronic peptic ulcers would mean gastric and duodenal ulcers, the two major forms of 'peptic ulcer disease' of the upper GI tract in which the acid-pepsin secretions are implicated in their pathogenesis. Peptic ulcers are common in the present-day life of the industrialised and civilised world.

Gastric and duodenal ulcers represent two distinct diseases as far as their etiology, pathogenesis and clinical features are concerned. However, pathological findings in both are similar and quite diagnostic. A comparative summary of features of gastric and duodenal peptic ulcers is presented in Table 18.3.

INCIDENCE. Peptic ulcers are more frequent in middle-aged adults. The peak incidence for duodenal ulcer is 5th decade, while for gastric ulcer it is a decade later (6th decade). Duodenal as well as gastric ulcers are more common in males than in females. Duodenal ulcer is almost four times more common than gastric ulcer.

ETIOLOGY. The immediate cause of peptic ulcer disease is disturbance in normal protective mucosal 'barrier' by acid-pepsin, resulting in digestion of the mucosa. However, in contrast to duodenal ulcers, *the patients of gastric ulcer have low-to-normal gastric acid secretions, though true achlorhydria in response to stimulants never occurs in benign gastric ulcer.* Thus, the etiology of peptic ulcers possibly may not be explained on the basis of a single factor but is multifactorial.

1. *Helicobacter pylori* gastritis. About 15-20% cases infected with *H. pylori* in the antrum develop duodenal ulcer in their life time while gastric colonisation by *H. pylori* never develops ulceration and remain asymptomatic. *H. pylori* can be identified in mucosal samples by histologic examination, culture, increased activity, and serology (IgG and IgA antibodies to *H. pylori*).

2. Acid-pepsin secretions. There is conclusive evidence that some level of acid-pepsin secretion is essential for the development of duodenal as well as gastric ulcer.

3. Mucus secretion. Any condition that decreases the quantity or quality of normal protective mucus 'barrier' predisposes to the development of peptic ulcer.

4. Gastritis. Some degree of gastritis is always present in the region of gastric ulcer, though it is not clear whether it is the cause or the effect of ulcer.

5. Local irritants. Pyloric antrum and lesser curvature of the stomach are the sites most exposed for longer periods to local irritants and thus are the common sites for occurrence of gastric ulcers. Some of the local irritating substances implicated in the etiology of peptic ulcers are heavily spiced foods, alcohol, cigarette smoking, unbuffered aspirin, non-steroidal anti-inflammatory drugs etc.

6. Dietary factors. Nutritional deficiencies have been regarded as etiologic factors in peptic ulcers e.g. occurrence of gastric ulcer in poor socioeconomic strata, higher incidence of duodenal ulcer in parts of South India.

7. Psychological factors. Psychological stress, anxiety, fatigue and ulcer-type personality may exacerbate as well as predispose to peptic ulcer disease.

TABLE 18.3: Distinguishing Features of Two Major Forms of Peptic Ulcers.

FEATURE	DUODENAL ULCER	GASTRIC ULCER
1. *Incidence*	i) Four times more common than gastric ulcers	Less common than duodenal ulcers
	ii) Usual age 25-50 years	Usually beyond 6th decade
	iii) More common in males than in females (4:1)	More common in males than in females (3.5:1)
2. *Etiology*	Most commonly as a result of *H. pylori* infection	Gastric colonisation with *H. pylori* asymptomatic but higher chances
	Other factors—hypersecretion of acid-pepsin, association with	of development of duodenal ulcer. Disruption of mucus barrier most
	alcoholic cirrhosis, tobacco, hyperparathyroidism, chronic	important factor. Association with gastritis, bile reflux, drugs,
	pancreatitis, blood group O, genetic factors	alcohol, tobacco
3. *Pathogenesis*	i) Mucosal digestion from hyperacidity most significant factor	Usually normal-to-low acid levels; hyperacidity if present is
		due to high serum gastrin
4. *Pathologic changes*	ii) Protective gastric mucus barrier may be damaged	Damage to mucus barrier significant factor
	i) Most common in the first part of duodenum	Most common along the lesser curvature and pyloric antrum
	ii) Often solitary, 1-2.5 cm in size, round to oval, punched out	Grossly similar to duodenal ulcer
	iii) Histologically, composed of 4 layers—necrotic, superficial	Histologically, indistinguishable from duodenal ulcer
	exudative, granulation tissue and cicatrisation	
5. *Complications*	Commonly haemorrhage, perforation, sometimes obstruction;	Perforation, haemorrhage and at times obstruction; malignant
	malignant transformation never occurs	transformation in less than 1% cases
6. *Clinical features*	i) Pain-food-relief pattern	Food-pain pattern
	ii) Night pain common	No night pain
	iii) No vomiting	Vomiting common
	iv) Melaena more common than haematemesis	Haematemesis more common
	v) No loss of weight	Significant loss of weight
	vi) No particular choice of diet fried foods, curries etc.	Patients choose bland diet devoid of
	vii) Deep tenderness in the right hypochondrium	Deep tenderness in the midline in epigastrium
	viii) Marked seasonal variation	No seasonal variation
	ix) Occurs more commonly in people at greater stress	More often in labouring groups

8. Genetic factors. People with blood group O appear to be more prone to develop peptic ulcers than those with other blood groups. Genetic influences appear to have greater role in duodenal ulcers as evidenced by their occurrence in families, monozygotic twins and association with HLA-B5 antigen.

9. Hormonal factors. Secretion of certain hormones by tumours is associated with peptic ulceration e.g. elaboration of gastrin by islet-cell tumour in Zollinger-Ellison syndrome.

10. Miscellaneous. Duodenal ulcers have been observed to occur in association with various other conditions such as alcoholic cirrhosis, chronic renal failure, hyperparathyroidism.

PATHOGENESIS. Although the role of various etiologic factors just described is well known in ulcerogenesis, two most important factors in peptic ulcer are:
- exposure of mucosa to gastric acid and pepsin secretion; and
- strong etiologic association with *H. pylori* infection.

Duodenal ulcer. There is conclusive evidence to support the role of high acid-pepsin secretions in the causation of duodenal ulcers.

1. There is generally *hypersecretion of gastric acid* into the fasting stomach at night which takes place under the influence of vagal stimulation.

2. Patients of duodenal ulcer have *rapid emptying* of the stomach so that the food which normally buffers and neutralises the gastric acid, passes down into the small intestine, leaving the duodenal mucosa exposed to the aggressive action of gastric acid.

3. *Helicobacter* gastritis caused by *H. pylori* is seen in 95-100% cases of duodenal ulcers.

Gastric ulcer. The pathogenesis of gastric ulcer is mainly explained on the basis of impaired gastric mucosal defenses against acid-pepsin secretions.

1. Hyperacidity may occur in gastric ulcer due to *increased serum gastrin* levels in response to ingested food in an atonic stomach.

2 However, many a patients of gastric ulcer have low-to-normal gastric acid levels. Ulcerogenesis in such patients is explained on the basis of damaging influence of *other factors* such as gastritis, bile reflux, cigarette smoke etc.

3. The normally protective *gastric mucus 'barrier'* against acid-pepsin is deranged in gastric ulcer. There is depletion in the quantity as well as quality of gastric mucus. One of the mechanisms for its depletion is colonisation of the gastric mucosa by *H. pylori* seen in 75-80% patients of gastric ulcer.

MORPHOLOGY. *Gastric ulcers* are found predominantly along the lesser curvature in the region of pyloric antrum, more commonly on the posterior than the anterior wall. Most *duodenal ulcers* are found in the first part of the duodenum, usually immediate post-pyloric, more commonly on the anterior than the posterior wall.

G/A Typical peptic ulcers are commonly solitary (80%), small (1-2.5 cm in diameter), round to oval and characteristically 'punched out'. Benign ulcers usually have flat margins in level with the surrounding mucosa. Vast majority of the peptic ulcers are benign. *Chronic duodenal ulcer never turns malignant.*

M/E Chronic peptic ulcers have 4 histological zones. From within outside, these are as under:

1. *Necrotic zone*—lies in the floor of the ulcer and is composed of fibrinous exudate containing necrotic debris and a few leucocytes.

2. *Superficial exudative zone*—lies underneath the necrotic zone. The tissue elements here show coagulative necrosis giving eosinophilic, smudgy appearance with nuclear debris.

3. *Granulation tissue zone*—is seen merging into the necrotic zone. It is composed of nonspecific inflammatory infiltrate and proliferating capillaries.

4. *Zone of cicatrisation*—is seen merging into thick layer of granulation tissue. It is composed of dense fibrocollagenic scar tissue over which granulation tissue rests.

COMPLICATIONS. Acute and subacute peptic ulcers usually heal without leaving any visible scar. However, healing of chronic, larger and deeper ulcers may result in complications:

1. Obstruction. Development of fibrous scar at or near the pylorus results in pyloric stenosis. In the case of healed duodenal ulcer, it causes duodenal stenosis. Healed ulcers along the lesser curvatures may produce 'hour glass' deformity due to fibrosis and contraction.

2. Haemorrhage. Minor bleeding by erosion of small blood vessels in the base of an ulcer occurs in all the ulcers and can be detected by testing the stool for occult blood. Chronic blood loss may result in iron deficiency anaemia.

3. Perforation. A perforated peptic ulcer is an acute abdominal emergency. Perforation occurs more commonly in chronic duodenal ulcers than chronic gastric ulcers.

4. Malignant transformation. The dictum *'cancers ulcerate but ulcers rarely cancerate'* holds true for most peptic ulcers. A chronic duodenal ulcer never turns malignant, while less than 1% of chronic gastric ulcers may transform into carcinoma.

HAEMATEMESIS AND MELAENA OF GASTRIC ORIGIN *(p. 568)*

i) Chronic peptic ulcers (gastric as well as duodenal). ii) Acute peptic ulcers (stress ulcers). iii) Multiple gastric and duodenal erosions. iv) Carcinoma of the stomach. v) Peptic ulcer in Meckel's diverticulum. vi) Mallory-Weiss syndrome. vii) Anaemias. viii) Purpuras. ix) Haemophilia.

A. TUMOUR-LIKE LESIONS (POLYPS) *(p. 568)*

Hyperplastic (Inflammatory) Polyps *(p. 568)*

Hyperplastic or inflammatory polyps are regenerative, non-neoplastic lesions which are the most common type (90%). They may be single or multiple and are more often located in the pyloric antrum.

G/A The lesions may be sessile or pedunculated, 1 cm or larger in size, smooth and soft. The surface may be ulcerated or haemorrhagic.

M/E They are composed of irregular hyperplastic glands, which may show cystic change. The lining epithelium is mostly superficial gastric type but antral glands, chief cells and parietal cells may be present.

Hamartomatous Polyps *(p. 569)*

Hamartomatous polyps are not true neoplasms but are malformations. They are of various types such as gastric polyps of the Peutz-Jeghers syndrome, juvenile polyp, pancreatic heterotopia, heterotopia of Brunner's glands and inflammatory fibroid polyps (eosinophilic granulomatous polyps).

Adenomas (Adenomatous or Neoplastic Polyps) *(p. 569)*

Adenomas, also, referred to as adenomatous or neoplastic polyps, are true benign epithelial neoplasms and are much rarer in the stomach than in the large intestine. They are also found more often in the region of pyloric antrum. They are commonly associated with atrophic gastritis and pernicious anaemia.

STROMAL TUMOURS *(p. 569)*

Stomach may be the site for occurrence of various uncommon benign tumours of stromal cell origin e.g. leiomyomas (being the most common); others are neurofibromas, schwannomas and lipomas. They are usually firm, circumscribed nodules, less than 4 cm in size and appear as submucosal nodules.

Currently, the term *gastrointestinal stromal tumours (GISTs)* is used for a group of uncommon benign tumours composed of spindle cells or stromal cells but lacking the true phenotypic features of smooth muscle cells, neural cells or Schwann cells. They are uncommon but as compared to other sites in the GIT, are most common in the stomach.

GASTRIC CARCINOMA *(p. 569)*

INCIDENCE. Carcinoma of the stomach comprises more than 90% of all gastric malignancies and is the leading cause of cancer-related deaths in countries where its incidence is high. The highest incidence is between 4th to 6th decades of life and is twice more common in men than in women.

ETIOLOGY. A number of etiologic factors have been implicated in causation of gastric cancer.

1. *H. pylori* infection. *H. pylori* infection of the stomach is an important risk factor for the development of gastric cancer. Epidemiologic studies throughout world have shown that a seropositivity with *H. pylori* is associated with 3 to 6 times higher risk of development of gastric cancer. It may be mentioned here that similar association of *H. pylori* infection exists with gastric lymphomas as well.

2. Dietary factors. The evidences in support of this are multifold:
i) Occurrence of gastric cancer in the region of gastric canal where irritating foods exert their maximum effect.
ii) Populations consuming certain foodstuffs have high risk of developing gastric cancer e.g. ingestion of smoked foods, high intake of salt, pickled raw vegetables, high intake of carcinogens as nitrates in foods and drinking water, nitrites as preservatives for certain meats etc.
iii) Tobacco smoke, tobacco juice and consumption of alcohol.

3. Geographical factors. There are geographic variations in the incidence of gastric cancer. Japan, Chile, Finland and Iceland have highest recorded death rate from gastric cancer, while the incidence is considerably low in the US, UK and Canada.

4. Racial factors. Within the country, different ethnic groups may have variations in incidence of gastric cancer e.g. incidence is higher in Blacks, American Indians, Chinese in Indonesia, North Wales than other parts of Wales.

5. Genetic factors. Not more than 4% of patients of gastric cancer have a family history of this disease. Individuals with blood group A have higher tendency to develop gastric cancer.

6. Pre-malignant changes in the gastric mucosa. There are some precancerous conditions of gastric mucosa implicated in the etiology of gastric cancer. These are:
i) Hypo- or achlorhydria in atrophic gastritis of gastric mucosa.
ii) Adenomatous (neoplastic) polyps of the stomach.
iii) Chronic gastric ulcer (ulcer-cancer), and its association with achlorhydria.
iv) Stump carcinoma in patients who have undergone partial gastrectomy.

LOCATION. Gastric carcinoma is most commonly located in the region of gastric canal (prepyloric region) formed by lesser curvature, pylorus and antrum.

MORPHOLOGY. Current studies indicate a pathogenetic evolution for all gastric carcinomas from an initial stage of *in situ* carcinoma confined to mucosal layers called early gastric carcinoma (EGC). *Based on this pathogenetic sequence,* gastric carcinomas are broadly classified into 2 main groups:

I. *Early gastric carcinoma (EGC).*

II. *Advanced gastric carcinoma,* which has 5 further major gross subtypes:
i) Ulcerative carcinoma. ii) Fungating (Polypoid) carcinoma. iii) Scirrhous carcinoma (Linitis plastica). iv) Colloid (Mucoid) carcinoma. v) Ulcer-cancer.

In addition to the above classification, gastric carcinomas have been classified, *on the basis of extent of invasion,* into 2 groups:

I. *Expanding (formerly intestinal type) carcinomas* that grow laterally by an invasive margin. The tumour cells are in the form of cohesive clusters.

II. *Infiltrating (formerly diffuse type) carcinomas* have poorly-defined invasive border. The tumour cells are loose and invade singly or in small group.

I.   EARLY GASTRIC CARCINOMA (EGC). EGC is the term used to describe cancer limited to the mucosa and submucosa. The diagnosis of this condition has been made possible by extensive work on histogenesis of gastric cancer by Japanese pathologists by the use of fibreoptic endoscope and gastrocamera. In Japan, EGC comprises 35% of newly-diagnosed cases of gastric cancer.

G/A The lesion of EGC may have 3 patterns—polypoid (protruded), superficial and ulcerated.

M/E EGC is a typical glandular adenocarcinoma, usually well-differentiated type.

II.   ADVANCED GASTRIC CARCINOMA. When the carcinoma crosses the basement membrane into the muscularis propria or beyond, it is referred to as advanced gastric carcinoma. Advanced gastric carcinoma has further 5 patterns:

i)   Ulcerative carcinoma. This is the most common pattern. The tumour appears as a flat, infiltrating and ulcerative growth with irregular necrotic base and raised margin. It is seen more commonly in the region of gastric canal.

M/E Ulcerative carcinomas are poorly-differentiated adenocarcinomas, which invade deeply into the stomach wall.

ii)   Fungating (polypoid) carcinoma. The second common pattern is a cauliflower growth projecting into the lumen, similar to what is commonly seen in the large intestine. It is seen more often in the fundus.

M/E Fungating or polypoid carcinomas are well-differentiated adenocarcinomas, commonly papillary type.

iii) Scirrhous carcinoma (Linitis plastica). In this pattern, the stomach wall is thickened due to extensive desmoplasia giving the appearance as 'leatherbottle stomach' or 'linitis plastica'. The involvement may be localised to pyloric antrum, or diffuse affecting whole of the stomach from the cardia to pylorus. The lumen of the stomach is reduced.

M/E It may be an adenocarcinoma or signet-ring cell carcinoma, extensively infiltrating the stomach wall, but due to marked desmoplasia cancer cells may be difficult to find.

iv)   Colloid (Mucoid) carcinoma. This pattern is usually seen in the fundus. The tumour grows like masses having gelatinous appearance due to secretion of large quantities of mucus.

M/E Mucoid carcinoma contains abundant pools of mucin in which are seen a small number of tumour cells, sometimes having signet-ring appearance.

v)   Ulcer-cancer. Development of cancer in chronic gastric ulcer is a rare occurrence (less than 1%). Majority of ulcer-cancers are malignant lesions from the beginning. For confirmation of cancer in a pre-existing gastric ulcer, the characteristic microscopic appearance of peptic ulcer should be demonstrable with one portion of the base or the margin of the ulcer showing carcinomatous changes. The differences between a benign and malignant gastric ulcer are summarised in Table 18.4.

TABLE 18.4: Differences between Benign and Malignant Gastric Ulcers.

	FEATURE	BENIGN ULCER	MALIGNANT ULCER
1.	*Age*	Younger age	Older age
2.	*Sex*	Markedly common in males	Slightly common in males
3.	*Duration of symptoms*	Weeks to years	Weeks to months
4.	*Location*	Commonly lesser curvature of pylorus and antrum	Commonly greater curvature of pylorus and antrum
5.	*Gross features*		
	a) *Size*	Small	Large
	b) *Shape*	Regular	Irregular
	c) *Mucosal folds*	Radiating	Interrupted
	d) *Ulcer bed*	Haemorrhagic	Necrotic
6.	*Barium studies*	Punched out ulcer	Irregular filling defect
7.	*Acidity*	Usually normal-to-low	May be normal-to-even achlorhydria
8.	*Therapy*	Responds well to medical therapy	Usually does not respond to medical therapy

SPREAD. 1. Direct spread. Direct spread by local extension is the most common feature of gastric carcinoma. The spread occurs mainly from the loose submucosal layer but eventually muscularis and serosa are also invaded. After the peritoneal covering of the stomach is involved, transcoelomic dissemination may occur in any other part of the peritoneal cavity but ovarian masses (one side or both-sided) occur more commonly, referred to as *Krukenberg tumours.*

2. Lymphatic spread. Metastases to regional lymph nodes occur early, especially in the scirrhous carcinoma. The groups of lymph nodes involved are along the lesser and greater curvature around the cardia and suprapancreatic lymph nodes. Involvement of left supraclavicular lymph node, *Virchow* or *Troisier's sign,* is sometimes the presenting feature of gastric carcinoma.

3. Haematogenous spread. Blood spread of gastric carcinoma may occur to the liver, lungs, brain, bones, kidneys and adrenals. It occurs more commonly with the poorly-differentiated carcinoma.

CLINICAL FEATURES. The usual clinical features are: i) Persistent abdominal pain, ii) gastric distension and vomiting, iii) loss of weight (cachexia), iv) loss of appetite (anorexia), and v) anaemia, weakness, malaise.

The most common complication of gastric cancer is haemorrhage (in the form of haematemesis and/or melaena); others are obstruction, perforation and jaundice.

Leiomyosarcoma *(p. 575)*

Leiomyosarcoma, though rare, is the commonest soft tissue sarcoma, the stomach being the more common site in the gastrointestinal tract.

G/A The tumour may be of variable size but is usually quite large, pedunculated and lobulated mass into the lumen.

M/E Leiomyosarcoma is characterised by high cellularity and presence of mitotic figures. Tumour is usually well-differentiated.

Leiomyoblastoma (Epithelioid Leiomyoma) *(p. 575)*

This is a rare tumour, the behaviour of which is intermediate between clearly benign and malignant tumour.

G/A The tumour is large, circumscribed and projects into the lumen.

M/E It is characterised by round to polygonal cells with clear perinuclear halos. The number of mitoses determines the biological behaviour of the tumour.

Carcinoid Tumour *(p. 575)*

Carcinoid tumours are rare in the stomach and are usually non-argentaffin type but argentaffinomas also occur. Their behaviour is usually malignant.

Lymphomas of Gut *(p. 575)*

Primary gastrointestinal lymphomas are defined as lymphomas arising in the gut without any evidence of systemic involvement at the time of presentation.

Secondary gastrointestinal lymphomas, on the other hand, appear in the gut after dissemination from other primary site. Gastric lymphomas constitute over 50% of all bowel lymphomas; other sites being small and large bowel in decreasing order of frequency. Prognosis of primary gastric lymphoma is better than for intestinal lymphomas. Primary lymphoma of stomach is the most common malignant gastric tumour (4%) next to carcinoma.

Age incidence for lymphomas of the gastrointestinal tract is usually lower than that for carcinoma (30-40 years as compared to 40-60 years in gastric carcinoma) and may occur even in childhood. Relationship with long-standing chronic *H. pylori* gastritis with lymphoid hyperplasia has been strongly suggested.

G/A Gastric lymphomas have 2 types of appearances:
1. *Diffusely infiltrating type,* producing thickening of the affected gut wall, obliteration of mucosal folds and ulcerations.
2. *Polypoid type,* which produces large protruding mass into the lumen with ulcerated surface.
   Lymph node involvement may occur in either of the two patterns.

M/E Gastric lymphomas are most often non-Hodgkin's lymphomas of the following types:
- *High-grade* large cell immunoblastic lymphoma being the most common.
- *Low-grade* small lymphocytic well-differentiated B-cell lymphoma referred to as *MALToma* is the next in frequency (arising from *Mucosa Associated Lymphoid Tissue*).

SMALL INTESTINE *(p. 575)*

NORMAL STRUCTURE *(p. 575)*

Anatomically, the small bowel includes the duodenum, jejunum and ileum and tends to become narrower throughout its course.

M/E The small bowel is identified by recognition of villi. The wall of the small intestine consists of 4 layers:
1. The **serosa** is the outer covering of the small bowel which is complete except over a part of the duodenum.
2. The **muscularis propria** is composed of 2 layers of smooth muscle tissue—outer thinner longitudinal and inner thicker circular layer.
3. The **submucosa** is composed of loose fibrous tissue with blood vessels and lacteals in it.

4. The **mucosa** consists of glandular epithelium overlying the lamina propria composed of loose connective tissue and contains phagocytic cells and abundance of lymphoid cells (Peyer's patches in the ileum) and plasma cells. It is supported externally by thin layer of smooth muscle fibres, *muscularis mucosae*. The absorptive surface is further increased by the intestinal villi. *Villi* are finger-like or leaf-like projections which contain 3 types of cells: i) *Simple columnar cells,* ii) *Goblet cells,* and iii) *endocrine cells*. These cells have various synonyms as under:

- *Kulchitsky cells,* after the name of its discoverer;
- *Enterochromaffin cells,* due to their resemblance to chromaffin cells of the adrenal medulla;
- *Argentaffin cells,* as the intracytoplasmic granules stain positively with silver salts by reduction reaction (argyrophil cells, on the other hand, require the addition of exogenous reducing substance for staining); and
- *Endocrine cells,* as these specialised cells are considered to be part of APUD cell system.

ANOMALIES *(p. 576)*

Intestinal Atresia and Stenosis *(p. 576)*

- **Intestinal atresia** is congenital absence of lumen, most commonly affecting the ileum or duodenum.
- **Intestinal stenosis** is congenital narrowing of the lumen affecting a segment of the small intestine.

Meckel's Diverticulum *(p. 576)*

Meckel's diverticulum is the most common congenital anomaly of the gastrointestinal tract, occurring in 2% of population. It is more common in males. The anomaly is commonly situated on the antimesenteric border of the ileum, about 1 metre above the ileocaecal valve. Like other true diverticula, Meckel's diverticulum is an outpouching containing all the layers of the intestinal wall in their normal orientation. It is almost always lined by small intestinal type of epithelium. Embryologic origin of Meckel's diverticulum is from incomplete obliteration of vitellointestinal duct.

The common *complications* of Meckel's diverticulum are perforation, haemorrhage and diverticulitis.

INTESTINAL OBSTRUCTION *(p. 577)*

Conditions which interfere with the propulsion of contents in the intestine are considered under the heading of intestinal obstruction. The causes of intestinal obstruction can be classified under the following 3 broad groups:

1. Mechanical obstruction. It can occur as a result of the following causes:

i) *Internal obstruction* (in the wall or the lumen): Inflammatory strictures (e.g. Crohn's disease), congenital stenosis, atresia, imperforate anus, tumours, meconium in mucoviscidosis, roundworms, gallstones, faecoliths, foreign bodies, and ulceration induced by potassium chloride tablets prescribed to counter hypokalaemia.

ii) *External compression*: Peritoneal adhesions and bands, strangulated hernias, intussusception, volvulus, and intra-abdominal tumour.

2. Neurogenic obstruction. It occurs due to paralytic ileus i.e. paralysis of muscularis of the intestine as a result of shock after abdominal operation or by acute peritonitis.

3. Vascular obstruction. Obstruction of the superior mesenteric artery or its branches may result in infarction causing paralysis. Its causes are thrombosis, embolism, and accidental ligation.

Chapter Eighteen

Peritoneal Adhesions and Bands *(p. 577)*

Adhesions and bands in the peritoneum composed of fibrous tissue result following healing in peritonitis. In either case, peritoneal bands and adhesions result in partial or complete intestinal obstruction by outside pressure on the bowel wall.

Hernias *(p. 577)*

Hernia is protrusion of portion of a viscus through an abnormal opening in the wall of its natural cavity.

- **External hernia** is the protrusion of the bowel through a defect or weakness in the peritoneum.
- **Internal hernia** is the term applied for herniation that does not present on the external surface.

Two major factors involved in the formation of a hernia are: i) *Local weakness,* ii) *increased intra-abdominal pressure.* Inguinal hernias may be:

- **direct** when hernia passes medial to the inferior epigastric artery and it appears through the external abdominal ring; and
- **indirect** when it follows the inguinal canal lateral to the inferior epigastric artery.

When the blood flow in the hernial sac is obstructed, it results in *strangulated hernia.*

Intussusception *(p. 578)*

Intussusception is the telescoping of a segment of intestine into the segment below due to peristalsis. The telescoped segment is called the *intussusceptum* and lower receiving segment is called the *intussuscipiens.* The condition occurs more commonly in infants and young children, more often in the ileocaecal region when the portion of ileum invaginates into the ascending colon.

The main *complications* of intussusception are intestinal obstruction, infarction, gangrene, perforation and peritonitis.

Volvulus *(p. 578)*

Volvulus is the twisting of loop of intestine upon itself through 180° or more. This leads to obstruction of the intestine as well as cutting off of the blood supply to the affected loop. The usual causes are bands and adhesions (congenital or acquired) and long mesenteric attachment. The condition is more common in the sigmoid colon than the small bowel.

ISCHAEMIC BOWEL DISEASE (ISCHAEMIC ENTEROCOLITIS) *(p. 578)*

Ischaemic lesions of the gastrointestinal tract may occur in the small intestine and/or colon; the latter is called *ischaemic colitis or ischaemic enterocolitis* and is commonly referred to as ischaemic bowel disease. In either case, the cause of ischaemia is compromised mesenteric circulation, while ischaemic effect is less likely to occur in the stomach, duodenum and rectum due to abundant collateral blood supply.

Depending upon the extent and severity of ischaemia, following 3 patterns of pathologic lesions can occur:

Transmural Infarction *(p. 578)*

Ischaemic necrosis of the full-thickness of the bowel wall is more common in the small intestine than the large intestine.

ETIOPATHOGENESIS. The common causes are:

i) *Mesenteric arterial thrombosis:* Atherosclerosis (most common), aortic aneurysm, vasospasm, fibromuscular hyperplasia, invasion by the tumour, use of oral contraceptives, and arteritis of various types.

ii) *Mesenteric arterial embolism*: Mural thrombi in the heart, endocarditis (infective and nonbacterial thrombotic), atherosclerotic plaques, and atrial myxoma

iii) *Mesenteric venous occlusion* is less common cause of full-thickness infarction of the bowel. The causes are: Intestinal sepsis (e.g. appendicitis), portal venous thrombosis in cirrhosis of the liver, tumour invasion, and use of oral contraceptives.

iv) *Miscellaneous causes*: Strangulated hernia, torsion, and fibrous bands and adhesions.

G/A Irrespective of the underlying etiology, infarction of the bowel is haemorrhagic (red) type. A varying length of the small bowel may be affected. In the case of colonic infarction, the distribution area of superior and inferior mesenteric arteries (i.e. *splenic flexure*) is more commonly involved.

M/E There is coagulative necrosis and ulceration of the mucosa and there are extensive submucosal haemorrhages.

The condition is clinically characterised by 'abdominal angina' in which the patient has acute abdominal pain, nausea, vomiting, and sometimes diarrhoea.

Mural and Mucosal Infarction (Haemorrhagic Gastroenteropathy, Membranous Colitis) *(p. 579)*

Mural and mucosal infarctions are limited to superficial layers of the bowel wall, sparing the deeper layer of the muscularis and the serosa. The condition is also referred to as *haemorrhagic gastroenteropathy,* and in the case of colon as *membranous colitis.*

ETIOPATHOGENESIS. Haemorrhagic gastroenteropathy results from conditions causing non-occlusive hypoperfusion (compared from transmural infarction which occurs from occlusive causes). The causes are: shock, cardiac failure, infections, and intake of drugs causing vasoconstriction e.g. digitalis, norepinephrine.

G/A The lesions affect variable length of the bowel. The affected segment of the bowel is red or purple but without haemorrhage and exudation on the serosal surface. The mucosa is oedematous at places, sloughed and ulcerated at other places. The lumen contains haemorrhagic fluid.

M/E There is patchy ischaemic necrosis of mucosa, vascular congestion, haemorrhages and inflammatory cell infiltrate.

Clinically, as in transmural infarction, the features of abdominal pain, nausea, vomiting and diarrhoea are present, but the changes are reversible and curable.

Ischaemic Stenosis *(p. 580)*

Although this condition affects primarily colon in the region of splenic flexure, it is described here due to its apparent pathogenetic relationship with ischaemic injury. The disease has 2 phases:

i) **Ischaemic colitis**—characterised by acute colonic necrosis as described above.

ii) **Ischaemic stricture**—occurring following segmental inflammation of the colon.

G/A There is fusiform or saccular external appearance.

M/E The ulcerated areas of the mucosa show granulation tissue. The submucosa is characteristically thickened due to inflammation and fibrosis.

NECROTISING ENTEROCOLITIS *(p. 580)*

Necrotising enterocolitis is an acute inflammation of the terminal ileum and ascending colon, occurring primarily in premature and low-birth-weight infants within the first week of life and less commonly in full-term infants.

ETIOLOGY. The condition has been considered as a variant of the spectrum of ischaemic bowel disease. Important factors in the etiology of this disorder, thus, are as follows:
1. Ischaemia. 2. Hypoxia/anoxia of the bowel due to bypassing of blood from the affected area. 3. Bacterial infection and endotoxins. 4. Establishment of feeding. 5. Infants fed on commercial formulae.

G/A The affected segment of the bowel is dilated, necrotic, haemorrhagic and friable. Bowel wall may contain bubbles of air (pneumatosis intestinalis).

M/E The changes are variable depending upon the stage. Initial changes are confined to mucosa and show oedema, haemorrhage and coagulative necrosis. A *pseudomembrane* composed of necrotic epithelium, fibrin and inflammatory cells may develop.

INFLAMMATORY BOWEL DISEASE (CROHN'S DISEASE AND ULCERATIVE COLITIS) *(p. 580)*

DEFINITION. The term 'inflammatory bowel disease (IBD)' is commonly used to include 2 idiopathic bowel diseases having many similarities but the conditions usually have distinctive morphological appearance:

1. Crohn's disease or Regional enteritis is an idiopathic chronic ulcerative IBD, characterised by transmural, non-caseating granulomatous inflammation, affecting most commonly the segment of terminal ileum and/or colon, though any part of the gastrointestinal tract may be involved.

2. Ulcerative colitis is an idiopathic form of acute and chronic ulcero-inflammatory colitis affecting chiefly the mucosa and submucosa of the rectum and descending colon, though sometimes it may involve the entire length of large bowel.

Both these disorders primarily affect the bowel but may have systemic involvement in the form of polyarthritis, uveitis, ankylosing spondylitis, skin lesions and hepatic involvement. Both diseases can occur at any age but are more common in 2nd and 3rd decades of life. Females are affected slightly more often.

ETIOPATHOGENESIS. The exact etiology of IBD remains unknown. The following observations, however, point towards multifactorial etiopathogenesis:

1. Genetic factors. Genetic factors are implicated in the etiopathogenesis of IBD is supported by the following evidences:
i) There is about 3 to 20 times higher incidence of occurrence of IBD in first-degree relatives.
ii) There is approximately 50% chance of development of IBD (particularly Crohn's disease) in monozygotic twins.
iii) Genomic search has revealed that disease-associated loci of IBD are present in chromosomes 16, 12, 7, 3 and 1 although there are no consistent genetic abnormalities.
iv) HLA studies show that ulcerative colitis is more common in DR2-related genes while Crohn's disease is more common in DR5 DQ1 alleles.

2. Immunologic factors. Defective immunologic regulation in IBD has been shown to play significant role in the pathogenesis of IBD:
i) *Defective regulation of immune suppression.* In a normal individual, there is lack of immune responsiveness to dietary antigens and commensal flora in the intestinal lumen. In IBD, this immune mechanism of suppression of inflammation is defective and thus results in uncontrolled inflammation.

ii) *Transgenic mouse experimental model studies.* Gene 'knock out' studies on colitis in mice have revealed that multiple immune abnormalities may be responsible for IBD.

iii) *Type of inflammatory cells.* In both types of IBD, activated CD4+ T cells are present in the lamina propria and in the peripheral blood. These cells either activate other inflammatory cells (e.g. macrophages and B cells), or recruit more inflammatory cells by stimulation of homing receptor on leucocytes and vascular endothelium.

3. Microbial factors. There has been some evidence, though not clear-cut, that IBD may have infectious etiology. Though at different times, different microorganisms (bacteria, viruses, protozoa and fungi) have been implicated by different workers, currently attention is focused on the three microbes: i) *Mycobacterium paratuberculosis* ii) *Measles virus* iii) *Helicobacter hepaticus.*

4. Psycosocial factors. It has been observed that individuals who are unduly sensitive, dependent on others and unable to express themselves, or some major life events such as illness or death in the family, divorce, interpersonal conflicts etc, suffer from irritable colon or have exacerbation of symptoms.

MORPHOLOGY. The morphologic features of Crohn's disease and ulcerative colitis are sufficiently distinctive so as to be classified separately. The distinguishing features of the two conditions are summarised in Table 18.5.

CROHN'S DISEASE. Crohn's disease may involve any portion of the gastrointestinal tract but affects most commonly 15-25 cm of the terminal ileum which may extend into the caecum and sometimes into the ascending colon:

G/A Characteristic feature is the multiple, well-demarcated segmental bowel involvement with intervening uninvolved 'skip areas'. The wall of the affected bowel segment is thick and hard, resembling a *'hose pipe'*. Serosa may be studded with minute granulomas. The lumen of the affected segment is markedly narrowed. The mucosa shows 'serpiginous ulcers', while intervening surviving mucosa is swollen giving 'cobblestone appearance'. There may be deep fissuring into the bowel wall.

M/E The characteristic features are:
1. *Transmural inflammatory cell infiltrate consisting* of chronic inflammatory cells (lymphocytes, plasma cells and macrophages) is the classical microscopic feature.
2. *Non-caseating, sarcoid-like granulomas* are present in all the layers of the affected bowel wall in 60% of cases.
3. There is *patchy ulceration* of the mucosa which may take the form of deep fissures.
4. There is *widening of the submucosa* due to oedema and foci of lymphoid aggregates.
5. In more *chronic cases,* fibrosis becomes increasingly prominent in all the layers.

   Complications of Crohn's disease are: 1. Malabsorption, 2. fistula formation, 3. stricture formation, and 4. development of malignancy.

ULCERATIVE COLITIS. Classically, ulcerative colitis begins in the rectum, and in continuity extends upwards into the sigmoid colon, descending colon, transverse colon, and sometimes may involve the entire colon. The colonic contents may rarely backflow into the terminal ileum in continuity, causing *'back-wash ileitis'* in about 10% of cases.

G/A The characteristic feature is the continuous involvement of rectum and colon without any uninvolved skip areas as seen in Crohn's disease. The

TABLE 18.5: Distinguishing Features of Crohn's Disease and Ulcerative Colitis.

	FEATURE	CROHN'S DISEASE	ULCERATIVE COLITIS
A.	**MACROSCOPIC FEATURES**		
1.	*Distribution*	Segmental with skip areas	Continuous without skip areas
2.	*Location*	Commonly terminal ileum and/or ascending colon	Commonly rectum, sigmoid colon and extending upwards
3.	*Extent*	Usually involves the entire thickness of the affected segment of bowel wall	Usually superficial, confined to mucosal layers
4.	*Ulcers*	Serpiginous ulcers, may develop into deep fissures	Superficial mucosal ulcers without fissures
5.	*Pseudopolyps*	Rarely seen	Commonly present
6.	*Fibrosis*	Common	Rare
7.	*Shortening*	Due to fibrosis	Due to contraction of muscularis
B.	**MICROSCOPIC FEATURES**		
1.	*Depth of inflammation*	Typically transmural	Mucosal and submucosal
2.	*Type of inflammation*	Non-caseating granulomas and infiltrate of mononuclear cells (lymphocytes, plasma cells and macrophages)	Crypt abscess and non-specific acute and chronic inflammatory cells (lympho-cytes, plasma cells, neutro-phils, eosinophils, mast cells)
3.	*Mucosa*	Patchy ulceration	Haemorrhagic mucosa with ulceration
4.	*Submucosa*	Widened due to oedema and lymphoid aggregates	Normal or reduced in width
5.	*Muscularis*	Infiltrated by inflammatory cells	Usually spared except in cases of toxic megacolon
6.	*Fibrosis*	Present	Usually absent
C.	**IMMUNOLOGIC FEATURES**		
1.	*Lymphocyte type*	CD4+ TH1	CD4+ TH2
2.	*Cytokines*	INF-γ, TNF, IL-12	TGF–β, IL-4, IL-5, IL-13
3.	*ANCA-P antibodies*	Positive in a few	Positive in most
D.	**COMPLICATIONS**		
1.	*Fistula formation*	Internal and external fistulae in 10% cases	Extremely rare
2.	*Malignant changes*	Rare	May occur infrequently in disease of more than 10 years' duration
3.	*Type of malignancy*	Lymphoma more than carcinoma	Carcinoma more than lymphoma
4.	*Fibrous strictures*	Common	Never

appearance of colon may vary depending upon the stage and intensity of the disease because of remissions and exacerbations. Mucosa shows linear and superficial ulcers, usually not penetrating the muscular layer. The intervening intact mucosa may form inflammatory 'pseudopolyps.' The muscle layer is thickened due to contraction, producing shortening and narrowing of the affected colon with loss of normal haustral folds giving 'garden-hose appear-ance'.

Chapter Eighteen

M/E Ulcerative colitis because of remission and exacerbations, is characterised by alternating 'active disease process' and 'resolving colitis.' The changes in the 'active disease process' are as under:

1. *Crypt distortion, cryptitis* and focal accumulations of neutrophils forming *crypt abscesses.*

2. *Marked congestion, dilatation and haemorrhages* from mucosal capillaries.

3. *Superficial mucosal ulcerations,* usually not penetrating into the muscle coat, except in severe cases.

4. *Goblet cells* are markedly *diminished.*

5. Areas of *mucosal regeneration and mucodepletion* of lining cells.

6. In long-standing cases, epithelial *cytologic atypia* ranging from mild to marked dysplasia and sometimes developing into carcinoma *in situ.*

Complications of ulcerative colitis are: 1. Toxic megacolon (Fulminant colitis), 2. perianal fistula, 3. carcinoma, and 4. stricture formation.

INFECTIVE ENTEROCOLITIS *(p. 584)*

These are a group of acute and chronic inflammatory lesions of small intestine and/or colon caused by microorganisms (bacteria, viruses, fungi, protozoa and helminths). All these are characterised by diarrhoeal syndromes. Pathogenetically speaking, these microorganisms can cause enterocolitis by 2 mechanisms—by *enteroinvasive bacteria* producing ulcerative lesions, and by *enterotoxin-producing bacteria* resulting in non-ulcerative lesions.

Intestinal Tuberculosis *(p. 584)*

Intestinal tuberculosis can occur in 3 forms—primary, secondary and hyperplastic caecal tuberculosis.

1. PRIMARY INTESTINAL TUBERCULOSIS. Though an uncommon disease in the Western world, primary tuberculosis of the ileocaecal region is quite common in India. It used to occur by ingestion of unpasteurised cow's milk infected with *Mycobacterium bovis.* But now-a-days due to control of tuberculosis in cattle and pasteurisation of milk, virtually all cases of intestinal tuberculosis are caused by *M. tuberculosis.* The predominant changes are in the mesenteric lymph nodes without any significant intestinal lesion.

G/A The affected lymph nodes are enlarged, matted and caseous (tabes mesenterica). Eventually, there is healing by fibrosis and calcification.

M/E In the initial stage, there is primary complex or Ghon's focus in the intestinal mucosa as occurs elsewhere in primary tuberculous infection. Subsequently, the mesenteric lymph nodes are affected which show typical tuberculous granulomatous inflammatory reaction with caseation necrosis.

2. SECONDARY INTESTINAL TUBERCULOSIS. Swallowing of sputum in patients with active pulmonary tuberculosis may cause secondary intestinal tuberculosis, most commonly in the terminal ileum and rarely in the colon.

G/A The intestinal lesions are prominent than the lesions in regional lymph nodes as in secondary pulmonary tuberculosis. The lesions begin in the Peyer's patches or the lymphoid follicles with formation of small ulcers that spread through the lymphatics to form large ulcers which are *transverse to the long axis of the bowel,* (*c.f.* typhoid ulcers of small intestine, described later).

M/E The tuberculous lesions in the intestine are similar to those observed elsewhere i.e. presence of tubercles. Mucosa and submucosa show ulceration and the muscularis may be replaced by variable degree of fibrosis. Tuberculous peritonitis may be observed.

3. HYPERPLASTIC CAECAL TUBERCULOSIS. This is a variant of secondary tuberculosis secondary to pulmonary tuberculosis.

G/A The caecum and/or ascending colon are thick-walled with mucosal ulceration. Clinically, the lesion is palpable and may be mistaken for carcinoma.

M/E The presence of caseating tubercles distinguishes the condition from Crohn's disease in which granulomas are non-caseating.

Enteric Fever (p. 586)

The term enteric fever is used to describe acute infection caused by *Salmonella typhi* (typhoid fever) or *Salmonella paratyphi* (paratyphoid fever). Besides these 2 salmonellae, *Salmonella typhimurium* causes food poisoning.

PATHOGENESIS. The typhoid bacilli are ingested through contaminated food or water. During the initial asymptomatic incubation period of about 2 weeks, the bacilli invade the lymphoid follicles and Peyer's patches of the small intestine and proliferate. Following this, the bacilli invade the bloodstream causing bacteraemia, and the characteristic clinical features of the disease like continuous rise in temperature and 'rose spots' on the skin are observed. Immunological reactions (Widal's test) begin after about 10 days and peak titres are seen by the end of the third week. Eventually, the bacilli are localised in the intestinal lymphoid tissue (producing typhoid intestinal lesions), in the mesenteric lymph nodes (leading to haemorrhagic lymphadenitis), in the liver (causing foci of parenchymal necrosis), in the gallbladder (producing typhoid cholecystitis), and in the spleen (resulting in splenic reactive hyperplasia).

MORPHOLOGY. The lesions are observed in the intestines as well as in other organs.

1.   INTESTINAL LESIONS. *G/A* Terminal ileum is affected most often, but lesions may be seen in the jejunum and colon. The Peyer's patches show oval typhoid ulcers with their *long axis along the length of the bowel*, (*c.f.* tuberculous ulcers of small intestine, described above). The base of the ulcers is black due to sloughed mucosa. The margins of the ulcers are slightly raised due to inflammatory oedema and cellular proliferation.

M/E There is hyperaemia, oedema and cellular proliferation consisting of phagocytic histiocytes (showing characteristic erythrophagocytosis), lymphocytes and plasma cells. Though enteric fever is an example of acute inflammation, neutrophils are invariably absent from the cellular infiltrate and this is reflected in the leucopenia with neutropenia and relative lymphocytosis in the peripheral blood.

The main **complications** of the intestinal lesions of typhoid are perforation of the ulcers and haemorrhage.

2.   OTHER LESIONS. Besides the intestinal involvement, various other organs and tissues showing pathological changes in enteric fever are as under:

i)   *Mesenteric lymph nodes*—haemorrhagic lymphadenitis. ii) *Liver*—foci of parenchymal necrosis. iii) *Gallbladder*—typhoid cholecystitis. iv) *Spleen*—splenomegaly with reactive hyperplasia. v) *Kidneys*—nephritis. vi) *Abdominal muscles*—Zenker's degeneration. vii) *Joints*—arthritis. viii) *Bones*—osteitis. ix) *Meninges*—Meningitis. x) *Testis*—Orchitis.

Bacterial Food Poisoning (p. 587)

This is a form of acute bacterial illness that occurs following ingestion of food or water contaminated with bacteria other than those that cause specific acute intestinal infections like typhoid, paratyphoid, cholera or dysentery bacilli.

1.   Staphylococcal food poisoning. *Staphylococcus aureus* infection acquired from contaminated food produces either *mild food poisoning* by enterotoxins, or may cause more severe form of the illness called *pseudomembranous enterocolitis* described below.

2. Clostridial food poisoning. Infection with anaerobic organisms *Clostridium welchii,* following consumption of contaminated meat results in acute food poisoning. The illness occurs both by bacterial invasion as well as by toxins.

3. Botulism. This is a severe form of paralysing illness caused by ingestion of organism, *Clostridium botulinum,* which produces neurotoxin.

4. Salmonella food poisoning (Salmonellosis). This is an infection (and not caused by toxins) occurring due to food contaminated by *S. typhimurium* or *S. enteritidis.*

Dysenteries *(p. 587)*

The term 'dysentery' is used to mean diarrhoea with abdominal cramps, tenesmus and passage of mucus in the stools, from any cause. There are 2 main forms of dysenteries—bacillary and amoebic.

1. BACILLARY DYSENTERY. Bacillary dysentery is the term used for infection by *shigella* species: *S. dysenteriae, S. flexneri, S. boydii* and *S. sonnei.* Infection occurs by foeco-oral route and is seen with poor personal hygiene, in densely populated areas, and with contaminated food and water. The common housefly plays a role in spread of infection.

2. AMOEBIC DYSENTERY. This is due to infection by *Entamoeba histolytica.* It is more prevalent in the tropical countries and primarily affects the large intestine. Infection occurs from ingestion of cyst form of the parasite. The cyst wall is dissolved in the small intestine from where the liberated amoebae pass into the large intestine. Here, they invade the epithelium of the mucosa, reach the submucosa and produce the characteristic flask-shaped ulcers.

G/A Early intestinal lesions appear as small areas of elevation on the mucosal surface. In advanced cases, typical flask-shaped ulcers having narrow neck and broad base are seen. They are more conspicuous in the caecum, rectum and in the flexures.

M/E The ulcerated area shows chronic inflammatory reaction consisting of lymphocytes, plasma cells, macrophages and eosinophils. The trophozoites of *Entamoeba* are seen in the inflammatory exudate and are concentrated at the advancing margin of the lesion.

Complications of intestinal amoebic ulcers are: amoebic liver abscess or amoebic hepatitis, perforation, haemorrhage and formation of amoeboma which is a tumour-like mass.

PSEUDOMEMBRANOUS ENTEROCOLITIS (ANTIBIOTIC-ASSOCIATED DIARRHOEA) *(p. 588)*

Pseudomembranous enterocolitis is a form of acute inflammation of colon and/or small intestine characterised by formation of '*pseudomembrane*' over the site of mucosal injury.

ETIOLOGY. Numerous studies have established the overgrowth of *Clostridium difficile* with production of its toxin in the etiology of antibiotic-associated diarrhoea culminating in pseudomembranous colitis. Oral antibiotics such as clindamycin, ampicillin and the cephalosporins are more often (20%) associated with antibiotic-associated diarrhoea, while development of pseudomembranous colitis may occur in 1-10% cases.

G/A The lesions may be confined, to the large intestine or small intestine, or both may be involved. The mucosa of the bowel is covered by patchy, raised yellow-white plaques.

M/E The '*pseudomembrane*' is composed of network of fibrin and mucus, in which are entangled inflammatory cells and mucosal epithelial cells. There is focal necrosis of surface epithelial cells.

MALABSORPTION SYNDROME *(p. 588)*

The malabsorption syndrome (MAS) is characterised by impaired intestinal absorption of nutrients especially of fat; some other substances are proteins, carbohydrates, vitamins and minerals. MAS is subdivided into 2 broad groups:

■ **Primary MAS,** which is due to primary deficiency of the absorptive mucosal surface and of the associated enzymes.

■ **Secondary MAS,** in which mucosal changes result secondary to other factors such as diseases, surgery, trauma and drugs.

Each of the two main groups has a number of causes listed in Table 18.6.

TABLE 18.6: Classification of Malabsorption Syndrome.

I.	**PRIMARY MALABSORPTION**
1.	Coeliac sprue
2.	Collagenous sprue
3.	Tropical sprue
4.	Whipple's disease
5.	Disaccharidase deficiency
6.	Allergic and eosinophilic gastroenteritis
II.	**SECONDARY MALABSORPTION**
1.	**Impaired digestion**
(i)	Mucosal damage e.g. in tuberculosis, Crohn's disease, lymphoma, amyloidosis, radiation injury, systemic sclerosis
(ii)	Hepatic and pancreatic insufficiency
(iii)	Resection of bowel
(iv)	Drugs e.g. methotrexate, neomycin, phenindione etc.
2.	**Impaired absorption**
(i)	Short or stagnant bowel (blind loop syndrome) from surgery or disease resulting in abnormal proliferation of microbial flora
(ii)	Acute infectious enteritis
(iii)	Parasitoses e.g. Giardia, Strongyloides, hookworms
3.	**Impaired transport**
(i)	Lymphatic obstruction e.g. in lymphoma tuberculosis, lymphangiectasia
(ii)	Abetalipoproteinaemia

Clinical Features *(p. 588)*

The clinical manifestations of MAS vary according to the underlying cause. However, some common symptoms are as follows:

1. Steatorrhoea (pale, bulky, foul-smelling stools), 2. chronic diarrhoea, 3. abdominal distension, 4. barborygmi and flatulence, 5. anorexia, 6. weight loss, 7. muscle wasting, 8. dehydration, 9. hypotension, and 10. specific malnutrition and vitamin deficiencies depending upon the cause.

Investigations *(p. 588)*

When MAS is suspected on clinical grounds, the following investigations may be carried out to confirm it:

I. LABORATORY TESTS. These are as under:

1. Tests for fat malabsorption: i) Faecal analysis for fat content. ii) Microscopic analysis for faecal fat. iii) Blood lipid levels after a fatty meal. iv) Tests based on absorption of radioactive-labelled fat.

2. Tests for protein malabsorption: i) Bile acid malabsorption. ii) Radioactive-labelled glycine breath test. iii) Prothrombin time (vitamin K deficiency). iv) Secretin and other pancreatic tests.

Chapter Eighteen

3. Tests for carbohydrate malabsorption: i) D-xylose tolerance test. ii) Lactose tolerance test. iii) Hydrogen breath test. iv) Bile acid breath test.

4. Vitamin B$_{12}$, malabsorption: i) Schilling test.

II. INTESTINAL BIOPSY: Per-oral small intestinal biopsy employing Crosby-Kugler capsule or endoscopic biopsy are widely used for investigation and diagnosis of MAS. The biopsy should first be examined under dissecting microscope before histologic sectioning.

Normal villous. Under the dissecting microscope, the normal jejunal mucosa has tall, slender, finger-shaped or leaf-shaped villi. It is lined by tall columnar absorptive epithelium and has scattered lymphocytes in the lamina propria.

Villous atrophy. Variable degree of flattening of intestinal mucosa in MAS is the commonest pathological change in mucosal pattern and is referred to as villous atrophy. It may be of 2 types—partial and subtotal/total type.

■ *Partial villous atrophy* is the mild form of the lesion in which villi fuse with each other and thus become short and broad, commonly called as convolutions and irregular ridges. The epithelial cells show compensatory hyperplasia suggesting a turnover of these cells. Lamina propria shows increased cellular infiltrate, predominantly of plasma cells.

Partial villous atrophy is commonly found in children and adults with diarrhoea, parasitic infestations, Crohn's disease, ulcerative colitis and malabsorption due to drugs and radiation injury.

■ *Subtotal/Total villous atrophy* is the severe form of the lesion in which there is flattening of mucosa due to more advanced villous fusion. The surface epithelium is cuboidal and there is increased plasma cell infiltrate in the lamina propria.

Subtotal and total villous atrophy is exhibited by a number of conditions such as nontropical sprue, tropical sprue, intestinal lymphomas, carcinoma, protein-calorie malnutrition etc.

Coeliac Sprue (Non-tropical Sprue, Gluten-Sensitive Enteropathy, Idiopathic Steatorrhoea) *(p. 589)*

This is the most important cause of primary malabsorption occurring in temperate climates. The condition is characterised by significant loss of villi in the small intestine and thence diminished absorptive surface area. The condition occurs in 2 forms:

Childhood form, seen in infants and children and is commonly referred to as *coeliac disease.*

Adult form, seen in adolescents and early adult life and used to be called *idiopathic steatorrhoea.*

In either case, there is genetic abnormality resulting in sensitivity to gluten (a protein) and its derivative, gliadin, present in diets such as grains of wheat, barley and rye. The symptoms are usually relieved on elimination of gluten from the diet. The role of heredity is further supported by the observation of familial incidence and HLA association of the disease.

M/E There is variable degree of flattening of the mucosa, particularly of the upper jejunum, and to some extent of the duodenum and ileum. The surface epithelial cells are cuboidal or low columnar type. There may be *partial villous atrophy* which is replacement of normal villous pattern by convolutions, or *subtotal villous atrophy* characterised by flat mucosal surface.

The major sequela of long-term coeliac sprue is increased incidence of intestinal carcinoma in these cases.

Collagenous Sprue *(p. 590)*

This entity is regarded as the end-result of coeliac sprue in which the villi are totally absent *(total villous atrophy)* and there are unique and diagnostic broad bands of collagen under the basal lamina of surface epithelium.

Tropical Sprue *(p. 590)*

This disease, as the name suggests, occurs in individuals living in or visiting tropical areas such as Caribbean countries, South India, Sri Lanka and Hong Kong. Pathogenesis of the condition is not clear but there is evidence to support enterotoxin production by some strains of *E. coli* which causes the intestinal injury.

M/E There is usually *partial villous atrophy* and sometimes *subtotal atrophy*.

Whipple's Disease (Intestinal Lipodystrophy) *(p. 591)*

This is an uncommon bacterial disease involving not only the intestines but also various other systems such as central nervous system, heart, blood vessels, skin, joints, lungs, liver, spleen and kidneys. Patients may present with features of malabsorption or may have atypical presentation in the form of migratory polyarthritis, neurological disturbances and focal hyperpigmentation of the skin.

M/E The affected tissues show presence of characteristic macrophages containing PAS-positive granules and rod-shaped micro-organisms (Whipple's bacilli). These macrophages are predominantly present in the lamina propria of the small intestine and mesenteric lymph nodes.

SMALL INTESTINAL TUMOURS *(p. 591)*

For obscure reasons, benign as well as malignant tumours of the small bowel are surprisingly rare. Most common *benign tumours,* in descending order of frequency, are: leiomyomas, adenomas and vascular tumours (haemangioma, lymphangioma). Amongst the *malignant tumours,* the most frequently encountered, in descending frequency, are: carcinoid tumours, lymphomas and adenocarcinoma.

Carcinoid Tumour (Argentaffinoma) *(p. 591)*

Carcinoid tumour or argentaffinoma is a generic term applied to tumours originating from endocrine cells *(synonyms:* argentaffin cells, Kulchitsky cells, enterochromaffin cells) belonging to APUD cell system and are therefore also called as apudomas. The endocrine cells are distributed throughout the mucosa of GI tract. These cells have secretory granules which stain positively with silver salts (argentaffin granules) or many stain after addition of exogenous reducing agent (non-argentaffin or argyrophil granules). Accordingly, carcinoid tumour may be argentaffin or argyrophil type. Depending upon the embryologic derivation of the tissues where the tumour is located, these are classified as foregut, midgut, and hindgut carcinoids.

■ **Midgut carcinoids,** seen in terminal ileum and appendix are the most common (60-80%) and are more often argentaffin positive.

■ **Hindgut carcinoids,** occurring in rectum and colon are more commonly argyrophil type, and comprise about 10-20% of carcinoids.

■ **Foregut carcinoids,** located in the stomach, duodenum and oesophagus are also argyrophil type and are encountered as frequently as in the hindgut (10-20%).

Other uncommon locations are bronchus, trachea, gallbladder, and Meckel's diverticulum.

Appendix and terminal ileum, the two most common sites for carcinoids, depict variation in their age and sex incidence and biologic behaviour:

■ **Appendiceal carcinoids,** occur more frequently in 3rd and 4th decades of life without any sex predilection, are often solitary and behave as locally malignant tumours.

■ **Ileal carcinoids,** on the other hand, are seen more often in later age (7th decade) with female preponderance, are more commonly multiple and behave like metastasising carcinomas.

G/A All carcinoids are small, button-like submucosal elevations with intact or ulcerated overlying mucosa. They are usually small; those larger than 2 cm are more often metastasising. Ileal and gastric carcinoids are commonly multiple, whereas appendiceal carcinoids commonly involve the tip of the organ and are solitary. Cut section of all the carcinoids is bright yellow.

M/E The tumour cells may be arranged in a variety of patterns—solid nests, sheets, cords, trabeculae and clusters, all of which show characteristic palisading of the peripheral cells. Acinar arrangement and rosettes are rarely seen. The tumour cells are classically small, monotonous, having uniform nuclei and poorly-defined cell boundaries.

CARCINOID SYNDROME. Carcinoid tumours that metastasise, especially to the liver, are sometimes associated with the carcinoid syndrome. The syndrome consists of the following features:
1. Intermittent attacks of flushing of the skin of face
2. Episodes of watery diarrhoea
3. Abdominal pain
4. Attacks of dyspnoea due to bronchospasm
5. Right-sided heart failure due to involvement of tricuspid and pulmonary valves and endocardium.

A number of *secretory products* in a functioning carcinoid tumour have been demonstrated: i) 5-Hydroxytryptamine (5-HT, serotonin), ii) 5-Hydroxytryptophan, iii) 5-Hydroxy-indole acetic acid (5-HIAA), iv) histamine, v) kallikrein, and vi) bradykinin.

However, 5-HT and its degradation product, 5-HIAA, are particularly significant in the production of *carcinoid syndrome*. 5-HT, a potent vasodilator and smooth muscle stimulant, is normally synthesised in the endocrine cells of the gut from dietary tryptophan.

APPENDIX *(p. 592)*

NORMAL STRUCTURE *(p. 592)*

Appendix is a vestigial organ which serves no useful purpose in man but instead becomes the site of trouble at times. It is like a diverticulum of the caecum, usually lying behind the caecum and varies in length from 4 to 20 cm (average 7 cm).

M/E Appendix has four layers in its wall—*mucosa, submucosa, muscularis* and *serosa*. The mucosa has patchy distribution of crypts and the submucosa has abundant lymphoid tissue. Argentaffin and non-argentaffin endocrine cells are present in the base of mucosal glands just as in the small intestine.

APPENDICITIS *(p. 593)*

Acute inflammation of the appendix, acute appendicitis, is the most common acute abdominal condition confronting the surgeon. The condition is seen more commonly in older children and young adults, and is uncommon at the extremes of age. The disease is seen more frequently in the West and in affluent societies which may be due to variation in diet—a diet with low bulk or cellulose and high protein intake more often causes appendicitis.

ETIOPATHOGENESIS. The most common etiological factor is obstruction of the lumen that leads to increased intraluminal pressure. This presses upon the blood vessels to produce ischaemic injury which in turn favours the bacterial proliferation and hence acute appendicitis. The common causes of appendicitis are as under:

A. Obstructive: 1. Faecolith, 2. calculi, 3. foreign body, 4. tumour, 5. worms (especially *Enterobius vermicularis),* and 6. diffuse lymphoid hyperplasia, especially in children.

B. Non-obstructive: 1. Haematogenous spread of generalised infection, 2. vascular occlusion, and 3. inappropriate diet lacking roughage.

G/A The appearance depends upon the stage at which the acutely-inflamed appendix is examined. In *early acute appendicitis,* the organ is swollen and serosa shows hyperaemia. In well-developed acute inflammation called *acute suppurative appendicitis,* the serosa is coated with fibrinopurulent exudate and engorged vessels on the surface. In further advanced cases called *acute gangrenous appendicitis,* there is necrosis and ulcerations of mucosa which extend through the wall.

M/E The most important diagnostic histological criteria is the *neutrophilic infiltration of the muscularis.* In early stage, the other changes besides acute inflammatory changes, are congestion and oedema of the appendiceal wall. In later stages, the mucosa is sloughed off, the wall becomes necrotic, the blood vessels may get thrombosed and there may be neutrophilic abscesses in the wall.

CLINICAL COURSE. The patient presents with features of acute abdomen as under:
1. Colicky pain, initially around umbilicus but later localised to right iliac fossa
2. Nausea and vomiting
3. Pyrexia of mild grade
4. Abdominal tenderness
5. Increased pulse rate
6. Neutrophilic leucocytosis.

An attack of acute appendicitis predisposes the appendix to repeated attacks *(recurrent acute appendicitis)* and thus surgery has to be carried out.

COMPLICATIONS 1. Peritonitis, 2. appendix abscess, 3. adhesions, 4. portal pylephlebitis, and 5. mucocele.

TUMOURS OF APPENDIX *(p. 594)*

CARCINOID TUMOUR. Both argentaffin and argyrophil types are encountered, the former being more common.

PSEUDOMYXOMA PERITONEI. Pseudomyxoma peritonei is appearance of gelatinous mucinous material around the appendix which may be from benign mucinous cystadenoma of the ovary or mucin-secreting carcinoma of the appendix.

ADENOCARCINOMA. It is an uncommon tumour in the appendix and is morphologically similar to adenocarcinoma elsewhere in the alimentary tract.

LARGE INTESTINE *(p. 595)*

NORMAL STRUCTURE *(p. 595)*

The large bowel consists of 6 parts—the caecum, ascending colon, transverse colon, descending colon, sigmoid colon and rectum, and in all measures about 1.5 meters in length. The serosal surface of the large intestine except the rectum is studded with *appendices epiploicae* which are small, rounded collections of fatty tissue covered by peritoneum.

M/E The wall of large bowel consists of 4 layers as elsewhere in the alimentary tract.

■ The **mucosa** lacks villi and there is preponderance of goblet cells over columnar epithelial cells.

■ The **muscularis propria** of the large intestine is quite peculiar—the inner circular muscle layer ensheaths whole length of the intestine, while the outer longitudinal muscle layer is concentrated into 3 muscle bands called *taenia coli*. The length of outer muscle layer is shorter than the length of the intestine and therefore, it forms the *sacculations or haustra* of the large intestine.

Anal canal, 3-4 cm long tubular structure, begins at the lower end of the rectum, though is not a part of large bowel, but is included here to cover simultaneously lesions pertaining to this region. It is lined by keratinised or nonkeratinised stratified squamous epithelium.

CONGENITAL AND MISCELLANEOUS CONDITIONS *(p. 595)*

Hirschsprung's Disease (Congenital Megacolon) *(p. 595)*

The term 'megacolon' is used for any form of marked dilatation of the entire colon or its segment and may occur as a congenital or acquired disorder. *Congenital form* characterised by congenital absence of ganglion cells in the bowel wall (enteric neurons) is called Hirschsprung's disease. As a result, the aganglionic segment remains contracted.

Clinically, the condition manifests shortly after birth with constipation, gaseous distension and sometimes with acute intestinal obstruction. Pathogenesis lies in the failure of neuroblasts to migrate to the rectum which normally occurs at about 12 weeks of gestation. Depending upon the length of the segment affected by aganglionosis in Hirschsprung's disease, 4 patterns are recognised:

1. *Short segment (rectal and recto-sigmoid) disease* as the most common form.
2. *Long segment or subtotal colonic disease,* involving colon from rectosigmoid to the ileo-caecal valve.
3. *Total colonic aganglionosis.*
4. *Ultra-short segment disease.*

G/A Typical case of Hirschsprung's disease shows 2 segments—a *distal narrow segment* that is aganglionic and a *dilated proximal segment* that contains normal number of ganglion cells.

M/E The distal narrow segment shows total absence of ganglion cells of all the three plexuses (Auerbach's or myenteric plexus present between the two layers of muscularis, deep submucosal or Henle's plexus, and superficial mucosal or Meissner's plexus) and prominence of non-myelinated nerve fibres. Histochemical staining for acetylcholine esterase activity provides confirmation for identifying ganglion cells and nerve trunks.

The various causes of **acquired megacolon** are as under:

1. *Obstructive* e.g. due to tumour, post-inflammatory strictures.
2. *Endocrine* e.g. in myxoedema, cretinism.
3. *CNS disorders* e.g. spina bifida, paraplegia, parkinsonism.
4. *Psychogenic* e.g. emotional disturbances, psychiatric disorders.
5. *Chagas' disease* due to infection with *Trypanosoma cruzi.*

Diverticulosis Coli *(p. 596)*

Diverticula are the outpouchings or herniations of the mucosa and submucosa of the colon through the muscle wall. *Diverticular disease,* as it is commonly known, is rare under 30 years of age and is seen more commonly as the age advances. Multiple diverticula of the colon are very common in the Western societies, probably due to ingestion of low-fibre diet but is seen much less frequently in tropical countries and in Japan. Diverticulosis is often asymptomatic and may be detected as an incidental finding at autopsy. However, a proportion of patients develop clinical symptoms such as low abdominal pain, distension, constipation and sometimes intermittent bleeding.

The etiologic role of the following 2 factors is generally accepted in the pathogenesis of diverticular disease of the colon: 1. Increased intraluminal pressure, and 2. muscular weakness.

G/A Diverticulosis is seen most commonly in the sigmoid colon (95%) but any other part of the entire colon may be involved. They may vary in number from a few to several hundred. They appear as small, spherical or flask-shaped outpouchings, usually less than 1 cm in diameter, commonly extend into appendices epiploicae and may contain inspissated faeces.

M/E The flask-shaped structures extend from the intestinal lumen through the muscle layer. The colonic wall in the affected area is thin and is composed of atrophic mucosa, compressed submucosa and thin or deficient muscularis.

The *complications* of diverticulosis and diverticulitis are perforation, haemorrhage, intestinal obstruction and fistula formation.

Melanosis Coli *(p. 597)*

Melanosis coli is a peculiar condition in which mucosa of the large intestine acquires brown-black coloration. The condition is said to occur in individuals who are habitual users of cathartics of anthracene type.

Haemorrhoids (Piles) *(p. 597)*

Haemorrhoids or piles are the varicosities of the haemorrhoidal veins. They are called *'internal piles'* if dilatation is of superior haemorrhoidal plexus covered over by mucous membrane, and *'external piles'* if they involve inferior haemorrhoidal plexus covered over by the skin. They are common lesions in elderly and pregnant women. They commonly result from increased venous pressure. The possible causes include the following:
1. Portal hypertension, 2. chronic constipation and straining at stool, 3. cardiac failure, 4. venous stasis of pregnancy, 5. hereditary predisposition, and 6. tumours of the rectum.

M/E Thin-walled and dilated tortuous veins are seen under the rectal mucosa *(internal piles)* or anal skin *(external piles)*.

Angiodysplasia *(p. 597)*

Angiodysplasia is a submucosal telangiectasia affecting caecum and right colon that causes recurrent acute and chronic haemorrhage. The condition is more common in the elderly past 6th decade. The pathogenesis is obscure but is possibly due to mechanical obstruction of the veins.

MISCELLANEOUS INFLAMMATORY CONDITIONS *(p. 597)*

■ **'Fistula-in-ano'** is a well known and common condition in which one or more fistulous tracts pass from the internal opening at the pectinate line through the internal sphincter on to the skin surface.

■ **'Anal fissure'** is an ulcer in the anal canal below the level of the pectinate line, mostly in midline and posteriorly.

■ **'Solitary rectal ulcer syndrome'** is a condition characterised usually by solitary, at times multiple, rectal ulcers with prolapse of rectal mucosa and development of proctitis.

COLORECTAL POLYPS *(p. 597)*

A polyp is defined as any growth or mass protruding from the mucous membrane into the lumen. Polyps are much more common in the large intestine than in the small intestine and are more common in the rectosigmoid colon than the proximal colon. Polyps are broadly classified into 2 groups—non-neoplastic and neoplastic. Non-neoplastic polyps have further subtypes indicating their mode of origin. Neoplastic polyps, on the other hand, include epithelial tumours, both benign and malignant (Table 18.7).

TABLE 18.7: Polyps and Tumours of the Large Intestine.

I.	**COLORECTAL POLYPS**
A.	**Non-neoplastic polyps**
	1. Hyperplastic (metaplastic) polyps
	2. Hamartomatous polyps
	(i) Peutz-Jeghers polyps and polyposis
	(ii) Juvenile (Retention) polyps and polyposis
	3. Inflammatory polyps (Pseudopolyps)
	4. Lymphoid polyps
B.	**Neoplastic polyps**
	1. Adenoma
	(i) Tubular adenoma (Adenomatous polyp)
	(ii) Villous adenoma (villous papilloma)
	(iii) Tubulovillous adenoma (Papillary adenoma, villoglandular adenoma)
	2. Polypoid carcinoma
C.	**Familial polyposis syndromes**
	1. Familial polyposis coli (Adenomatosis)
	2. Gardner's syndrome
	3. Turcot's syndrome
	4. Juvenile polyposis syndrome
II.	**OTHER BENIGN COLORECTAL TUMOURS**
	(Leiomyomas, leiomyoblastoma, neurilemmoma, lipoma and vascular tumours)
III.	**MALIGNANT COLORECTAL TUMOURS**
A.	**Carcinoma**
	1. Adenocarcinoma
	2. Other carcinomas
	(Mucinous adenocarcinoma, signet-ring cell carcinoma, adenosquamous carcinoma, undifferentiated carcinoma)
B.	**Other malignant tumours**
	(Leiomyosarcoma, malignant lymphoma, carcinoid tumours)
IV.	**TUMOURS OF THE ANAL CANAL**
A.	**Benign** (viral warts or condyloma acuminata)
B.	**Malignant** (squamous cell carcinoma, basaloid carcinoma, mucoepidermoid carcinoma, adenocarcinoma, undifferentiated carcinoma, malignant melanoma)

A. NON-NEOPLASTIC POLYPS *(p. 597)*

Hyperplastic (Metaplastic) Polyps *(p. 597)*

The hyperplastic or metaplastic polyps are the most common amongst all epithelial polyps, particularly in the rectosigmoid. They are called *'hyperplastic'* because there is epithelial hyperplasia at the base of the crypts, and *'metaplastic'* as there are areas of cystic metaplasia.

G/A Hyperplastic polyps are generally multiple, sessile, smooth-surfaced and small (less than 0.5 cm).

M/E They are composed of long and cystically dilated glands and crypts lined by normal epithelial cells. Their lining is partly flat and partly papillary. The luminal border of the lining epithelium is often serrated or saw-toothed.

Hyperplastic polyps are usually symptomless and have no malignant potential unless there is a coexistent adenoma.

Hamartomatous Polyps (p. 598)

These are tumour-like lesions composed of abnormal mixture of tissues indigenous to the part. They are further of 2 types:

I) PEUTZ-JEGHERS POLYPS AND POLYPOSIS. Peutz-Jeghers syndrome is autosomal dominant defect, characterised by hamartomatous intestinal polyposis and melanotic pigmentation of lips, mouth and genitalia. The polyps may be located in the stomach, small intestine or colon but are most common in the jejunum and ileum.

G/A These polyps are of variable size but are often large, multiple and pedunculated and more commonly situated in the small intestine.

M/E The most characteristic feature is the tree-like branching of muscularis mucosae. The lining epithelium is by normal-appearing epithelial cells.

Peutz-Jeghers polyps do not undergo malignant transformation unless a coexistent adenoma is present.

II) JUVENILE (RETENTION) POLYPS. Juvenile or retention polyps, another form of hamartomatous polyps, occur more commonly in children below 5 years of age.

G/A Juvenile polyps are spherical, smooth-surfaced, about 2 cm in diameter and are often pedunculated.

M/E The classical appearance is of cystically dilated glands containing mucus and lined by normal mucus-secreting epithelium.

Most cases, on becoming symptomatic in the form of rectal bleeding, are removed. In common with other non-neoplastic polyps, they are also not precancerous.

Inflammatory Polyps (Pseudopolyps) (p. 599)

Inflammatory polyps or pseudopolyps appear due to re-epithelialisation of the undermined ulcers and overhanging margins in inflammatory bowel disease, most frequently in ulcerative colitis (colitis polyposa) and sometimes in Crohn's disease.

G/A They are usually multiple, cylindrical to rounded overgrowths of mucosa and may vary from minute nodules to several centimeters in size.

M/E The centre of inflammatory polyp consists of connective tissue core that shows some inflammatory cell infiltrate and is covered superficially by regenerating epithelial cells and some cystically-dilated glands.

These lesions have no malignant potential; carcinomas seen in long-standing cases of ulcerative colitis arise in the region of epithelial dysplasia and not from the polyps.

Lymphoid Polyps (p. 599)

Reactive hyperplasia of lymphoid tissue that is normally also more prominent in the rectum and terminal ileum, gives rise to localised or diffuse lymphoid polyps. Localised form occurs more often in the rectum in elderly, while diffuse form is seen at younger age and in children.

G/A They are solitary or multiple, tiny elevated lesions.

M/E They are composed of prominent lymphoid follicles with germinal centres located in the submucosa and mucosa, and are covered by epithelium that may be inflamed.

Chapter Eighteen

They are benign lesions and have to be distinguished from malignant lymphoma.

B. NEOPLASTIC POLYPS *(p. 599)*

Tubular Adenoma (Adenomatous Polyp) *(p. 599)*

Tubular adenomas or adenomatous polyps are the most common neoplastic polyps (75%). They are common beyond 3rd decade of life and have slight male preponderance. They occur most often in the distal colon and rectum. They may be found singly as sporadic cases, or multiple tubular adenomas as part of familial polyposis syndrome with autosomal dominant inheritance pattern.

G/A Adenomatous polyps may be single or multiple, sessile or pedunculated, vary in size from less than 1 cm to large, spherical masses with an irregular surface.

M/E The usual appearance is of benign tumour overlying muscularis mucosa and is composed of branching tubules which are embedded in the lamina propria. The lining epithelial cells are of large intestinal type with diminished mucus secreting capacity, large nuclei and increased mitotic activity. However, tubular adenomas may show variable degree of cytologic atypia ranging from atypical epithelium restricted within the glandular basement membrane called as 'carcinoma *in situ*' to invasion into the fibrovascular stromal core referred to as frank 'adenocarcinoma'.

Malignant transformation is present in about 5% of tubular adenomas; the incidence being higher in larger adenomas.

Villous Adenoma (Villous Papilloma) *(p. 600)*

Villous adenomas or villous papillomas of the colon are much less common than tubular adenomas. The mean age at which they appear is 6th decade of life with approximatey equal sex incidence.

G/A Villous adenomas are round to oval exophytic masses, usually sessile, varying in size from 1 to 10 cm or more in diameter. Their surface may be haemorrhagic or ulcerated.

M/E The characteristic histologic feature is the presence of many slender, finger-like villi, which appear to arise directly from the area of muscularis mucosae. Each of the papillae has fibrovascular stromal core that is covered by epithelial cells varying from apparently benign to anaplastic cells.

Villous adenomas are invariably symptomatic; rectal bleeding, diarrhoea and mucus being the common features. The presence of severe atypia, carcinoma *in situ* and invasive carcinoma are seen more frequently. Invasive carcinoma has been reported in 30% of villous adenomas.

Tubulovillous Adenoma
(Papillary Adenoma, Villoglandular Adenoma) *(p. 600)*

Tubulovillous adenoma is an intermediate form of pattern between tubular adenoma and villous adenoma. It is also known by other names like papillary adenoma and villo-glandular adenoma.

G/A Tubulovillous adenomas may be sessile or pedunculated and range in size from 0.5-5 cm.

M/E They show intermediate or mixed pattern, characteristic vertical villi and deeper part showing tubular pattern.

The behaviour of tubulovillous adenoma is intermediate between tubular and villous adenomas.

C. FAMILIAL POLYPOSIS SYNDROMES *(p. 601)*

Familial Polyposis Coli (Adenomatosis) *(p. 601)*

This hereditary disease is defined as the presence of more than 100 neoplastic polyps (adenomas) on the mucosal surface of the colon; the average number is about 1000. Adenomatosis can be distinguished from multiple adenomas in which the number of adenomas is fewer, not exceeding 100. The condition has autosomal dominant transmission and is due to germline mutations in *APC* gene which results in occurrence of hundreds of adenomas which progress to invasive cancer. The average age at diagnosis is 2nd and 3rd decades of life with equal incidence in both the sexes.

G/A and M/E The commonest pattern is that of adenomatous polyps (tubular adenomas) discussed above.

The malignant potential of familial polyposis coli is very high. Colorectal cancer develops virtually in 100% of cases over a period of several years if not treated with colectomy.

Gardner's Syndrome *(p. 601)*

Gardner's syndrome is combination of familial polyposis coli and certain extra-colonic lesions such as multiple osteomas (particularly of the mandible and maxilla), sebaceous cysts and connective tissue tumours.

Turcot's Syndrome *(p. 601)*

Turcot's syndrome is combination of familial polyposis coli and malignant neoplasms of the central nervous system.

Juvenile Polyposis Syndrome *(p. 601)*

Juvenile polyposis is appearance of multiple juvenile polyps in the colon, stomach and small intestine but their number is not as high as in familial polyposis coli. Family history in some cases may show autosomal dominant inheritance pattern.

MALIGNANT COLORECTAL TUMOURS *(p. 601)*

A. Colorectal Carcinoma *(p. 601)*

Colorectal cancer comprises 98% of all malignant tumours of the large intestine. It is the commonest form of visceral cancer, next only to lung cancer in the United States. The incidence of carcinoma of the large intestine rises with age; average age of patients is about 60 years.

ETIOLOGY. A few etiological factors have been implicated:

1. Geographic variations. The incidence of large bowel carcinoma shows wide variation throughout the world. Colorectal cancer is generally thought to be a disease of affluent societies because its incidence is directly correlated with the socioeconomic status of the countries. In Japan, however, colon cancer is much less common than in the US but the incidence of rectal cancer is similar.

2. Dietary factors. The following factors are implicated.
i)   A low intake of vegetable fibre-diet leading to low stool bulk is associated with higher risk of colorectal cancer.
ii) Consumption of large amounts of fatty foods by populations results in excessive cholesterol and their metabolites which may be carcinogenic.
iii) Excessive consumption of refined carbohydrates that remain in contact with the colonic mucosa for prolonged duration changes the bacterial flora of the bowel.

3. Adenoma-carcinoma sequence. There is strong evidence to suggest that colonic adenocarcinoma arises from pre-existing adenomas, referred to as adenoma-carcinoma sequence. The following evidences are cited to support this hypothesis:

i) In a case with early invasive cancer, the surounding tissue often shows *preceding changes* of evolution from adenoma → hyperplasia → dysplasia → carcinoma *in situ* → invasive carcinoma.

ii) *Incidence* of adenomas in a population is directly proportionate to the prevalence of colorectal cancer.

iii) The risk of adenocarcinoma colon declines with *endoscopic removal* of all identified adenomas.

iv) The peak incidence of adenomas generally *precedes* by some years to a few decades the peak incidence for colorectal cancer.

v) The risk of malignancy increases with the following *adenoma-related factors:*

a) *Number of adenomas*: familial polyposis syndromes almost certainly evolve into malignancy.

b) *Size of adenomas*: large size increases the risk.

c) *Type of adenomas*: greater villous component associated with higher prevalence.

4. Other diseases. Presence of certain pre-existing diseases such as inflammatory bowel disease (especially ulcerative colitis) and diverticular disease for long duration increases the risk of developing colorectal cancer subsequently.

GENETIC BASIS OF COLORECTAL CARCINOGENESIS. Studies by molecular genetics have revealed that there are sequential multistep mutations in evolution of colorectal cancer from adenomas by one of the following two mechanisms:

1. APC mutation/ β-catenin mechanism. This pathway of multiple mutations is generally associated with morphologically identifiable changes as described above in adenoma-carcinoma sequence. These changes are as under:

i) Loss of tumour suppressor APC (adenomatous polyposis coli) gene. ii) Point mutation in K-RAS gene. iii) Deletion of DCC gene. iv) Loss of TP53 tumour suppressor gene.

2. Microsatellite instability mechanism. In this pathway also, there are multiple mutations but of different genes, and unlike APC mutation/β–catenin mechanism there are no morphologically identifiable changes. Basic mutation is loss of DNA repair gene. This results in a situation in which repetitive DNA sequences (i.e. microsatellites) become unstable during replication cycle, termed microsatellite instability, which is the hallmark of this pathway. The significant DNA repair genes which are mutated in colon cancer as under:

i) TGF-β receptor gene, ii) BAX gene.

LOCATION. *Distribution* of the primary colorectal cancer reveals that about 60% of the cases occur in the rectum, followed in descending order, by sigmoid and descending colon (25%), caecum and ileocaecal valve (10%); ascending colon, hepatic and splenic flexures (5%); and quite uncommonly in the transverse colon.

G/A There are distinct differences between the growth on the right and left half of the colon:

■　The **right-sided growths** tend to be large, cauliflower-like, soft and friable masses projecting into the lumen *(fungating polypoid carcinoma)*.

■　**Growths in the left colon,** on the other hand, have napkin-ring configuration i.e. they encircle the bowel wall circumferentially with increased fibrous tissue forming annular ring, and have central ulceration on the surface with slightly elevated margins *(carcinomatous ulcers)*.

M/E The appearance of right and left-sided growths is similar. About 95% of colorectal carcinomas are adenocarcinomas of varying grades of differentiation, out of which approximately 10% are mucin-secreting colloid carcinomas. The remaining 5% tumours include uncommon microscopic patterns like undifferentiated carcinoma, signet-ring cell carcinoma, and adeno-squamous carcinomas seen in more distal colon near the anus. The histologic grades indicating the degree of differentiation are: well-differentiated, moderately-differentiated and poorly-differentiated.

SPREAD. The tumour may spread by following routes:

1. Direct spread. The tumour spreads most commonly by direct extension in both ways— *circumferentially* into the bowel wall as well as *directly* into the depth of the bowel wall to the serosa, pericolic fat, and sometimes into peritoneal cavity.

2. Lymphatic spread. Spread via lymphatics occurs rather commonly and involves, firstly the regional lymph nodes in the vicinity of the tumour, and then into other groups of lymph nodes like preaortic, internal iliac and the sacral lymph nodes.

3. Haematogenous spread. Blood spread of large bowel cancer occurs relatively late and involves the liver, lungs, brain, bones and ovary.

CLINICAL FEATURES. i) Occult bleeding (melaena). ii) Change in bowel habits, more often in left-sided growth.iii) Loss of weight (cachexia). iv) Loss of appetite (anorexia). v) Anaemia, weakness, malaise.

The most common *complications* are obstruction and haemorrhage; less often perforation and secondary infection may occur. Aside from the diagnostic methods like stool test for occult blood, PR examination, procto-scopy, radiographic contrast studies and CT scan, recently the role of tumourmarkers has been emphasised. Of particular importance is the estimation of carcinoembryonic antigen (CEA) level which is elevated in 100% cases of metastatic colorectal cancers, while it is positive in 20-40% of early lesions, and 60-70% of advanced primary lesions.

The **prognosis** of colorectal cancer depends upon a few variables: i) Extent of the bowel involvement. ii) Presence or absence of metastases. iii) Histologic grade of the tumour. iv) Location of the tumour.

The most important prognostic factor in colorectal cancer is, however, the stage of the disease at the time of diagnosis. Three staging systems are in use:

1. *Dukes' ABC staging* (modified Duke's includes stage D as well).

2. *Astler-Coller staging* which is a further modification of Duke's staging and is most widely used.

3. *TNM staging* described by American Joint committee is also used.

IV. TUMOURS OF THE ANAL CANAL *(p. 605)*

Amongst the *benign tumours* of the anal canal, multiple viral warts called as condyloma acuminata are the only tumours of note. *Malignant tumours* of the anal canal include: 1. Squamous cell carcinoma. 2. Basaloid carcinoma. 3. Mucoepidermoid carcinoma. 4. Adenocarcinoma (rectal, of anal glands, within anorectal fistulas) 5. Undifferentiated carcinoma. 6. Malignant melanoma.

CAUSES OF GASTROINTESTINAL BLEEDING *(p. 606)*

Gastrointestinal bleeding from upper (haematemesis), middle (small intestinal) and lower (melaena) is a major presenting clinical feature of a variety of gastrointestinal diseases. Table 18.8 summarises the main causes of gastrointestinal bleeding.

TABLE 18.8: Causes of Gastrointestinal (G.I.) Bleeding.

UPPER G.I. BLEEDING	SMALL INTESTINAL BLEEDING	LOWER G.I. BLEEDING
1. Oesophageal varices	Vascular ectasias	Inflammatory bowel disease (IBD)
2. Mallory-Weiss tear	Tumours (adenocarcinoma, lymphoma, leiomyoma)	Carcinoma colon
3. Haemorrhagic/ erosive gastritis	NSAIDs	Carcinoma rectosigmoid
4. Duodenal ulcer	Meckel's diverticulum	Haemorroids
5. Gastric ulcer	Intussusception	Anal fissure
6. Cancer stomach	Crohn's disease	Diverticulosis

PERITONEUM *(p. 606)*

The peritoneal cavity is lined by a layer of surface mesothelium derived from mesoderm.

PERITONITIS *(p. 606)*

1. Chemical peritonitis can be caused by:

■ *Bile* extravasated due to trauma or diseases of the gallbladder.

■ *Pancreatic secretions* released from pancreas in acute haemorrhagic pancreatitis.

■ *Gastric juice* leaked from perforation of stomach.

■ *Barium sulfate* from perforation of bowel during radiographic studies.

Chemical peritonitis is localised or generalised sterile inflammation of the peritoneum.

2. Bacterial peritonitis may be primary or secondary; the latter being more common.

Primary form is caused by streptococcal infection, especially in children. *Secondary* bacterial peritonitis may occur from the following disorders:

Appendicitis, cholecystitis, salpingitis, rupture of peptic ulcer, gangrene of bowel, and tuberculosis (specific inflammation).

IDIOPATHIC RETROPERITONEAL FIBROSIS *(p. 606)*

Also known as Ormond's disease or sclerosing retroperitonitis, this rare entity of unknown etiology is characterised by diffuse fibrous overgrowth and chronic inflammation. The condition is, therefore, more like inflammatory rather than of neoplastic origin.

MESENTERIC CYSTS *(p. 606)*

Mesenteric cysts of unknown etiology and varying size may be found in the peritoneal cavity. On the basis of their possible origin, they are of various types:

■ *Chylous cyst* is a thin-walled cyst arising from lymph vessels and lined by endothelium.

■ *Pseudocysts* are those which are formed following walled-off infection or pancreatitis.

■ *Neoplastic cysts* occur due to cystic change in tumours.

TUMOURS *(p. 607)*

Peritoneum may be involved in malignant tumours—primary and metastatic.

■ **Mesothelioma** is an example of primary peritoneal tumour (benign and malignant) and is similar in morphology as in pleural cavity.

■ **Intra-abdominal desmoplastic small cell tumour** is a recently described highly malignant tumour belonging to the group of other round cell or blue cell tumours such as small cell carcinoma lung, Ewing's sarcoma, rhabdo-myosarcoma, neuroblastoma and others.

■ **Metastatic peritoneal tumours** are quite common and may occur from dissemination from any intra-abdominal malignancy.

■ **SELF ASSESSMENT**

1. The distance from the incisor teeth to the gastro-oesophageal junction is:
   A. 25 cm
   B. 30 cm
   C. 35 cm
   D. 40 cm

2. Oesophageal webs have the following features *except*:
   A. They are located at lower oesophagus
   B. They are associated with dysphagia
   C. They are associated with chronic atrophic glossitis
   D. They are associated with iron deficiency anaemia

3. Some of the common causes of haematemesis of oesophageal origin are as follows *except*:
   A. Oesophageal varices
   B. Mallory-Weiss syndrome
   C. Reflux oesophagitis
   D. Oesophageal rupture

4. Some common conditions predisposing to reflux oesophagitis are as follows *except*:
   A. Hiatus hernia
   B. Mallory-Weiss syndrome
   C. Peptic ulcers
   D. Persistent vomiting

5. The nature of lesion in Barrett's oesophagus is:
   A. Congenital anomaly
   B. Inflammatory disease
   C. Metaplastic process
   D. Neoplastic lesion

6. Barrett's oesophagus predisposes to development of:
   A. Reflux oesophagitis
   B. Oesophageal varices
   C. Squamous cell carcinoma
   D. Adenocarcinoma

7. The most frequent anatomic site for squamous cell carcinoma of the oesophagus is:
   A. Upper third
   B. Middle third
   C. Lower third
   D. Gastro-oesophageal junction

8. *H. pylori* gastritis has the following features *except*:
   A. *H. pylori* is seen on the epithelial layer of the luminal surface
   B. *H. pylori* is seen on areas with intestinal metaplasia
   C. *H. pylori* does not invade the mucosa
   D. *H. pylori* gastritis may lead to malignant transformation

9. Patients of benign gastric ulcer generally have:
   A. High gastric acid
   B. Normal-to-high gastric acid
   C. Normal-to-low gastric acid
   D. Absence of gastric acid

10. Duodenal ulcers are found most commonly at:
    A. First part, anterior surface
    B. First part, posterior surface
    C. Second part, anterior surface
    D. Second part, posterior surface

11. The most common location for gastric colloid carcinoma is:
    A. Cardia
    B. Fundus
    C. Body
    D. Pylorus

12. The most common gross growth pattern of gastric carcinoma is:
    A. Scirrhous
    B. Fungating
    C. Ulcerative
    D. Colloid

13. **Meckel's diverticulum is commonly located at:**
   A. Mesenteric border of small intestine one meter above ileocaecal valve
   B. Mesenteric border of small intestine two meter above ileocaecal valve
   C. Antimesenteric border of small intestine one meter above ileocaecal valve
   D. Antimesenteric border of small intestine two meter above ileocaecal valve

14. **The remnants of vitellointestinal duct are in the form of following lesions *except*:**
   A. Vitelline sinus   B. Vitelline cyst
   C. Omphalocele   D. Meckel's diverticulum

15. **Following humoral factors are implicated in the etiology of inflammatory bowel disease *except*:**
   A. Anti-colon antibodies to *E. coli*
   B. Decreased synthesis of IgG
   C. IgE-mediated hypersensitivity
   D. Circulating immune complexes

16. **Crohn's disease is characterised by the following histopathologic features *except*:**
   A. Non-caseating sarcoid like granulomas
   B. Superficial mucosal ulceration
   C. Stricture formation in chronic cases
   D. Widening of submucosa due to oedema

17. **The following features characterise ulcerative colitis *except*:**
   A. Formation of crypt abscess and cryptitis
   B. Superficial mucosal ulceration
   C. Depletion of goblet cells and mucus
   D. Stricture formation in chronic cases

18. **Long-standing cases of Crohn's disease may develop the following complications *except*:**
   A. Malabsorption   B. Toxic megacolon
   C. Fistula formation   D. Stricture formation

19. **Tuberculous ulcers in bowel have the following features *except*:**
   A. They begin in the Peyer's patches
   B. They are transverse to the long axis
   C. Advanced cases may cause intestinal obstruction
   D. Tuberculous ulcers often cause intestinal perforation

20. **The major complication of typhoid ulcer is:**
   A. Intestinal obstruction   B. Intestinal perforation
   C. Malabsorption   D. Fistula formation

21. **Pseudomembranous enterocolitis occurs most often in association with the following:**
   A. Shigella dysentery   B. Candida enterocolitis
   C. Cephalosporin antibiotics   D. Clostridial food poisoning

22. **Common causes of total/subtotal villous atrophy are as follows *except*:**
   A. Crohn's disease   B. Tropical sprue
   C. Nontropical sprue   D. Intestinal lymphoma

23. **The nature of Whipple's disease is:**
   A. Genetic defect   B. Familial occurrence
   C. Bacterial infection   D. Hypersensitivity reaction

24. **The most common location for carcinoid tumour is:**
   A. Foregut
   B. Midgut
   C. Hindgut
   D. Equal at all these three sites

25. **The histologic hallmark of diagnosis of acute appendicitis is:**
    - A. Mucosal ulceration
    - B. Impacted foreign body
    - C. Neutrophilic infiltrate in muscularis
    - D. Thrombosed blood vessels

26. **Out of various patterns of Hirschsprung's disease, the most common is:**
    - A. Total colonic aganglionosis
    - B. Long segment disease
    - C. Short segment disease
    - D. Ultra short segment disease

27. **The following type of colorectal polyps has highest malignant transformation:**
    - A. Hyperplastic polyp
    - B. Adenomatous
    - C. Villous adenoma
    - D. Tubulovillous adenoma

28. **The most common location for primary colorectal carcinoma is:**
    - A. Rectum
    - B. Sigmoid and descending colon
    - C. Caecum and ileocaecal valve
    - D. Ascending colon

29. **Elevation of carcinoembryonic antigen (CEA) level is particularly significant in:**
    - A. Early lesion of colorectal carcinoma
    - B. Advanced primary colorectal carcinoma
    - C. Metastatic colorectal carcinoma
    - D. Ulcerative colitis

30. **Intra-abdominal desmoplastic small cell tumour is a:**
    - A. Benign tumour
    - B. Fibromatosis
    - C. Tumour-like lesion
    - D. Highly malignant tumour

31. **The significant genetic mutations in adenoma-carcinoma sequence are all the following *except:***
    - A. Loss of *APC* gene
    - B. Deletion of *DCC* gene
    - C. Mutated *RB* gene
    - D. Mutation in *K-RAS* gene

32. ***H. pylori* colonisation of gastric mucosa is implicated in the following diseases *except:***
    - A. Gastritis
    - B. Gastric carcinoma
    - C. MALT lymphoma
    - D. Intestinal metaplasia

KEY

1 = D	2 = A	3 = C	4 = B
5 = C	6 = D	7 = B	8 = B
9 = C	10 = A	11 = B	12 = C
13 = C	14 = C	15 = B	16 = B
17 = D	18 = B	19 = D	20 = B
21 = C	22 = A	23 = C	24 = B
25 = C	26 = C	27 = C	28 = A
29 = C	30 = D	31 = C	32 = D

19

The Liver, Biliary Tract and Exocrine Pancreas

LIVER *(p. 608)*

NORMAL STRUCTURE *(p. 608)*

ANATOMY. The liver is the largest organ in the body weighing 1400-1600 gm in the males and 1200-1400 gm in the females. There are 2 main anatomical lobes—right and left, the right being about six times the size of the left lobe. The right lobe has quadrate lobe on its inferior surface and a caudate lobe on the posterior surface. The right and left lobes are separated anteriorly by a fold of peritoneum called the *falciform ligament,* inferiorly by the fissure for the *ligamentum teres,* and posteriorly by the fissure for the *ligamentum venosum.*

The *porta hepatis* is the region on the inferior surface of the right lobe where blood vessels, lymphatics and common hepatic duct form the hilum of the liver. A firm smooth layer of connective tissue called *Glisson's capsule* encloses the liver and is continuous with the connective tissue of the porta hepatis forming a sheath around the structures in the porta hepatis. The liver has a double blood supply—the portal vein brings the venous blood from the intestines and spleen, and the hepatic artery coming from the coeliac axis supplies arterial blood to the liver. This dual blood supply provides sufficient protection against infarction in the liver. The venous drainage from the liver is into the right and left hepatic veins which enter the inferior vena cava. Lymphatics and the nerve fibres accompany the hepatic artery into their branchings and terminate around the porta hepatis.

HISTOLOGY. The hepatic parenchyma is composed of numerous hexagonal or pyramidal *classical lobules;* each with a diameter of 0.5 to 2 mm. Each classical lobule has a central tributary from the hepatic vein and at the periphery are 4 to 5 portal tracts or triads containing branches of bile duct, portal vein and hepatic artery. Cords of hepatocytes and blood-containing sinusoids radiate from the central vein to the peripheral portal triads.

The blood supply to the liver parenchyma flows from the portal triads to the central veins. Accordingly, the hepatic parenchyma of liver lobule is divided into 3 zones:

■ **Zone 1** or the *periportal (peripheral) area* is closest to the arterial and portal blood supply and hence bears the brunt of all forms of toxic injury.

■ **Zone 3** or the *centrilobular area* surrounds the central vein and is most remote from the blood supply and thus suffers from the effects of hypoxic injury.

■ **Zone 2** is the intermediate *midzonal area.*

The **hepatocytes** are polygonal cells with a round single nucleus and a prominent nucleolus. The liver cells have a remarkable capability to undergo mitosis and regeneration.

The *space of Disse* is the space between hepatocytes and sinusoidal lining endothelial cells. A few scattered fat storing *Ito cells* lie within the space of Disse.

The *portal triad or tract* besides containing portal vein radicle, the hepatic arteriole and bile duct, has a few mononuclear cells and a little connective tissue considered to be extension of Glisson's capsule. The portal triads are surrounded by a limiting plate of hepatocytes.

The *intrahepatic biliary system* begins with the bile canaliculi interposed between the adjacent hepatocytes.

LIVER FUNCTION TESTS *(p. 610)*

A battery of liver function tests are employed for accurate diagnosis, to assess the severity of damage, to judge prognosis and to evaluate therapy (Table 19.1).

JAUNDICE—GENERAL *(p. 613)*

Jaundice or icterus refers to the yellow pigmentation of the skin or sclerae by bilirubin. Bilirubin pigment has high affinity for elastic tissue and hence jaundice is particularly noticeable in tissues rich in elastin content. Jaundice is the result of elevated levels of bilirubin in the blood termed hyperbilirubinaemia. Normal serum bilirubin concentration ranges from 0.2-0.8 mg/dl, about 80% of which is unconjugated. Jaundice becomes clinically evident when the total serum bilirubin exceeds 2 mg/dl. A rise of serum bilirubin between the normal and 2 mg/dl is generally not accompanied by visible jaundice and is called *latent jaundice*.

Normal Bilirubin Metabolism *(p. 613)*

Normal metabolism of bilirubin can be conveniently described under 4 main headings.

1. SOURCE OF BILIRUBIN. About 80-85% of the bilirubin is derived from the catabolism of haemoglobin present in senescent red blood cells. The destruction of effete erythrocytes at the end of their normal life-span of 120 days takes place in the reticuloendothelial system in the bone marrow, spleen and liver. The remaining 15-20% of the bilirubin comes partly from non-haemoglobin haem-containing pigments such as myoglobin, catalase and cytochromes, and partly from ineffective erythropoiesis.

2. TRANSPORT OF BILIRUBIN. Bilirubin on release from macrophages circulates as unconjugated bilirubin in plasma tightly bound to albumin. Certain drugs such as sulfonamides and salicylates compete with bilirubin for albumin binding and displace bilirubin from albumin, thus facilitating bilirubin to enter into the brain in neonates and increase the risk of *kernicterus*.

3. HEPATIC PHASE. On coming in contact with the hepatocyte surface, unconjugated bilirubin is preferentially metabolised which involves 3 steps.

i) Hepatic uptake: Albumin-bound unconjugated bilirubin upon entry into the hepatocyte, is dissociated into bilirubin and albumin. The bilirubin gets bound to cytoplasmic protein *glutathione-S-transferase (GST)* (earlier called ligandin).

ii) Conjugation: Unconjugated bilirubin is not water-soluble but is alcohol-soluble and is converted into water-soluble compound by conjugation. Conjugation occurs in endoplasmic reticulum and involves conversion to bilirubin diglucuronide by the action of microsomal enzyme, *bilirubin-UDP-glucuronosyl transferase*, to mono- and diglucuronides.

Conjugated bilirubin is bound to albumin in two forms: reversible and irreversible. Reversible binding is similar to that of unconjugated bilirubin. However, when present in serum for a long time (e.g. in cholestasis, long-standing biliary obstruction, chronic active hepatitis), conjugated bilirubin is bound to albumin irreversibly and is termed *delta bilirubin* or *biliprotein*.

iii) Secretion into bile: Conjugated (water soluble) bilirubin is rapidly transported directly into bile canaliculi by energy-dependent process and then excreted into the bile.

4. INTESTINAL PHASE. Appearance of conjugated bilirubin in the intestinal lumen is followed by either direct excretion in the stool as stercobilinogen

TABLE 19.1: Liver Function Tests.

TESTS	SIGNIFICANCE
I.	**TESTS FOR MANUFACTURE AND EXCRETION OF BILE**
1.	**Bilirubin:**
i) Serum bilirubin	Increased in hepatocellular, obstructive and haemolytic disease, Gilbert's disease
ii) In faeces	Absent in biliary obstruction
iii) In urine	Conjugated bilirubinuria in patients of hepatitis
2.	**Urobilinogen:**	Increased in hepatocellular and haemolytic diseases, absent in biliary obstruction
3.	**Bile acid (Bile salts):**	Increased in serum and detectable in urine in cholestasis
II.	**SERUM ENZYME ASSAYS**
1.	**Alkaline phosphatase:**	Increased in hepatobiliary disease (highest in biliary obstruction), bone diseases, pregnancy
2.	**γ-Glutamyl transpeptidase (γ-GT):**	Rise parallels alkaline phosphatase but is specific for hepatobiliary diseases
3.	**Transaminases:**
i) SGOT (AST)	Increased in tissue injury to liver as well as to other tissues like in myocardial infarction
ii) SGPT (ALT)	Increase is fairly specific for liver cell injury
4.	**Other enzymes:**
i) 5'-Nucleotidase	Rise parallels alkaline phosphatase but more specific for diseases of hepatic origin
ii) Lactic dehydrogenase	Increased in tumours involving the liver
iii) Cholinesterase	Decreased in hepatocellular disease, malnutrition
III.	**TESTS FOR METABOLIC FUNCTIONS**
1.	**Amino acid and protein metabolism:**
i) Serum proteins (total, A/G ratio, protein electrophoresis)	Hypoalbuminaemia in hepatocellular diseases; hyperglobulinaemia in cirrhosis and chronic active hepatitis
ii) Immunoglobulins	Nonspecific alterations in IgA, IgG and IgM
iii) Clotting factors	Prothrombin time and partial thromboplastin time prolonged in patients with hepatocellular disease
iv) Serum ammonia	Increased in acute fulminant hepatitis, cirrhosis, hepatic encephalopathy
v) Aminoaciduria	In fulminant hepatitis
2.	**Lipid and lipoprotein metabolism:**
Blood lipids (total serum cholesterol, triglycerides and lipoprotein fractions)	Increased in cholestasis, decreased in acute and chronic diffuse liver disease and in malnutrition
3.	**Carbohydrate metabolism:**
Blood glucose and GTT	Decreased in hepatic necrosis
IV.	**IMMUNOLOGIC TESTS**
1.	**Nonspecific immunologic reactions:**
i) Smooth muscle antibody	In hepatic necrosis
ii) Mitochondrial antibody	In primary biliary cirrhosis
iii) Antinuclear antibody and LE cell test	In chronic active hepatitis
2.	**Antibodies to specific etiologic agents:**
i) Antibodies to hepatitis B (HBsAg, HBc, HBeAg)	In hepatitis B
ii) Amoeba antibodies	Amoebic liver abscess
V.	**ANCILLARY DIAGNOSTIC TESTS**
1.	**Ultrasound examination**	Cholestasis of various etiologies; SOLs, US-guided-FNAC/liver biopsy
2.	**FNAC and/ or percutaneous liver biopsy**	Unknown cause of hepatocellular disease, hepatomegaly and splenomegaly; long-standing hepatitis; PUO and SOLs of the liver

which imparts the normal yellow colour to stool, or may be metabolised to urobilinogen by the action of intestinal bacteria. Conjugated bilirubin is normally not reabsorbable whereas its metabolic product, urobilinogen, is reabsorbed from the small intestine and reaches enterohepatic circulation.

The major differences between unconjugated and conjugated bilirubin are summarised in Table 19.2.

TABLE 19.2: Major Differences between Unconjugated and Conjugated Bilirubin.

	FEATURE	UNCONJUGATED	CONJUGATED
1.	*Normal serum level*	More	Less (less than 0.25 mg/dl)
2.	*Water solubility*	Absent	Present
3.	*Affinity to lipids (alcohol solubility)*	Present	Absent
4.	*Serum albumin binding*	High	Low
5.	*van den Bergh reaction*	Indirect (Total minus direct)	Direct
6.	*Renal excretion*	Absent	Present
7.	*Bilirubin albumin covalent complex formation*	Absent	Present
8.	*Affinity to brain tissue*	Present (Kernicterus)	Absent

CLASSIFICATION AND FEATURES OF JAUNDICE *(p. 615)*

Jaundice may result from one or more of the following mechanisms (Table 19.3):
1. Increased bilirubin production
2. Decreased hepatic uptake
3. Decreased hepatic conjugation
4. Decreased excretion of bilirubin into bile

Hyperbilirubinaemia due to first three mechanisms is *mainly unconjugated* while the last variety yields *mainly conjugated* hyperbilirubinaemia. A simple test to determine whether hyperbilirubinaemia is of unconjugated or conjugated variety is to determine whether bilirubin is present in urine or not; its absence in urine suggests unconjugated hyperbilirubinaemia since unconjugated bilirubin is not filtered by the glomerulus.

Predominantly Unconjugated Hyperbilirubinaemia *(p. 615)*

1. INCREASED BILIRUBIN PRODUCTION (HAEMOLYTIC, ACHOLURIC OR PREHEPATIC JAUNDICE). This results from excessive red cell destruction as occurs in intra- and extravascular haemolysis or due to ineffective erythropoiesis. There is increased release of haemoglobin from excessive breakdown of red cells that leads to overproduction of bilirubin. Hyperbilirubinaemia develops when the capacity of the liver to conjugate large amount of bilirubin is exceeded. In premature infants, the liver is deficient in enzyme necessary for conjugation while the rate of red cell destruction is high. This results in *icterus neonatorum* which is particularly severe in haemolytic disease of the newborn due to maternal isoantibodies. Since there is predominantly unconjugated hyperbilirubinaemia in such cases, there is danger of permanent brain damage in these infants from kernicterus when the serum level of unconjugated bilirubin exceeds 20 mg/dl.

Bile pigment being unconjugated type is absent from urine (acholuric jaundice). However, there is dark brown colour of stools due to excessive faecal excretion of bile pigment and increased urinary excretion of urobilinogen.

TABLE 19.3: Pathophysiologic Classification of Jaundice.

I.   PREDOMINANTLY UNCONJUGATED HYPERBILIRUBINAEMIA

1.   Increased bilirubin production (Haemolytic, acholuric or prehepatic jaundice)

- Intra- and extravascular haemolysis
- Ineffective erythropoiesis

2.   Decreased hepatic uptake

- Drugs
- Prolonged starvation
- Sepsis

3.   Decreased bilirubin conjugation

- Hereditary disorders (e.g. Gilbert's syndrome, Crigler-Najjar syndrome)
- Acquired defects (e.g. drugs, hepatitis, cirrhosis)
- Neonatal jaundice

II.   PREDOMINANTLY CONJUGATED HYPERBILIRUBINAEMIA (CHOLESTASIS)

1.   Intrahepatic cholestasis (Impaired hepatic excretion)

- Hereditary disorders or *'pure cholestasis'* (e.g. Dubin-Johnson syndrome, Rotor's syndrome, fibrocystic disease of pancreas, benign familial recurrent cholestasis, intrahepatic atresia, cholestatic jaundice of pregnancy)
- Acquired disorders or *'hepatocellular cholestasis'* (e.g. viral hepatitis, drugs, alcohol-induced injury, sepsis, cirrhosis)

2.   Extrahepatic cholestasis (Extrahepatic biliary obstruction)

- Mechanical obstruction (e.g. gallstones, inflammatory strictures, carcinoma head of pancreas, tumours of bile ducts, sclerosing cholangitis, congenital atresia of extrahepatic ducts)

---

2.   DECREASED HEPATIC UPTAKE. The uptake of bilirubin by the hepatocyte that involves dissociation of the pigment from albumin and its binding to cytoplasmic protein, GST or ligandin, may be deranged in certain conditions e.g. due to drugs, prolonged starvation and sepsis.

3.   DECREASED BILIRUBIN CONJUGATION. This mechanism involves deranged hepatic conjugation due to defect or deficiency of the enzyme, glucuronosyl transferase. This can occur in certain inherited disorders of the enzyme (e.g. Gilbert's syndrome and Crigler-Najjar syndrome), or acquired defects in its activity (e.g. due to drugs, hepatitis, cirrhosis). However, hepato-cellular damage causes deranged excretory capacity of the liver more than its conjugating capacity *(see below)*.

II. Predominantly Conjugated Hyperbilirubinaemia (Cholestasis) *(p. 616)*

This form of hyperbilirubinaemia is defined as failure of normal amounts of bile to reach the duodenum. Morphologically, cholestasis means accumulation of bile in liver cells and biliary passages. The defect in excretion may be within the biliary canaliculi of the hepatocyte and in the microscopic bile ducts *(intrahepatic cholestasis or medical jaundice)*, or there may be mechanical obstruction to the extrahepatic biliary excretory apparatus *(extrahepatic cholestasis or obstructive jaundice)*. It is important to distinguish these two forms of cholestasis since extrahepatic cholestasis or obstructive jaundice is often treatable with surgery, whereas the intrahepatic cholestasis or medical jaundice cannot be benefitted by surgery.

1.   INTRAHEPATIC CHOLESTASIS. Intrahepatic cholestasis is due to impaired hepatic excretion of bile and may occur from hereditary or acquired disorders.

The **features** of intrahepatic cholestasis include: predominant conjugated hyperbilirubinaemia due to regurgitation of conjugated bilirubin into blood, bilirubinuria, elevated levels of serum bile acids and consequent pruritus, elevated serum alkaline phosphatase, hyperlipidaemia and hypoprothrombinaemia. 'Pure cholestasis' can be distinguished from 'hepatocellular cholestasis' by elevated serum levels of transaminases in the latter due to liver cell injury.

■ **Liver biopsy** in cases with intrahepatic cholestasis reveals milder degree of cholestasis than the extrahepatic disorders. The biliary canaliculi of the hepatocytes are dilated and contain characteristic elongated green-brown *bile plugs*.

2. EXTRAHEPATIC CHOLESTASIS. Extrahepatic cholestasis results from mechanical obstruction to large bile ducts outside the liver or within the porta hepatis. The common causes are gallstones, inflammatory strictures, carcinoma head of pancreas, tumours of bile duct, sclerosing cholangitis and congenital atresia of extrahepatic ducts.

The **features** of extrahepatic cholestasis (obstructive jaundice), like in intrahepatic cholestasis, are predominant conjugated hyperbilirubinaemia, bilirubinuria, elevated serum bile acids causing intense pruritus, high serum alkaline phosphatase and hyperlipidaemia. However, there are certain features which help to distinguish extrahepatic from intrahepatic cholestasis. In obstructive jaundice, there is malabsorption of fat-soluble vitamins (A,D,E and K) and steatorrhoea resulting in vitamin K deficiency. Prolonged prothrombin time in such cases shows improvement following parenteral administration of vitamin K, whereas hypoprothrombinaemia due to hepatocellular disease shows no such improvement in prothrombin time with vitamin K administration. The stools of such patients are clay-coloured due to absence of bilirubin metabolite, stercobilin, in faeces and there is virtual disappearance of urobilinogen from the urine.

■ **Liver biopsy** in cases with extrahepatic cholestasis shows more marked changes of cholestasis. Since the obstruction is in the extrahepatic bile ducts, there is progressive retrograde extension of bile stasis into intrahepatic duct system. This results in dilatation of bile ducts and rupture of canaliculi with extravasation of bile producing *bile lakes*. Since bile is toxic, the regions of bile lakes are surrounded by focal necrosis of hepatocytes.

HEREDITARY NON-HAEMOLYTIC HYPERBILIRUBINAEMIAS *(p. 618)*

Hereditary non-haemolytic hyperbilirubinaemias are a small group of uncommon familial disorders of bilirubin metabolism when haemolytic causes have been excluded. The commonest is Gilbert's syndrome; others are Crigler-Najjar syndrome, Dubin-Johnson syndrome, Rotor's syndrome and benign familial recurrent cholestasis. The features common to all these conditions are presence of icterus but almost normal liver function tests and no well-defined morphologic changes except in Dubin-Johnson syndrome. Gilbert's syndrome and Crigler-Najjar syndrome are examples of *hereditary non-haemolytic unconjugated hyperbilirubinaemia,* whereas Dubin-Johnson syndrome, Rotor's syndrome and benign familial recurrent cholestasis are conditions with *hereditary conjugated hyperbilirubinaemia.* Their distinguishing features are summarised in Table 19.4.

NEONATAL HEPATITIS *(p. 619)*

Neonatal hepatitis, also termed giant cell hepatitis or neonatal hepatocellular cholestasis, is a general term used for the constant morphologic change seen in conjugated hyperbilirubinaemia as a result of known infectious and metabolic

Chapter Nineteen

TABLE 19.4: Contrasting Features of Major Hereditary Non-haemolytic Hyperbilirubinaemias.

FEATURE	GILBERT'S SYNDROME	TYPE 1 CRIGLER-NAJJAR SYNDROME	TYPE 2 CRIGLER-NAJJAR SYNDROME	DUBIN-JOHNSON SYNDROME	ROTOR SYNDROME
1. *Inheritance*	Autosomal dominant	Autosomal recessive	Autosomal dominant	Autosomal recessive	Autosomal recessive
2. *Predominant hyperbilirubinaemia*	Unconjugated	Unconjugated	Unconjugated	Conjugated	Conjugated
3. *Intensity of jaundice*	Mild (<5mg/dl)	Marked (>20 mg/dl)	Mild to moderate (<20 mg/dl)	Mild (<5 mg/dl)	Mild (< 5 mg/dl)
4. *Basic defect*	↓ UDP-glucuronosyl transferase activity	Absence of UDP-glucuronosyl transferase	↓ UDP-glucuronosyl transferase	Defect in canalicular excretion (Prolonged BSP excretion test)	Deranged hepatic uptake
5. *Hepatic morphology*	Normal (except slightly increased lipofuscin)	Normal (except mild canalicular stasis)	Normal	Greenish-black pigment	Normal
6. *Prognosis*	Excellent	Poor (due to kernicterus)	Good	Excellent	Excellent

causes or may have an idiopathic etiology. The 'idiopathic' neonatal hepatitis is more common and accounts for 75% of cases. The condition usually presents in the first week of birth with jaundice, bilirubinuria, pale stools and high serum alkaline phosphatase.

M/E 1. Loss of normal lobular architecture of the liver.
2. Presence of prominent multinucleate giant cells derived from hepatocytes.
3. Mononuclear inflammatory cell infiltrate in the portal tracts with some periportal fibrosis.
4. Haemosiderosis.
5. Cholestasis in small proliferated ductules in the portal tract and between necrotic liver cells.

BILIARY ATRESIAS *(p. 620)*

Biliary atresias, also called as *infantile cholangiopathies*, are a group of intrauterine developmental abnormalities of the biliary system. Though they are often classified as congenital, the abnormality of development in most instances is extraneous infection during the intrauterine development or shortly after birth that brings about inflammatory destruction of the bile ducts. The condition may, therefore, have various grades of destruction ranging from complete absence of bile ducts termed *atresia,* to reduction in their number called *paucity of bile ducts.*

Depending upon the portion of biliary system involved, biliary atresias may be extrahepatic or intrahepatic.

Extrahepatic Biliary Atresia *(p. 620)*

The extrahepatic bile ducts fail to develop normally so that in some cases the bile ducts are *absent* at birth, while in others the ducts may have been formed but start undergoing sclerosis in the perinatal period. It is common to have multiple defects and other congenital lesions. Extrahepatic biliary atresia is found in 1 per 10,000 livebirths. Cholestatic jaundice appears by the first week after birth. The baby has severe pruritus, pale stools, dark urine and elevated serum transaminases. In some cases, the condition is correctable by surgery, while in vast majority the atresia is not correctable and in such cases hepatic portoenterostomy (Kasai procedure) or hepatic transplantation must be considered.

G/A The liver is enlarged and dark green. The atretic segments of biliary system are reduced to cord-like structures.

M/E 1. Inflammation and fibrous obliteration of the extrahepatic ducts with absence of bile in them.
2. Ductular proliferation and periductular inflammation.
3. Cholestasis and bile thrombi in the portal area.
4. Periportal fibrosis and later secondary biliary cirrhosis.
5. Transformation of hepatic parenchyma to neonatal (giant cell) hepatitis in 15% of cases.

Intrahepatic Biliary Atresia *(p. 620)*

Intrahepatic biliary atresia is characterised by biliary hypoplasia so that there is *paucity of bile ducts* rather than their complete absence. The condition probably has its origin in viral infection acquired during intrauterine period or in the neonatal period. Cholestatic jaundice usually appears within the first few days of birth and is characterised by high serum bile acids with associated pruritus, and hypercholesterolaemia with appearance of xanthomas by first year of life.

M/E 1. Paucity of intrahepatic bile ducts.
2. Cholestasis.
3. Increased hepatic copper.
4. Inflammation and fibrosis in the portal area, leading to cirrhosis.

REYE'S SYNDROME *(p. 620)*

Reye's syndrome is defined as an acute postviral syndrome of encephalopathy and fatty change in the viscera. The syndrome may follow almost any known viral disease but is most common after influenza A or B and varicella. Viral infection may act singly, or more often its effect is modified by certain exogenous factors such as by administration of salicylates, aflatoxins and insecticides. These effects cause mitochondrial injury and decreased activity of mitochondrial enzymes in the liver. This eventually leads to rise in blood ammonia and accumulation of triglycerides within hepatocytes.

The patients are generally children between 6 months and 15 years of age. Characteristic laboratory findings are elevated blood ammonia, serum transaminases, bilirubin and prolonged prothrombin time.

G/A The liver is enlarged and yellowish-orange.

M/E The hepatocytes show small droplets of neutral fat in their cytoplasm (microvesicular fat). Similar fatty change is seen in the renal tubular epithelium and in the cells of skeletal muscles and heart.

HEPATIC FAILURE *(p. 621)*

Though the liver has a marked regenerative capacity and a large functional reserve, hepatic failure may develop from severe acute and fulminant liver injury with massive necrosis of liver cells *(acute hepatic failure)*, or from advanced chronic liver disease *(chronic hepatic failure)*. Acute hepatic failure develops suddenly with severe impairment of liver functions whereas chronic liver failure comes insidiously. The prognosis is much worse in acute hepatic failure than that in chronic liver failure.

ETIOLOGY. The two types of hepatic failure result from different causes:

■ **Acute (fulminant) hepatic failure** occurs most frequently in severe viral hepatitis. Other causes are hepatotoxic drug reactions (e.g. anaesthetic agents, nonsteroidal anti-inflammatory drugs, anti-depressants), carbon tetrachloride poisoning, acute alcoholic hepatitis, mushroom poisoning and pregnancy complicated with eclampsia.

■ **Chronic hepatic failure** is most often due to cirrhosis. Other causes include chronic active hepatitis, chronic cholestasis (cholestatic jaundice) and Wilson's disease.

MANIFESTATIONS. The major manifestations are as under:

1. **Jaundice.** Jaundice usually reflects the severity of liver cell damage. In acute failure such as in viral hepatitis, jaundice nearly parallels the extent of liver cell damage, while in chronic failure such as in cirrhosis jaundice appears late and is usually of mild degree.

2. **Hepatic encephalopathy (Hepatic coma).** Neuropsychiatric syndrome may complicate liver disease of both acute and chronic types. The features include disturbed consciousness, personality changes, intellectual deterioration, low slurred speech, flapping tremors, and finally, coma and death.

3. **Hyperkinetic circulation.** All forms of hepatic failure are associated with a hyperkinetic circulation characterised by peripheral vasodilatation, increased splanchnic blood flow and increased cardiac output.

4. **Hepatorenal syndrome.** The term hepatorenal syndrome is applied to patients of both acute and chronic hepatic failure who develop renal failure as

well, in the absence of clinical, laboratory or morphologic evidence of other causes of renal dysfunction. The acute renal failure is usually associated with oliguria and uraemia but with good tubular function. The histology of kidney is virtually normal, suggesting functional defect for the renal failure.

5. Hepatopulmonary syndrome. The pulmonary changes in chronic hepatic failure such as in cirrhosis consist of pulmonary vasodilatation with intra-pulmonary arteriovenous shunting. This results in ventilation-perfusion inequality that may lead to impaired pulmonary function, clubbing of fingers and sometimes cyanosis.

6. Coagulation defects. Impaired synthesis of a number of coagulation factors by the diseased liver may result in coagulation disorders. These include disseminated intravascular coagulation (consumption coagulopathy), thrombocytopenia and presence of fibrin degradation products in the blood.

7. Ascites and oedema. Chronic liver failure due to cirrhosis may result in portal hypertension and ascites. Decreased synthesis of albumin by the liver resulting in hypoproteinaemia and consequent fall in plasma oncotic pressure, increased hydrostatic pressure due to portal hypertension and secondary hyperaldosteronism, contribute to the development of ascites and oedema in these patients.

8. Endocrine changes. Endocrine changes may be found in association with chronic hepatic failure. The changes are more common in alcoholic cirrhosis in active reproductive life. In the male, the changes are towards feminisation such as gynaecomastia and hypogonadism. In the female, the changes are less towards masculinisation but atrophy of gonads and breasts occurs.

9. Skin changes. In alcoholic cirrhosis 'arterial spiders' having radiating small vessels from a central arteriole are frequent in the vascular region drained by superior vena cava such as in the neck, face, forearms and dorsum of hands.

10. Foetor hepaticus. A sweetish pungent smell of the breath is found in severe cases of acute and chronic hepatocellular diseases. It appears to be of intestinal origin, possibly due to failure of the liver to detoxify sulfur-containing substances absorbed from the gut.

CIRCULATORY DISTURBANCES (p. 622)

Vascular disorders of general nature involving the liver such as chronic passive congestion and infarction have already been discussed in Chapter 5. Hepatic and portal venous obstruction and hepatic arterial obstruction are considered here.

I. Hepatic Venous Obstruction (p. 622)

The central veins of lobules of the liver are tributaries of the hepatic veins. In the normal liver, there are no anastomoses between hepatic vein and portal vein but in cirrhotic liver there are such anastomoses.

Diseases produced by obstruction of the hepatic veins are Budd-Chiari syndrome (hepatic vein thrombosis) and hepatic veno-occlusive disease.

Budd-Chiari Syndrome (Hepatic Vein Thrombosis) (p. 622)

Budd-Chiari syndrome in its pure form consists of slowly developing thrombosis of the hepatic veins and the adjacent inferior vena cava.

ETIOLOGY. The etiology of hepatic venous thrombosis in about one-third of cases is unknown (idiopathic), while in the remaining cases various causes associated with increased thrombotic tendencies are attributed such as due to polycythaemia vera, paroxysmal nocturnal haemoglobinuria, oral contraceptives, pregnancy, postpartum state, intra-abdominal cancers (e.g. hepatocellular carcinoma), chemotherapy, radiation and myeloproliferative diseases.

G/A The liver is enlarged, swollen, red-purple and has a tense capsule.

M/E The changes in sudden hepatic vein occlusion are those of centrilobular congestion, necrosis and rupture of sinusoids into the space of Disse.

CLINICAL FEATURES. Budd-Chiari syndrome is clinically characterised by either an acute form or chronic form.

■ In the *acute form,* the features are abdominal pain, vomiting, enlarged liver, ascites and mild icterus.

■ In the more usual *chronic form,* the patients present with pain over enlarged tender liver, ascites and other features of portal hypertension.

Hepatic Veno-occlusive Disease *(p. 623)*

Hepatic veno-occlusive disease consists of intimal thickening, stenosis and obliteration of the terminal central veins and medium-sized hepatic veins. The venous occlusion results in pathologic changes similar to those of Budd-Chiari syndrome and can be distinguished from the latter by demonstration of absence of thrombosis in the major hepatic veins.

The cause and stimulus for hepatic veno-occlusive disease are obscure. The condition is more widespread in countries such as Africa, India and certain other tropical countries where 'bush tea' (medicinal tea) is consumed that contains hepatotoxic alkaloids. More recently, the disease has been found in association with administration of antineoplastic drugs and immunosuppressive therapy.

II. Portal Venous Obstruction *(p. 623)*

■ **Intrahepatic cause** of portal venous occlusion is hepatic cirrhosis as the commonest and most important, followed in decreasing frequency by tumour invasion, congenital hepatic fibrosis and schistosomiasis.

■ **Extrahepatic causes** of portal vein obstruction are intra-abdominal cancers, intra-abdominal sepsis, direct invasion by tumour, myeloproliferative disorders and upper abdominal surgical procedure followed by thrombosis.

The **effects** of portal venous obstruction depend upon the site of obstruction. The most important effect, irrespective of the site of occlusion or cause, is portal hypertension and its manifestations. If the obstruction is in the extrahepatic portal vein alongwith extension of occlusion into splenic vein, it may result in venous infarction of the bowel.

III. Hepatic Arterial Obstruction *(p. 623)*

Diseases from obstruction of the hepatic artery are uncommon. Rarely, accidental ligation of the main hepatic artery or its branch to right lobe may be followed by fatal infarction.

LIVER CELL NECROSIS *(p. 623)*

All forms of injury to the liver such as microbiologic, toxic, circulatory or traumatic, result in necrosis of liver cells. The extent of involvement of hepatic lobule in necrosis varies. Accordingly, liver cell necrosis is divided into 3 types:

1. DIFFUSE (SUBMASSIVE TO MASSIVE) NECROSIS. When there is extensive and diffuse necrosis of the liver involving all the cells in groups of lobules, it is termed diffuse, or submassive to massive necrosis. It is most commonly caused by viral hepatitis or drug toxicity.

2. ZONAL NECROSIS. Zonal necrosis is necrosis of hepatocytes in 3 different zones of the hepatic lobule. Accordingly, it is of 3 types; each type affecting respective zone is caused by different etiologic factors:

i) Centrilobular necrosis is the commonest type involving hepatocytes in zone 3 (i.e. located around the central vein). Centrilobular necrosis is characteristic feature of ischaemic injury such as in shock and CHF since zone 3 is farthest from the blood supply. Besides, it also occurs in poisoning with chloroform, carbon tetrachloride and certain drugs.

ii) Midzonal necrosis is uncommon and involves zone 2 of the hepatic lobule. This pattern of necrosis is seen in yellow fever and viral hepatitis. In viral hepatitis, some of the necrosed hepatocytes of the mid-zone are transformed into acidophilic, rounded Councilman bodies.

iii) Periportal (peripheral) necrosis is seen in zone 1 involving the parenchyma closest to the arterial and portal blood supply. Since zone 1 is most well perfused, it is most vulnerable to the effects of circulating hepato-toxins e.g. in phosphorus poisoning and eclampsia.

3. FOCAL NECROSIS. This form of necrosis involves small groups of hepatocytes irregularly distributed in the hepatic lobule. Focal necrosis is most often caused by microbiologic infections. These include viral hepatitis, miliary tuberculosis, typhoid fever and various other forms of bacterial, viral and fungal infections. Focal necrosis may also occur in drug-induced hepatitis.

VIRAL HEPATITIS *(p. 624)*

The term viral hepatitis is used to describe infection of the liver caused by hepatotropic viruses. Currently there are 5 main varieties of these viruses and a sixth poorly-characterised virus, causing distinct types of viral hepatitis:

■ *Hepatitis A virus (HAV)*, causing a faecally-spread self-limiting disease;

■ *Hepatitis B virus (HBV)*, causing a parenterally transmitted disease that may become chronic;

■ *Hepatitis C virus (HCV)*, previously termed non-A, non-B (NANB) hepatitis virus involved chiefly in transfusion-related hepatitis;

■ *Hepatitis delta virus (HDV)* which is sometimes associated as superinfection with hepatitis B infection;

■· *Hepatitis E virus (HEV)*, causing water-borne infection; and

■ *Hepatitis G virus (HGV)*, is a recently discovered parenterally transmitted hepatotropic virus.

All these human hepatitis viruses are RNA viruses except HBV which is a DNA virus. Their contrasting features are given in Table 19.5.

Though a number of other viral diseases such as infection with Epstein-Barr virus (in infectious mononucleosis), arbovirus (in yellow fever), cytomegalovirus, herpes simplex and several others affect the liver but the changes produced by them are nonspecific and the term 'viral hepatitis' is strictly applied to infection of the liver by the hepatitis viruses.

Hepatitis A *(p. 624)*

Hepatitis A is responsible for 20-25% of clinical hepatitis in the developing countries of the world but the incidence is much lower in the developed countries. Hepatitis A is usually a benign, self-limiting disease and has an incubation period of 15-45 days. The disease occurs in epidemic form as well as sporadically. It is usually spread by faeco-oral route. Most frequently affected age is 5-14 years; adults are often infected by spread from children.

PATHOGENESIS. An immunologic basis is suspected but the evidence in support is indirect in the form of immunologic markers but not direct demonstration of the etiologic agent in the affected hepatocytes. These markers are:

1. *IgM anti-HAV antibody* appears in the serum at the onset of symptoms of acute hepatitis A.

2. *IgG anti-HAV antibody* is detected in the serum after IgM antibody and gives life-long protective immunity against reinfection with HAV.

Hepatitis B *(p. 624)*

Hepatitis B (serum hepatitis) caused by HBV infection has a longer incubation period (30-180 days) and is transmitted parenterally such as in recipients of blood and blood products, intravenous drug addicts, patients treated by renal dialysis and hospital workers exposed to blood, and by intimate physical contact such as from mother to child and sexually. The disease may occur at any age.

HEPATITIS B VIRUS (HBV). The etiologic agent for hepatitis B, HBV, is a DNA virus which has been extensively studied. Electron microscopic studies on serum of patients infected with HBV show 3 forms of viral particles of 2 sizes—small (spheres and tubules/filaments) and large (spheres) as under:

i) *Small particles* are most numerous and are in 2 forms: as 22 nm spheres, and as tubules 22 nm in diameter and 100 nm long. These are antigenically identical to envelope protein of HBV and represent excess of viral envelope protein referred as hepatitis B surface antigen (HBsAg).

ii) *Large particles,* 42 nm in diameter, are double-shelled spherical particles, also called as *Dane particles.* These are about 100 to 1000 times less in number in serum compared to small 22 nm particles and represent intact virion of HBV.

The genomic structure of HBV is quite compact and complex. The HBV DNA consists of 4 overlapping genes which encode for multiple proteins:

1. *S gene* codes for the major surface envelope protein, hepatitis B surface antigen (HBsAg). HBsAg is present on the outer surface of the large spherical particles as well as in small spherical and tubular structures. *Pre-S1 and pre-S2* regions of genome which are upstream of S gene, code for two other large proteins.

2. *P gene* is the largest and codes for DNA polymerase.

3. *C gene* codes for two nucleocapsid proteins, HBeAg and a core protein termed HBcAg.

4. *X gene* codes for HBxAg having a role in activation and transcription of viral and cellular genes and may actually contribute to carcinogenesis by binding with *TP53.*

PATHOGENESIS. The evidence linking immuno-pathogenetic mechanism with hepatocellular damage is much stronger in HBV infection than with HAV infection.

Serologic and viral markers. Various immunological markers indicative of presence of HBV infection can be demonstrated in the sera as well as in the hepatocytes of infected individuals. These are as under:

1. **HBsAg.** In 1965, Blumberg and colleagues in Philadelphia found a lipoprotein complex in the serum of a multiple-transfused haemophiliac of Australian aborigine which was subsequently shown by them to be associated with serum hepatitis. This antigen was termed *Australia antigen* by them (In 1977, Blumberg was awarded the Nobel Prize for his discovery). The term Australia antigen is now used synonymous with hepatitis B surface antigen (HBsAg). HBsAg appears early in the blood after about 6 weeks of infection and its detection is an indicator of active HBV infection. It usually disappears in 3-6 months.

2. **Anti-HBs.** Specific antibody to HBsAg in serum called anti-HBs appears late, about 3 months after the onset. Anti-HBs response may be both IgM and IgG type.

TABLE 19.5: Features of Various Types of Hepatitis Viruses.

FEATURE	HEPATITIS A	HEPATITIS B	HEPATITIS C	HEPATITIS D	HEPATITIS E	HEPATITIS G
1. *Agent*	HAV	HBV	HCV	HDV	HEV	HGV
2. *Year identified*	1973	1965	1989	1977	1980	1995
3. *Viral particle*	27 nm	42 nm	30-60 nm	35-37 nm	32-34 nm	?
4. *Genome*	RNA, ss, linear	DNA, ss/ds	RNA, ss, linear circular	RNA, ss, circular	RNA, ss, linear	RNA, ss, linear
5. *Morphology*	Icosahedral non-enveloped	Double-shelled, enveloped	Enveloped	Enveloped, replication defective	Icosahedral, non-enveloped	?
6. *Spread*	Faeco-oral	Parenteral, close contact	Parenteral, close contact	Parenteral, close contact	Water-borne	Parenteral
7. *Incubation period*	15-45 days	30-180 days	20-90 days	30-50 days (In superinfection)	15-60 days	?
8. *Antigen(s)*	HAV	HBsAg HBcAg HBeAg HBxAg	HCV RNA C 100-3 C 33c NS5	HBsAg HDV	HEV	?
9. *Antibodies*	anti-HAV	anti-HBs anti-HBc anti-HBe	anti-HCV	anti-HBs anti-HDV	anti-HEV	?
10. *Severity*	Mild	Occasionally severe	Moderate	Occasionally severe	Mild	?
11. *Chronic hepatitis*	None	Occasional	Common	Common	None	?
12. *Carrier state*	None	<1%	<1%	1-10%	Unknown	1-2%
13. *Hepatocellular carcinoma*	No	+	+	±	None	?
14. *Prognosis*	Excellent	Worse with age	Moderate	Acute good; chronic poor	Good	?

ss= single-stranded; ss/ds= partially single-stranded partially double-stranded.

3. HBeAg. HBeAg derived from core protein is present transiently (3-6 weeks) during an acute attack.

4. Anti-HBe. Antibody to HBeAg called anti-HBe appears after disappearance of HBeAg.

5. HBcAg. HBcAg derived from core protein cannot be detected in the blood. But HBcAg can be demonstrated in the nuclei of hepatocytes in carrier state and in chronic hepatitis patients by Orcein staining but not in the liver cells during acute stage.

6. Anti-HBc. Antibody to HBcAg called anti-HBc can, however, be detected in the serum of acute hepatitis B patients during pre-icteric stage. Anti-HBc may be IgM or IgG class antibody.

7. HBV-DNA. Detection of HBV-DNA by molecular hybridisation using the Southern blot technique is the most sensitive index of hepatitis B infection. It is present in pre-symptomatic phase and transiently during early acute stage.

Hepatitis D *(p. 627)*

Infection with delta virus (HDV) in the hepatocyte nuclei of HBsAg-positive patients is termed hepatitis D. HDV is a defective virus for which HBV is the helper. Thus, hepatitis D develops when there is concomitant hepatitis B infection.

▪ With **coinfection**, acute hepatitis D may range from mild to fulminant hepatitis but fulminant hepatitis is more likely in such simultaneous delta infection. Chronicity rarely develops in coinfection.

▪ With **superinfection**, (incubation period 30-35 days), chronic HBV infection gets worsened indicated by appearance of severe and fulminant acute attacks, progression of carrier stage to chronic delta hepatitis or acceleration towards cirrhosis. Hepatocellular carcinoma is, however, less common in HBsAg carriers with HDV infection.

HEPATITIS DELTA VIRUS (HDV). The etiologic agent, HDV, is a small single-stranded RNA particle with a diameter of 36 nm. It is double-shelled—the outer shell consists of HBsAg and the inner shell consists of delta antigen provided by a circular RNA strand.

PATHOGENESIS. HDV, unlike HBV, is thought to cause direct cytopathic effect on hepatocytes. However, there are examples of transmission of HDV infection from individuals who themselves have not suffered from any attack of hepatitis, suggesting that it may not be always cytopathic.

Hepatitis C *(p. 628)*

The diagnosis of a third major category of hepatitis was earlier made after exclusion of infection with other known hepatitis viruses and was designated non-A, non-B (NANB) hepatitis. However, now this third type has been characterised and is called hepatitis C.

Hepatitis C infection is acquired by blood transfusions, blood products, haemodialysis, parenteral drug abuse and accidental cuts and needle-pricks in health workers. About 90% of post-transfusion hepatitis is of hepatitis C type. About 1-2% of volunteer blood donors and up to 5% of professional blood donors are carriers of HCV. Hepatitis C has an incubation period of 20-90 days (mean 50 days). Clinically, acute HCV hepatitis is milder than HBV hepatitis but HCV has a higher rate of progression to chronic hepatitis than HBV. Persistence of infection and chronic hepatitis are the key features of HCV. Currently, HCV is considered more important cause of chronic liver disease worldwide than HBV.

HEPATITIS C VIRUS (HCV). HCV is a single-stranded, enveloped RNA virus, having a diameter of 30-60 nm. HCV genome has about 3000 amino acids. The genomic organisation of HCV shows a 5'- terminal end, C (capsid) region and the envelope regions E1 and E2 in the exons.

The viral proteins result in corresponding serologic and virologic markers for HCV infection as under:

1. *Anti-HCV antibodies.* Three generations of anti-HCV IgG assays are available:

i) First generation antibodies are against C100-3 region proteins and appear 1 to 3 months after infection.

ii) Second generation antibodies are against C200 and C33c proteins and appear about one month earlier than the first generation.

iii) Third generation antibodies are against C22-3 and NS-5 region proteins and are detected even earlier.

2. *HCV-RNA.* HCV infection is, however, confirmed by HCV-RNA employing PCR technique which can be detected within a few days after exposure to HCV infection, much before appearance of anti-HCV and persists for the duration of HCV infection.

PATHOGENESIS. How HCV causes liver cell injury is not yet clearly established. HCV virions have not been identified in hepatocytes. Cell-mediated immune mechanism certainly play a role in hepatocytic injury due to HCV. Perhaps, HCV infection of lymphoid cells may play a role in immunologic injury to hepatocytes. In patients with chronic HCV hepatitis, HCV-specific CD4+ T cells and HLA-restricted CD8+ T cells have been identified.

Hepatitis E *(p. 629)*

Hepatitis E is an enterically-transmitted virus, previously labelled as epidemic or enterically transmitted type of non-A non-B hepatitis. The infection occurs in young or middle-aged individuals, primarily in India, other Asian countries, Africa and central America. The infection is generally acquired by contamination of water supplies such as after monsoon flooding.

HEPATITIS E VIRUS (HEV). HEV is a single-stranded 32-34 nm, icosahedral non-enveloped virus. The virus has been isolated from stools, bile and liver of infected persons. Serologic markers for HEV include the following:

1. Anti-HEV antibodies of both IgM and IgG class.

2. HEV-RNA.

Hepatitis G *(p. 629)*

A virus distinct from the foregoing hepatitis viruses has been designated separately by two groups of workers as hepatitis G (HGV) and hepatitis F (HFV) virus. Like HCV, HGV is a blood-borne infection and may cause acute and chronic viral hepatitis.

HEPATITIS G VIRUS (HGV). HGV is a single-stranded RNA virus. At present HGV infection has been found in blood donors and is transmitted by blood transfusion. The virus has been identified by PCR amplification technique.

CLINICOPATHOLOGIC SPECTRUM *(p. 629)*

Among of the various etiologic types of hepatitis, evidence linking HBV and HCV infection with the spectrum of clinicopathologic changes is stronger than with other hepatotropic viruses. The typical pathologic changes of hepatitis by all hepatotropic viruses are virtually similar. HAV and HEV, however, do not have a carrier stage or cause chronic hepatitis. The various clinical patterns and pathologic consequences of different hepatotropic viruses can be considered under the following headings:

i) Carrier state. ii) Asymptomatic infection. iii) Acute hepatitis. iv) Chronic hepatitis. v) Fulminant hepatitis (Submassive to massive necrosis).

I. Carrier State *(p. 630)*

An asymptomatic individual without manifest disease, harbouring infection with hepatotropic virus and capable of transmitting it is called carrier state. There can be 2 types of carriers:

1. An *'asymptomatic healthy carrier'* who does not suffer from ill-effects of the virus infection.

2. An *'asymptomatic carrier with chronic disease'* capable of transmitting the organisms.

Hepatitis A and E do not produce the carrier state. Hepatitis B is responsible for the largest number of carriers in the world, while concomitant infection with HDV more often causes progressive disease rather than an asymptomatic carrier state. An estimated 2-3% of the general population are asymptomatic carriers of HCV. Data on HBV carrier state reveal role of 2 important factors rendering the individual more vulnerable to harbour the organisms—*early age at infection* and *impaired immunity*.

Clinical recognition of carrier state of HBV is more frequently done by detection of HBsAg in the serum and less often by other markers. Concomitant infection of HDV with HBV depends upon the demonstration of anti-HD.

M/E Carriers of HBV may or may not show changes on liver biopsy:

■ *Healthy HBV carriers* may show no changes or minor hepatic change such as presence of finely granular, ground-glass, eosinophilic cytoplasm as evidence of HBsAg.

■ *Asymptomatic carriers with chronic disease* may show changes of chronic hepatitis and even cirrhosis.

II. Asymptomatic Infection *(p. 630)*

These are cases who are detected incidentally to have infection with one of the hepatitis viruses as revealed by their raised serum transaminases or by detection of the presence of antibodies but are otherwise asymptomatic.

III. Acute Hepatitis *(p. 630)*

The most common consequence of all hepatotropic viruses is acute inflammatory involvement of the entire liver. In general, type A, B, C, D and E run similar clinical course and show identical pathologic findings.

Clinically, acute hepatitis is categorised into 4 phases:

1. **Incubation period:** The patient remains asymptomatic during incubation period but the infectivity is highest during the last days of incubation period.

2. **Pre-icteric phase:** This phase is marked by prodromal constitutional symptoms that include anorexia, nausea, vomiting, fatigue, malaise, distaste for smoking, arthralgia and headache. There may be low-grade fever preceding the onset of jaundice, especially in hepatitis A. The earliest laboratory evidence of hepatocellular injury in pre-icteric phase is the elevation of transaminases.

3. **Icteric phase:** The prodromal period is heralded by the onset of clinical jaundice and the constitutional symptoms diminish. Other features include dark-coloured urine due to bilirubinuria, clay-coloured stools due to cholestasis, pruritus as a result of elevated serum bile acids, loss of weight and abdominal discomfort due to enlarged, tender liver.

4. **Post-icteric phase:** The icteric phase lasting for about 1 to 4 weeks is usually followed by clinical and biochemical recovery in 2 to 12 weeks.

G/A The liver is slightly enlarged, soft and greenish.

M/E The changes are as under:

1. **Hepatocellular injury:** There may be variation in the degree of liver cell injury but it is most marked in zone 3 (centrilobular zone):

i)   Mildly injured hepatocytes appear swollen with granular cytoplasm which tends to condense around the nucleus *(ballooning degeneration).*

ii)   Others show acidophilic degeneration in which the cytoplasm becomes intensely eosinophilic, the nucleus becomes small and pyknotic and is eventually extruded from the cell, leaving behind necrotic, acidophilic mass called *Councilman body* or *acidophil body* by the process known as apoptosis.

iii)   Another type of hepatocellular necrosis is *dropout necrosis* in which isolated or small clusters of hepatocytes undergo lysis.

iv)   *Bridging necrosis* is a more severe form of hepatocellular injury in acute viral hepatitis and may progress to fulminant hepatitis or chronic hepatitis. Bridging necrosis is characterised by bands of necrosis linking portal tracts to central hepatic veins, one central hepatic vein to another, or a portal tract to another tract.

2.   Inflammatory infiltrate: There is infiltration by mononuclear inflammatory cells, usually in the portal tracts, but may permeate into the lobules.

3.   Kupffer cell hyperplasia: There is reactive hyperplasia of Kupffer cells many of which contain phagocytosed cellular debris, bile pigment and lipofuscin granules.

4.   Cholestasis: Biliary stasis is usually not severe in viral hepatitis and may be present as intracytoplasmic bile pigment granules.

5.   Regeneration: As a result of necrosis of hepatocytes, there is lobular disarray. Surviving adjacent hepatocytes undergo regeneration and hyperplasia.

In general, it is not possible to distinguish histologically between viral hepatitis of various etiologies, the following morphologic features may help in giving an etiologic clue:

■   **HAV hepatitis** is a panlobular involvement by heavy inflammatory infiltrate compared to other types.

■   **HCV hepatitis** causes milder necrosis, with fatty change in hepatocytes, presence of lymphoid aggregates in the portal triads and degeneration of bile duct epithelium.

IV.   Chronic Hepatitis *(p. 631)*

Chronic hepatitis is defined as continuing or relapsing hepatic disease for more than 6 months with symptoms alongwith biochemical, serologic and histopathologic evidence of inflammation and necrosis. Majority of cases of chronic hepatitis are the result of infection with hepatotropic viruses—hepatitis B, hepatitis C and combined hepatitis B and hepatitis D infection.

Until recent years, prediction of prognosis of chronic hepatitis used to be made on the basis of morphology which divided it into 2 main types—*chronic persistent* and *chronic active (aggressive) hepatitis.* Subsequent studies have revealed that morphologic subtypes do not necessarily correlate with the prognosis since the disease is not essentially static but may vary from mild form to severe and *vice versa.* Besides, two other factors which determine the vulnerability of a patient of viral hepatitis to develop chronic hepatitis are: *impaired immunity* and *extremes of age* at which the infection is first contracted.

Currently, chronic hepatitis is classified on the basis of etiology. The frequency and severity with which hepatotropic viruses cause chronic hepatitis varies with the organisms as under:

■   *HCV* infection accounts for 40-60% cases of chronicity in adults. HCV infection is particularly associated with progressive form of chronic hepatitis that may evolve into cirrhosis.

■   *HBV* causes chronic hepatitis in 90% of infected infants and in about 5% adult cases of hepatitis B.

■   *HDV* superinfection on HBV carrier state may be responsible for chronic hepatitis in 10-40% cases.

■   *HAV and HEV* do not produce chronic hepatitis.

M/E The pathologic features are common to both HBV and HCV infection and include the following lesions:

1. Piecemeal necrosis. Piecemeal necrosis is defined as periportal destruction of hepatocytes at the limiting plate (*piecemeal* = piece by piece). Its features in chronic hepatitis are:

i)   Necrosed hepatocytes at the limiting plate in periportal zone.

ii) Interface hepatitis due to expanded portal tract by infiltration of lymphocytes, plasma cells and macrophages.

iii) Expanded portal tracts are often associated with proliferating bile ductules as a response to liver cell injury.

2. Portal tract lesions. All forms of chronic hepatitis are characterised by variable degree of changes in the portal tract.

i)   Inflammatory cell infiltration by lymphocytes, plasma cells and macrophages (triaditis).

ii) Proliferated bile ductules in the expanded portal tracts.

iii) Additionally, chronic hepatitis C may show lymphoid aggregates or follicles with reactive germinal centre and infiltration of inflammatory cells in the damaged bile duct epithelial cells.

3. Intralobular lesions. Generally, the architecture of lobule is retained in mild to moderate chronic hepatitis.

i)   There are focal areas of necrosis and inflammation within the hepatic parenchyma.

ii) Scattered acidophilic bodies in the lobule.

iii) Kupffer cell hyperplasia.

iv) More severe form of injury shows bridging necrosis (i.e. bands of necrosed hepatocytes that may bridge portal tract-to-central vein, central vein-to-central vein, and portal tract-to-portal tract).

v)   Regenerative changes in hepatocytes in cases of persistent hepatocellular necrosis.

vi) Cases of chronic hepatitis C show moderate fatty change.

vii) Cases of chronic hepatitis B show scattered ground-glass hepatocytes indicative of abundance of HBsAg in the cytoplasm.

4. Bridging fibrosis. The onset of fibrosis in chronic hepatitis from the area of interface hepatitis and bridging necrosis is a feature of irreversible damage.

i)   At first, there is periportal fibrosis at the sites of interface hepatitis giving the portal tract stellate-shaped appearance.

ii) Progressive cases show bridging fibrosis connecting portal tract-to-portal tract or portal tract-to-central vein traversing the lobule.

iii) End stage of chronic hepatitis is characterised by dense collagenous septa destroying lobular architecture and forming nodules resulting in postnecrotic cirrhosis.

   As prognostic indicator of chronic hepatitis, criteria have been evolved to classify chronic hepatitis by giving *activity score* (Table 19.6).

TABLE 19.6: Correlation of Older Classification and Activity Score in Chronic Hepatitis.

OLD CLASSIFICATION	ACTIVITY SCORE
Chronic persistent hepatitis	Mild activity, no or minimal fibrosis
Chronic lobular hepatitis	Mild to moderate activity, mild fibrosis
Chronic active hepatitis	Moderate to severe activity and fibrosis

CLINICAL FEATURES. The clinical features of chronic hepatitis are quite variable ranging from mild disease to full blown picture of cirrhosis.

i) Mild chronic hepatitis shows only slight but persistent elevation of transaminases ('transaminitis') with fatigue, malaise and loss of appetite.

ii) Other cases may show mild hepatomegaly, hepatic tenderness and mild splenomegaly.

iii) Laboratory findings may reveal prolonged prothrombin time, hyperbilirubinaemia, hyperglobulinaemia and markedly elevated alkaline phosphatase.

iv) Systemic features of circulating immune complexes due to HBV and HCV infection may produce features of immune complex vasculitis, glomerulonephritis and cryoglobulinaemia in a proportion of cases.

V. Fulminant Hepatitis (Submassive to Massive Necrosis) *(p. 633)*

Fulminant hepatitis is the most severe form of acute hepatitis in which there is rapidly progressive hepatocellular failure. Two patterns are recognised— *submassive necrosis* having a less rapid course extending up to 3 months; and *massive necrosis* in which the liver failure is rapid and fulminant occurring in 2-3 weeks. Fulminant hepatitis of either of the two varieties can occur from viral and non-viral etiologies:

■ *Acute viral hepatitis* accounts for about half the cases, most often from HBV and HCV; less frequently from combined HBV-HDV and rarely from HAV. However, HEV infection is a serious complication in pregnant women. In addition, herpesvirus can also cause serious viral hepatitis.

■ *Non-viral causes* include acute hepatitis due to drug toxicity (e.g. acetaminophen, non-steroidal anti-inflammatory drugs, isoniazid, halothane and anti-depressants), poisonings, hypoxic injury and massive infiltration of malignant tumours into the liver.

The patients present with features of hepatic failure with hepatic encephalopathy. The mortality rate is high if hepatic transplantation is not undertaken.

G/A The liver is small and shrunken, often weighing 500-700 gm. The capsule is loose and wrinkled. The sectioned surface shows diffuse or random involvement of hepatic lobes. There are extensive areas of muddy-red and yellow necrosis (previously called *acute yellow atrophy*) and patches of green bile staining.

M/E Two forms of fulminant necrosis are distinguished:

i) In **submassive necrosis,** large groups of hepatocytes in zone 3 (centrilobular area) and zone 2 (mid zone) are wiped out leading to a collapsed reticulin framework. Regeneration in submassive necrosis is more orderly and may result in restoration of normal architecture.

ii) In **massive necrosis,** the entire liver lobules are necrotic. As a result of loss of hepatic parenchyma, all that is left is the collapsed and condensed reticulin framework and portal tracts with proliferated bile ductules plugged with bile. Inflammatory infiltrate is scanty. Regeneration, if it takes place, is disorderly forming irregular masses of hepatocytes.

IMMUNOPROPHYLAXIS AND HEPATITIS VACCINES *(p. 634)*

Immunoprophylaxis and a few hepatitis vaccines have been developed and some more are under development:

1. Hepatitis A. Passive immunisation with immune globulin as well as active immunisation with a killed vaccine are available.

2. Hepatitis B. Earlier, only passive immunoprophylaxis with standard immune globulin was used. Later, active immunisation against HBsAg was introduced.

■ *Pre-exposure prophylaxis* is done for individuals at high-risk e.g. health care workers, haemodialysis patients and staff, haemophiliacs, intravenous drug users etc.

■ *Post-exposure prophylaxis* is carried out for unvaccinated persons exposed to HBV infection and includes prophylaxis with combination of hepatitis B immune globulin and hepatitis B vaccine.

3. Hepatitis D. Hepatitis D infection can also be prevented by hepatitis B vaccine.

4. Hepatitis C. Currently, hepatitis C vaccine has yet not been feasible though antibodies to HCV envelope have been developed.

5. Hepatitis E. It is not certain whether immune globulin (like for HAV) prevents hepatitis E infection or not but a vaccine against HEV is yet to be developed.

OTHER INFECTIONS AND INFESTATIONS *(p. 635)*

Pyogenic Cholangitis *(p. 635)*

Cholangitis occurring secondary to obstruction of a major extrahepatic duct causes pyogenic cholangitis. Most commonly, the obstruction is from impacted gallstone; other causes are carcinoma arising in the extrahepatic ducts, carcinoma head of pancreas, acute pancreatitis and inflammatory strictures in the bile duct.

M/E The affected ducts show small beaded abscesses accompanied by bile stasis along their course and larger abscesses within the liver. The abscesses are composed of acute inflammatory cells which in time are replaced by chronic inflammatory cells and enclosed by fibrous capsule.

Pyogenic Liver Abscess *(p. 635)*

Most liver abscesses are of bacterial (pyogenic) origin; less often they are amoebic, hydatid and rarely actinomycotic. Pyogenic liver abscesses are becoming uncommon due to improved diagnostic facilities and the early use of antibiotics. However, their incidence is higher in old age and in immuno-suppressed patients such as in AIDS, transplant recipients and those on intensive chemotherapy.

Pyogenic liver abscesses are classified on the basis of the mode of entry:
1. *Ascending cholangitis* through ascending infection in the biliary tract.
2. *Portal pyaemia* by means of spread of pelvic or gastrointestinal infection.
3. *Septicaemia* through spread by hepatic artery.
4. *Direct infection* resulting in solitary liver abscess.
5. *Iatrogenic causes* include liver biopsy, percutaneous biliary drainage and accidental surgical trauma.
6. *Cryptogenic* from unknown causes.

Liver abscesses are clinically characterised by pain in the right upper quadrant, fever, tender hepatomegaly and sometimes jaundice. Laboratory examination reveals leucocytosis, elevated serum alkaline phosphatase, hypoalbuminaemia and a positive blood culture.

G/A Depending upon the cause for pyogenic liver abscess, they occur as single or multiple yellow abscesses, 1 cm or more in diameter, in an enlarged liver. A single abscess generally has a thick fibrous capsule. The abscesses are particularly common in right lobe of the liver.

M/E Typical features of abscess are seen. There are multiple small neutrophilic abscesses with areas of extensive necrosis of the affected liver parenchyma. The adjacent viable area shows pus and blood clots in the portal vein, inflammation, congestion and proliferating fibroblasts.

Amoebic Liver Abscess *(p. 636)*

Amoebic liver abscesses are less common than pyogenic liver abscesses and have many similar features. They are caused by the spread of *Entamoeba histolytica* from intestinal lesions. The trophozoite form of amoebae in the colon invade the colonic mucosa forming flask-shaped ulcers from where they are carried to the liver in the portal venous system. Amoebae multiply and block small intrahepatic portal radicles resulting in infarction necrosis of the adjacent liver parenchyma.

The patients, generally from tropical and subtropical countries, may give history of amoebic dysentery in the past.

G/A Amoebic liver abscesses are usually solitary and more often located in the right lobe in the posterosuperior portion. Amoebic liver abscess may vary greatly in size but is generally of the size of an orange. The centre of the abscess contains large necrotic area having reddish-brown, thick pus resembling anchovy or chocolate sauce.

M/E The necrotic area consists of degenerated liver cells, leucocytes, red blood cells, strands of connective tissue and debris. Amoebae are most easily found in the liver tissue at the margin of abscess. PAS-staining is employed to confirm the trophozoites of *E. histolytica*.

Hepatic Tuberculosis *(p. 636)*

Tuberculosis of the liver occurs as a result of miliary dissemination from primary complex or from chronic adult pulmonary tuberculosis. The diagnosis is possible by liver biopsy. The patients may have unexplained fever, jaundice, hepatomegaly or hepatosplenomegaly.

M/E The basic lesion is the epithelioid cell granuloma characterised by central caseation necrosis with destruction of the reticulin framework and peripheral cuff of lymphocytes. Ziehl-Neelsen staining for AFB or culture of the organism from the biopsy tissue is confirmatory.

Hydatid Disease (Echinococcosis) *(p. 636)*

Hydatid disease occurs as a result of infection by the larval cyst stage of the tapeworm, *Echinococcus granulosus*. The dog is the common definite host, while man, sheep and cattle are the intermediate hosts. The dog is infected by eating the viscera of sheep containing hydatid cysts. The infected faeces of the dog contaminate grass and farmland from where the ova is ingested by sheep, pigs and man. About 70% of hydatid cysts develop in the liver which acts as the first filter for ova. However, ova which pass through the liver enter the right side of the heart and are caught in the pulmonary capillary bed and form pulmonary hydatid cysts. Some ova which enter the systemic circulation give rise to hydatid cysts in the brain, spleen, bone and muscles.

Complications of hydatid cyst include its rupture (e.g. into the peritoneal cavity, bile ducts and lungs), secondary infection and hydatid allergy due to sensitisation of the host with cyst fluid.

G/A Hydatid cyst grows slowly and may eventually attain a size over 10 cm in diameter in about 5 years. *E. granulosus* generally causes unilocular hydatid cyst while *E. multilocularis* results in multilocular or alveolar hydatid disease in the liver.

M/E The cyst wall is composed of 3 distinguishable zones:

1. Pericyst is the outer host inflammatory reaction consisting of fibroblastic proliferation, mononuclear cells, eosinophils and giant cells.

2. Ectocyst is the intermediate layer composed of characteristic acellular, chitinous, laminated hyaline material.

3. Endocyst is the inner germinal layer bearing daughter cysts (brood-capsules) and scolices.

Hydatid sand is the grain-like material composed of numerous scolices present in the hydatid fluid. Hydatid fluid, in addition, contains antigenic proteins so that its liberation into circulation gives rise to pronounced eosinophilia or may cause anaphylaxis.

CHEMICAL AND DRUG INJURY *(p. 637)*

HEPATIC DRUG METABOLISM. The liver plays a central role in the metabolism of a large number of organic and inorganic chemicals and drugs which gain access to the body by inhalation, injection, or most commonly, via the intestinal tract. The main drug metabolising system resides in the microsomal fraction of the smooth endoplasmic reticulum of the liver cells via P-450 cytochrome and cytochrome reductase enzyme systems. Other steps involved in the drug metabolism are its conjugation with an endogenous molecule, its active transport from the hepatocytes and ultimately its excretion in the bile or in urine depending upon the molecular weight of the substance.

HEPATOTOXICITY. Toxic liver injury produced by drugs and chemicals may virtually mimic any form of naturally-occurring liver disease. In fact, any patient presenting with liver disease or unexplained jaundice is thoroughly questioned about history of drug intake or exposure to chemicals. Hepatotoxicity from drugs and chemicals is the commonest form of iatrogenic disease. Severity of hepatotoxicity is greatly increased if the drug is continued after symptoms develop.

Among the various *inorganic compounds* producing hepatotoxicity are arsenic, phosphorus, copper and iron. *Organic agents* include certain naturally-occurring plant toxins such as pyrrolizidine alkaloids, mycotoxins and bacterial toxins.

In general, drug reactions affecting the liver are divided into two main classes:

1. Direct or predictable, when the drug or one of its metabolites is either directly toxic to the liver or it lowers the host immune defense mechanism. The adverse effects occur in most individuals who consume them and their hepatotoxicity is dose-dependent e.g. carbon tetrachloride.

2. Indirect or unpredictable or idiosyncratic, when the drug or one of its metabolites acts as a hapten and induces hypersensitivity in the host. The hepatotoxicity by this group does not occur regularly in all individuals and the effects are usually not dose-related e.g. acetaminophen.

The pathologic changes by hepatotoxins include 2 large categories:

1 *Acute liver disease* characterised by cholestasis, hepatocellular necrosis, fatty change, granulomatous reaction or vascular disease.

2. *Chronic liver disease* characterised by variable degree of fibrosis, cirrhosis or neoplasia.

CIRRHOSIS *(p. 638)*

Cirrhosis of the liver is a diffuse disease having the following 4 features:

1. It involves the entire liver.

2. The normal lobular architecture of hepatic parenchyma is disorganised.

3. There is formation of nodules separated from one another by irregular bands of fibrosis.

4. It occurs following hepatocellular necrosis of varying etiology so that there are alternate areas of necrosis and regenerative nodules.

Pathogenesis *(p. 639)*

Continued destruction of hepatocytes causes collapse of normal lobular hepatic parenchyma followed by *fibrosis* around necrotic liver cells and proliferated ductules and there is formation of compensatory *regenerative nodules*.

FIBROGENESIS. The mechanism of fibrosis that may be portal-central, portal-portal, or both, is by increased synthesis of all types of collagen and increase in the number of collagen-producing cells. Development of fibrosis leads to proliferation of fat-storing Ito cells underlying the sinusoidal epithelium which become transformed into myofibroblasts and fibrocytes.

REGENERATIVE NODULE. The cause of compensatory proliferation of hepatocytes to form regenerative nodules is obscure. Possibly, growth factors, chalones and hormonal imbalance, play a role in regeneration.

Classification *(p. 639)*

Cirrhosis can be classified on the basis of morphology and etiology:

A. MORPHOLOGIC CLASSIFICATION. There are 3 morphologic types of cirrhosis—micronodular, macronodular and mixed. Each of these forms may have an active and inactive form.

1. In **micronodular cirrhosis**, the nodules are usually regular and small, *less than 3 mm* in diameter.

2. In **macronodular cirrhosis**, the nodules are of variable size and are generally *larger than 3 mm* in diameter.

3. In **mixed cirrhosis**, some parts of the liver show micronodular appearance while other parts show macronodular pattern.

B. ETIOLOGIC CLASSIFICATION. Based on the cause for cirrhosis, the etiologic categories of cirrhosis are given in Table 19.7.

TABLE 19.7: Classification of Cirrhosis.

A. MORPHOLOGIC	B. ETIOLOGIC
I. Micronodular (nodules less than 3 mm)	1. Alcoholic cirrhosis (the most common, 60-70%)
II. Macronodular (nodules more than 3 mm)	2. Post-necrotic cirrhosis (10%)
III. Mixed	3. Biliary cirrhosis (5-10%)
	4. Pigment cirrhosis in haemochromatosis (5%)
	5. Cirrhosis in Wilson's disease
	6. Cirrhosis in α-1-antitrypsin deficiency
	7. Cardiac cirrhosis
	8. Indian childhood cirrhosis (ICC)
	9. Miscellaneous forms of cirrhosis
	10. Cryptogenic cirrhosis

Alcoholic Liver Disease and Cirrhosis *(p. 639)*

Alcoholic liver disease is the term used to describe the spectrum of liver injury associated with acute and chronic alcoholism. There are three stages in alcoholic liver disease: *alcoholic steatosis (fatty liver), alcoholic hepatitis* and *alcoholic cirrhosis.*

ETHANOL METABOLISM. Ethanol after ingestion and absorption from the small bowel circulates through the liver where about 90% of it is oxidised to acetate by a *two-step enzymatic process* involving two enzymes: *alcohol dehydrogenase (ADH)* present in the cytosol, and *acetaldehyde dehydrogenase (ALDH)* in the mitochondria of hepatocytes. The remaining 10% of ethanol is oxidised elsewhere in the body.

Most of the acetate on leaving the liver is finally oxidised to carbon dioxide and water, or converted by the citric acid cycle to other compounds including fatty acids. Simultaneously, the same cofactor, NAD, is reduced to NADH resulting in *increased NADH: NAD redox ratio* which is the basic biochemical alteration occurring during ethanol metabolism.

ETIOLOGY. All those who indulge in alcohol abuse do not develop liver damage. The incidence of cirrhosis among alcoholics at autopsy is about 10-15%. The following factors are implicated:

1. Drinking patterns. Most epidemiologic studies have attributed alcoholic cirrhosis to chronic alcoholism. The quantity and duration of drinking necessary to cause cirrhosis is largely unknown but it is generally agreed that continued daily imbibing of more than 80 gm of any type of alcoholic beverage for at least 10 years is likely to result in alcoholic cirrhosis.

2. Malnutrition. Absolute or relative malnutrition of proteins and vitamins is regarded as a contributory factor in the evolution of cirrhosis. The combination of chronic alcohol ingestion and impaired nutrition leads to alcoholic liver disease and not malnutrition *per se*.

3. Infections. Intercurrent bacterial infections are common in cirrhotic patients and may accelerate the course of the disease.

4. Genetic factors. The rate of ethanol metabolism is under genetic control. Various HLA histocompatibility types have been associated with susceptibility of different populations to alcoholic liver damage.

PATHOGENESIS. Following mechanisms are implicated:

1. Hepatotoxicity by ethanol. There is some evidence to suggest that ethanol ingestion for a period of 8-10 days regularly may cause direct hepatotoxic effect on the liver and produce fatty change.

2. Hepatotoxicity by ethanol metabolites. The major hepatotoxic effects of ethanol are exerted by its metabolites, chiefly acetaldehyde.

3. Free radicals. Oxidation of ethanol by the cytochrome-450 oxidases (MEOS) leads to generation of free radicals which attack the membrane and proteins.

4. Increased redox ratio. Marked increase in the NADH:NAD redox ratio in the hepatocytes results in increased redox ratio of lactate-pyruvate, leading to lactic acidosis. This altered redox potential has been implicated in a number of metabolic consequences such as in fatty liver, collagen formation, occurrence of gout, impaired gluconeogenesis and altered steroid metabolism.

5. Retention of liver cell water and proteins. Alcohol is inhibitory to secretion of newly-synthesised proteins by the liver leading to their retention in the hepatocytes.

6. Hypoxia. Chronic ingestion of alcohol results in increased oxygen demand by the liver resulting in a hypoxic state which causes hepatocellular necrosis in centrilobular zone (zone 3).

7. Increased liver fat. In chronic alcoholism, there is rise in the amount of fat available to the liver which could be from exogenous (dietary) sources, excess mobilisation from adipose tissue or increased lipid synthesis by the liver itself.

8. Immunological mechanism. Cell-mediated immunity is impaired in alcoholic liver disease. Ethanol causes direct immunologic attack on hepatocytes. In a proportion of cases, alcohol-related liver cell injury continues unabated despite cessation of alcohol consumption which is attributed to immunologic mechanisms.

9. Fibrogenesis and inflammation. The mechanisms of fibrosis and inflammatory response in alcoholic liver disease are uncertain but the possible mediators are lymphokines and monokines. The major stimulus for fibrogenesis is cell necrosis.

MORPHOLOGY. Three types of morphologic lesions are described in alcoholic liver disease.

1. ALCOHOLIC STEATOSIS (FATTY LIVER). It is regarded as the forerunner of subsequent stages.

G/A The liver is enlarged, yellow, greasy and firm with a smooth and glistening capsule.

M/E The features consist of initial *microvesicular* droplets of fat in the hepatocyte cytoplasm followed by more common and pronounced feature of *macrovesicular* large droplets of fat displacing the nucleus to the periphery. *Fat cysts* may develop due to coalescence and rupture of fat-containing hepatocytes. Less often, *lipogranulomas* consisting of collection of lymphocytes, macrophages and some multinucleate giant cells may be found.

2. ALCOHOLIC HEPATITIS. Alcoholic hepatitis develops acutely, usually following a bout of heavy drinking. Repeated episodes of alcoholic hepatitis superimposed on pre-existing fatty liver are almost certainly a forerunner of alcoholic cirrhosis.

M/E Characteristic features are as under:

i) Hepatocellular necrosis: Single or small clusters of hepatocytes, especially in the centrilobular area (zone 3), undergo ballooning degeneration and necrosis.

ii) Mallory bodies or alcoholic hyalin: These are eosinophilic, intracytoplasmic inclusions seen in perinuclear location within swollen and balloned hepatocytes. They represent aggregates of cytoskeletal intermediate filaments (prekeratin). Mallory bodies are also found in certain other conditions such as: primary biliary cirrhosis, Indian childhood cirrhosis, cholestatic syndromes, Wilson's disease, intestinal bypass surgery, focal nodular hyperplasia and hepatocellular carcinoma.

iii) Inflammatory response: The areas of hepatocellular necrosis and regions of Mallory bodies are associated with an inflammatory infiltrate, chiefly consisting of polymorphs and some scattered mononuclear cells.

iv) Fibrosis: Most cases of alcoholic hepatitis are accompanied by pericellular and perivenular fibrosis, producing a web-like or chickenwire-like appearance. This is also termed as *creeping collagenosis*.

3. ALCOHOLIC CIRRHOSIS. Alcoholic cirrhosis is the most common form of lesion, constituting 60-70% of all cases of cirrhosis.

G/A Alcoholic cirrhosis classically begins as micronodular cirrhosis (nodules less than 3 mm diameter), the liver being large, fatty and weighing usually above 2 kg. The nodules of the liver due to their fat content are tawny-yellow, on the basis of which Laennec in 1818 introduced the term *cirrhosis* first of all (from Greek *kirrhos* = tawny). The surface of liver in alcoholic cirrhosis is studded with diffuse nodules which vary little in size, producing hobnail liver.

M/E Alcoholic cirrhosis is a progressive alcoholic liver disease.

i) Lobular architecture: No normal lobular architecture can be identified and central veins are hard to find.

ii) Fibrous septa: The fibrous septa that divide the hepatic parenchyma into nodules are initially delicate and extend from central vein to portal regions, or portal tract to portal tract, or both.

iii) Hepatic parenchyma: The hepatocytes in the islands of surviving parenchyma undergo slow proliferation forming regenerative nodules having disorganised masses of hepatocytes. There is an inverse relationship between the amount of fat and the amount of fibrous scarring in the nodules.

iv) Necrosis, inflammation and bile duct proliferation: The etiologic clue to diagnosis in the form of Mallory bodies is hard to find in a fully-developed alcoholic cirrhosis. The fibrous septa usually contain sparse infiltrate of mononuclear cells with some bile duct proliferation.

Post-necrotic Cirrhosis *(p. 644)*

Post-necrotic cirrhosis, also termed *post-hepatitic cirrhosis, macronodular cirrhosis* and *coarsely nodular cirrhosis,* is characterised by large and irregular nodules with broad bands of connective tissue and occurring most commonly after previous viral hepatitis.

ETIOLOGY. Following factors are implicated:

1. Viral hepatitis. About 25% of patients give history of recent or remote attacks of acute viral hepatitis followed by chronic hepatitis. Most common association is with hepatitis B and C.

2. Drugs and chemical hepatotoxins. A small percentage of cases may have origin from toxicity due to chemicals and drugs such as phosphorus, carbon tetrachloride, mushroom poisoning, acetaminophen and α-methyl dopa.

3. Others. Certain infections (e.g. brucellosis), parasitic infestations (e.g. clonorchiasis), metabolic diseases (e.g. Wilson's disease or hepatolenticular degeneration) and advanced alcoholic liver disease may produce a picture of post-necrotic cirrhosis.

4. Idiopathic. After all these causes have been excluded, a group of cases remain in which the etiology is unknown.

G/A The liver is usually small, weighing less than 1 kg, having distorted shape with irregular and coarse scars and nodules of varying size. Sectioned surface shows scars and nodules varying in diameter from 3 mm to a few centimeters.

M/E The features are as follows:

1. Lobular architecture: The normal lobular architecture of hepatic parenchyma is not completely lost. Instead, uninvolved portal tracts and central veins in the hepatic lobules can still be seen.

2. Fibrous septa: The fibrous septa dividing the variable-sized nodules are generally thick.

3. Necrosis, inflammation and bile duct proliferation: Active liver cell necrosis is usually inconspicuous. Fibrous septa contain prominent mono-nuclear inflammatory cell infiltrate which may even form follicles. Often there is extensive proliferation of bile ductules.

4. Hepatic parenchyma: Liver cells vary considerably in size and multiple large nuclei are common in regenerative nodules.

Biliary Cirrhosis *(p. 644)*

Biliary cirrhosis is defined as a chronic disorder characterised by clinical, biochemical and morphological features of long-continued cholestasis of intrahepatic or extrahepatic origin. Accordingly, biliary cirrhosis is of 2 main types:

■ *Primary biliary cirrhosis* in which the destructive process of unknown etiology affects intrahepatic bile ducts.

■ *Secondary biliary cirrhosis* resulting from prolonged mechanical obstruction of the extrahepatic biliary passages.

■ In addition, a third cause for biliary cirrhosis is *primary sclerosing cholangitis* discussed at the end of this discussion.

ETIOLOGY. The etiology of the two forms of biliary cirrhosis is distinctive:

A. Primary biliary cirrhosis. It is largely idiopathic. However, following observations have been made:

1. The condition is predominant in middle-aged women (male: female ratio = 1:9) and has led to the suggestion of a possible *endocrine origin.*

2. *Familial incidence* has been observed suggesting the role of some genetic influence and certain HLA types.

3. There is *elevated cholesterol* level with appearance of xanthoma and xanthelasma.

4. However, presently the most widely accepted hypothesis is *autoimmune origin* of the disease. In support are the following observations:

■ increased incidence of associated autoimmune diseases (e.g. scleroderma, Sjögren's syndrome, CREST syndrome, and autoimmune thyroiditis);

■ circulating anti-mitochondrial antibody of IgG class detected in more than 90% cases;

■ elevated levels of immunoglobulins, particularly of IgM;

■ increased levels of circulating immune complexes;

■ decreased number of circulating T cells; and

■ accumulation of T cells around bile ducts.

B. Secondary biliary cirrhosis. Most cases of secondary biliary cirrhosis result from prolonged obstruction of extrahepatic biliary passages e.g.:

1. Extrahepatic cholelithiasis, most common
2. Biliary atresia
3. Cancer of biliary tree and of head of pancreas
4. Postoperative strictures with superimposed ascending cholangitis.

G/A In both primary and secondary biliary cirrhosis, the liver is initially enlarged and greenish-yellow in appearance, but later becomes smaller, firmer and coarsely micronodular.

M/E The salient features are as under:

A. Primary biliary cirrhosis: The diagnostic histologic feature is a chronic, non-suppurative, destructive cholangitis involving intrahepatic bile ducts. The disease evolves through the following 4 histologic states: florid bile duct lesions, ductular proliferation, fibrous scarring, and micronodular pattern.

B. Secondary biliary cirrhosis: Prolonged obstruction of extrahepatic bile ducts may produce the following histologic changes:

1. *Bile stasis,* degeneration and focal areas of centrilobular necrosis of hepatocytes.

2. Proliferation, dilatation and rupture of bile ductules in the portal area with formation of *bile lakes.*

3. *Cholangitis,* sterile or pyogenic, with accumulation of polymorphs around the bile ducts.

4. *Progressive expansion* of the portal tract by fibrosis and evolution into micronodular cirrhosis.

CLINICAL FEATURES. Clinical features of primary and secondary biliary cirrhosis are variable:

■ **Primary biliary cirrhosis** may remain asymptomatic for months to years. Symptoms develop insidiously. Basically, it is a cholestatic disorder. The patients present with persistent pruritus, dark urine, pale stools, steatorrhoea, jaundice and skin pigmentation. The earliest laboratory finding is a markedly elevated serum alkaline phosphatase level.

■ The diagnosis of **secondary biliary cirrhosis** is considered in patients with previous history of gallstones, biliary tract surgery or clinical features of ascending cholangitis.

PRIMARY SCLEROSING CHOLANGITIS. Primary or idiopathic sclerosing cholangitis is characterised by progressive, inflammatory, sclerosing and obliterative process affecting mainly extra-hepatic, and sometimes intrahepatic ducts as well. The disease occurs in 3rd to 5th decade of life with two fold preponderance in males.

ETIOLOGY. Though idiopathic, the condition coexists with the following:

1. Inflammatory bowel disease, particularly idiopathic. 2. Multifocal fibrosclerosis syndromes. 3. AIDS.

G/A There is characteristic beading of intra- and extrahepatic bile ducts due to irregular strictures and dilatation.

M/E 1. *Fibrosing cholangitis* with lymphocytic infiltrate around bile ducts with segmental involvement.

2. *Periductal fibrosis* with eventual obliteration of lumen of affected bile ducts.

3. *Intervening bile ducts* are dilated, tortuous and inflamed.

4. Late cases show *cholestasis* and full blown picture of biliary cirrhosis.

Clinically, the patients may remain asymptomatic or may show features of cholestatic jaundice (raised alkaline phosphatase, pruritus, fatigue). Late cases show manifestations of chronic liver disease.

Pigment Cirrhosis in Haemochromatosis *(p. 647)*

Haemochromatosis is an iron-storage disorder in which there is excessive accumulation of iron in parenchymal cells with eventual tissue damage and functional insufficiency of organs such as the liver, pancreas, heart and pituitary gland. The condition is characterised by a triad of features—*micronodular pigment cirrhosis, diabetes mellitus* and *skin pigmentation*. On the basis of the last two features, the disease has also come to be termed as '*bronze diabetes*'.

1. *Idiopathic (primary, genetic) haemochromatosis* is an autosomal recessive disorder of excessive accumulation of iron associated with susceptible gene, linked to HLA-A3 complex on chromosome 6.

2. *Secondary (acquired) haemochromatosis* is gross iron overload with tissue injury arising secondary to other diseases such as thalassaemia, sideroblastic anaemias, alcoholic cirrhosis or multiple transfusions.

ETIOPATHOGENESIS. Normally, the body iron content is 3-4 gm which is maintained in such a way that intestinal mucosal absorption of iron is equal to its loss. This amount is approximately 1 mg/day in men and 1.5 mg/day in menstruating women. In haemochromatosis, however, this amount goes up to 4 mg/day or more, as evidenced by elevated serum iron (normal about 125µg/dl) and increased serum transferrin saturation (normal 30%).

■ In **idiopathic haemochromatosis,** the primary mechanism of disease appears to be the genetic basis in which the defect may either lie at the intestinal mucosal level causing excessive iron absorption, or at the postabsorption excretion level leading to excessive accumulation of iron. The excess iron in primary haemochromatosis is deposited mainly in the cytoplasm of parenchymal cells of organs such as the liver, pancreas, spleen, heart and endocrine glands.

■ In **secondary haemochromatosis,** there is excessive accumulation of iron due to acquired causes like ineffective erythropoiesis, defective haemoglobin synthesis, multiple blood transfusions and enhanced absorption of iron due to alcohol consumption. The last-named phenomenon is observed in *Bantu siderosis* affecting South African Bantu tribals.

MORPHOLOGY. The organs most frequently affected are the liver and pancreas, and to a lesser extent, the heart, endocrine glands, skin, synovium and testis.

■ In the **liver,** excess of pigment accumulates in the hepatocytes, and less often Kupffer cells and in bile duct epithelium. The deposits in the initial stage may be prominent in the periportal liver cells alongwith increased fibrosis in the portal zone. But eventually, micronodular cirrhosis develops. The deposits may produce grossly chocolate brown colour of the liver and nodular surface.

■ In the **pancreas,** pigmentation is less intense and is found in the acinar and islet cells. The deposits in pancreas produce diffuse interstitial fibrosis and atrophy of parenchymal cells leading to occurrence of diabetes mellitus.

Cirrhosis in Wilson's Disease *(p. 648)*

Wilson's disease, also termed by a more descriptive designation of *hepatolenticular degeneration,* is an autosomal recessive inherited disease of copper metabolism, characterised by toxic accumulation of copper in many tissues, chiefly the liver, brain and eye. These accumulations lead to the *triad* of features:

1. Cirrhosis of the liver.
2. Bilateral degeneration of the basal ganglia of the brain.
3. Greenish-brown pigmented rings in the periphery of the cornea (Kayser-Fleischer rings).

The disease manifests predominantly in children and young adults (5-30 years). Initially, the clinical manifestations are referable to liver involvement such as jaundice and hepatomegaly *(hepatic form)* but later progressive *neuropsychiatric changes* and *Kayser-Fleischer rings* in the cornea appear.

PATHOGENESIS. It is described in relation to normal copper metabolism.

■ **Normally,** dietary copper is more than body's requirement. Excess copper so absorbed through the stomach and duodenum is transported to the liver where it is incorporated into α_2-globulin to form ceruloplasmin, which is excreted by the liver via bile normally. Most of the plasma copper circulates as ceruloplasmin.

■ **In Wilson's disease,** the initial steps of dietary absorption and transport of copper to the liver are normal but copper accumulates in the liver rather than being excreted by the liver. Eventually, capacity of hepatocytes to store copper is exceeded and copper is released into circulation which then gets deposited in extrahepatic tissues such as the brain, eyes and others.

Biochemical abnormalities in Wilson's disease include the following:

1. *Decreased serum ceruloplasmin.*
2. *Increased hepatic copper* in liver biopsy
3. *Increased urinary excretion* of copper.
4. However, *serum copper levels* are of no diagnostic help and may vary from low-to-normal-to-high depending upon the stage of disease.

MORPHOLOGY. The **liver** shows varying grades of changes that include fatty change, acute and chronic active hepatitis, submassive liver necrosis and macronodular cirrhosis. Mallory bodies are present in some cases. Copper is usually deposited in the periportal hepatocytes in the form of reddish granules in the cytoplasm.

Involvement of basal ganglia in **brain** is in the form of toxic injury to neurons, in the **cornea** as greenish-brown deposits of copper in Descemet's membrane, and in the **kidney** as fatty and hydropic change.

Cirrhosis in α-1-Antitrypsin Deficiency *(p. 648)*

Alpha-1-antitrypsin deficiency is an autosomal codominant condition in which the homozygous state produces liver disease (cirrhosis), pulmonary disease (emphysema), or both. α-1-antitrypsin is a glycoprotein normally synthesised in the rough endoplasmic reticulum of the hepatocytes and is the most potent protease inhibitor (Pi). PiMM is the most common normal phenotype, while the most frequent abnormal phenotype in α-1-antitrypsin deficiency leading to liver and/or lung disease is PiZZ in homozygote form.

The patients may present with respiratory disease due to the development of emphysema, or may develop liver dysfunction, or both.

M/E The hepatic changes vary according to the age at which the deficiency becomes apparent. At birth or in neonates, the histologic features consist of neonatal hepatitis that may be acute or 'pure' cholestasis. Micronodular or macronodular cirrhosis may appear in childhood or in adolescence in which the diagnostic feature is the presence of intracellular, acidophilic, PAS-positive globules in the periportal hepatocytes.

Chapter Nineteen

Cardiac Cirrhosis *(p. 649)*

Cardiac cirrhosis is an uncommon complication of severe right-sided congestive heart failure of long-standing duration. The common causes culminating in cardiac cirrhosis are cor pulmonale, tricuspid insufficiency or constrictive pericarditis. The pressure in the right ventricle is elevated which is transmitted to the liver via the inferior vena cava and hepatic veins.

G/A The liver is enlarged and firm with stretched Glisson's capsule.

M/E Severe and more prolonged heart failure results in delicate fibrous strands radiating from the central veins. These fibrous strands may form interconnections leading to cardiac cirrhosis and regenerative nodules.

Indian Childhood Cirrhosis *(p. 649)*

Indian childhood cirrhosis (ICC) is an unusual form of cirrhosis seen in children between the age of 6 months and 3 years in rural, middle class, Hindus in India and in parts of South-East Asia and the Middle-East. There is no role of viral infection in its etiology. Instead, a combination of some common toxic effects and inherited abnormality of copper metabolism has been suggested.

ME Five histologic types of ICC have been distinguished of which type II is the most common. This form is characterised by the following features:

i) Liver cell injury ranging from ballooning degeneration to significant damage to hepatocytes.

ii) Prominent Mallory bodies in some hepatocytes without fatty change.

iii) Neutrophilic and sometimes alongwith lymphocytic infiltrate.

iv) Creeping pericellular fibrosis which may eventually lead to fine micro-macro-nodular cirrhosis.

v) There is significant deposition of copper and copper-associated proteins in hepatocytes.

NON-CIRRHOTIC PORTAL FIBROSIS *(p. 650)*

Non-cirrhotic portal fibrosis (NCPF) is a group of congenital and acquired diseases in which there is localised or generalised hepatic fibrosis without nodular regenerative activity and there is absence of clinical and functional evidence of cirrhosis. Besides, the patients of NCPF are relatively young as compared to those of cirrhosis and develop repeated bouts of haematemesis in the course of disease. One of the types associated with increased portal fibrosis without definite cirrhosis is seen in *idiopathic(primary) portal hypertension with splenomegaly,* reported from India and Japan. Another variant is *congenital hepatic fibrosis* seen in polycystic disease of the liver. The type common in India, particularly in young males, is related to *chronic arsenic ingestion* in drinking water and intake of orthodox medicines.

G/A The liver is small, fibrous and shows prominent fibrous septa on both external as well as on cut surface.

M/E The salient features are as under:
i) Standing out of portal tracts due to their fibrous thickening without significant inflammation.

ii) Obliterative sclerosis of portal vein branches in the portal tracts (obliterative portovenopathy).

CLINICAL MANIFESTATIONS AND COMPLICATIONS OF CIRRHOSIS *(p. 650)*

The range of clinical features in cirrhosis varies widely, from an asymptomatic state to progressive liver failure and death. The onset of disease is insidious.

1. *Portal hypertension* and its major effects such as ascites, splenomegaly and development of collaterals (e.g. oesophageal varices, spider naevi etc.).

2. *Progressive hepatic failure* and its manifestations.

3. Development of *hepatocellular carcinoma*, more often in post-necrotic cirrhosis (HBV and HCV more often) than following alcoholic cirrhosis.

4. *Chronic relapsing pancreatitis*, especially in alcoholic liver disease.

5. *Steatorrhoea* due to reduced hepatic bile secretion.

6. *Gallstones* usually of pigment type.

7. *Infections* are more frequent in patients with cirrhosis.

8. *Haematologic derangements* such as bleeding disorders and anaemia.

9. *Cardiovascular complications* such as atherosclerosis of coronaries and aorta and myocardial infarction.

10. *Musculoskeletal abnormalities* like digital clubbing, hypertrophic osteoarthropathy.

11. In males these consist of feminisation such as gynaecomastia, changes in pubic hair pattern, testicular atrophy and impotence, whereas in cirrhotic women amenorrhoea is a frequent abnormality.

12. *Hepatorenal syndrome* leading to renal failure may occur in late stages of cirrhosis.

The ultimate *causes of death* are hepatic coma, massive gastrointestinal haemorrhage from oesophageal varices (complication of portal hypertension), intercurrent infections, hepatorenal syndrome and development of hepatocellular carcinoma.

PORTAL HYPERTENSION *(p. 650)*

Increase in pressure in the portal system usually follows obstruction to the portal blood flow anywhere along its course. Portal veins have no valves and thus obstruction anywhere in the portal system raises pressure in all the veins proximal to the obstruction. However, unless proved otherwise, portal hypertension means obstruction to the portal blood flow by cirrhosis of the liver. The normal portal venous pressure is quite low (10-15 mm saline). Portal hypertension occurs when the portal pressure is above 30 mm saline.

CLASSIFICATION. Based on the site of obstruction to portal venous blood flow, portal hypertension is categorised into 3 main types—*intrahepatic, posthepatic* and *prehepatic* (Table 19.8).

TABLE 19.8: Major Causes of Portal Hypertension.

A. INTRAHEPATIC
1. Cirrhosis
2. Metastatic tumours
3. Budd-Chiari syndrome
4. Hepatic veno-occlusive disease
5. Diffuse granulomatous diseases
6. Extensive fatty change

B. POSTHEPATIC
1. Congestive heart failure
2. Constrictive pericarditis
3. Hepatic veno-occlusive disease
4. Budd-Chiari syndrome

C. PREHEPATIC
1. Portal vein thrombosis
2. Neoplastic obstruction of portal vein
3. Myelofibrosis
4. Congenital absence of portal vein

MAJOR SEQUELAE OF PORTAL HYPERTENSION. Irrespective of the mechanisms involved in the pathogenesis of portal hypertension, there are 4 major clinical consequences:

1. Ascites. Ascites is the accumulation of excessive volume of fluid within the peritoneal cavity. It frequently accompanies cirrhosis and other diffuse liver diseases. The development of ascites is associated with haemodilution, oedema and decreased urinary output.

Pathogenesis. The ascites becomes clinically detectable when more than 500 ml of fluid has accumulated in the peritoneal cavity. The systemic and local factors favouring ascites formation are as under.

A. SYSTEMIC FACTORS: i) Decreased plasma colloid oncotic pressure. ii) Hyperaldosteronism. iii) Impaired renal excretion.

B. LOCAL FACTORS: i) Portal hypertension. ii) Increased hepatic lymph formation.

2. Varices (Collateral channels or Porto-systemic shunts). As a result of rise in portal venous pressure and obstruction in the portal circulation within or outside the liver, the blood tends to bypass the liver and return to the heart by development of porto-systemic collateral channels (or shunts or varices). These varices develop at sites where the systemic and portal circulations have common capillary beds. The principal sites: i) Oesophageal varices. ii) Haemorrhoids. iii) Caput medusae. iv) Retroperitoneal anastomoses.

3. Splenomegaly. The enlargement of the spleen in prolonged portal hypertension is called congestive splenomegaly. The spleen may weigh 500-1000 gm and is easily palpable. The spleen is larger in young people and in macronodular cirrhosis than in micronodular cirrhosis.

4. Hepatic encephalopathy. Porto-systemic venous shunting may result in a complex metabolic and organic syndrome of the brain characterised by disturbed consciousness, neurologic signs and flapping tremors.

TUMOURS AND TUMOUR-LIKE LESIONS *(p. 653)*

A histogenetic classification of benign and malignant tumours is presented in Table 19.9.

TABLE 19.9: Classification of Primary Hepatic Tumours.

	BENIGN	MALIGNANT
A.	**Hepatocellular tumours** Hepatocellular (liver cell) adenoma	Hepatocellular (liver cell) carcinoma Hepatoblastoma (Embryoma)
B.	**Biliary tumours** Bile duct adenoma (Cholangioma)	Cholangiocarcinoma Combined hepatocellular and cholangiocarcinoma Cystadenocarcinoma
C.	**Mesodermal tumours** Haemangioma	Angiosarcoma Embryonal sarcoma

Hepatic Cysts *(p. 653)*

Cysts in the liver may be single or multiple.

1. CONGENITAL CYSTS. These are uncommon. They are usually small (less than 1 cm in diameter) and are lined by biliary epithelium. On occasions, these cysts have abundant connective tissue and numerous ducts, warranting the designation of *congenital hepatic fibrosis.*

2. SIMPLE (NON-PARASITIC) CYSTS. Simple cysts are solitary non-parasitic cysts seen more frequently in middle-aged women. The cyst is usually large (up to 20 cm in diameter), lying underneath the Glisson's capsule and filled with serous fluid.

Focal Nodular Hyperplasia *(p. 653)*

G/A Focal nodular hyperplasia is a well-demarcated tumour-like nodule occurring underneath the Glisson's capsule. The nodules may be single or multiple, measuring about 5 cm in diameter.

M/E It is composed of collagenous septa radiating from the central fibrous scar which separate nodules of normal hepatocytes without portal triads or central hepatic veins.

Hepatocellular (Liver Cell) Adenoma *(p. 654)*

Adenomas arising from hepatocytes are rare and are reported in women in reproductive age group in association with use of oral contraceptives, sex hormone therapy and with pregnancy.

G/A The tumour usually occurs singly but about 10% are multiple. It is partly or completely encapsulated and slightly lighter in colour than adjacent liver or may be bile-stained. The tumours vary from a few centimetres up to 30 cm in diameter.

M/E Liver cell adenomas are composed of sheets and cords of hepatocytes which may be normal-looking or may show slight variation in size and shape but no mitoses.

Bile Duct Adenoma (Cholangioma) *(p. 654)*

Intrahepatic or extrahepatic bile duct adenoma is a rare benign tumour. The tumour may be small, composed of acini lined by biliary epithelium and separated by variable amount of connective tissue.

Haemangioma *(p. 654)*

Haemangioma is the commonest benign tumour of the liver. Majority of them are asymptomatic and discovered incidentally. Rarely, a haemangioma may rupture into the peritoneal cavity.

G/A Haemangiomas appear as solitary or multiple, circumscribed, red-purple lesions, commonly subcapsular and varying from a few millimetres to a few centimetres in diameter. They are commonly cavernous type giving the sectioned surface a spongy appearance.

M/E Characteristic cavernous blood-filled spaces lined by flattened endothelium are seen.

Hepatocellular Carcinoma *(p. 654)*

Hepatocellular or liver cell carcinoma (HCC), sometimes termed hepatoma, is the most common primary malignant tumour of the liver. The tumour shows marked geographic variations in incidence which is closely related to hepatitis B virus infection in the region. Whereas the prevalence of HCC is less than 1% of all autopsies in the United States and Europe, the incidence in Africa and South-East Asia is 2-8%. Liver cell cancer is 4-6 times more common in males than in females. The peak incidence occurs in 5th to 6th decades of life but in high incidence areas where HBV infection is prevalent, it occurs a decade or two earlier. The tumour supervenes on cirrhosis, usually post-necrotic macro-nodular type, in 70-80% of cases.

ETIOPATHOGENESIS. Following factors are implicated:

1. Relation to HBV infection. Genesis of HCC is linked to prolonged infection with HBV. The evidence in support is both epidemiologic and direct.

2. Relation to HCV infection. More recent evidence points to long-standing HCV infection as a major factor in the etiology of HCC.

3. Relation to cirrhosis. Cirrhosis of all etiologic types is more commonly associated with HCC but the most frequent association is with macronodular post-necrotic cirrhosis. The mechanism of progression to HCC appears to be chronic regenerative activity in cirrhosis, or that the damaged liver in cirrhosis is rendered vulnerable to carcinogenic influences.

4. Relation to alcohol. It has been observed that alcoholics have about four-fold increased risk of developing HCC.

5. Mycotoxins. An important mycotoxin, aflatoxin B1, produced by a mould *Aspergillus flavus,* can contaminate stored grains or groundnuts, especially in less developed countries. Aflatoxin B1 is carcinogenic.

6. Chemical carcinogens. A number of chemical carcinogens can induce liver cancer in experimental animals. These include butter-yellow and nitrosamines used as common food additives.

7. Miscellaneous factors. Limited role of various other factors in HCC has been observed. These include:

i) haemochromatosis;
ii) α-1-antitrypsin deficiency;
iii) prolonged immunosuppressive therapy in renal transplant patients;
iv) other types of viral hepatitis;
v) tobacco smoking; and
vi) parasitic infestations such as clonorchiasis and schistosomiasis.

G/A The HCC may form one of the following 3 patterns of growth, in decreasing order of frequency:

i) *Expanding type:* Most frequently, it forms a *single,* yellow-brown, *large mass,* most often in the right lobe of the liver with central necrosis, haemorrhage and occasional bile-staining.

ii) *Multifocal type:* Less often, *multifocal, multiple masses,* 3-5 cm in diameter, scattered throughout the liver are seen.

iii) *Infiltrating (Spreading) type:* Rarely, the HCC forms diffusely infiltrating tumour mass.

M/E The tumour cells in the typical HCC resemble hepatocytes but vary with the degree of differentiation, ranging from well-differentiated to highly anaplastic lesions. Most of the HCC have trabecular growth pattern.

1. Histologic patterns: These include the following:

i) *Trabecular or sinusoidal pattern* is the most common. The trabeculae are made up of 2-8 cell wide layers of tumour cells separated by vascular spaces.

ii) *Pseudoglandular or acinar pattern* is seen sometimes.

iii) *Compact pattern* resembles trabecular pattern but the tumour cells form large solid masses with inconspicuous sinusoids.

iv) *Scirrhous pattern* is characterised by more abundant fibrous stroma.

2. Cytologic features: The typical cytologic features in the HCC consist of cells resembling hepatocytes having vesicular nuclei with prominent nucleoli. The cytoplasm is granular and eosinophilic but becomes increasingly basophilic with increasing malignancy. Aside from these features, a few other cytologic variants are: pleomorphism, bizarre giant cell formation, spindle-shaped cells, tumour cells with clear cytoplasm, presence of bile within dilated canaliculi, and intracytoplasmic Mallory's hyalin.

FIBROLAMELLAR CARCINOMA. A clinicopathologic variant of the HCC is fibrolamellar carcinoma of the liver found in young people of both sexes. The tumour forms a single large mass which may be encapsulated and occurs in the absence of cirrhosis.

M/E The tumour is composed of eosinophilic polygonal cells (oncocytes) forming cords and nests which are separated by bands of fibrous stroma.

The prognosis of fibrolamellar carcinoma is better than other forms of HCC.

CLINICAL FEATURES. Hepatic cancer may remain undetected initially because it often occurs in patients with underlying cirrhosis. The usual features consist of hepatomegaly with palpable mass in the liver, right upper quadrant pain or tenderness, and less often, jaundice, fever and haemorrhage from oesophageal varices. Ascites with RBCs and malignant cells is found in about half the patients. Rarely, systemic endocrine manifestations such as hypercalcaemia, hypoglycaemia, gynaecomastia and acquired porphyria are encountered.

Laboratory findings yield nonspecific results like anaemia, markedly elevated serum alkaline phosphatase as found in cirrhosis, and high serum alpha-foetoprotein (AFP).

SPREAD. The tumour spreads by following routes.

■ **Intrahepatic spread** occurs by haematogenous route and forms multiple metastases in the liver.

■ **Extrahepatic spread** occurs via hepatic or portal veins to different sites, chiefly to lungs and bones, and by lymphatic route to regional lymph nodes at the porta hepatis and to mediastinal and cervical lymph nodes.

The causes of death from the HCC are cachexia, massive bleeding from oesophageal varices, and liver failure with hepatic coma.

Cholangiocarcinoma *(p. 657)*

Cholangiocarcinoma is the designation used for carcinoma arising from bile duct epithelium within the liver *(peripheral cholangiocarcinoma).* Carcinomas arising from the large hilar ducts *(hilar cholangiocarcinoma)* and from extrahepatic ducts are termed *bile duct carcinomas.* None of the etiologic factors related to HCC have any role in the genesis of cholangiocarcinoma. However, the etiological factors involved in it are exposure to radio-opaque dye thorotrast, anabolic steroids, clonorchiasis and fibrocystic disease.

G/A The tumour is firm to hard and whitish.

M/E The tumour has glandular structure. The tumour cells resemble biliary epithelium but without bile secretion. They form various patterns such as tubular, ductular or papillary.

Hepatoblastoma (Embryoma) *(p. 657)*

Hepatoblastoma is a rare malignant tumour arising from primitive hepatic parenchymal cells. It presents before the age of 2 years as progressive abdominal distension with anorexia, failure to thrive, fever and jaundice. It is more common in boys. The concentration of serum AFP is high. The tumour grows rapidly.

G/A The tumour is circumscribed and lobulated mass measuring 5-25 cm in size, having areas of cystic degeneration, haemorrhage and necrosis.

M/E Hepatoblastoma consists of 2 components:

i) Epithelial component contains 2 types of cells—*'embryonal'* hepatocytes are small with dark-staining, hyperchromatic nuclei and scanty cytoplasm, and *'foetal'* hepatocytes are larger with more cytoplasm that may be granular or clear.

ii) Mesenchymal component includes fibrous connective tissue, cartilage and osteoid of variable degree of maturation.

Secondary Hepatic Tumours *(p. 657)*

Metastatic tumours in the liver are more common than the primary hepatic tumours. Most frequently, they are blood-borne metastases, irrespective of whether the primary tumour is drained by portal vein or systemic veins. Most frequent primary tumours metastasising to the liver, in descending order of frequency, are those of stomach, breast, lungs, colon, oesophagus, pancreas, malignant melanoma and haematopoietic malignancies. Sarcomas rarely metastasise to the liver. There is little hepatic dysfunction until late in the course of hepatic metastatic disease.

BILIARY SYSTEM (p. 658)

NORMAL STRUCTURE (p. 658)

ANATOMY. The gallbladder is a pear-shaped organ, 9 cm in length and has a capacity of approximately 50 ml. It consists of the *fundus, body* and *neck* that tapers into the cystic duct. The common bile duct enters the second part of the duodenum posteriorly.

M/E The gallbladder, unlike the rest of gastrointestinal tract, lacks the muscularis mucosae and submucosa. The wall of the gallbladder is composed of the following 4 layers: 1. Mucosal layer. 2. Smooth muscle layer. 3. Perimuscular layer. 4. Serosal layer.

CONGENITAL ANOMALIES (p. 658)

Several uncommon congenital anomalies of the biliary system have been described. These include: agenesis, duplication and heterotopic tissue. However, *congenital cystic lesions* of the bile ducts (as also of the liver) are more frequently being diagnosed. These conditions include: congenital intrahepatic biliary dilatation (Caroli's disease), choledochal cysts, polycystic liver disease and congenital hepatic fibrosis.

CHOLELITHIASIS (GALLSTONES) (p. 658)

Gallstones are formed from constituents of the bile (viz. cholesterol, bile pigments and calcium salts) alongwith other organic components. Accordingly, the gallstones commonly contain cholesterol, bile pigment and calcium salts in varying proportions.

RISK FACTORS. These factors which largely pertain to cholesterol stones can be summed up in the old saying that gallstones are common in 4F's—'*fat, female, fertile (multipara)* and *forty*'. Some of the risk factors in lithogenesis are explained below:

1. **Geography.** Gallstones are quite prevalent in almost the entire Western world.

2. **Genetic factors.** There is increased frequency of gallstones in first-degree relatives of patients with cholelithiasis.

3. **Age.** There is steady increase in the prevalence of gallstones with advancing age which may be related to increased cholesterol content in the bile.

4. **Sex.** Gallstones are twice more frequent in women than in men.

5. **Drugs.** Women on oestrogen therapy or on birth control pills have higher incidence of gallstones.

6. **Obesity.** Obesity is associated with increased cholesterol synthesis and excretion resulting in higher incidence of gallstones in obese patients.

7. **Diet.** Deficiency of dietary fibre content is linked to higher prevalence of gallstones.

8. **Gastrointestinal diseases.** Certain gastrointestinal disorders such as Crohn's disease, ileal resection, ileal bypass surgery etc are associated with interruption in enterohepatic circulation followed by gallstone formation.

9. Factors in pigment gallstones. All the above factors apply largely to cholesterol stones. Pigment stones, whether pure or mixed type, are more frequently associated with haemolytic anaemias.

PATHOGENESIS. The mechanism of gallstone formation or lithogenesis is explained separately below under 2 headings:

PATHOGENESIS OF CHOLESTEROL, MIXED GALLSTONES AND BILIARY SLUDGE. Cholesterol is essentially insoluble in water and can be solublised by another lipid. Normally, cholesterol and phospholipids (lecithin) are secreted into bile as 'bilayered vesicles' but are converted into 'mixed miscelles' by addition of bile acids, the third constituent. If there is excess of cholesterol compared to the other two constituents, unstable cholesterol-rich vesicles remain behind which aggregate and form cholesterol crystals. Formation of such lithogenic (stone-forming) bile is explained by the following mechanisms:

1. Supersaturation of bile: Several etiologic factors listed above favour increased secretion of cholesterol in the presence of normal bile acids and lecithin in the bile as the major mechanism for initiation of gallstone formation. Additional factors include:
i) Reduced bile acid pool, and ii) Increased conversion of cholic acid to deoxycholic acid

Although supersaturation of the bile with cholesterol is an important pre-requisite for lithogenesis, this in itself is not sufficient for cholesterol precipitation.

2. Cholesterol nucleation. Initiation of cholesterol stones occurs by nucleation of cholesterol monohydrate crystals. Accelerated nucleation of cholesterol monohydrate may occur either from pro-nucleating factors or from deficiency of anti-nucleating factors.

3. Gallbladder hypomotility. Normally, the gallbladder is capable of emptying and clearing any sludge or debris which might initiate stone formation.

PATHOGENESIS OF PIGMENT GALLSTONES. The mechanism of pigment stone formation is explained on the basis of following factors:
i) Chronic haemolysis resulting in increased level of unconjugated bilirubin in the bile.
ii) Alcoholic cirrhosis.
iii) Chronic biliary tract infection e.g. by parasitic infestations of the biliary tract such as by *Clonorchis sinensis* and *Ascaris lumbricoides*.
iv) Demographic and genetic factors e.g. in rural setting and prevalence in Asian countries.

TYPES OF GALLSTONES. As stated before, gallstones contain cholesterol, bile pigment and calcium carbonate, either in pure form or in various combinations. Accordingly, gallstones are of 3 major types—pure gallstones, mixed gallstones and combined gallstones.

The salient features of various types of gallstones are summarised in Table 19.10.

CLINICAL MANIFESTATIONS AND COMPLICATIONS. Symptomatic gall-stone disease appears only when complications develop. These are:
1. Cholecystitis. 2. Choledocholithiasis. 3. Mucocele. 4. Biliary fistula.
5. Gallstone ileus. 6. Gallbladder cancer.

CHOLECYSTITIS *(p. 661)*

Cholecystitis or inflammation of the gallbladder may be acute, chronic, or acute superimposed on chronic.

Acute Cholecystitis *(p. 661)*

ETIOPATHOGENESIS. Based on the initiating mechanisms, acute cholecystitis occurs in two types of situations.

TABLE 19.10: Features of Gallstones.

TYPE	FREQU-ENCY	COMPOSITION	GALL-BLADDER CHANGES	APPEARANCE
1. *Pure gallstones*	10%	i) Cholesterol	Cholesterolosis	Solitary, oval, large, smooth, yellow-white; on C/S radiating glistening crystals
		ii) Bile pigment	No change	Multiple, small, jet-black, mulberry-shaped; on C/S soft black
		iii) Calcium carbonate	No change	Multiple, small, grey-white, faceted; C/S hard
2. *Mixed gallstones*	80%	Cholesterol, bile pigment and calcium carbonate invarying combination	Chronic cholecystitis	Multiple, multifaceted, variable size, on C/S laminated alternating dark-pigment layer and pale-white layer
3. *Combined gallstones*	10%	Pure gallstone nucleus with mixed gallstone shell, or mixed gallstone nucleus with pure gallstone shell	Chronic cholecystitis	Solitary, large, smooth; on C/S central nucleus of pure gallstone with mixed shell or vice versa

■ **Acute calculous cholecystitis.** In 90% of cases, acute cholecystitis is caused by obstruction in the neck of the gallbladder or in the cystic duct by a gallstone.

■ **Acute acalculous cholecystitis.** The remaining 10% cases of acute cholecystitis do not contain gallstones. In such cases, a variety of causes have been assigned such as previous nonbiliary surgery, multiple injuries, burns, recent childbirth, severe sepsis, dehydration, torsion of the gallbladder and diabetes mellitus.

G/A The gallbladder is distended and tense. The serosal surface is coated with fibrinous exudate with congestion and haemorrhages. The mucosa is bright red.

M/E Wall of the gallbladder shows marked inflammatory oedema, congestion and neutrophilic exudate. There may be frank abscesses in the wall and gangrenous necrosis with rupture into the peritoneal cavity (*gangrenous cholecystitis*).

CLINICAL FEATURES. The patients of acute cholecystitis of either type have similar clinical features. They present with severe pain in the upper abdomen with features of peritoneal irritation such as guarding and hyperaesthesia. The gallbladder is tender and may be palpable. Fever, leucocytosis with neutrophilia and slight jaundice are generally present.

Chronic Cholecystitis *(p. 662)*

Chronic cholecystitis is the commonest type of clinical gallbladder disease.

ETIOPATHOGENESIS. The association of chronic cholecystitis with mixed and combined gallstones is virtually always present.

G/A The gallbladder is generally contracted but may be normal or enlarged. The wall of the gallbladder is thickened which on cut section is grey-white due to dense fibrosis or may be even calcified. The mucosal folds may be intact, thickened, or flattened and atrophied. The lumen commonly contains multiple mixed stones or a combined stone.

M/E The features are as under:

1. Thickened and congested mucosa but occasionally mucosa may be totally destroyed.

2. Penetration of the mucosa deep into the wall of the gallbladder up to muscularis layer to form *Rokitansky-Aschoff'sinuses.*

3. Variable degree of chronic inflammatory reaction, consisting of lymphocytes, plasma cells and macrophages, present in the lamina propria and subserosal layer.

4. Variable degree of fibrosis in the subserosal and subepithelial layers.

A few morphologic variants of chronic cholecystitis are considered below:

■ **Cholecystitis glandularis,** when the mucosal folds fuse together due to inflammation and result in formation of crypts of epithelium buried in the gallbladder wall.

■ **Porcelain gallbladder** is the pattern when the gallbladder wall is calcified and cracks like an egg-shell.

■ **Acute on chronic cholecystitis** is the term used for the morphologic changes of acute cholecystitis superimposed on changes of chronic cholecystitis.

CLINICAL FEATURES. Chronic cholecystitis has ill-defined and vague symptoms. Generally, the patient—*a fat, fertile, female of forty or fifty*, presents with abdominal distension or epigastric discomfort, especially after a fatty meal. There is a constant dullache in the right hypochondrium and epigastrium and tenderness over the right upper abdomen.

CARCINOMA OFTHE GALLBLADDER *(p. 663)*

Primary carcinoma of the gallbladder is more prevalent than other cancers of the extrahepatic biliary tract. Like cholelithiasis and cholecystitis, it is more frequent in women than in men with a peak incidence in 7th decade of life. It is usually slow-growing and may remain undetected until the time it is widely spread and rendered inoperable.

ETIOLOGY. A number of etiologic factors have been implicated:

1. **Cholelithiasis and cholecystitis.** The most significant association of cancer of the gallbladder is with cholelithiasis and cholecystitis. Porcelain gallbladder is particularly likely to become cancerous.

2. **Chemical carcinogens.** These include methyl cholanthrene, various nitrosamines and pesticides. Workers engaged in rubber industry have higher incidence of gallbladder cancer.

3. **Genetic factors.** There is higher incidence of cancer of the gallbladder in certain populations living in the same geographic region suggesting a strong genetic component in the disease.

4. **Miscellaneous.** Patients who have undergone previous surgery on the biliary tract have higher incidence of subsequent gallbladder cancer.

G/A Cancer of the gallbladder is of 2 types—

1. *Infiltrating type* appears as an irregular area of diffuse thickening and induration of the gallbladder wall. It may have deep ulceration causing direct invasion of the gallbladder wall and liver bed.

2. *Fungating type* grows like an irregular, friable, papillary or cauliflower-like growth into the lumen as well as into the wall of the gallbladder and beyond.

M/E The following patterns are observed:

1. Most gallbladder cancers are *adenocarcinomas* (90%). They may be papillary or infiltrative, well-differentiated or poorly-differentiated.

2. About 5% of gallbladder cancers are *squamous cell carcinomas* arising from squamous metaplastic epithelium.

3. A few cases show both squamous and adenocarcinoma pattern of growth called *adenosquamous carcinoma*.

CLINICAL FEATURES. Carcinoma of the gallbladder is slow-growing and causes symptoms late in the course of disease. Quite often, the diagnosis is made when gallbladder is removed for cholelithiasis. The symptomatic cases have pain, jaundice, noticeable mass, anorexia and weight loss.

CARCINOMA OF EXTRAHEPATIC BILE DUCTS AND AMPULLA OF VATER *(p. 665)*

Unlike other diseases of the biliary passages, it is more common in males with peak incidence in 6th decade of life.

ETIOLOGY. There is no association between bile duct carcinoma and gallstones. Bile duct cancers are associated with a number of other conditions such as ulcerative colitis, sclerosing cholangitis, parasitic infestations of the bile ducts with *Fasciola hepatica* (liver fluke), *Ascaris lumbricoides* and *Clonorchis sinensis*.

Extrahepatic bile duct carcinoma may arise anywhere in the biliary tree but the most frequent sites, in descending order of frequency, are: the ampulla of Vater, lower end of common bile duct, hepatic ducts, and the junction of hepatic ducts to form common bile duct.

G/A Bile duct carcinoma is usually small, extending for 1-2 cm along the duct, producing thickening of the affected duct.

M/E The tumour is usually well-differentiated adenocarcinoma which may or may not be mucin-secreting. Perineural invasion is frequently present.

EXOCRINE PANCREAS *(p. 665)*

NORMAL STRUCTURE *(p. 665)*

The human pancreas, though anatomically a single organ, histologically and physiologically has 2 distinct parts—the *exocrine* and *endocrine parts*.

ANATOMY. The pancreas lies obliquely in the concavity of the duodenum as an elongated structure about 15 cm in length and 100 gm in weight. It is subdivided into 3 topographic zones:

1. The *head* lying in the concavity of the duodenum and the *uncinate process* projecting from the head.

2. The *body* comprises the main part of the gland.

3. The *tail* is the thin, tapering part of the gland towards the hilum of the spleen.

HISTOLOGY. The exocrine pancreas constitutes 80 to 85% of the total gland, while the endocrine pancreas comprises the remaining part. The exocrine part is divided into rhomboid lobules separated by thin fibrous tissue septa containing blood vessels, lymphatics, nerves and ducts. Each lobule is composed of numerous acini. The acini are lined by pyramid-shaped columnar epithelial cells.

CYSTIC FIBROSIS *(p. 665)*

Cystic fibrosis of the pancreas or fibrocystic disease is a hereditary disorder characterised by viscid mucous secretions in all the exocrine glands of the body *(mucoviscidosis)* and associated with increased concentrations of electrolytes in the eccrine glands. The terms 'cystic fibrosis' and 'fibrocystic disease' are preferable over 'mucoviscidosis' in view of the main pathologic change of fibrosis produced as a result of obstruction of the passages by viscid mucous secretions. The disease is transmitted as an *autosomal recessive trait* with apparent clinical features in homozygotes only. The clinical manifestations may appear at birth or later in adolescence and pertain to multiple organs and systems.

MORPHOLOGY. Most of the changes are produced as a result of obstruction by viscid mucous.

1. **Pancreas.** The pancreas is almost invariably involved in cystic fibrosis.

G/A Pancreatic lobules are ovoid rather than rhomboid. Fatty replacement of the pancreas and grossly visible cysts may be seen.

M/E The lobular architecture of pancreatic parenchyma is maintained. There is increased interlobular fibrosis. The acini are atrophic and many of the acinar ducts contain laminated, eosinophilic concretions.

2. **Liver.** The bile canaliculi are plugged by viscid mucous which may cause diffuse fatty change, portal fibrosis and ductular proliferation. More severe involvement may cause biliary cirrhosis.

3. **Respiratory tract.** Changes in the respiratory passages are seen in almost all typical cases of cystic fibrosis. The viscid mucous secretions of the submucosal glands of the respiratory tract cause obstruction, dilatation and infection of the airways. The changes include chronic bronchitis, bronchiectasis, bronchiolitis, bronchiolectasis, peribronchiolar pneumonia and inflammatory nasal polyps.

4. **Salivary glands.** Pathologic changes in the salivary glands are similar to those in pancreas and include obstruction of the ducts, dilatation, fibrosis and glandular atrophy.

5. **Sweat glands.** Hypersecretion of sodium and chloride in the sweat observed in these patients may be reflected pathologically by diminished vacuolation of the cells of eccrine glands.

PANCREATITIS *(p. 666)*

It is classified into acute and chronic forms.

Acute Pancreatitis *(p. 666)*

Acute pancreatitis is an acute inflammation of the pancreas presenting clinically with 'acute abdomen'. The severe form of the disease associated with macroscopic haemorrhages and fat necrosis in and around the pancreas is termed *acute haemorrhagic pancreatitis* or *acute pancreatic necrosis*. The condition occurs in adults between the age of 40 and 70 years and is commoner in females than in males.

The onset of acute pancreatitis is sudden, occurring after a bout of alcohol or a heavy meal. The patient presents with abdominal pain, vomiting and collapse. Characteristically, there is elevation of *serum amylase* level within the first 24 hours and of *serum lipase* level after 3 to 4 days; the latter being more specific for pancreatic disease.

ETIOLOGY. The two leading causes associated with acute pancreatitis are *alcoholism* and *cholelithiasis,* both of which are implicated in more than 80% of cases. Less common causes of acute pancreatitis include trauma, ischaemia, shock, extension of inflammation from the adjacent tissues, blood-borne bacterial infection, viral infections, certain drugs (e.g. thiazides, sulfonamides, oral contraceptives), hyperthermia.

PATHOGENESIS. The destructive changes in the pancreas are attributed to the liberation and activation of pancreatic enzymes. Though more than 20 enzymes are secreted by exocrine pancreas, 3 main groups of enzymes which bring about destructive effects on the pancreas are: 1. Proteases 2. Lipases and phospholipases 3. Elastases.

The activation and release of these enzymes is brought about by: 1. Acinic cell damage 2. Duct obstruction 3. Block in exocytosis.

G/A In the early stage, the pancreas is swollen and oedematous. Subsequently, in a day or two, the characteristic variegated appearance of grey-white pancreatic necrosis, chalky-white fat necrosis and blue-black haemorrhages are seen. In typical case, the peritoneal cavity contains blood-stained ascitic fluid and white flecks of fat necrosis in the omentum, mesentry and peripancreatic tissue.

M/E 1. Necrosis of pancreatic lobules and ducts.
2. Necrosis of the arteries and arterioles with areas of haemorrhages.
3. Fat necrosis.
4. Inflammatory reaction, chiefly by polymorphs, around the areas of necrosis and haemorrhages.

COMPLICATIONS. Systemic complications. 1. Chemical and bacterial peritonitis. 2. Endotoxic shock. 3. Acute renal failure.

Local sequelae. 1. Pancreatic abscess. 2. Pancreatic pseudocyst. 3. Duodenal obstruction.

Mortality in acute pancreatitis is high (20-30%). Patients succumb to hypotensive shock, infection, acute renal failure, and DIC.

Chronic Pancreatitis *(p. 667)*

Chronic pancreatitis or *chronic relapsing pancreatitis* is the progressive destruction of the pancreas due to repeated mild and subclinical attacks of acute pancreatitis. Most patients present with recurrent attacks of severe abdominal pain at intervals of months to years. Weight loss and jaundice are often associated.

ETIOLOGY. Most cases of chronic pancreatitis are caused by the same factors as for acute pancreatitis. Thus, most commonly, chronic pancreatitis is related to *chronic alcoholism* with protein-rich diet, and less often by *biliary tract disease. Familial hereditary pancreatitis,* though uncommon, is more frequently chronic than the acute form.

PATHOGENESIS. Acute haemorrhagic pancreatitis seldom develops into chronic pancreatitis, but instead develops pancreatic pseudocysts following recovery. Pathogenesis of alcoholic and non-alcoholic chronic pancreatitis is explained by different mechanisms:
1. Chronic pancreatitis due to *chronic alcoholism* accompanied by a high-protein diet results in increase in protein concentration in the pancreatic juice which obstructs the ducts and causes damage.
2. *Non-alcoholic cases* of chronic pancreatitis seen in tropical countries (tropical chronic pancreatitis) result from protein-calorie malnutrition. Genetic factors play a role in some cases of chronic pancreatitis.

G/A The pancreas is enlarged, firm and nodular. The cut surface shows a smooth grey appearance with loss of normal lobulation. Foci of calcification and tiny pancreatic concretions to larger visible stones are frequently found. Pseudocysts may be present.

M/E 1. Obstruction of the ducts by fibrosis in the wall and protein plugs or stones in the lumina.
2. Squamous metaplasia and dilatation of some inter- and intralobular ducts.
3. Chronic inflammatory infiltrate around the lobules as well as the ducts.
4. Atrophy of the acinar tissue with marked increase in interlobular fibrous tissue.
5. Islet tissue is involved in late stage only.

COMPLICATIONS. Late stage of chronic pancreatitis may be complicated by diabetes mellitus, pancreatic insufficiency with steatorrhoea and malabsorption and formation of pancreatic pseudocysts.

PANCREATIC PSEUDOCYST *(p. 668)*

Pancreatic pseudocyst is a localised collection of pancreatic juice, necrotic debris and haemorrhages. It develops following either acute pancreatitis or trauma.

G/A The pseudocyst may be present within or adjacent to the pancreas. Usually it is solitary, unilocular, measuring up to 10 cm in diameter with thin or thick wall.

M/E The cyst wall is composed of dense fibrous tissue with marked inflammatory reaction. There is evidence of preceding haemorrhage and necrosis in the form of deposits of haemosiderin pigment, calcium and cholesterol crystals.

CARCINOMA OF PANCREAS *(p. 668)*

Pancreatic cancer is the term used for cancer of the exocrine pancreas. It is one of the common cancers, particularly in the Western countries and Japan. In the United States, cancer of the pancreas is the second most common cancer of the alimentary tract after colorectal cancer, and accounts for 5% of all cancer deaths in that country. It is commoner in males than in females and the incidence increases progressively after the age of 50 years.

ETIOLOGY. Following factors have been implicated in its etiology. 1. Smoking 2. Diet and obesity 3. Chemical carcinogens 4. Diabetes mellitus 5. Chronic pancreatitis.

However, excessive consumption of alcohol or coffee, and cholelithiasis are not risk factors for pancreatic cancer. A mutation in *RAS* gene has been found in more than 85% cases of cancer of the pancreas.

The most common location of pancreatic cancer is the head of pancreas (70%), followed in decreasing frequency, by the body and the tail of pancreas.

G/A Carcinoma of the head of pancreas is generally small, homogeneous, poorly-defined, grey-white mass without any sharp demarcation between the tumour and the surrounding pancreatic parenchyma. The tumour of the head extends into the ampulla of Vater, common bile duct and duodenum, producing obstructive biliary symptoms and jaundice early in the course of illness.

M/E Most pancreatic carcinomas arise from the ductal epithelium which normally comprises less than 4% of total pancreatic cells, whereas carcinoma of the acini constitutes less than 1% of pancreatic cancers. The following histologic patterns of pancreatic carcinoma are seen: 1. Well-differentiated adenocarcinoma 2. Adenoacanthoma 3. Rarely, peculiar tumour giant cell formation 4. Acinar cell carcinoma.

CLINICAL FEATURES. Generally, the following features are present: 1. Obstructive jaundice. 2. Other features.

The prognosis of pancreatic cancer is dismal: median survival is 6 months from the time of diagnosis.

Chapter Nineteen

■ SELF ASSESSMENT

1. **The following zone/area of liver lobule is more prone to all forms of toxic injury:**
   A. Zone 1 (periportal area)   B. Zone 2 (midzonal area)
   C. Zone 3 (centrilobular area)   D. Subcapsular area
2. **The following enzyme assay in serum is most specific of liver cell injury:**
   A. SGOT (aspartate transaminase) B. SGPT (alanine transaminase)
   C. γ-GT (γ-Glutamyl transpeptidase) D. Alkaline phosphatase
3. **The form of bilirubin which remains detectable in serum for sufficient time after recovery from the disease is:**
   A. Biliverdin   B. Unconjugated bilirubin
   C. Unbound conjugated bilirubin D. Delta bilirubin

4. **Acute viral hepatitis by the following hepatotropic virus is characterised by fatty change in liver:**
   - A. HAV
   - B. HBV
   - C. HCV
   - D. HDV

5. **Extrahepatic cholestasis can be distinguished from intrahepatic cholestasis by the following tests in the former:**
   - A. Bilirubinuria
   - B. Hypoprothrombinaemia showing improvement following parenteral administration of vitamin K
   - C. Elevated serum alkaline phosphatase
   - D. Elevated serum bile acids

6. **The following conditions have unconjugated hyperbilirubinaemia** *except:*
   - A. Dubin-Johnson syndrome
   - B. Crigler-Najjar syndrome
   - C. Jaundice of prematurity
   - D. Gilbert syndrome

7. **Kernicterus often develops in the following type of hereditary hyperbilirubinaemia:**
   - A. Gilbert syndrome
   - B. Crigler-Najjar syndrome, type I
   - C. Dubin-Johnson syndrome
   - D. Rotor syndrome

8. **Reye's syndrome is characterised by the following features** *except:*
   - A. It is a form of hereditary hyperbilirubinaemia
   - B. There is microvesicular fatty change in hepatocytes
   - C. Patients have a rapidly downhill course
   - D. There is decreased activity of mitochondrial enzymes in the liver

9. **Hepatic encephalopathy is due to:**
   - A. Hypoxic damage from ischaemia
   - B. Toxic damage from ammonia
   - C. Thromboembolic phenomena
   - D. Hepatopulmonary syndrome

10. **Some etiologic factors implicated in Budd-Chiari syndrome are as under** *except:*
    - A. Pulmonary embolism
    - B. Hepatocellular carcinoma
    - C. Polycythaemia vera
    - D. Pregnancy

11. **Councilman bodies in viral hepatitis are a form of apoptosis commonly at the following site:**
    - A. Submassive
    - B. Centrilobular
    - C. Midzonal
    - D. Periportal

12. **The following hepatotropic virus is a DNA virus:**
    - A. HAV
    - B. HBV
    - C. HCV
    - D. HEV

13. **Chronic carrier state of the following hepatotropic virus infection is observed in the following** *except:*
    - A. HAV
    - B. HBV
    - C. HCV
    - D. HDV

14. **In hepatitis A, life-long protective immunity against reinfection is given by the following class of antibody:**
    - A. IgA
    - B. IgE
    - C. IgG
    - D. IgM

15. **Hepatitis B surface antigen (HBsAg) is present as the following structures** *except:*
    - A. Viral spheres
    - B. Viral tubules
    - C. Surface envelope of Dane particle
    - D. Inner core of Dane particle

16. **HBsAg can be demonstrated at the following sites** *except:*
    A. Serum of HBV-infected patient
    B. Carrier state of HBV
    C. Hepatocyte cell membrane in acute stage of illness
    D. Hepatocyte cell membrane in chronic hepatitis B

17. **In chronic hepatitis B and carrier state of HBV infection, the following antigen is detected on the nuclei of infected hepatocytes:**
    A. HBsAg
    B. HBeAg
    C. HBcAg
    D. HBV-DNA

18. **In an HDV-infected individual, HDV antigen is detected at the following sites** *except:*
    A. Serum in acute illness
    B. Serum in carrier state
    C. Hepatocyte cell membrane
    D. Hepatocyte nuclei

19. **Vast majority (more than 90%) of cases of post-transfusion hepatitis are caused by:**
    A. HBV
    B. HCV
    C. HDV
    D. HGV

20. **The most progressive form of chronic hepatitis is caused by:**
    A. Hepatitis A
    B. Hepatitis B
    C. Hepatitis C
    D. Hepatitis D

21. **The following genetic component of HBV is considered responsible for its carcinogenic influence:**
    A. HBsAg
    B. HBeAg
    C. HBcAg
    D. HBxAg

22. **In amoebic liver abscess, trophozoites of** *E.histolytica* **are best demonstrated at:**
    A. Necrotic centre of abscess
    B. Margin of abscess with viable liver tissue
    C. Granulation tissue in the abscess wall
    D. Fibrous wall of the abscess

23. **The most common site for hydatid cyst is:**
    A. Liver
    B. Lungs
    C. Spleen
    D. Brain

24. **Micronodular cirrhosis includes the following etiologic types** *except:*
    A. Laennec's cirrhosis
    B. Nutritional cirrhosis
    C. Post-necrotic cirrhosis
    D. Portal cirrhosis

25. **The major hepatotoxic effect of ethanol is exerted by:**
    A. Direct hepatotoxicity of ethanol
    B. Free radical injury
    C. Hepatotoxicity of acetaldehyde
    D. Immunologic mechanisms

26. **Mallory's hyalin is seen in the following conditions** *except:*
    A. Alcoholic hepatitis
    B. Hepatocellular carcinoma
    C. Post-necrotic cirrhosis
    D. Primary biliary cirrhosis

27. **Primary biliary cirrhosis has the following features** *except:*
    A. There is elevated cholesterol level in blood
    B. It has familial occurrence
    C. The condition is more common in men
    D. The disease has autoimmune origin

28. **Patients of following type of cirrhosis more often may develop hepatocellular carcinoma as a late complication:**
    A. Biliary cirrhosis
    B. Haemochromatosis-induced cirrhosis
    C. Cirrhosis in α1 antitrypsin deficiency
    D. Cardiac cirrhosis

Chapter Nineteen

29. **Biochemical abnormalities in Wilson's disease include the following *except*:**
    A. Increased serum ceruloplasmin
    B. Increased urinary copper excretion
    C. Increased hepatic copper
    D. Serum copper low-to-normal-to-high

30. **Intrahepatic causes of portal hypertension include the following *except*:**
    A. Cirrhosis
    B. Budd-Chiari syndrome
    C. Portal vein thrombosis
    D. Metastatic tumours

31. **In developed countries the major risk factor in the pathogenesis of hepatocellular carcinoma is:**
    A. Long-standing HBV infection
    B. Long-standing HCV infection
    C. Alcoholic cirrhosis
    D. Aflatoxin B1

32. **Risk factors implicated in the etiology of cholesterol gallstones include the following *except*:**
    A. Family history
    B. Obesity
    C. Haemolytic anaemia
    D. Oral contraceptives

33. **The following type of gallstones are generally unassociated with changes in the gallbladder wall:**
    A. Cholesterol
    B. Mixed
    C. Combined
    D. Pigment

34. **The most common site for cancer of the gallbladder is:**
    A. Fundus
    B. Body
    C. Neck
    D. Cystic duct

35. **Pancreatic carcinoma of the following site more often produces obstructive jaundice:**
    A. Head
    B. Body
    C. Tail
    D. Uncinate process

KEY

1 = A	2 = B	3 = D	4 = C
5 = B	6 = A	7 = B	8 = A
9 = B	10 = A	11 = C	12 = B
13 = A	14 = C	15 = D	16 = C
17 = C	18 = C	19 = B	20 = C
21 = D	22 = B	23 = A	24 = C
25 = C	26 = C	27 = C	28 = B
29 = A	30 = C	31 = C	32 = C
33 = D	34 = A	35 = A	

20

The Kidney and Lower Urinary Tract

KIDNEY (p. 670)

NORMAL STRUCTURE (p. 670)

ANATOMY. The kidneys are bean-shaped paired organs, each weighing about 150 gm in the adult male and about 135 gm in the adult female.

Cut surface of the kidney is made up of well-demarcated *peripheral cortex and inner medulla*. The pelvis is the funnel-shaped, dilated proximal part of the ureter formed by the union of 2 to 3 *major calyces,* each of which is further subdivided into 3 to 4 minor calyces into which the papillae project.

HISTOLOGY. The parenchyma of each kidney is composed of approximately one million microstructures called nephrons. A nephron, in turn, consists of 5 major parts, each having a functional role in the formation of urine: the glomerular capsule (glomerulus and Bowman's capsule), the proximal convoluted tubule (PCT), the loop of Henle, the distal convoluted tubule (DCT), and the collecting ducts. From point of view of diseases of the kidneys, 4 components of renal parenchyma require further elaboration : renal vasculature, glomeruli, tubules and interstitium.

1. Renal vasculature. Each kidney is supplied with blood by a main *renal artery* which arises from the aorta at the level of the 2nd lumbar vertebra. It usually divides into *anterior and posterior divisions* at the hilum although occasionally these divisions may even arise directly from the aorta. The anterior and posterior divisions divide into *segmental branches* from which interlobar arteries arise which course between the lobes. Along their course, they give off the *arcuate arteries* which arch between the cortex and medulla. The arcuate arteries, in turn, give off *interlobular arteries* which lie in the cortex perpendicular to the capsular surface in the part overlying the pyramids and, therefore, are also called *straight arteries*. It is from the interlobular arteries that the *afferent arterioles* take their origin, each one supplying a single glomerulus.

The following important derivations can be made from the peculiarities of the renal vasculature:

i)   The renal cortex receives about 90% of the total renal blood supply and that the pressure in the glomerular capillaries is high. Therefore, renal cortex is more prone to the effects of hypertension.

ii)   The renal medulla, on the other hand, is poorly perfused and any interference in blood supply to it results in medullary necrosis.

iii) The divisions and subdivisions of the renal artery up to arterioles are end-arteries and have no anastomoses. Thus, occlusion of any of the branches results in infarction of the renal parenchyma supplied by it.

iv)   Since the tubular capillary beds are derived from the efferent arterioles leaving the glomeruli, diseases affecting the blood flow through glomerular tuft have significant effects on the tubules as well.

2. Glomerulus. The glomerulus consists of invagination of the blind end of the proximal tubule and contains a *capillary tuft* fed by the afferent arteriole and drained by efferent arteriole. The capillary tuft is covered by visceral epithelial cells (podocytes) which are continuous with those of the parietal epithelium at the *vascular pole.* The transition to proximal tubular cells occurs at the *urinary pole* of the glomerulus. The visceral and parietal epithelial cells are separated by the urinary space or *Bowman's space,* into which glomerular filtrate passes.

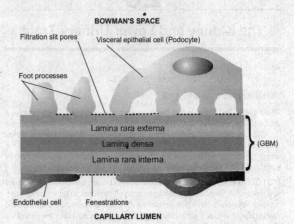

BOWMAN'S SPACE

Filtration slit pores   Visceral epithelial cell (Podocyte)

Foot processes

Lamina rara externa
Lamina densa   (GBM)
Lamina rara interna

Endothelial cell   Fenestrations

CAPILLARY LUMEN

Fig. 20.1: Ultrastructure of glomerular filtration barrier.

Subdivisions of capillaries derived from the afferent arterioles result in the formation of *lobules* of which there are not more than eight within a glomerulus. Each lobule of a glomerular tuft consists of a centrilobular supporting stalk composed of mesangium containing *mesangial cells* and *mesangial matrix*.

The major *function* of glomerulus is complex filtration from the capillaries to the urinary space. The barrier to glomerular filtration consists of the following 3 components (Fig. 20.1):
i)   Fenestrated endothelial cells lining the capillary loops.
ii) Glomerular basement membrane (GBM) on which the endothelial cells rest and consists of 3 layers—the central lamina densa, bounded by lamina rara interna and lamina rara externa.
iii) Filtration slit pores between the foot processes of the visceral epithelial cells (podocytes) external to GBM.

The barrier to filtration of macromolecules of the size and molecular weight of albumin and larger depends upon the following:
■ A normal lamina densa.
■ Maintenance of negative charge on both lamina rarae.
■ A healthy covering of glomerular epithelial cells.

Juxtaglomerular apparatus. The juxtaglomerular apparatus (JGA) is situated at the vascular pole of the glomerulus and is made up of 3 parts: (i) The *juxtaglomerular cells* (ii) The *macula densa* (iii) The *lacis cells* or *non-granular cells*.

The JGA is intimately concerned with sodium metabolism and is the principal source of renin production.

3. Tubules. The tubules of the kidney account for the greatest amount of the renal parenchyma. The structure of renal tubular epithelium varies in different parts of the nephron and is correlated with the functional capacity of that part of the tubule.
i)   *Proximal convoluted tubule (PCT).* This is the first part arising from the glomerulus and is highly specialised part functionally.
ii) *Loop of Henle.* The PCT drains into the straight part of loop of Henle that consists of thin, descending and ascending limbs and the actual loop, all of which are found in the medulla.

iii) Distal convoluted tubule (DCT). The DCT represents a transition from thick ascending limb from the point where the ascending limb meets the vascular pole of the glomerulus of its origin, to the early collecting ducts.

iv) Collecting ducts. The system of collecting ducts is the final pathway by which urine reaches the tip of renal papilla.

4. Interstitium. In health, the renal cortical interstitium is scanty and consists of a small number of fibroblast-like cells. But the medullary interstitium is more plentiful and contains stellate interstitial cells which are considered to produce an anti-hypertensive agent and are involved in the metabolism of prostaglandins.

Renal function tests are broadly divided into 4 groups (Table 20.1):
1. Urine analysis. 2. Concentration and dilution tests. 3. Blood chemistry. 4. Renal clearance tests.

TABLE 20.1: Renal Function Tests.

1. **Urine analysis:**
   i) Physical examination (output, colour, specific gravity, pH, osmolality)
   ii) Chemical constituents (protein, glucose, red cells, haemoglobin)
   iii) Bacteriologic examination
   iv) Microscopy

2. **Concentration and dilution tests:**
   i) Concentration test (fluid deprivation test)
   ii) Dilution test (excess fluid intake test)

3. **Blood chemistry:**
   i) Urea
   ii) Blood urea nitrogen (BUN)
   iii) Creatinine

4. **Renal clearance test:**
   i) Inulin or mannitol clearance test
   ii) Creatinine clearance
   iii) Urea clearance
   iv) Para-aminohippuric acid (PAH) clearance

In addition, renal biopsy is performed to confirm the diagnosis of renal disease. Renal biopsy is ideally fixed in alcoholic Bouin's solution and examined morphologically supported by special stains and further studies as under:
1. *Periodic acid-Schiff* stain for highlighting glomerular basement membrane.
2. *Silver impregnation* to outline the glomerular and tubular basement membrane.
3. *Immunofluorescence* to localise the antigens, complements and immunoglobulins.
4. *Electron microscopy* to see the ultrastructure of glomerular changes.

PATHOPHYSIOLOGY OF RENAL DISEASE (RENAL FAILURE) *(p. 675)*

Traditionally, diseases of the kidneys are divided into 4 major groups according to the predominant involvement of corresponding morphologic components:

1. Glomerular diseases 2. Tubular diseases 3. Interstitial diseases 4. Vascular diseases.

In addition, other diseases described in this chapter include: congenital anomalies, obstructive uropathy (including urolithiasis) and tumours of the kidneys.

The major morphologic involvements of the kidneys in the initial stage is confined to one component (glomeruli, tubules, interstitium or blood vessels), but eventually all components are affected leading to *end-stage kidneys*.

Acute Renal Failure (ARF) *(p. 676)*

Acute renal failure (ARF) is a syndrome characterised by rapid onset of renal dysfunction, chiefly oliguria or anuria, and sudden increase in metabolic waste-products (urea and creatinine) in the blood with consequent development of uraemia.

ETIOPATHOGENESIS. The causes of ARF may be classified as pre-renal, intra-renal and post-renal in nature.

1. Pre-renal causes. Pre-renal diseases are those which cause sudden decrease in blood flow to the nephron. These causes include inadequate cardiac output and hypovolaemia or vascular disease causing reduced perfusion of the kidneys.

2. Intra-renal causes. Intra-renal disease is characterised by disease of renal tissue itself. These include vascular disease of the arteries and arterioles within the kidney, diseases of glomeruli, acute tubular necrosis due to ischaemia, or the effect of a nephrotoxin, acute tubulointerstitial nephritis and pyelonephritis.

3. Post-renal causes. Post-renal disease is characteristically caused by obstruction to the flow of urine anywhere along the renal tract distal to the opening of the collecting ducts. This may be caused by a mass within the lumen or from wall of the tract, or from external compression anywhere along the tract—ureter, bladder neck or urethra.

CLINICAL FEATURES. One of the following three major patterns usually emerge:

1. Syndrome of acute nephritis. This is most frequently associated with acute post-streptococcal glomerulonephritis and rapidly progressive glomerulonephritis. The characteristic features are: mild proteinuria, haematuria, oedema and mild hypertension.

2. Syndrome accompanying tubular pathology. When the ARF is caused by destruction of the tubular cells of the nephron as occurs in acute tubular necrosis the disease typically progresses through 3 characteristic stages from oliguria to diuresis to recovery.

i) *Oliguric phase:* The initial oliguric phase lasting on an average from 7 to 10 days is characterised by urinary output of less than 400 ml per day.

ii) *Diuretic phase:* With the onset of healing of tubules, there is improvement in urinary output.

iii) *Phase of recovery:* Full recovery with healing of tubular epithelial cells occurs in about half the cases, while others terminate in death.

3. Pre-renal syndrome. The ARF occurring secondary to disorders in which neither the glomerulus nor the tubules are damaged, results in pre-renal syndrome.

Chronic Renal Failure (CRF) *(p. 677)*

Chronic renal failure is a syndrome characterised by progressive and irreversible deterioration of renal function due to slow destruction of renal parenchyma, eventually terminating in death when sufficient number of nephrons have been damaged.

ETIOPATHOGENESIS. All chronic nephropathies can lead to CRF. The diseases leading to CRF can generally be classified into two major groups: *those causing glomerular pathology,* and *those causing tubulointerstitial pathology.*

1. Diseases causing glomerular pathology. A number of glomerular diseases associated with CRF have their pathogenesis in immune mechanisms.

i) *Primary glomerular pathology:* The major cause of CRF is chronic glomerulonephritis, usually initiated by various types of *glomerulonephritis* such as membranous glomerulonephritis, membranoproliferative glomerulonephritis, lipoid nephrosis (minimal change disease) and anti-glomerular basement membrane nephritis.

ii) *Systemic glomerular pathology:* Certain conditions originate outside the renal system but induce changes in the nephrons secondarily. Major examples of this type are systemic lupus erythematosus, serum sickness nephritis and diabetic nephropathy.

2. Diseases causing tubulointerstitial pathology. Damage to tubulo-interstitial tissues results in alterations in reabsorption and secretion of important constituents leading to excretion of large volumes of dilute urine. Tubulointer-stitial diseases can be categorised according to initiating etiology into 4 groups: vascular, infectious, toxic and obstructive.

i) *Vascular causes:* Long-standing primary or essential hypertension produces characteristic changes in renal arteries and arterioles referred to as nephrosclerosis.

ii) *Infectious causes:* A good example of chronic renal infection causing CRF is chronic pyelonephritis.

iii) *Toxic causes:* Some toxic substances induce slow tubular injury, eventually culminating in CRF. The most common example is intake of high doses of analgesics such as phenacetin, aspirin and acetaminophen (chronic analgesic nephritis).

iv) *Obstructive causes:* Chronic obstruction in the urinary tract leads to progressive damage to the nephron due to fluid back-pressure. The examples of this type of chronic injury are stones, blood clots, tumours, strictures and enlarged prostate.

CLINICAL FEATURES. Clinical manifestations of full-blown CRF culminating in uraemic syndrome are thus described under 2 main headings: primary (renal) uraemic manifestations and secondary (systemic or extra-renal) uraemic manifestations.

A. Primary uraemic (renal) manifestations. Primary symptoms of uraemia develop when there is slow and progressive deterioration of renal function. The resulting imbalances cause the following manifestations:

1. Metabolic acidosis. As a result of renal dysfunction, acid-base balance is progressively lost. Excess of hydrogen ions occurs, while bicarbonate level declines in the blood, resulting in metabolic acidosis.

2. Hyperkalaemia. A decreased GFR results in excessive accumulation of potassium in the blood since potassium is normally excreted mainly in the urine. Hyperkalaemia is further worsened by metabolic acidosis.

3. Sodium and water imbalance. As GFR declines, sodium and water cannot pass sufficiently into Bowman's capsule leading to their retention. The main symptoms referable to sodium and water retention are: hypervolaemia and circulatory overload with congestive heart failure.

4. Hyperuricaemia. Decreased GFR results in excessive accumulation of uric acid in the blood.

5. Azotaemia. The waste-products of protein metabolism fail to be excreted resulting in elevation in the blood levels of urea, creatinine, phenols and guanidines causing biochemical abnormality, azotaemia.

B. Secondary uraemic (extra-renal) manifestations. A number of extra-renal systemic manifestations develop secondarily following fluid-electrolyte and acid-base imbalances.

1. Anaemia. Decreased production of erythropoietin by diseased kidney results in decline in erythropoiesis and anaemia.

2. **Integumentary system.** Deposit of urinary pigment such as urochrome in the skin causes sallow-yellow colour.

3. **Cardiovascular system.** Fluid retention secondarily causes cardiovascular symptoms such as increased workload on the heart due to the hypervolaemia.

4. **Respiratory system.** Hypervolaemia and heart failure cause pulmonary congestion and pulmonary oedema due to back pressure.

5. **Digestive system.** Azotaemia directly induces mucosal ulcerations in the lining of the stomach and intestines.

6. **Skeletal system.** The skeletal manifestations of renal failure are referred to as *renal osteodystrophy*. Two major types of skeletal disorders may occur:
i) *Osteomalacia* occurs from deficiency of a form of vitamin D which is normally activated by the kidney.
ii) *Osteitis fibrosa* occurs due to elevated levels of parathormone. How parathormone excess develops in CRF is complex.

CYSTIC DISEASES OF KIDNEY *(p. 679)*

Cystic lesions of the kidney may be *congenital or acquired, non-neoplastic or neoplastic*. Majority of these lesions are congenital non-neoplastic. Cystic lesions in the kidney may occur at any age, extending from foetal (detected on ultrasonography) to old age. Their clinical presentation may include: abdominal mass, infection, respiratory distress (due to accompanied pulmonary hypoplasia), haemorrhage, and neoplastic transformation.

A simple classification including all cystic lesions of the kidney is given in Table 20.2.

TABLE 20.2: Classification of Cystic Lesions of the Kidney.

A. NON-NEOPLASTIC CYSTIC LESIONS

   I. Renal cystic dysplasia (Potter type II)

   II. Polycystic kidney disease (PKD)
      1. Adult (autosomal dominant) polycystic kidney disease (ADPKD) (Potter type III)
      2. Infantile (autosomal recessive) polycystic kidney disease (ARPKD) (Potter type I)

   III. Glomerulocystic kidney disease

   IV. Medullary cystic disease
      1. Medullary sponge kidney (MSK)
      2. Nephronophthiasis-medullary cystic disease complex

   V. Simple renal cysts

   VI. Acquired renal cysts

   VII. Para-renal cysts

B. NEOPLASTIC CYSTIC LESIONS

   I. Cystic nephroma

   II. Cystic partially-differentiated nephroblastoma (CPDN)

   III. Multifocal cystic change in Wilms' tumour

I. Renal Cystic Dysplasia *(p. 679)*

The term 'renal cystic dysplasia' or Potter type II is used for defective renal differentiation with persistence of structures in the kidney not represented in normal nephrogenesis such as presence of undifferentiated mesenchyme containing smooth muscle or cartilage and immature collecting ducts. Renal dysplasia is thus diagnosed on the basis of histologic features. The condition is fairly common in the newborn and infants.
G/A The dysplastic kidney is almost always cystic. The kidney is replaced by disorderly mass of multiple cysts that is not reniform but resembles a bunch of

grapes. No normal renal parenchyma is recognisable. The ureter is invariably abnormal, being either absent or atretic.

M/E The characteristic feature is the presence of undifferentiated mesenchyme that contains smooth muscle or cartilage. The cysts are dilated tubules lined by flattened epithelium surrounded by concentric layers of connective tissue. Glomeruli are scanty or absent.

CLINICAL FEATURES. Often, renal dysplasia is associated with other congenital malformations and syndromes such as ventricular septal defect, tracheo-esophageal fistula, lumbosacral meningomyelocele and Down's syndrome.

II. Polycystic Kidney Disease *(p. 680)*

Polycystic disease of the kidney (PKD) is a disorder in which major portion of the renal parenchyma is converted into cysts of varying size. The disease occurs in two forms:

A. An *adult type* inherited as an *autosomal dominant* disease; and

B. An *infantile type* inherited as an *autosomal recessive* disorder.

A. ADULT POLYCYSTIC KIDNEY DISEASE *(p. 680)*

Adult (autosomal dominant) polycystic kidney disease (ADPKD) is relatively common and is the cause of end-stage renal failure in approximately 10% of haemodialysis patients. The pattern of inheritance is *autosomal dominant* having high penetrance with variable expressivity. Family history of renal disease may be present. The condition occurs due to mutation in chromosome 16. The true adult polycystic renal disease is always bilateral and diffuse. Though the kidneys are abnormal at birth, renal function is retained, and symptoms appear in adult life, mostly between the age of 30 and 50 years.

G/A Kidneys in ADPKD are always bilaterally enlarged, usually symmetrically, heavy (weighing up to 4 kg) and cystic. The cut surface shows cysts throughout the renal parenchyma varying in size from tiny cysts to 4-5 cm in diameter. The renal pelvis and calyces are present but are greatly distorted by the cysts. The cysts, however, do not communicate with the pelvis of the kidney—a feature that helps to distinguish polycystic kidney from hydronephrotic kidney on sectioned surface.

M/E The cysts arise from all parts of nephron. It is possible to find some cysts containing recognisable glomerular tufts reflecting their origin from Bowman's capsule, while others have epithelial lining like that of distal or proximal tubules or collecting ducts. The intervening tissue between the cysts shows some normal renal parenchyma.

CLINICAL FEATURES. The condition may become clinically apparent at any age but most commonly manifests in 3rd to 5th decades of life. The most frequent and earliest presenting feature is a dull-ache in the lumbar regions. In others, the presenting complaints are haematuria or passage of blood clots in urine, renal colic, hypertension, urinary tract infections and progressive CRF with polyuria and proteinuria.

B. INFANTILE POLYCYSTIC KIDNEY DISEASE *(p. 680)*

The infantile (autosomal recessive) form of polycystic kidney disease (ARPKD) is distinct from the adult form. Infantile polycystic kidney disease is rare. It is transmitted as an *autosomal recessive* trait and the family history of similar disease is usually not present. The condition occurs due to a mutation in chromosome 6. It is invariably bilateral. The age at presentation may be perinatal, neonatal, infantile or juvenile, but frequently serious manifestations are present at birth and result in death from renal failure in early childhood.

G/A The kidneys are bilaterally enlarged with smooth external surface and retained normal shape. Cut surface reveals small, fusiform or cylindrical cysts formed from dilatation of collecting tubules which extend radially to the outer cortex. This gives the sectioned surface of the kidney *sponge-like appearance*. No normal renal parenchyma is grossly recognised. Pelvis, calyces and ureters are normal.

M/E The total number of nephrons is normal but all the collecting tubules show cylindrical or saccular dilatations and are lined by cuboidal to low columnar epithelium. Many of the glomeruli are also cystically dilated.

CLINICAL FEATURES. The clinical manifestations depend on age of the child. In severe form, the gross bilateral cystic renal enlargement may interfere with delivery. In infancy, renal failure may manifest early. Almost all the cases of infantile polycystic kidney disease have associated multiple epithelium-lined cysts in the liver or proliferation of portal bile ductules.

III. Glomerulocystic Kidney Disease *(p. 681)*

Many cystic diseases of kidney may have both glomerular as well as tubular cysts e.g. in renal cystic dysplasia, ADPKD. In glomerulocystic kidney disease, exclusive glomerular cysts appear due to dilatation of Bowman's space.

IV. Medullary Cystic Disease *(p. 681)*

Cystic disease of the renal medulla has two main types:

A. MEDULLARY SPONGE KIDNEY *(p. 682)*

Medullary sponge kidney consists of multiple cystic dilatations of the papillary ducts in the medulla. The condition occurs in adults and may be recognised as an incidental radiographic finding in asymptomatic cases, or the patients may complain of colicky flank pain, dysuria, haematuria and passage of sandy material in the urine.

G/A The kidneys may be enlarged, normal or shrunken in size depending upon the extent of secondary pyelonephritis. On cut surface, the characteristic feature is the presence of several, small (less than 0.5 cm diameter), cystically dilated papillary ducts, which may contain spherical calculi.

M/E The cysts are lined by tall columnar, cuboidal, transitional or squamous epithelium. Renal cortex may show secondary pyelonephritis but cortical cysts are never a component of medullary sponge kidney.

B. NEPHRONOPHTHIASIS-MEDULLARY CYSTIC DISEASE COMPLEX *(p. 682)*

This form of medullary cystic disease, also called *juvenile nephronophthiasis or uraemic sponge kidney,* is a progressive renal disease that makes its appearance in childhood. Familial occurrence is common and both patterns of inheritance occur, recessive transmission being more common than dominant transmission.

G/A The kidneys are moderately reduced in size and granular and have narrow cortices. Cut surface reveals minute cysts, majority of which are present at the cortico-medullary junction.

M/E The cysts are lined by flattened or cuboidal epithelium. There is widespread nonspecific chronic inflammatory infiltrate and interstitial fibrosis. Many glomeruli are hyalinised but tubular atrophy is more pronounced due to marked thickening of tubular basement membrane.

V. Simple Renal Cysts *(p. 682)*

Simple renal cysts are a very common postmortem finding. They are seen in about half of all persons above the age of 50 years. Since these cysts are rare in infants and children, they appear to be acquired rather than congenital lesions.

G/A Simple renal cysts are usually solitary but may be multiple. They are commonly located in the cortex. Their size varies from a few millimeters to 10 cm in diameter.

M/E The lining of the cyst is by flattened epithelium.

GLOMERULAR DISEASES (p. 683)

Glomerular diseases encompass a large and clinically significant group of renal diseases. Glomerulonephritis (GN) or Bright's disease is the term used for diseases that primarily involve the renal glomeruli. It is convenient to classify glomerular diseases into 2 broad groups:

I.   *Primary glomerulonephritis* in which the glomeruli are the predominant site of involvement.

II.   *Secondary glomerular diseases* include certain systemic and hereditary diseases which secondarily affect the glomeruli.

Though this division is widely followed, it is somewhat arbitrary since many primary forms of glomerulonephritis have systemic effects, and many systemic diseases may initially present with glomerular involvement. Most widely accepted classification is based on clinical presentation and pathologic changes in the glomeruli given in Table 20.3.

TABLE 20.3: Clinicopathologic Classification of Glomerular Diseases.

I.	**Primary Glomerulonephritis**
1.	Acute GN
	i) Post-streptococcal
	ii) Non-streptococcal
2.	Rapidly progressive GN
3.	Minimal change disease
4.	Membranous GN
5.	Membrano-proliferative GN
6.	Focal proliferative GN
7.	Focal segmental glomerulosclerosis (FSGS)
8.	IgA nephropathy
9.	Chronic glomerulonephritis
II.	**Secondary Systemic Glomerular Diseases**
1.	Lupus nephritis (SLE)
2.	Diabetic nephropathy
3.	Amyloidosis
4.	Polyarteritis nodosa
5.	Wegener's granulomatosis
6.	Goodpasture's syndrome
7.	Henoch-Schönlein purpura
8.	Systemic infectious diseases (*bacterial* e.g. bacterial endocarditis, syphilis, leprosy; *viral* e.g. HBV, HCV, HIV; *parasitic* e.g. falciparum malaria, filariasis)
9.	Idiopathic mixed cryoglobulinaemia
III.	**Hereditary Nephritis**
1.	Alport's syndrome
2.	Fabry's disease
3.	Nail-patella syndrome

CLINICAL MANIFESTATIONS (p. 683)

The clinical presentation of glomerular disease is quite variable but in general four features—proteinuria, haematuria, hypertension and disturbed excretory function, are present in varying combinations depending upon the underlying condition. A firm diagnosis, however, can be established by examination of renal biopsy under light, electron and immunofluorescence microscopy.

A number of clinical syndromes are recognised in glomerular diseases.

I.   ACUTE NEPHRITIC SYNDROME. This is the acute onset of haematuria, proteinuria, hypertension, oedema and oliguria following an infective illness about 10 to 20 days earlier.

1.   The **haematuria** is generally slight giving the urine smoky appearance and erythrocytes are detectable by microscopy or by chemical testing for haemoglobin.

2.   The **proteinuria** is mild (less than 3 gm per 24 hrs) and is usually non-selective *(nephritic range proteinuria).*

3.   **Hypertension** is variable depending upon the severity of the glomerular disease but is generally mild.

4.   **Oedema** in nephritic syndrome is usually mild and results from sodium and water retention.

5.   **Oliguria** is variable and reflects the severity of glomerular involvement.

The underlying causes of acute nephritic syndrome may be primary glomerulonephritic diseases (classically acute glomerulonephritis and rapidly progressive glomerulonephritis) or certain systemic diseases (Table 20.4).

TABLE 20.4: Causes of Acute Nephritic Syndrome.

I.	**Primary Glomerulonephritis**
1.	Acute GN
	i) Post-streptococcal
	ii) Non-streptococcal
2.	Rapidly progressive GN
3.	Membranoproliferative GN
4.	Focal GN
5.	IgA nephropathy
II.	**Systemic Diseases**
1.	SLE
2.	Polyarteritis nodosa
3.	Wegener's granulomatosis
4.	Henoch-Schonlein purpura
5.	Cryoglobulinaemia

II.   NEPHROTIC SYNDROME Nephrotic syndrome is a group of diseases having different pathogenesis and characterised by clinical findings of massive proteinuria, hypoalbuminaemia, oedema, hyperlipidaemia, lipiduria, and hypercoagulability.

1.   **Heavy proteinuria** (protein loss of more than 3 gm per 24 hrs) is the chief characteristic of nephrotic syndrome *(nephrotic range proteinuria).* In children, protein loss is correspondingly less. Another feature of protein loss is its 'selectivity'. A *highly-selective proteinuria* consists mostly of loss of low molecular weight proteins, while a *poorly-selective proteinuria* is loss of high molecular weight proteins in the urine. In nephrotic syndrome, proteinuria mostly consists of loss of albumin in the urine.

2.   **Hypoalbuminaemia** is produced primarily consequent to urinary loss of albumin, and partly due to increased renal catabolism and inadequate hepatic synthesis of albumin. Often, the plasma albumin level is 1 to 3 gm/dl (normal 3.5 to 5.5 gm/dl) and there is reversed albumin-globulin ratio.

3.   **Oedema** in nephrotic syndrome appears due to fall in colloid osmotic pressure consequent upon hypoalbuminaemia. Sodium and water retention further contribute to oedema.

4. Hyperlipidaemia is a frequent accompaniment of nephrotic syndrome. It is hypothesised that the liver faced with the stress of massive protein synthesis in response to heavy urinary protein loss, also causes increased synthesis of lipoproteins.

5. Lipiduria occurs following hyperlipidaemia due to excessive leakiness of glomerular filtration barrier.

6. Hypercoagulability. Patients with nephrotic syndrome may develop spontaneous arterial or venous thrombosis, renal vein thrombosis and pulmonary embolism as a result of various factors.

The causes of nephrotic syndrome are diverse and are listed in Table 20.5. But it must be mentioned here that:

■ in *children,* primary glomerulonephritis is the cause in majority of cases of the nephrotic syndrome, most frequently *lipoid nephrosis (65%); and*

■ in *adults,* on the other hand, systemic diseases (diabetes, amyloidosis and SLE) are more frequent causes of nephrotic syndrome. The most common primary glomerular disease in adults is *membranous glomerulonephritis* (40%).

TABLE 20.5: Causes of Nephrotic Syndrome.

I.	**Primary Glomerulonephritis**
1.	Minimal change disease *(most common in children)*
2.	Membranous GN *(most common in adults)*
3.	Membranoproliferative GN
4.	Focal segmental glomerulosclerosis
5.	Focal GN
6.	IgA nephropathy
II.	**Systemic Diseases**
1.	Diabetes mellitus
2.	Amyloidosis
3.	SLE
III.	**Systemic Infections**
1.	Viral infections (HBV, HCV, HIV)
2.	Bacterial infections (bacterial endocarditis, syphilis, leprosy)
3.	Protozoa and parasites (*P. falciparum* malaria, filariasis)
IV.	**Hypersensitivity Reactions**
1.	Drugs (heavy metal compounds like gold and mercury, other drugs like penicillamine, trimethadione and tolbutamide, heroin addiction)
2.	Bee stings, snake bite, poison ivy
V.	**Malignancy**
1.	Carcinomas
2.	Myeloma
3.	Hodgkin's disease
VI.	**Pregnancy**
	Toxaemia of pregnancy
VII.	**Circulatory Disturbances**
1.	Renal vein thrombosis
2.	Constrictive pericarditis
VIII.	**Hereditary Diseases**
1.	Alport's disease
2.	Fabry's disease
3.	Nail-patella syndrome

III. ACUTE RENAL FAILURE. As already described above, acute renal failure (ARF) is characterised by rapid decline in renal function. ARF has many causes including glomerular disease, principally rapidly progressive GN and acute diffuse proliferative GN.

IV. CHRONIC RENAL FAILURE. Glomerular causes of chronic renal failure (CRF) have already been described above. These cases have advanced renal impairment progressing over years and is detected by significant proteinuria, haematuria, hypertension and azotaemia.

V. ASYMPTOMATIC PROTEINURIA. Presence of proteinuria unexpectedly in a patient may be unrelated to renal disease (e.g. exercise-induced, extreme lordosis and orthostatic proteinuria), or may indicate an underlying mild glomerulonephritis.

VI. ASYMPTOMATIC HAEMATURIA. Glomerular haematuria is indicated by the presence of red blood cells, red cell casts and haemoglobin in the urine. Glomerular haematuria is frequently associated with asymptomatic proteinuria.

PATHOGENESIS OF GLOMERULAR INJURY (p. 685)

Most forms of primary GN and many of the secondary glomerular diseases in human beings have immunologic pathogenesis.

The consequences of injury at different sites within the glomerulus in various glomerular diseases can be assessed when compared with the normal physiologic role of the main cells involved i.e. *endothelial, mesangial, visceral epithelial,* and *parietal epithelial cells* as well as of the *GBM* (Table 20.6).

TABLE 20.6: Relationship of Physiologic Role of Glomerular Components with Consequences in Glomerular Injury.

COMPONENT	PHYSIOLOGIC FUNCTION	CONSEQUENCE OF INJURY	RELATED GLOME-RULAR DISEASE
1. Endothelial cells	i) Maintain glome-rular perfusion	Vasoconstriction	Acute renal failure
	ii) Prevent leucocyte adhesion	Leucocyte infiltration	Focal/diffuse proliferative GN
	iii) Prevent platelet aggregation	Intravascular microthrombi	Thrombotic microangiopathies
2. Mesangial cells	Control glomerular filtration	Proliferation and increased matrix	Membrano-proliferative GN
3. Visceral epithelial cells	Prevent plasma protein filtration	Proteinuria	Minimal change disease, FSGS
4. GBM	Prevents plasma protein filtration	Proteinuria	Membranous GN
5. Parietal epithelial cells	Maintain Bowman's space	Crescent formation	RPGN.

Immunologic mechanisms underlying glomerular injury are primarily *antibody-mediated* (immune-complex disease). There is evidence to suggest that *cell-mediated immune reactions* in the form of delayed type hypersensitivity can also cause glomerular injury. In addition, a few secondary mechanisms and some non-immunologic mechanisms are involved (Table 20.7).

I. IMMUNOLOGIC MECHANISMS (p. 685)

A. Antibody-Mediated Glomerular Injury (p. 685)

1. IMMUNE COMPLEX DISEASE. Majority of cases of glomerular disease result from deposits of immune complexes (antigen-antibody complexes). The immune complexes are represented by *irregular or granular glomerular deposits*

TABLE 20.7: Pathogenetic Mechanisms in Glomerular Diseases.

MECHANISM	RELATED GLOMERULAR DISEASE
I. IMMUNOLOGIC MECHANISMS	
A. *Antibody-mediated glomerular injury*	
1. Immune-complex disease	Immune-complex mediated GN (Acute diffuse proliferative GN, membranous GN, membrano-proliferative GN, IgA nephropathy; secondary glomerular disease in SLE, malaria etc.)
2. Anti-glomerular basement membrane (Anti-GBM) disease	Goodpasture's disease
3. Alternate pathway disease	Membranoproliferative GN type II
4. Other mechanisms (anti-neutrophil cytoplasmic antibodies ANCA, anti-endothelial cell antibodies AECA)	Focal segmental GS
B. *Cell-mediated glomerular injury*	Pauci-immune GN (type III RPGN)
C. *Secondary pathogenetic mechanisms*	Mediate glomerular injury in various primary and secondary glomerular diseases
II. NON-IMMUNOLOGIC MECHANISMS	
1. Metabolic	Diabetic nephropathy, Fabry's disease
2. Haemodynamic	Hypertensive nephrosclerosis, FSGS
3. Deposition	Amyloid nephropathy
4. Infectious	HIV-nephropathy, immune-complex GN in SABE
5. Drugs	NSAIDs-associated minimal change disease
6. Inherited	Alport's syndrome, nail-patella syndrome

of immunoglobulins (IgG, IgM and IgA) and complement (mainly C3). Based on the experimental models and studies in human beings, the following 3 patterns of glomerular deposits of immune complexes in various glomerular diseases have been observed:

i) *Exclusive mesangial deposits* are characterised by very mild form of glomerular disease.

ii) *Extensive subendothelial deposits* along the GBM are accompanied by severe hypercellular sclerosing glomerular lesions.

iii) *Subepithelial deposits* are seen between the outer surface of the GBM and the podocytes.

Deposits may be located at one or more of the above sites in any case of glomerular injury.

It was widely believed earlier that glomerular deposits result from circulating immune complexes. Now, it has been shown that glomerular deposits are formed by one of the following two mechanisms:

i) Local immune complex deposits.

ii) Circulating immune complex deposits.

Immune complex GN is observed in the following human diseases:

i) *Primary GN* e.g. acute diffuse proliferative GN, membranous GN, membranoproliferative GN, IgA nephropathy and some cases of rapidly progressive GN and focal GN.

ii) *Systemic diseases* e.g. glomerular disease in SLE, malaria, syphilis, hepatitis, Henoch-Schonlein purpura and idiopathic mixed cryoglobulinaemia.

2.   ANTI-GBM DISEASE. Less than 5% cases of human GN are associated with anti-GBM antibodies. The constituent of GBM acting as antigen appears to be a component of collagen IV of the basement membrane.

Anti-GBM disease is classically characterised by *interrupted linear deposits* of anti-GBM antibodies (mostly IgG; rarely IgA and IgM) and complement (mainly C3) along the glomerular basement membrane. These deposits are detected by immunofluorescence microscopy or by electron microscopy.

Anti-GBM disease is characteristically exemplified by glomerular injury in Goodpasture's syndrome in some cases of rapidly progressive GN.

3. ALTERNATE PATHWAY DISEASE. Deposits of C3 are associated with the early components C1, C2 and C4 which are evidence of classic pathway activation of complement. But in alternate pathway activation, there is decreased serum C3 level, decreased serum levels of factor B and properdin, normal serum levels of C1, C2 and C4 but C3 and properdin are found deposited in the glomeruli without immunoglobulin deposits, reflecting activation of alternate pathway of complement.

The deposits in alternate pathway disease are characteristically electron-dense under electron microscopy, glomerular lesions in such cases are referred to as *dense-deposit disease.*

Alternate pathway disease occurs in most cases of type II membrano-proliferative GN, some patients of rapidly progressive GN, acute diffuse proliferative GN, IgA nephropathy and in SLE.

4. OTHER MECHANISMS OF ANTIBODY-MEDIATED INJURY. A few autoantibodies have been implicated in some patients of focal segmental glomerulosclerosis and few other types of GN. These antibodies include:

i) **Anti-neutrophil cytoplasmic antibodies (ANCA).** About 40% cases of rapidly progressive GN are deficient in immunoglobulins in glomeruli and are positive for ANCA against neutrophil cytoplasmic antigens in their circulation.

ii) **Anti-endothelial cell antibodies (AECA).** Autoantibodies against endothelial antigens have been detected in circulation in several inflammatory vasculitis and glomerulonephritis.

B. Cell-mediated Glomerular Injury
   (Delayed-type Hypersensitivity) *(p. 688)*

Recent evidence suggests that cell-mediated immune reactions may be involved in causing glomerular injury, particularly in cases with deficient immunoglobulins (e.g. in pauci-immune type glomerulonephritis in RPGN). Cytokines and other mediators released by activated T cells stimulate cytotoxicity, recruitment of more leucocytes and fibrogenesis. CD4+ T lymphocytes recruit more macrophages while CD8+ cytotoxic T lymphocytes and natural killer cells cause further glomerular cell injury.

C. Secondary Pathogenetic Mechanisms
   (Mediators of Immunologic Injury) *(p. 688)*

1. NEUTROPHILS. Neutrophils are conspicuous in certain forms of glomerular disease such as in acute diffuse proliferative GN, and may also be present in membranoproliferative GN and lupus nephritis. Neutrophils can mediate glomerular injury by activation of complement as well as by release of proteases, arachidonic acid metabolites and oxygen-derived free radicals.

2. MONONUCLEAR PHAGOCYTES. Many forms of human and experimental proliferative GN are associated with glomerular infiltration by monocytes and macrophages. Accumulation of mononuclear phagocytes is considered an important constituent of hypercellularity in these forms of GN aside from proliferation of mesangial and endothelial cells.

3. COMPLEMENT SYSTEM. Besides the components of complement which mediate glomerular injury via neutrophils C5b9 is capable of inducing damage to GBM directly.

4. PLATELETS. Platelet aggregation and release of mediators play a role in the evolution of some forms of GN.

5. MESANGIAL CELLS. There is evidence to suggest that mesangial cells present in the glomeruli may be stimulated to produce mediators of inflammation and take part in glomerular injury.

6. COAGULATION SYSTEM. The presence of fibrin in early crescents in certain forms of human and experimental GN suggests the role of coagulation system in glomerular damage.

II. NON-IMMUNOLOGIC MECHANISMS *(p. 688)*

1. *Metabolic glomerular injury* e.g. in diabetic nephropathy (due to hyperglycaemia), Fabry's disease (due to sialdosis).
2. *Haemodynamic glomerular injury* e.g. systemic hypertension, intraglomerular hypertension in FSGS.
3. *Deposition diseases* e.g. amyloidosis.
4. *Infectious diseases* e.g. HBV, HCV, HIV, *E. coli*-derived nephrotoxin.
5. *Drugs* e.g. minimal change disease due to NSAIDs.
6. *Inherited glomerular diseases* e.g. Alport's syndrome, nail-patella syndrome.

SPECIFIC TYPES OF GLOMERULAR DISEASES *(p. 689)*

I. PRIMARY GLOMERULONEPHRITIS *(p. 689)*

Acute Glomerulonephritis *(Synonyms: Acute Diffuse Proliferative GN, Diffuse Endocapillary GN) (p. 689)*

Acute GN is known to follow acute infection and characteristically presents as acute nephritic syndrome. Based on etiologic agent, acute GN is subdivided into 2 main groups: acute post-streptococcal GN and acute non-streptococcal GN, the former being more common.

Acute Post-streptococcal GN *(p. 689)*

Acute post-streptococcal GN is fairly common form of GN, seen most commonly in children 6 to 16 years of age but adolescents and adults may also be affected. The onset of disease is generally sudden after 1-2 weeks of streptococcal infection, most frequently of the throat (e.g. streptococcal pharyngitis) and sometimes of the skin (e.g. streptococcal impetigo).

ETIOPATHOGENESIS. The relationship between streptococcal infection and this form of GN is now well established. Particularly nephritogenic are types 12,4,1 and Red Lake of group A β-haemolytic streptococci. The glomerular lesions appear to result from deposition of immune complexes in the glomeruli.

Streptococcal infection may be identified by *culture* or may be inferred from elevated titres of *antibodies* against streptococcal antigens. These include:

- anti-streptolysin O (ASO);
- anti-deoxyribonuclease B (anti-DNAse B);
- anti-streptokinase (ASKase);
- anti-nicotinyl adenine dinucleotidase (anti-NADase); and
- anti-hyaluronidase (AHase).

iv) There is usually *hypocomplementaemia* indicating involvement of complement in the glomerular deposits.

v) More recently, it has been possible to identify antigenic component of streptococci which is cytoplasmic antigen, *endostreptosin*.

G/A The kidneys are symmetrically enlarged, weighing one and a half to twice the normal weight. The cortical as well as sectioned surface show petechial haemorrhages giving the characteristic appearance of flea-bitten kidney.

M/E Light microscopic findings are:

i) Glomeruli—The glomeruli are affected diffusely. They are enlarged and hypercellular. The diffuse hypercellularity of the tuft is due to proliferation of mesangial, endothelial and occasionally epithelial cells *(acute proliferative lesions)* as well as by infiltration of leucocytes, chiefly polymorphs and sometimes monocytes *(acute exudative lesion)*.

ii) Tubules—Tubular changes are not very striking. There may be swelling and hyaline droplets in tubular cells.

iii) Interstitium—There may be some degree of interstitial oedema and leucocytic infiltration.

iv) Vessels—Changes in arteries and arterioles are seldom present in acute GN.

EM Shows the characteristic electron-dense irregular deposits *('humps')* on the epithelial side of the GBM. These deposits represent the immune complexes.

IF Reveals that the irregular deposits along the GBM consist principally of IgG and complement C3.

CLINICAL FEATURES. Typically, the patient is a young child, presenting with acute nephritic syndrome having sudden and abrupt onset following an episode of sore throat 1-2 weeks prior to the development of symptoms. The features include microscopic or intermittent haematuria, red cell casts, mild non-selective proteinuria (less than 3 gm per 24 hrs), hypertension, periorbital oedema and variably oliguria. In adults, the features are atypical and include sudden hypertension, oedema and azotaemia. Development of hypertension in either case is a poor prognostic sign.

Prognosis varies with the age of the patient. Children almost always (95%) recover completely with reversal of proliferative glomerular changes. Complications arise more often in adults and occasionally in children. These include development of rapidly progressive GN, chronic GN, uraemia and chronic renal failure.

Acute Non-streptococcal GN *(p. 690)*

About one-third cases of acute GN are caused by organisms other than haemolytic streptococci. These include other bacteria (e.g. staphylococci, pneumococci, meningococci, *Salmonella* and *Pseudomonas*), viruses (e.g. hepatitis B virus, mumps, infectious mononucleosis and varicella), parasitic infections (e.g. malaria, toxoplasmosis and schistosomiasis) and syphilis. The appearance of renal biopsy by light microscopy, EM and immunofluorescence microscopy is similar to that seen in acute post-streptococcal GN.

Rapidly Progressive Glomerulonephritis (Synonyms; RPGN, Crescentic GN, Extracapillary GN) *(p. 690)*

RPGN presents with an acute reduction in renal function resulting in acute renal failure in a few weeks or months. It is characterised by formation of 'crescents' *(crescentic GN)* outside the glomerular capillaries *(extracapillary GN)*. 'Crescents' are formed from the proliferation of parietal epithelial cells lining Bowman's capsule with contribution from visceral epithelial cells and the invading mononuclear cells. The stimulus for crescent formation appears to be the presence of fibrin in the capsular space. RPGN occurs most frequently in adults, with a slight male preponderance. Prognosis of RPGN in general is dismal.

ETIOPATHOGENESIS. Based on the etiologic agents and pathogenetic mechanism, patients with RPGN are divided into 3 groups (Table 20.8):

Type I RPGN: Anti-GBM disease. A number of systemic diseases such as Goodpasture's syndrome, SLE, vasculitis, Wegener's granulomatosis, Henoch-

TABLE 20.8: Distinguishing Features of Three Main Categories of Rapidly Progressive Glomerulonephritis.

	FEATURE	TYPE I RPGN (ANTI-GBM DISEASE)	TYPE II RPGN (IMMUNE COMPLEX DISEASE)	TYPE III RPGN (PAUCI-IMMUNE GN)
1.	*Clinical syndrome*	Nephritic	Nephritic	Nephritic
2.	*Pathogenetic type*	Anti-GBM	Immune-complex	Pauci-immune
3.	*Immunofluorescence*	Linear Ig and C3	Granular Ig and C3	Sparse or absent Ig and C3
4.	*Serologic markers*			
	i) *Serum C3 level*	Normal	Low-to-normal	Normal
	ii) *Anti-GBM antibody*	Positive	Negative	Negative
	iii) *ANCA*	Negative	Negative	Positive
5.	*Underlying cause*	Idiopathic	Idiopathic	Idiopathic
		Goodpasture's syndrome, SLE, vasculitis, Wegener's granulomatosis, Henoch-Schonlein purpura	Post-infectious (post-strepto-coccal GN)	Polyarteritis nodosa, Wegener's granulomatosis

Schonlein purpura and idiopathic mixed cryoglobulinaemia are associated with crescentic GN. Goodpasture's syndrome is the characteristic example of anti-GBM disease and is described below:

Goodpasture's syndrome. Goodpasture's syndrome is characterised by acute renal failure due to RPGN and pulmonary haemorrhages. The condition is more common in males in 3rd decade of life. The disease results from damage to the glomeruli by anti-GBM antibodies which cross-react with alveolar basement membrane and hence, produce renal as well as pulmonary lesions. Pulmonary lesions can be experimentally induced if the lungs are previously injured by viral or bacterial infection or exposed to hydrocarbons. The Goodpasture's antigen appears to be a component of collagen type IV.

Type II RPGN: Immune complex disease. A small proportion of cases of post-streptococcal GN, particularly in adults and sometimes of non-streptococcal origin, develop RPGN. The evidences in support of post-infectious RPGN having immune complex pathogenesis are granular deposits of immune complexes of IgG and C3 along the glomerular capillary walls, lowering of blood complement levels and demonstration of circulating complexes.

Type III RPGN: Pauci-immune GN. These include cases of Wegener's granulomatosis and microscopic polyarteritis nodosa. The pathogenesis of pauci-immune GN is yet not fully defined. However, majority of these patients are ANCA-positive, implying a defect in humoral immunity. There is little or no glomerular immune deposit (i.e. pauci-immune).

G/A The kidneys are usually enlarged and pale with smooth outer surface *(large white kidney)*. Cut surface shows pale cortex and congested medulla.

M/E

i) **Glomeruli**—Irrespective of the underlying etiology, all forms of RPGN show pathognomonic *'crescents'* on the inside of Bowman's capsules. These are collections of pale-staining polygonal cells which commonly tend to be elongated. Eventually, crescents obliterate the Bowman's space and compress the glomerular tuft. Fibrin thrombi are frequently present in the glomerular tufts.

ii) Tubules—Tubular epithelial cells may show hyaline droplets.

iii) Interstitium—The interstitium is oedematous and may show early fibrosis.

iv) Vessels—Arteries and arterioles may show no change, but cases associated with hypertension usually show severe vascular changes.

EM Post-infectious RPGN cases show electron-dense subepithelial granular deposits similar to those seen in acute GN, while cases of RPGN in Goodpasture's syndrome show characteristic linear deposits along the GBM.

IF shows:

■ linear pattern of RPGN in Goodpasture's syndrome (type I RPGN), containing IgG accompanied by C3 along the capillaries

■ granular pattern of post-infectious RPGN (type II RPGN) consisting of IgG and C3 along the capillary wall; and

■ scanty or no deposits of immunoglobulin and C3 in pauci-immune GN (type III RPGN).

CLINICAL FEATURES. Generally, the features of post-infectious RPGN are similar to those of acute GN, presenting as acute renal failure. The patients of Goodpasture's syndrome may present as acute renal failure and/or associated intrapulmonary haemorrhage producing recurrent haemoptysis. Prognosis of all forms of RPGN is poor.

Minimal Change Disease *(Synonyms:* MCD, *Lipoid Nephrosis, Foot Process Disease, Nil Deposit Disease) (p. 692)*

Minimal change disease (MCD) is a condition in which the nephrotic syndrome is accompanied by no apparent change in glomeruli by light microscopy. Minimal change disease accounts for 80% cases of nephrotic syndrome in children under 16 years of age with preponderance in boys (ratio of boys to girls 2:1).

ETIOPATHOGENESIS. The etiology of MCD remain elusive. However, following two groups have been identified:

i) Idiopathic (majority of cases).

ii) Cases associated with systemic diseases (Hodgkin's disease, HIV infection) and drug therapy (e.g. NSAIDs, rifampicin, interferon-α).

The following features point to possible immunologic pathogenesis for MCD:

i) Absence of deposits by electron microscopy.

ii) Normal circulating levels of complement but presence of circulating immune complexes in many cases.

iii) Universal satisfactory response to steroid therapy.

iv) Evidence of increased suppressor T cell activity with elaboration of cytokines (interleukin-8, tumour necrosis factor) which probably cause foot process flattening.

v) Recent detection of a mutation in nephrin gene in cases of congenital MCD has focused attention on genetic basis.

The Nephrotic syndrome in MCD *in children* is characterised by *selective proteinuria* containing mainly albumin, and minimal amounts of high molecular weight proteins such as α2-macroglobulin.

Adults having MCD, however, have *non-selective proteinuria,* suggesting more extensive membrane permeability defect.

G/A The kidneys are of normal size and shape.

M/E The features are as under:

i) Glomeruli—The most characteristic feature is no apparent abnormality in the glomeruli.

ii) Tubules—There is presence of fine lipid vacuolation and hyaline droplets in the cells of proximal convoluted tubules and, hence, the older name of the condition as 'lipoid nephrosis'.

iii) Interstitium—There may be oedema of the interstitium.

iv) Vessels—Blood vessels do not show any significant change (minimal change).

EM The most characteristic feature of the disease is identified which is diffuse flattening of foot processes of the visceral epithelial cells (podocytes). Unlike other forms of GN, no deposits are seen and the GBM is normal.

IF No deposits of complement or immunoglobulins are recognised (nil deposit disease).

CLINICAL FEATURES. The classical presentation of MCD is of fully-developed nephrotic syndrome with massive and *highly selective proteinuria,* but hypertension is unusual. Most frequently, the patients are children under 16 years (peak incidence at 6-8 years of age).

The disease characteristically responds to steroid therapy.

Membranous Glomerulonephritis
(Synonym: Epimembranous Nephropathy) (p. 693)

Membranous GN is characterised by wide-spread thickening of the glomerular capillary wall and is the most common cause of nephrotic syndrome in adults. In about 15% of cases, membranous GN is *secondary* to an underlying condition (e.g. SLE, malignancies, infections such as chronic hepatitis B and C, syphilis, malaria and drugs), while in the majority of cases (85%) it is truly *idiopathic*.

ETIOPATHOGENESIS. *Idiopathic membranous GN* is an immune complex disease. The deposits of immune complex are formed locally because circulating immune complexes are detected in less than a quarter of cases. While nephritogenic antigen against which autoantibodies are formed in *idiopathic membranous GN* is not known yet, the antigen in cases of *secondary membranous GN* is either an endogenous (e.g. DNA in SLE) or exogenous one (e.g. hepatitis B virus, tumour antigen, treponema antigen, drug therapy with penicillamine).

G/A The kidneys are enlarged, pale and smooth.

M/E The features are as under:

i) Glomeruli—The characteristic finding is diffuse thickening of the glomerular capillary walls with all the glomeruli being affected more or less uniformly. As the disease progresses, the deposits are incorporated into enormously thickened basement membrane, producing 'duplication' of GBM which is actually formation of a new basement membrane. These basement membrane changes are best appreciated by silver impregnation stains (black colour) or by periodic acid-Schiff stain (pink colour). There is no cellular proliferation in the glomerular tufts.

ii) Tubules—The renal tubules remain normal except in the early stage when lipid vacuolation of the proximal convoluted tubules may be seen.

iii) Interstitium—The interstitium may show fine fibrosis and scanty chronic inflammatory cells.

iv) Vessels—In the early stage, vascular changes are not prominent, while later hypertensive changes of arterioles may occur.

ChapterTwenty

EM Shows electron-dense deposits situated in the epithelial side of the GBM. The basement membrane material protrudes between deposits as *'spikes'*.

IF Reveals granular deposits of immune complexes consisting of IgG associated with complement C3.

CLINICAL FEATURES. The presentation in majority of cases is insidious onset of nephrotic syndrome in an adult. The proteinuria is usually of *non-selective* type. In addition, microscopic haematuria and hypertension may be present at the onset or may develop during the course of the disease. The changes in membranous GN are irreversible in majority of patients.

Membranoproliferative Glomerulonephritis
(Synonyms: MPGN, Mesangiocapillary GN) (p. 695)

Membranoproliferative GN is another important cause of nephrotic syndrome in children and young adults. As the name implies, it is characterised by two histologic features—increase in cellularity of the mesangium associated with increased lobulation of the tuft, and irregular thickening of the capillary wall.

ETIOPATHOGENESIS. Based on ultrastructural, immunofluorescence and pathogenetic mechanisms, three types of MPGN are recognised:

■ **Type I or classic form** is an example of immune complex disease and comprises more than 70% cases. It is characterised by immune deposits in the subendothelial position. Immune-complex MPGN is seen in association with systemic immune-complex diseases (e.g. SLE, mixed cryoglobulinaemia, Sjögren's syndrome), chronic infections (e.g. bacterial endocarditis, HIV, hepatitis B and C) and malignancies (e.g. lymphomas and leukaemias).

■ **Type II or dense deposit disease** is the example of alternate pathway disease and constitutes about 30% cases. The capillary wall thickening is due to the deposition of electron-dense material in the lamina densa of the GBM. Type II MPGN is an autoimmune disease in which patients have IgG autoantibody termed C3 nephritic factor.

■ **Type III** is rare and shows features of type I MPGN and membranous nephropathy in association with systemic diseases or drugs.

G/A The kidneys are usually pale in appearance and firm in consistency.

M/E The features are as under:

i) **Glomeruli**—Glomeruli show highly characteristic changes. They are enlarged with accentuated lobular pattern. The enlargement is due to variable degree of mesangial cellular proliferation and increase in mesangial matrix. The GBM is considerably thickened, which with silver stains shows two basement membranes with a clear zone between them. This is commonly referred to as *'double contour', splitting, or 'tram track'* appearance.

ii) **Tubules**—Tubular cells may show vacuolation and hyaline droplets.

iii) **Interstitium**—There may be scattered chronic inflammatory cells and some finely granular foam cells in the interstitium.

iv) **Vessels**—Vascular changes are prominent in cases in which hypertension develops.

EM & IF The features are as under:

Type I: It shows *electron-dense deposits* in subendothelial location conforming to immune-complex character of the disease. These deposits reveal positive fluorescence for C3 and slightly fainter staining for IgG.

Type II: The hallmark of type II MPGN is the presence of *dense amorphous deposits* within the lamina densa of the GBM and in the mesangium. Immuno-fluorescence studies reveal the universal presence of C3 and properdin in the deposits.

Type III: This rare form has *electron-dense deposits* within the GBM as well as in subendothelial and subepithelial regions of the GBM. Immunofluorescence studies show the presence of C3, IgG and IgM.

CLINICAL FEATURES. The most common age at diagnosis is between 15 and 20 years. Approximately 50% of the patients present with nephrotic syndrome; about 30% have asymptomatic proteinuria; and 20% have nephritic syndrome at presentation. The proteinuria is non-selective. Haematuria and hypertension are frequently present.

Focal Glomerulonephritis
(Synonyms: Focal Segmental GN, Mesangial Proliferative GN) (p. 696)

Focal GN is characterised by pathologic changes in certain number of glomeruli *(focal)*, and often confined to one or two lobules of the affected glomeruli *(segmental)*, while other glomeruli are normal. Focal GN is, thus, a pathologic diagnosis.

ETIOPATHOGENESIS. It may occur under following diverse clinical settings:

■ As an early manifestation of a number of *systemic diseases* such as SLE, Henoch-Schonlein purpura, subacute bacterial endocarditis, Wegener's granulomatosis, and polyarteritis nodosa, Goodpasture's syndrome.

■ As a component of a known *renal disease* such as in IgA nephropathy.

■ As a primary *idiopathic* glomerular disease unrelated to systemic or other renal disease.

The diverse settings under which focal GN is encountered make it unlikely that there are common etiologic agents or pathogenetic mechanisms.

M/E The single most important feature in focal GN is the abnormality seen in certain number of glomeruli and generally confined to one or two lobules of the affected glomeruli i.e. *focal and segmental glomerular involvement*. The pathologic change most frequently consists of focal and segmental cellular proliferation of mesangial cells and endothelial cells but sometimes necrotising changes can be seen.

IF Widespread mesangial deposits of immunoglobulins (mainly IgA with or without IgG), complement (C3) and fibrin are demonstrated in most cases of focal GN.

CLINICAL FEATURES. The clinical features vary according to the condition causing it. Haematuria is one of the most common clinical manifestation. Proteinuria is frequently mild to moderate but hypertension is uncommon.

Focal Segmental Glomerulosclerosis
(Synonyms: Focal Sclerosis, Focal Hyalinosis) (p. 696)

Focal segmental glomerulosclerosis (FSGS) is a condition in which there is sclerosis and hyalinosis of some glomeruli and portions of their tuft (less than 50% in a tissue section), while the other glomeruli are normal by light microscopy i.e. involvement is focal and segmental. The incidence of FSGS has increased over the last decades and is currently responsible for about one-third cases of nephrotic syndrome in the adults.

ETIOPATHOGENESIS. Currently, the condition is divided into 3 groups:

i) Idiopathic type. This group comprises majority of cases. It is found in children and young adults with presentation of nephrotic syndrome. It differs from minimal change disease in having non-selective proteinuria, in being steroid-resistant, and may progress to chronic renal failure.

ii) With superimposed primary glomerular disease. There may be cases of FSGS with superimposed MCD or IgA nephropathy. Those associated with MCD show good response to steroid therapy and progression to chronic renal failure may occur after a long time.

iii) Secondary type. This group consists of focal segmental sclerotic lesions as a secondary manifestation of certain diseases such as HIV, diabetes mellitus, reflux nephropathy, heroin abuse and analgesic nephropathy. Infection with HIV, particularly in blacks, has been found associated with a variant of FSGS which is characterised by *collapsing sclerosis*.

M/E Variable number of glomeruli are affected focally and segmentally, while others are normal. The affected glomeruli show solidification or *sclerosis* of one or more lobules of the tuft. *Hyalinosis* refers to collection of eosinophilic, homogeneous, PAS-positive, hyaline material present on the inner aspect of a sclerotic peripheral capillary loop. Mesangial hypercellularity is present in appreciable number of cases.

HIV-associated nephropathy in FSGS is characterised by focal sclerosis that may be segmental or global, having collapsed capillaries in the tuft. Besides glomerular changes, there is interstitial fibrosis and infiltration by mononuclear leucocytes, and tubular epithelial cell atrophy and degeneration.

EM Diffuse loss of foot processes as seen in minimal change disease is evident but, in addition, there are electron-dense deposits in the region of hyalinosis and sclerosis.

IF The deposits in the lesions are shown to contain IgM and C3.

CLINICAL FEATURES. The condition may affect all ages including children and has male preponderance. The most common presentation is in the form of nephrotic syndrome with heavy proteinuria.

IgA Nephropathy
(Synonyms: Berger's Disease, IgA GN) (p. 697)

IgA nephropathy is another common form of glomerulopathy worldwide and is characterised by aggregates of IgA, deposited principally in the mesangium.

ETIOPATHOGENESIS. The etiology of IgA nephropathy remains unclear:
i) It is idiopathic in most cases.
ii) Seen as part of Henoch-Schonlein purpura.
iii) Association with chronic inflammation in various body systems (e.g. chronic liver disease, inflammatory bowel disease, interstitial pneumonitis, leprosy, dermatitis herpetiformis, uveitis, ankylosing spondylitis, Sjögren's syndrome, monoclonal IgA gammopathy).

M/E The pattern of involvement varies. These include: focal proliferative GN, focal segmental glomerulosclerosis, membranoproliferative GN, and rarely RPGN.

EM Finely granular electron-dense deposits are seen in the mesangium.

IF The diagnosis is firmly established by demonstration of mesangial deposits of IgA, with or without IgG, and usually with C3 and properdin.

CLINICAL FEATURES. The disease is common in children and young adults. The clinical picture is usually characterised by recurrent bouts of haematuria that are often precipitated by mucosal infections. Mild proteinuria is usually present and occasionally nephrotic syndrome may develop.

Chronic Glomerulonephritis
(Synonym: End-Stage Kidney) (p. 698)

Chronic GN is the final stage of a variety of glomerular diseases which result in irreversible impairment of renal function. The conditions which may progress to chronic GN, in descending order of frequency, are as under:
i) Rapidly progressive GN (90%) ii) Membranous GN (50%) iii) Membrano-proliferative GN (50%) iv) Focal segmental glomerulosclerosis (50%) v) IgA nephropathy (40%) vi) Acute post-streptococcal GN (1%)

However, about 20% cases of chronic GN are *idiopathic* without evidence of preceding GN of any type.

G/A The kidneys are usually small and contracted weighing as low as 50 gm each. The capsule is adherent to the cortex. The cortical surface is generally diffusely granular. On cut section, the cortex is narrow and atrophic, while the medulla is unremarkable.

M/E The features are as under:

i) Glomeruli—Glomeruli are reduced in number and most of those present show completely hyalinised tufts, giving the appearance of acellular, eosinophilic masses which are PAS-positive.

ii) Tubules—Many tubules completely disappear and there may be atrophy of tubules close to scarred glomeruli.

iii) Interstitium—There is fine and delicate fibrosis of the interstitial tissue and varying number of chronic inflammatory cells are often seen.

iv) Vessels—Advanced cases which are frequently associated with hypertension show conspicuous arterial and arteriolar sclerosis.

CLINICAL FEATURES. The patients are usually adults. The terminal stage of chronic GN is characterised by hypertension, uraemia and progressive deterioration of renal function.

The salient features of various types of primary glomerulonephritis are summarised in Table 20.9.

II. SECONDARY GLOMERULAR DISEASES *(p. 699)*

Lupus Nephritis *(p. 699)*

Renal manifestations of systemic lupus erythematosus (SLE) are termed lupus nephritis. The incidence of renal involvement in SLE ranges from 40 to 75%. The two cardinal clinical manifestations of lupus nephritis are proteinuria and haematuria. In addition, hypertension and casts of different types such as red cell casts, fatty casts and leucocyte casts in the urinary sediment are found.

Morphology According to the WHO, six patterns of mutually-merging renal lesions are seen in lupus nephritis:

Class I: Minimal lesions. On light microscopy, these cases do not show any abnormality. But examination by electron microscopy and immunofluorescence microscopy shows deposits within the mesangium which consist of IgG and C3.

Class II: Mesangial lupus nephritis. These cases have mild clinical manifestations. By light microscopy, there is increase in the number of mesangial cells and of mesangial matrix. Ultrastructural and immunofluorescence studies reveal granular mesangial deposits of IgG and C3; sometimes IgA and IgM are also present in the deposits.

Class III: Focal segmental lupus nephritis. This is characterised by focal and segmental proliferation of endothelial and mesangial cells, together with infiltration by macrophages and sometimes neutrophils. Subendothelial and subepithelial deposits of IgG, often with IgM or IgA and C3, are seen.

Class IV: Diffuse proliferative lupus nephritis. In this type, all the morphologic manifestations of lupus are present in most advanced form. This is the most severe and the most common form of lupus nephritis. There is diffuse proliferation of endothelial, mesangial, and sometimes epithelial cells, involving most or all glomeruli. Electron microscopy shows large electron-dense deposits in the mesangium and in the subendothelial region which on immunofluorescence are positive for IgG; sometimes also for IgA or IgM, and C3.

ChapterTwenty

ChapterTwenty

TABLE 20.9: Comparative Features of Major Forms of Primary Glomerulonephritis.

TYPE	CLINICAL FEATURES	PATHOGENESIS	PATHOLOGY		
			LM	EM	IFM
1. *Acute GN*	Acute nephrotic syndrome	Immune complex disease (local or circulating)	Diffuse proliferation, leucocytic infiltration	Subepithelial deposits ('humps')	Irregular IgG, C3
2. *RPGN*	Acute renal failure	i) Type I: anti-GBM type ii) Type II: immune complex type iii) Type III: pauci-immune RPGN	Proliferation, crescents	i) Linear deposits along GBM ii) Subepithelial deposits iii) No deposits	i) Linear IgG, C3 ii) Granular IgG, C3 iii) Negative
3. *Minimal change disease*	Nephrotic syndrome (highly selective proteinuria)	Reduction of normal negative charge on GBM ?Cell-mediated mechanism	Normal glomeruli, lipid vacuolation in tubules	Loss of foot processes, no deposits	Negative
4. *Membranous GN*	Nephrotic syndrome	Immune complex disease (local)	Diffuse thickening of capillary wall	Subepithelial deposits ('spikes')	Granular IgG, C3

Contd...

Table 20.9 Contd...

TYPE	CLINICAL FEATURES	PATHOGENESIS	PATHOLOGY			IFM
			LM	EM		
5. **Membrano-proliferative GN**	Nephrotic syndrome	Type I: immune complex disease Type II: dense deposit disease (alternate pathway activation) Type III: rare, with systemic diseases and drugs	Lobular proliferation of mesangial cells, increased mesangial matrix, double contour of GBM	Type I: Subendothelial deposits Type II: Dense intramembranous deposits Type III: Subendothelial and subepithelial deposits		Type I: IgG, C3 Type II: C3 properdin Type III: C3 IgG, IgM
6. **Focal GN**	Variable, haema-turia common	Variable, possibly immune complex disease	Focal and segmental proliferation	Mesangial deposits		IgA ± IgG, C3 and fibrin
7. **Focal Segmental glomerulo-sclerosis**	Nephrotic syndrome	i) Idiopathic ii) With superimposed primary glomerular disease iii) Secondary type	Focal and segmental sclerosis and hyalinosis	Loss of foot processes, electron dense deposits in regions of sclerosis and hyalinosis		IgM, C3
8. **IgA nephropathy**	Recurrent haematuria, mild proteinuria	Unknown, possibly alternate pathway disease	Variable, commonly focal proliferative GN	Mesangial electron-dense deposits		IgA ± IgG, C3, properdin
9. **Chronic GN**	Chronic renal failure	Variable	Hyalinised glomeruli	Variable		Variable

GN = glomerulonephritis; LM = light microscopy; EM = electron microscopy; IFM = immunofluorescence microscopy.

Class V: Membranous lupus nephritis. These lesions resemble those of idiopathic membranous GN. These consist of diffuse thickening of glomerular capillary wall on light microscopy and show subendothelial deposits of immune complexes containing IgG, IgM and C3 on ultrastructural studies.

Class VI: Sclerosing lupus nephritis. This is end-stage kidney of SLE, akin to chronic GN.

Diabetic Nephropathy *(p. 701)*

Renal involvement is an important complication of diabetes mellitus. End-stage kidney with renal failure accounts for deaths in more than 10% of all diabetics. Renal complications are more severe, develop early and more frequently in type 1 (i.e. insulin-dependent) diabetes mellitus (30-40% cases) than in type 2 (non-insulin-dependent) diabetics (about 20% cases). A variety of clinical syndromes are associated with diabetic nephropathy that includes asymptomatic proteinuria, nephrotic syndrome, progressive renal failure and hypertension. Cardiovascular disease is 40 times more common in patients of end-stage renal disease in diabetes mellitus than in non-diabetics and more diabetics die from cardiovascular complications than from uraemia.

MORPHOLOGY. Diabetic nephropathy is the term that encompasses 4 types of renal lesions in diabetes mellitus:

1. DIABETIC GLOMERULOSCLEROSIS. Glomerular lesions in diabetes mellitus are particularly common and account for majority of abnormal findings referable to the kidney.

Pathogenesis of these lesions in diabetes mellitus is explained by following sequential changes: hyperglycaemia → glomerular hypertension → renal hyperperfusion → deposition of proteins in the mesangium → glomerulosclerosis → renal failure.

Glomerulosclerosis in diabetes may take one of the 2 forms: diffuse or nodular lesions.

i) Diffuse glomerulosclerosis. Diffuse glomerular lesions are the most common. There is involvement of all parts of glomeruli. The pathologic changes consist of thickening of the GBM and diffuse increase in mesangial matrix with mild proliferation of mesangial cells. Various exudative lesions such as capsular hyaline drops and fibrin caps may also be present. *Capsular drop* is an eosinophilic hyaline thickening of the parietal layer of Bowman's capsule and bulges into the glomerular space. *Fibrin cap* is homogeneous, brightly eosinophilic material appearing on the wall of a peripheral capillary of a lobule.

ii) Nodular glomerulosclerosis. Nodular lesions of diabetic glomerulo-sclerosis are also called as *Kimmelstiel-Wilson (KW) lesions* or *intercapillary glomerulosclerosis*. These lesions are specific for juvenile-onset diabetes or islet cell antibody-positive diabetes mellitus. The pathologic changes consist of one or more nodules in a few or many glomeruli. *Nodule* is an ovoid or spherical, laminated, hyaline, acellular mass located within a lobule of the glomerulus. The nodules are surrounded peripherally by glomerular capillary loops which may have normal or thickened GBM. The nodules are PAS-positive and contain lipid and fibrin.

2. VASCULAR LESIONS. *Atheroma* of renal arteries is very common and severe in diabetes mellitus. *Hyaline arteriolosclerosis* affecting the afferent and efferent arterioles of the glomeruli is also often severe in diabetes.

3. DIABETIC PYELONEPHRITIS. Poorly-controlled diabetics are particularly susceptible to bacterial infections. Papillary necrosis (necrotising papillitis) is an important complication of diabetes that may result in acute pyelonephritis. Chronic pyelonephritis is 10 to 20 times more common in diabetics than in others.

4. TUBULAR LESIONS (ARMANNI-EBSTEIN LESIONS). In untreated diabetics who have extremely high blood sugar level, the epithelial cells of the proximal convoluted tubules develop extensive glycogen deposits appearing as vacuoles. These are called Armanni-Ebstein lesions.

Hereditary Nephritis *(p. 701)*

1. Alport's syndrome. Out of various hereditary nephritis, Alport's syndrome is relatively more common and has been extensively studied. This is an X-linked dominant disorder having mutation in α–5 chain of type IV collagen located on X-chromosome. It affects males more severely than females. The syndrome consists of sensori-neural deafness and ophthalmic complications (lens dislocation, posterior cataracts and corneal dystrophy) associated with hereditary nephritis.

M/E The glomeruli have predominant involvement and show segmental proliferation of mesangial cells with increased mesangial matrix and occasional segmental sclerosis. Another prominent feature is the presence of *lipid-laden foam cells* in the interstitium.

EM Reveals characteristic basement membrane splitting or lamination in the affected parts of glomeruli.

IF Fail to show deposits of immunoglobulins or complement components.

2. Fabry's disease, another hereditary nephritis is characterised by accumulation of neutral glycosphingolipids in lysosomes of glomerular, tubular, vascular and interstitial cells.

3. Nail-patella syndrome or osteonychodysplasia is a rare hereditary disease having abnormality in α-1 chain of collagen V on chromosome 9 associated with multiple osseous defects of elbows, knees and nail dysplasia.

ACUTE TUBULAR NECROSIS *(p. 703)*

Acute tubular necrosis (ATN) is the term used for acute renal failure (ARF) resulting from destruction of tubular epithelial cells. ATN is the most common and most important cause of ARF characterised by sudden cessation of renal function. Two forms of ATN—ischaemic and toxic, are distinguished on etiology and morphology but both have a somewhat common pathogenesis.

Pathogenesis of ATN *(p. 703)*

The pathogenesis of both types of ATN resulting in ARF is explained on the basis of the following sequential mechanism:

■ *Tubular damage* in ischaemic ATN is initiated by arteriolar vasoconstriction induced by renin-angiotensin system, while in toxic ATN by direct damage to tubules.

■ This is followed by *tubular obstruction* by desquamated epithelium and casts in the lumina or by interstitial oedema.

■ This causes *increased intratubular pressure* resulting in damage to tubular basement membrane.

■ Due to increased intratubular pressure, there is *tubular rupture*.

■ This leads to *back-leakage* of tubular fluid into the interstitium which increases interstitial pressure.

■ Increased interstitial pressure causes *compression of tubules and blood vessels* and hence further accentuates ischaemia and necrosis.

Ischaemic ATN *(p. 703)*

Ischaemic ATN, also called tubulorrhectic ATN, lower nephron nephrosis, or shock kidney, occurs due to hypoperfusion of the kidneys resulting in focal damage to the tubules.

ETIOLOGY. Ischaemic ATN is more common than toxic ATN and accounts for more than 80% cases of tubular injury. Ischaemia may result from a variety of causes such as:

1. Shock (post-traumatic, surgical, burns, dehydration, obstetrical and septic type).
2. Crush injuries.
3. Non-traumatic rhabdomyolysis induced by alcohol, coma, muscle disease or extreme muscular exertion (myoglobinuric nephrosis).
4. Mismatched blood transfusions, black-water fever (haemoglobinuric nephrosis).

G/A The kidneys are enlarged and swollen. On cut section, the cortex is often widened and pale, while medulla is dark.

M/E Predominant changes are seen in the tubules, while glomeruli are normal. Interstitium shows oedema and mild chronic inflammatory cell infiltrate. Tubular changes are as follows:

1. Dilatation of the proximal and distal convoluted tubules.
2. Focal tubular necrosis at different points along the nephron.
3. Flattened epithelium lining the tubules suggesting epithelial regeneration.
4. Eosinophilic hyaline casts or pigmented haemoglobin and myoglobin casts in the tubular lumina.
5. Disruption of tubular basement membrane adjacent to the cast (tubulorrhexis).

In general, cases that follow severe trauma, surgical procedures, extensive burns and sepsis have much worse outlook than the others.

Toxic ATN *(p. 703)*

Toxic or nephrotoxic ATN occurs as a result of direct damage to tubular cells by ingestion, injection or inhalation of a number of toxic agents.

ETIOLOGY. The toxic agents causing toxic ATN are as under:

1. General poisons such as mercuric chloride, carbon tetrachloride, ethylene glycol, mushrooms and insecticides.
2. Heavy metals (mercury, lead, arsenic, phosphorus and gold).
3. Drugs such as sulfonamides, certain antibiotics (gentamycin, cephalosporin), anaesthetic agents (methoxyflurane, halothane), barbiturates, salicylates.
4. Radiographic contrast material.

Poisoning with mercuric chloride provides the best example that produces widespread and readily discernible tubular necrosis *(acute mercury nephropathy).*

G/A The kidneys are enlarged and swollen. On cut section, the cortex is pale and swollen, while the medulla is slightly darker than normal.

M/E The appearance varies according to the cause of toxic ATN but, in general, involves the segment of tubule diffusely (unlike ischaemic ATN where the involvement of nephron is focal). In mercuric chloride poisoning, the features are as follows:

1. Epithelial cells of mainly proximal convoluted tubules are necrotic and desquamated into the tubular lumina.
2. The desquamated cells may undergo dystrophic calcification.
3. Tubular basement membrane is generally intact.
4. The regenerating epithelium, which is flat and thin with few mitoses, may be seen lining the tubular basement membrane.

Prognosis of toxic ATN is good if there is no serious damage to other organs such as heart and liver.

TUBULOINTERSTITIAL DISEASE *(p. 704)*

The term tubulointerstitial nephritis is used for inflammatory process that predominantly involves the renal interstitial tissue and is usually accompanied by some degree of tubular damage. The term *interstitial nephritis* is reserved for those cases where there is no primary involvement of glomeruli, tubules or blood vessels. The older nomenclature, interstitial nephritis, is currently used synonymously with *tubulointerstitial nephritis or tubulointerstitial nephropathy.*

A number of bacterial and non-bacterial, acute and chronic conditions may produce tubulointerstitial nephritis and are listed in Table 20.10.

TABLE 20.10: Tubulointerstitial Diseases.

A.   Infective
1. Acute pyelonephritis
2. Chronic pyelonephritis
3. Tuberculous pyelonephritis
4. Other infections (viruses, parasites etc)

B.   Non-infective
1. Acute hypersensitivity interstitial nephritis
2. Analgesic abuse (phenacetin) nephropathy
3. Myeloma nephropathy
4. Balkan nephropathy
5. Urate nephropathy
6. Gout nephropathy
7. Radiation nephritis
8. Transplant rejection
9. Nephrocalcinosis
10. Idiopathic interstitial nephritis

Acute Pyelonephritis *(p. 704)*

Acute pyelonephritis is an acute suppurative inflammation of the kidney caused by pyogenic bacteria.

ETIOPATHOGENESIS. Most cases of acute pyelonephritis follow infection of the lower urinary tract. The most common pathogenic organism in urinary tract infection (UTI) is *Escherichia coli* (in 90% of cases), followed in decreasing frequency, by *Enterobacter, Klebsiella, Pseudomonas* and *Proteus.* The bacteria gain entry into the urinary tract, and thence into the kidney by one of the two routes: ascending infection and haematogenous infection.

G/A Well-developed cases of acute pyelonephritis show enlarged and swollen kidney that bulges on section. The cut surface shows small, yellow-white abscesses with a haemorrhagic rim.

M/E Acute pyelonephritis is characterised by extensive acute inflammation involving the interstitium and causing destruction of the tubules. Generally, the glomeruli and renal blood vessels show considerable resistance to infection and are spared.

CLINICAL FEATURES. Classically, acute pyelonephritis has an acute onset with chills, fever, loin pain, lumbar tenderness, dysuria and frequency of micturition. Urine will show bacteria in excess of 100,000/ml, pus cells and pus cell casts in the urinary sediment.

COMPLICATIONS. Complications of acute pyelonephritis are encountered more often in patients with diabetes mellitus or with urinary tract obstruction.

1.   Papillary necrosis. Papillary necrosis or necrotising papillitis develops more commonly in analgesic abuse nephropathy and in sickle cell disease but may occur as a complication of acute pyelonephritis as well. It may affect one or both kidneys.

2. Pyonephrosis. Rarely, the abscesses in the kidney in acute pyelonephritis are extensive, particularly in cases with obstruction. This results in inability of the abscesses to drain and this transforms the kidney into a multilocular sac filled with pus called as pyonephrosis or renal carbuncle.

3. Perinephric abscess. The abscesses in the kidney may extend through the capsule of the kidney into the perinephric tissue and form perinephric abscess.

Chronic Pyelonephritis *(p. 706)*

Chronic pyelonephritis is a chronic tubulointerstitial disease resulting from repeated attacks of inflammation and scarring.

ETIOPATHOGENESIS. Depending upon the etiology and pathogenesis, two types of chronic pyelonephritis are described—reflux nephropathy and obstructive pyelonephritis.

1. Reflux nephropathy. Reflux of urine from the bladder into one or both the ureters during micturition is the major cause of chronic pyelonephritis. *Vesicoureteric reflux* is particularly common in children, especially in girls, due to congenital absence or shortening of the intravesical portion of the ureter so that ureter is not compressed during the act of micturition.

2. Obstructive pyelonephritis. Obstruction to the outflow of urine at different levels predisposes the kidney to infection. Recurrent episodes of such obstruction and infection result in renal damage and scarring.

G/A The kidneys show rather characteristic appearance. The kidneys are usually small and contracted (weighing less than 100 gm) showing unequal reduction so as to distinguish it from other forms of contracted kidney. The surface of the kidney is irregularly scarred; the capsule can be stripped off with difficulty due to adherence to scars. These scars are of variable size and show characteristic U-shaped depressions on the cortical surface.

M/E Predominant changes are seen in interstitium and tubules.

i)   **Interstitium**—There is chronic interstitial inflammatory reaction, chiefly composed of lymphocytes, plasma cells and macrophages with pronounced interstitial fibrosis.

ii)   **Tubules**—The tubules show varying degree of atrophy and dilatation. Dilated tubules may contain eosinophilic colloid casts producing thyroidisation of tubules.

iii)   **Pelvicalyceal system**—The renal pelvis and calyces are dilated. The walls of pelvis and calyces show marked chronic inflammation and fibrosis.

iv)   **Blood vessels**—Blood vessels entrapped in the scarred areas show obliterative endarteritis.

v)   **Glomeruli**—Though glomerular tuft in the scarred area is usually intact, there is often periglomerular fibrosis.

CLINICAL FEATURES. Chronic pyelonephritis often has an insidious onset. The patients present with clinical picture of chronic renal failure or with symptoms of hypertension. Sometimes, the patients may present with features of acute recurrent pyelonephritis with fever, loin pain, lumbar tenderness, dysuria, pyouria, bacteriuria and frequency of micturition.

Tuberculous Pyelonephritis *(p. 707)*

Tuberculosis of the kidney occurs due to haematogenous spread of infection from another site, most often from the lungs. Less commonly, it may result from ascending infection from tuberculosis of the genitourinary system such as from epididymis or Fallopian tubes.

G/A The lesions in tuberculous pyelonephritis are often bilateral, usually involving the medulla with replacement of the papillae by caseous tissue.

M/E Typical granulomatous reaction is seen. Acid-fast bacilli can often be demonstrated in the lesions.

CLINICAL FEATURES. Most patients are young to middle-aged adults. There is persistent sterile pyuria, microscopic haematuria and mild proteinuria.

Myeloma Nephropathy *(p. 708)*

Renal involvement in multiple myeloma is referred to as myeloma nephropathy or myeloma kidney. Functional renal impairment in multiple myeloma is a common manifestation, developing in about 50% of patients. The pathogenesis of myeloma kidney is related to excess filtration of Bence Jones proteins through the glomerulus, usually *kappa (κ)* light chains. These light chain proteins are precipitated in the distal convoluted tubules in combination with Tamm-Horsfall proteins, the urinary glycoproteins.

G/A The kidneys may be normal or small and shrunken.

M/E There are some areas of tubular atrophy while many other tubular lumina are dilated and contain characteristic bright pink laminated casts. These casts are surrounded by peritubular interstitial inflammatory reaction including the presence of nonspecific inflammatory cells and some multinucleate giant cells induced by tubular casts.

Nephrocalcinosis *(p. 708)*

Nephrocalcinosis is a diffuse deposition of calcium salts in renal tissue in a number of renal diseases, in hypercalcaemia, hyperphosphataemia and renal tubular acidosis. Most commonly, it develops as a complication of severe hypercalcaemia such as due to hyperparathyroidism, hypervitaminosis D, excessive bone destruction in metastatic malignancy, hyperthyroidism, excessive calcium intake such as in milk-alkali syndrome and sarcoidosis.

M/E Nephrocalcinosis due to hypercalcaemia characteristically shows deposition of calcium in the tubular epithelial cells in the basement membrane, within the mitochondria and the cytoplasm.

HYPERTENSIVE VASCULAR DISEASE *(p. 708)*

An elevated arterial blood pressure is a major health problem, particularly in developed countries. A persistent and sustained high blood pressure has damaging effects on the heart (e.g. hypertensive heart disease), brain (e.g. cerebrovascular accident) and kidneys (benign and malignant nephrosclerosis).

Definition and Classification *(p. 708)*

Arterial or systemic hypertension in a patient is defined clinically as *'borderline'* if the systolic blood pressure is more than 140 mm Hg, and diastolic pressure is above 90 mm Hg (currently labelled as *mild hypertension*), and *'hypertensive'* when the elevation of systolic and diastolic pressure exceeds 160 and 95 mm Hg respectively (now termed as *moderate hypertension*). The diastolic pressure is often considered more significant. A clinically useful classification of hypertension has been recently described by the Joint National Committee of the WHO/International Society of Hypertension (Table 20.11). By means of these criteria, the prevalence of hypertension is observed in about 25% of population.

Hypertension is generally classified into 2 types:

1. Primary or essential hypertension in which the cause of increase in blood pressure is unknown. Essential hypertension constitutes about 90-95% patients of hypertension.

TABLE 20.11: Clinical Classification of Hypertension.*

CATEGORY	SYSTOLIC (mm Hg)	DIASTOLIC (mm Hg)
Normal	< 130	< 85
High normal	130-139	85-89
Hypertension		
mild (stage 1)	140-159	90-99
moderate (stage 2)	160-179	100-109
severe (stage 3)	180-209	110-119
very severe (stage 4)	≥ 210	≥ 120
Malignant hypertension	> 200	≥ 140

*WHO/International Society of Hypertension (ISH) Special Report, 1995.

2. Secondary hypertension, in which the increase in blood pressure is caused by diseases of the kidneys, endocrines or some other organs. Secondary hypertension comprises 5-10% cases of hypertension.

According to the clinical course, both essential and secondary hypertension may be benign or malignant.

▪ **Benign hypertension** is moderate elevation of blood pressure and the rise is slow over the years. About 90-95% patients of hypertension have benign hypertension.

▪ **Malignant hypertension** is marked and rapid increase of blood pressure to 200/140 mm Hg or more and the patients have papilloedema, retinal haemorrhages and hypertensive encephalopathy. Less than 5% of hypertensive patients develop malignant hypertension and life expectancy after diagnosis in these patients is generally less than 2 years if not treated effectively.

Etiology and Pathogenesis *(p. 709)*

The etiology and pathogenesis of secondary hypertension that comprises less than 10% cases has been better understood, whereas the mechanism of essential hypertension that constitutes about 90% of cases remains largely obscure (Table 20.12).

TABLE 20.12: Etiologic Classification of Hypertension.

A. ESSENTIAL HYPERTENSION (90%)
1. Genetic factors
2. Racial and environmental factors
3. Risk factors modifying the course

B. SECONDARY HYPERTENSION (10%)
1. *Renal*
   i) Renovascular
   ii) Renal parenchymal diseases
2. *Endocrine*
   i) Adrenocortical hyperfunction
   ii) Hyperparathyroidism
   iii) Oral contraceptives
3. *Coarctation of Aorta*
4. *Neurogenic*

In general, normal blood pressure is regulated by 2 haemodynamic forces—*cardiac output* and *total peripheral vascular resistance.* Factors which alter these two factors result in hypertension. The role of kidney in hypertension, particularly in secondary hypertension, by elaboration of renin and subsequent formation of angiotensin II, is well established (renin-angiotensin system).

ESSENTIAL (PRIMARY) HYPERTENSION. By definition, the cause of essential hypertension is unknown but a number of factors are related to its development. These are as under:

1. Genetic factors. The role of heredity in the etiology of essential hypertension has long been suspected. The evidences in support are the familial aggregation, occurrence of hypertension in twins, epidemiologic data.

2. Racial and environmental factors. Surveys in the US have revealed higher incidence of essential hypertension in blacks than in whites. A number of environmental factors have been implicated in the development of hypertension including salt intake, obesity, skilled occupation, higher living standards and patients in high stress.

3. Risk factors modifying the course of essential hypertension. There is sufficient evidence to show that the course of essential hypertension that begins in middle life is modified by a number of factors:

i) Age. Younger the age at which hypertension is first noted but left untreated, lower the life expectancy.

ii) Sex. Females with hypertension appear to do better than males.

iii) Atherosclerosis. Accelerated atherosclerosis invariably accompanies essential hypertension.

iv) Other risk factors. Other factors which alter the prognosis in hypertension include: smoking, excess of alcohol intake, diabetes mellitus, persistently high diastolic pressure above 115 mm Hg.

SECONDARY HYPERTENSION. Mechanisms underlying hypertension with identifiable cause have been studied more extensively. Based on the etiology, these are described under four headings:

1. RENAL HYPERTENSION. Hypertension produced by renal diseases is called renal hypertension. Renal hypertension is subdivided into 2 groups:

i) Renal vascular hypertension e.g. in occlusion of a major renal artery, pre-eclampsia, eclampsia, polyarteritis nodosa and fibromuscular dysplasia of renal artery.

ii) Renal parenchymal hypertension e.g. in various types of glomerulonephritis, pyelonephritis, interstitial nephritis, diabetic nephropathy, amyloidosis, polycystic kidney disease and renin-producing tumours.

In either case, renal hypertension can be produced by one of the 3 inter-related pathogenetic mechanisms:

- activation of renin-angiotensin system,
- sodium and water retention, and
- decreased release of vasodepressor materials.

a) Activation of renin-angiotensin system. Renin is a proteolytic enzyme produced and stored in the granules of the juxtaglomerular cells surrounding the afferent arterioles of glomerulus. Released renin is transported through blood stream to the liver where it acts upon substrate angiotensinogen, an α_2-globulin synthesised in the liver, to form angiotensin I, a decapeptide. Angiotensin I is converted into angiotensin II, an octapeptide, by the action of convertase in the lungs. Angiotensin II is the most potent naturally-occurring vasoconstrictor substance and its pressor action is mainly attributed to peripheral arteriolar vasoconstriction.

Thus, the renin-angiotensin system is concerned mainly with 3 functions:

i)   Control of blood pressure by altering plasma concentration of angiotensin II and aldosterone.

ii) Regulation of sodium and water content.

iii) Regulation of potassium balance.

b) Sodium and water retention. Blood volume and cardiac output, both of which have a bearing on blood pressure, are regulated by blood levels of sodium which is significant for maintaining extracellular fluid volume. Blood concentration of sodium is regulated by 3 mechanisms: i) Release of aldosterone ii) Reduction in GFR iii) Release of atriopeptin hormone.

c) Release of vasodepressor material. A number of vasodepressor materials and antihypertensives counterbalance the vasopressor effect of angiotensin II. These substances include: prostaglandins (PGE2, PGF2, PGA or medullin) released from interstitial cells of the medulla, urinary kallikrein-kinin system and platelet-activating factor.

2. ENDOCRINE HYPERTENSION. A number of hormonal secretions may produce secondary hypertension.

i) *Adrenal gland*—e.g. in primary aldosteronism, Cushing's syndrome, adrenal virilism and pheochromocytoma.

ii) *Parathyroid gland*—e.g. hypercalcaemia in hyperparathyroidism.

iii) *Oral contraceptives*—Oestrogen component in the oral contraceptives stimulates hepatic synthesis of renin substrate.

3. COARCTATION OF AORTA. Coarctation of the aorta causes systolic hypertension in the upper part of the body due to constriction itself. Diastolic hypertension results from changes in circulation.

4. NEUROGENIC. Psychogenic, polyneuritis, increased intracranial pressure and section of spinal cord are all uncommon causes of secondary hypertension.

EFFECTS OF HYPERTENSION *(p. 711)*

Systemic hypertension causes major effects in three main organs—heart and its blood vessels, nervous system, and kidneys. The renal effects in the form of benign and malignant nephrosclerosis.

Benign Nephrosclerosis *(p. 711)*

Benign nephrosclerosis is the term used to describe the kidney of benign phase of hypertension. Mild benign nephrosclerosis is the most common form of renal disease in persons over 60 years of áge but its severity increases in the presence of hypertension and diabetes mellitus.

G/A Both the kidneys are affected equally and are reduced in size and weight, often weighing about 100 gm or less. The capsule is often adherent to the cortical surface. The surface of the kidney is finely granular and shows V-shaped areas of scarring.*

M/E There are primarily diffuse vascular changes which produce parenchymal changes secondarily as a result of ischaemia.

i) **Vascular changes:** There are 2 types of changes in these blood vessels:

a) *Hyaline arteriolosclerosis* that results in homogeneous and eosinophilic thickening of the wall of small blood vessels.

b) *Intimal thickening* due to proliferation of smooth muscle cells in the intima.

ii) **Parenchymal changes:** As a consequence of ischaemia, there is variable degree of atrophy of parenchyma. This includes: glomerular shrinkage, deposition of collagen in Bowman's space, periglomerular fibrosis, tubular atrophy and fine interstitial fibrosis.

---

*The various acquired causes of *'small contracted kidney'* and their characteristic gross macroscopic appearance may be recollected here. These are: 1. Chronic GN (granular appearance); 2. Chronic pyelonephritis (U-shaped scars) and 3. Benign nephrosclerosis (V-shaped scars). Although granular, U- and V-shaped scars correspond to the respective macroscopic patterns, an easy way to remember is: *'granular'* for glomerular scars of chronic GN; *'U-scars'* for uneven scars of chronic pyelonephritis; and *'V-scars'* for vascular scars of benign nephrosclerosis. Less common causes are: amyloidosis of the kidney, myeloma kidney and diabetic nephropathy.

Malignant Nephrosclerosis *(p. 712)*

Malignant nephrosclerosis is the form of renal disease that occurs in malignant or accelerated hypertension. Malignant nephrosclerosis is uncommon and usually occurs as a superimposed complication in 5% cases of pre-existing benign essential hypertension or in those having secondary hypertension with identifiable cause such as in chronic renal diseases.

G/A The appearance of the kidney varies. In a case of malignant hypertension superimposed on pre-existing benign nephrosclerosis, the kidneys are small in size, shrunken and reduced in weight and have finely granular surface. However, the kidneys of a patient who develops malignant hypertension in pure form are enlarged, oedematous and have petechial haemorrhages on the surface producing so called *'flea-bitten kidney'*.*

M/E Most commonly the changes are superimposed on benign nephrosclerosis. These changes are as under:

i) **Vascular changes:** The two characteristic vascular changes seen are as under:
a) Necrotising arteriolitis
b) Hyperplastic intimal sclerosis or onionskin proliferation

ii) **Ischaemic changes:** The effects of vascular narrowing on the parenchyma include tubular loss, fine interstitial fibrosis and foci of infarction necrosis.

THROMBOTIC MICROANGIOPATHY *(p. 713)*

Thrombotic renal disease encompasses a group of diseases having in common the formation of thrombi composed by platelets and fibrin in arterioles and glomeruli of the kidney and culminating clinically in acute renal failure. Causes of thrombotic microangiopathy of renal microvasculature are listed in Table 20.13.

TABLE 20.13: Causes of Thrombotic Microangiopathy.

1.	Infections *(E.coli, Shigella, Pseudomonas)*
2.	Drugs (e.g. mitomycin, cisplatin, cyclosporine)
3.	Autoimmune disease (scleroderma, SLE)
4.	Thrombotic thrombocytopenic purpura
5.	Haemolytic-uraemic syndrome
6.	Pregnancy and pre-eclampsia
7.	Malignant hypertension

The common clinical manifestations include microangiopathic haemolytic anaemia, thrombocytopenia, DIC, and eventually renal failure.

PATHOGENESIS In all such cases, endothelial injury appears to be the trigger for vascular changes. The injured endothelial surface causes the following effects:
■ Passage of plasma constituents to the subendothelial zone of microvasculature.
■ Promotes thrombosis.

RENAL CORTICAL NECROSIS *(p. 714)*

Renal cortical necrosis is infarction of renal cortex varying from microscopic foci to a situation where most of the renal cortex is destroyed. The medulla, the

---
*Recall the other causes of *flea-bitten kidney:* acute post-streptococcal GN, rapidly progressive GN, haemolytic-uraemic syndrome, thrombotic thrombocytopenic purpura and Henoch-Schonlein purpura.

juxtamedullary cortex and a rim of cortex under the capsule are usually spared. The condition develops most commonly as an obstetrical emergency (e.g. in eclampsia, pre-eclampsia, premature separation of the placenta). Other causes include septic shock, poisoning, severe trauma etc.

The lesions may be present focally, patchily or diffusely. The gross and microscopic characteristics of infarcts of cortex are present.

OBSTRUCTIVE UROPATHY *(p. 714)*

Obstruction in the urinary tract is common and important because it increases the susceptibility to infection and stone formation. Obstruction can occur at any age and in either sex. The cause of obstruction may lie at any level of the urinary tract—renal pelvis, ureters, urinary bladder and urethra. The obstruction at any of these anatomic locations may be intraluminal, intramural or extramural. Important causes are listed in Table 20.14.

TABLE 20.14: Causes of Obstructive Uropathy.

A.	**Intraluminal**
1.	Calculi
2.	Tumours (e.g. cancer of kidney and bladder)
3.	Sloughed renal papilla
4.	Blood clots
5.	Foreign body
B.	**Intramural**
1.	Pelvi-ureteric junction (PUJ) obstruction
2.	Vesicoureteric obstruction
3.	Urethral stricture
4.	Urethral valves
5.	Inflammation (e.g. phimosis, cystitis etc)
6.	Neuromuscular dysfunction
C.	**Extramural**
1.	Pregnant uterus
2.	Retroperitoneal fibrosis
3.	Tumours (e.g. carcinoma of cervix, rectum, colon, caecum etc)
4.	Prostatic enlargement, prostatic carcinoma and prostatitis
5.	Trauma

The obstruction may be unilateral or bilateral, partial or complete, sudden or insidious. Complete bilateral obstruction may result in irreversible renal failure, whereas long-standing chronic partial obstruction may cause various functional abnormalities and anatomic changes. There are three important anatomic sequelae of obstruction, namely: *hydronephrosis, hydroureter and hypertrophy of the bladder.*

UROLITHIASIS *(p. 714)*

Urolithiasis or formation of urinary calculi at any level of the urinary tract is a common condition. Urinary calculi are worldwide in distribution but are particularly common in some geographic locales such as in parts of the United States, South Africa, India and South-East Asia. It is estimated that approximately 2% of the population experiences renal stone disease at sometime in their life with male-female ratio of 2:1. The peak incidence is observed in 2nd to 3rd decades of life. Renal calculi are characterised clinically by colicky pain *(renal colic)* as they pass down along the ureter and manifest by haematuria.

Types of Urinary Calculi (p. 714)

There are 4 main types of urinary calculi—calcium containing, mixed (struvite), uric acid and cystine stones, and a small number of rare types (Table 20.15).

TABLE 20.15: Salient Features of Urinary Calculi.

	TYPE	INCIDENCE	ETIOLOGY	PATHOGENESIS
1.	*Calcium stones*	75%	Hypercalciuria with or without hypercalcaemia; idiopathic	Supersaturation of ions in urine, alkaline pH of urine; low urinary volume, oxaluria and hyperuricosuria
2.	*Mixed (struvite) stones*	15%	Urinary infection with urea-splitting organisms like *Proteus*	Alkaline urinary pH produced by ammonia from splitting of urea by bacterially produced urease
3.	*Uric acid stones*	6%	Hyperuricosuria with or without hyperuricaemia (e.g. in primary and secondary gout)	Acidic urine (pH below 6) decreases the solubility of uric acid in urine and favours its precipitation
4.	*Cystine stones*	2%	Genetically-determined defect in cystine transport	Cystinuria containing least soluble cystine precipitates as cystine crystals
5.	*Other types*	< 2%	Inherited abnormalities of amino acid metabolism	Xanthinuria

1. CALCIUM STONES. Calcium stones are the most common comprising about 75% of all urinary calculi. They may be pure stones of calcium oxalate (50%) or calcium phosphate (5%), or mixture of calcium oxalate and calcium phosphate (45%).

Etiology. Etiology of calcium stones is variable.

i) About 50% of patients with calcium stones have *idiopathic hypercalciuria without hypercalcaemia*.

ii) Approximately 10% cases are associated with *hypercalcaemia* and *hypercalciuria*.

iii) About 15% of patients with calcium stones have *hyperuricosuria with a normal blood uric acid level* and without any abnormality of calcium metabolism.

iv) In about 25% of patients with calcium stones, the cause is unknown as there is no abnormality in urinary excretion of calcium, uric acid or oxalate and is referred to as *'idiopathic calcium stone disease'*.

Pathogenesis. The mechanism of calcium stone formation is explained on the basis of imbalance between the degree of supersaturation of the ions forming the stone and the concentration of inhibitors in the urine.

Morphology. Calcium stones are usually small (less than a centimeter), ovoid, hard, with granular rough surface. They are dark brown due to old blood pigment deposited in them as a result of repeated trauma caused to the urinary tract by these sharp-edged stones.

2. MIXED (STRUVITE) STONES. About 15% of urinary calculi are made of magnesium-ammonium-calcium phosphate, often called *struvite*. That is why mixed stones are also called as *'struvite stones'* or 'triple phosphate stones'.

Etiology. Struvite stones are formed as a result of infection of the urinary tract with urea-splitting organisms that produce urease such as by species of *Proteus,* and occasionally *Klebsiella, Pseudomonas* and *Enterobacter.*

Morphology. Struvite stones are yellow-white or grey. They tend to be soft and friable and irregular in shape. 'Staghorn stone' which is a large, solitary stone that takes the shape of the renal pelvis where it is often formed is an example of struvite stone.

3. URIC ACID STONES. Approximately 6% of urinary calculi are made of uric acid. Uric acid calculi are radiolucent unlike radio-opaque calcium stones.

Etiology. Uric acid stones are frequently formed in cases with hyperuricaemia and hyperuricosuria such as due to primary gout or secondary gout due to myeloproliferative disorders (e.g. in leukaemias).

Pathogenesis. The solubility of uric acid at pH of 7 is 200 mg/dl while at pH of 5 is 15 mg/dl. Thus, as the urine becomes more acidic, the solubility of uric acid in urine decreases and precipitation of uric acid crystals increases favouring the formation of uric acid stones.

Morphology. Uric acid stones are smooth, yellowish-brown, hard and often multiple. On cut section, they show laminated structure.

4. CYSTINE STONES. Cystine stones comprise less than 2% of urinary calculi.

Etiology. Cystine stones are associated with cystinuria due to a genetically-determined defect in the transport of cystine and other amino acids across the cell membrane of the renal tubules and the small intestinal mucosa.

Pathogenesis. The resultant excessive excretion of cystine which is least soluble of the naturally-occurring amino acids leads to formation of crystals and eventually cystine calculi.

Morphology. Cystine stones are small, rounded, smooth and often multiple. They are yellowish and waxy.

5. OTHER CALCULI. Less than 2% of urinary calculi consist of other rare types such as due to inherited abnormality of xanthine metabolism resulting in xanthinuria and consequently xanthine stones.

HYDRONEPHROSIS *(p. 716)*

Hydronephrosis is the term used for dilatation of renal pelvis and calyces due to partial or intermittent obstruction to the outflow of urine. Hydronephrosis develops if one or both the pelviureteric sphincters are incompetent, as otherwise there will be dilatation and hypertrophy of the urinary bladder but no hydronephrosis. Hydroureter nearly always accompanies hydronephrosis. Hydronephrosis may be *unilateral or bilateral*.

Unilateral Hydronephrosis *(p. 716)*

This occurs due to some form of ureteral obstruction at the level of pelviureteric junction (PUJ). The causes are:

1. **Intraluminal** e.g. a calculus in the ureter or renal pelvis.

2. **Intramural** e.g. congenital PUJ obstruction, atresia of ureter, inflammatory stricture, trauma, neoplasm of ureter or bladder.

3. **Extramural** e.g. obstruction of upper part of ureter by inferior renal artery or vein, pressure on ureter from outside such as carcinoma cervix, prostate, rectum, colon or caecum and retroperitoneal fibrosis.

Bilateral Hydronephrosis *(p. 716)*

This is generally the result of some form of urethral obstruction but can occur from the various causes listed above if the lesions involve both sides. The causes are:

1. **Congenital** e.g. atresia of the urethral meatus, congenital posterior urethral valve.

2. Acquired e.g. bladder tumour involving both ureteric orifices, prostatic enlargement, prostatic carcinoma and prostatitis, bladder neck stenosis, inflammatory or traumatic urethral stricture and phimosis.

G/A The kidneys may have moderate to marked enlargement. Initially, there is *extrarenal hydronephrosis* characterised by dilatation of renal pelvis medially in the form of a sac. As the obstruction persists, there is progressive dilatation of pelvis and calyces and pressure atrophy of renal parenchyma. Eventually, the dilated pelvi-calyceal system extends deep into the renal cortex so that a thin rim of renal cortex is stretched over the dilated calyces and the external surface assumes lobulated appearance. This advanced stage is called as *intrarenal hydronephrosis.*

M/E The wall of hydronephrotic sac is thickened due to fibrous scarring and chronic inflammatory cell infiltrate. There is progressive atrophy of tubules and glomeruli alongwith interstitial fibrosis.

TUMOURS OF KIDNEY *(p. 717)*

Table 20.16 provides a list of kidney tumours; the important forms of renal neoplasms are described below.

TABLE 20.16: Classification of Kidney Tumours.

BENIGN	MALIGNANT
A. EPITHELIAL TUMOURS OF RENAL PARENCHYMA	
Adenoma	Adenocarcinoma
Oncocytoma	(hypernephroma, renal cell carcinoma)
B. EPITHELIAL TUMOURS OF RENAL PELVIS	
Transitional cell papilloma	Transitional cell carcinoma
	Others (squamous cell carcinoma, adenocarcinoma of renal pelvis, undifferentiated carcinoma of renal pelvis)
C. EMBRYONAL TUMOURS	
Mesoblastic nephroma	Wilms' tumour (nephroblastoma)
Multicystic nephroma	
D. NON-EPITHELIAL TUMOURS	
Angiomyolipoma	Sarcomas (rare)
Medullary interstitial tumour (fibroma)	
E. MISCELLANEOUS	
Juxtaglomerular cell tumour (Reninoma)	
F. METASTATIC TUMOURS	

Cortical Adenoma *(p. 717)*

Cortical tubular adenomas are more common than other benign renal neoplasms. They are frequently multiple and associated with chronic pyelonephritis or benign nephrosclerosis.

G/A These tumours may form tiny nodules up to 3 cm in diameter. They are encapsulated and white or yellow.

M/E They are composed of tubular cords or papillary structures projecting into cystic space. The cells of the adenoma are usually uniform, cuboidal with no atypicality or mitosis. Those larger than 3 cm in diameter are potentially malignant and metastasising.

Oncocytoma *(p. 718)*

Oncocytoma is a benign epithelial tumour arising from collecting ducts.

G/A The tumour is encapsulated and has variable size. Cut section is homogeneous and has characteristic mahogany-brown or tan colour.

M/E The tumour cells are plump with abundant, finely granular, acidophilic cytoplasm and round nuclei.

Other Benign Tumours *(p. 718)*

■ **Angiomyolipoma** is a hamartoma of the kidney that contains differentiated tissue element derived from blood vessels, smooth muscle and fat.

■ **Mesoblastic nephroma** is a congenital benign tumour.

■ **Multicystic nephroma** is another uncommon tumour of early infancy.

■ **Medullary interstitial cell tumour** is a tiny nodule in the medulla composed of fibroblast-like cells in hyalinised stroma.

■ **Juxtaglomerular tumour or reninoma** is a rare tumour of renal cortex consisting of sheets of epithelioid cells with many small blood vessels.

Adenocarcinoma of Kidney *(Synonyms: Renal cell carcinoma, Hypernephroma, Grawitz tumour) (p. 718)*

Hypernephroma is an old misnomer under the mistaken belief that the tumour arises from adrenal rests because of the resemblance of the tumour cells with clear cells of the adrenal cortex. It is now known that the renal cell carcinoma (RCC) is an adenocarcinoma arising from tubular epithelium. This cancer comprises 70 to 80% of all renal cancers and occurs most commonly in 50 to 70 years of age with male preponderance (2:1).

ETIOLOGY AND PATHOGENESIS. Various etiologic factors implicated in the etiology of RCC are as follows:

1. Tobacco. Tobacco is the major risk factor for RCC, whether chewed or smoked. Cigarette smokers have 2-times higher risk of developing RCC.

2. Additional risk factors. These include:
i) Exposure to asbestos, heavy metals and petrochemical products.
ii) In women, obesity and oestrogen therapy.
iii) Hereditary and acquired cystic diseases of the kidney.
iv) Analgesic nephropathy.
v) Hereditary and family history are associated with 4-5 times higher risk.
vi) Hypertension.

Majority of cases of RCC are sporadic but about 5% cases are inherited in which *carcinogenesis* has been studied in detail. Carcinongenesis in RCC is explained on the basis of following:

1. *von Hippel-Lindau (VHL) disease:* It is an autosomal dominant cancer syndrome that includes: haemangioblastoma of the cerebellum, retinal angiomas, multiple RCC (clear cell type), pheochromocytoma and cysts in different organs.

2. *Hereditary clear cell RCC:* These are cases of clear cell type RCC confined to the kidney without other manifestations of VHL but having autosomal dominant inheritance.

3. *Papillary RCC:* This form of RCC is characterised by bilateral and multifocal cancer with papillary growth pattern.

4. *Chromophobe RCC*: These cases have genetic defects in the form of multiple losses of whole chromosomes i.e. they have extreme degree of hypodiploidy.

CLASSIFICATION. Based on cytogenetics of sporadic and familial tumours, RCC has been reclassified into clear cell, papillary, granular cell, chromophobe, sarcomatoid and collecting duct type (Table 20.17).

TABLE 20.17: Classification of Renal Cell Carcinoma

TYPE	INCIDENCE	GENETICS	MAIN HISTOLOGY
1. **Clear cell type** (non-papillary)	70%	Sporadic and familial (Homozygous loss of *VHL* gene located on chromosome 3)	Clear cytoplasm (due to glycogen and lipid), well differentiated
2. **Papillary type**	15%	Familial and sporadic (Familial cases: mutation in *MET* gene on chromosome 7; sporadic cases trisomy of chromosome 7, 16, 17 and loss of Y chromosome)	Papillary pattern, psammoma bodies
3. **Granular cell type**	8%	Sporadic and familial	Abundant acidophilic cytoplasm, marked atypia
4. **Chromophobe type**	5%	Multiple chromosome losses, hypodiploidy	Mixture of pale clear cells with perinuclear halo and granular cells
5. **Sarcomatoid type**	1.5%	—	Whorls of atypical anaplastic spindle cells
6. **Collecting duct type**	0.5%	—	Tubular and papillary pattern

G/A The RCC commonly arises from the poles of the kidney as a solitary and unilateral tumour, more often in the upper pole. The tumour is generally large, golden yellow and circumscribed. Papillary tumours may be multifocal and bilateral, besides grossly visible papillae. Cut section of the tumour commonly shows large areas of ischaemic necrosis, cystic change and foci of haemorrhages. Another significant characteristic is the frequent presence of tumour thrombus in the renal vein which may extend into the vena cava.

M/E The features of various types of RCC are as under:

1. *Clear cell type RCC (70%):* This is the most common pattern. The clear cytoplasm of tumour cells is due to removal of glycogen and lipid from the cytoplasm during processing of tissues. The tumour cells have a variety of patterns: solid, trabecular and tubular, separated by delicate vasculature. Majority of clear cell tumours are well differentiated.

2. *Papillary type RCC (15%):* The tumour cells are arranged in papillary pattern over the fibrovascular stalks. The tumour cells are cuboidal with small round nuclei. Psammoma bodies may be seen.

3. *Granular cell type RCC (8%):* The tumour cells have abundant acidophilic cytoplasm. These tumours have more marked nuclear pleomorphism, hyperchromatism and cellular atypia.

4. *Chromophobe type RCC (5%):* This type shows admixture of pale clear cells with perinuclear halo and acidophilic granular cells. The cytoplasm of these tumour cells contains many vesicles.

5. *Sarcomatoid type RCC (1.5%):* This is the most anaplastic and poorly differentiated form. The tumour is characterised by whorls of atypical spindle tumour cells.

6. *Collecting duct type RCC (0.5%):* This is a rare type that occurs in the medulla. It is composed of a single layer of cuboidal tumour cells arranged in tubular and papillary pattern.

CLINICAL FEATURES. Renal cell carcinoma is generally a slow-growing tumour and the tumour may have been present for years before it is detected. The classical evidence for diagnosis of renal cell carcinoma is the triad of *gross haematuria, flank plain* and *palpable abdominal mass.* The most common presenting abnormality is haematuria that occurs in about 60% of cases. By the time the tumour is detected, it has spread to distant sites via haematogenous route to lungs, brain and bone, and locally to liver and perirenal lymph nodes.

A number of paraneoplastic syndromes due to ectopic hormone production by the renal cell carcinoma have been described. These include *polycythaemia* (by erythropoietin), *hypercalcaemia* (by parathyroid hormone and prostaglandins), *hypertension* (by renin), effects of *feminisation* or *masculinisation* (by gonadotropins) and *Cushing's syndrome* (by glucocorticoids).

Wilms' Tumour *(Synonym: Nephroblastoma)* *(p. 721)*

Nephroblastoma or Wilms' tumour is an embryonic tumour derived from primitive renal epithelial and mesenchymal components. It is the most common abdominal malignant tumour of young children, seen most commonly between 1 to 6 years of age with equal sex incidence.

G/A The tumour is usually quite large, spheroidal, replacing most of the kidney. It is generally solitary and unilateral but 5-10% cases may have bilateral tumour. On cut section, the tumour shows characteristic variegated appearance—soft, fishflesh-like grey-white to cream-yellow tumour with foci of necrosis and haemorrhages and grossly identifiable myxomatous or cartilaginous elements.

M/E Nephroblastoma shows mixture of primitive epithelial and mesenchymal elements. Most of the tumour consists of small, round to spindled, anaplastic, sarcomatoid tumour cells. In these areas are present abortive tubules and poorly-formed glomerular structures. Sometimes, mesenchymal elements such as smooth and skeletal muscle, cartilage and bone, fat cells and fibrous tissue, may be seen.

CLINICAL FEATURES. The most common presenting feature is a palpable abdominal mass in a child. Other common abnormalities are haematuria, pain, fever and hypertension. The tumour rapidly spreads via blood, especially to lungs.

Secondary Tumours *(p. 721)*

Leukaemic infiltration of the kidneys is a common finding, particularly in chronic myeloid leukaemia. Kidney is a common site for blood-borne metastases from different primary sites, chiefly from cancers of lungs, breast and stomach.

LOWER URINARY TRACT *(p. 721)*

NORMAL STRUCTURE *(p. 721)*

The lower urinary tract consists of *ureters, urinary bladder* and *urethra.*

URETERS are tubular structures, 30 cm in length and half a centimeter in diameter, and extend from the renal pelvis (pelvi-ureteric junction) to the urinary bladder (vesico-ureteric junction).

M/E Ureter has an outer fibrous investing layer which overlies a thick muscular layer and is lined internally by transitional epithelium or urothelium similar to the lining of the renal pelvis above and bladder below.

URINARY BLADDER lies extraperitoneally and the peritoneum is reflected on its superior surface. Normally, the capacity of bladder is about 400 to 500 ml without over-distension. Micturition is partly a reflex and partly a voluntary act under the control of sympathetic and parasympathetic innervation.

M/E The greater part of the bladder wall is made up of muscular layer (detrusor muscle) having 3 coats—internal, middle and external. The inner layer of bladder consists of urothelium up to 6 layers in thickness.

URETHRA runs from the bladder up to the external meatus. The *male urethra* consists of 3 parts—prostatic, membranous and penile. It is lined in the prostatic part by urothelium but elsewhere by stratified columnar epithelium except near its orifice where the epithelium is stratified squamous. There are numerous small mucous glands in the urethral mucosa. The *female urethra* is shorter and runs from the bladder parallel with the anterior wall of the vagina.

CONGENITAL ANOMALIES *(p. 722)*

Vesicoureteric reflux is the most common anomaly described already. A few others are considered below.

DOUBLE URETER. This is a condition in which the entire ureter or only the upper part is duplicated. Double ureter is invariably associated with a double renal pelvis, *one* in the upper part and the *other* in the lower part of the kidney.

URETEROCELE. Ureterocele is cystic dilatation of the terminal part of the ureter which lies within the bladder wall. The cystic dilatation lies beneath the bladder mucosa and can be visualised by cystoscopy.

ECTOPIA VESICAE (EXSTROPHY). This is a rare condition owing to congenital developmental deficiency of anterior wall of the bladder and is associated with splitting of the overlying anterior abdominal wall. This results in exposed interior of the bladder. The condition in males is often associated with *epispadias* in which the urethra opens on the dorsal aspect of penis. If the defect is not properly repaired, the exposed bladder mucosa gets infected repeatedly and may undergo squamous metaplasia with increasing tendency to develop carcinoma of the bladder.

URACHAL ABNORMALITIES. Rarely, there may be persistence of urachus in which urine passes from the bladder to the umbilicus. More often, part of urachus remains patent which may be the umbilical end, bladder end, or central portion. Persistence of central portion gives rise to *urachal cyst* lined by transitional or squamous epithelium. Adenocarcinoma may develop in urachal cyst.

INFLAMMATIONS *(p. 722)*

Urinary tract infection (UTI) is common, especially in females and has been described already alongwith its morphologic consequences. Inflammation of the tissues of urinary tract (ureteritis, cystitis and urethritis) are considered here.

Ureteritis *(p. 722)*

Infection of the ureter is almost always secondary to pyelitis above, or cystitis below. Ureteritis is usually mild but repeated and longstanding infection may give rise to chronic ureteritis.

Cystitis *(p. 722)*

Inflammation of the urinary bladder is called cystitis. Primary cystitis is rare since the normal bladder epithelium is quite resistant to infection. Cystitis may occur by spread of infection from upper urinary tract as seen following renal tuberculosis, or may spread from the urethra such as in instrumentation. Cystitis is caused by a variety of bacterial and fungal infections as discussed in the etiology of pyelonephritis. The most common pathogenic organism in urinary tract infection is *E. coli*, followed in decreasing frequency by *Enterobacter*, *Klebsiella*, *Pseudomonas* and *Proteus*. Infection with *Candida albicans* may occur in the bladder in immunosuppressed patients.

G/A The bladder mucosa is red, swollen and haemorrhagic. There may be suppurative exudate or ulcers on the bladder mucosa.

M/E This form of cystitis is characterised by intense neutrophilic exudate admixed with lymphocytes and macrophages. There is oedema and congestion of mucosa.

CHRONIC CYSTITIS. Repeated attacks of acute cystitis lead to chronic cystitis.

G/A The mucosal epithelium is thickened, red and granular with formation of polypoid masses.

M/E There is patchy ulceration of the mucosa with formation of granulation tissue in the regions of polypoid masses. Submucosa and muscular coat show fibrosis and infiltration by chronic inflammatory cells. A form of chronic cystitis characterised by formation of lymphoid follicles in the bladder mucosa is termed *cystitis follicularis*.

A few other special forms of cystitis having distinct clinical and morphological appearance are described below.

INTERSTITIAL CYSTITIS (HUNNER'S ULCER). This variant of cystitis occurs in middle-aged women. The patients get repeated attacks of severe and excruciating pain on distension of the bladder, frequency of micturition and great decrease in bladder capacity. Cystoscopy often reveals a localised ulcer. The *etiology* of the condition is unknown but it is thought to be neurogenic in origin.

CYSTITIS CYSTICA. As a result of long-standing chronic inflammation, there occurs a downward projection of epithelial nests known as *Brunn's nests* from the deeper layer of bladder mucosa.

MALAKOPLAKIA. This is a rare condition most frequently found in the urinary bladder but can occur in the ureters, kidney, testis and prostate, and occasionally in the gut. The *etiology* of the condition is unknown but probably results from persistence of chronic inflammation with defective phagocytic process by the macrophages.

M/E The plaques are composed of massive accumulation of foamy macrophages with occasional multinucleate giant cells and some lymphocytes. These macrophages have granular PAS-positive cytoplasm and some of them contain cytoplasmic laminated concretions of calcium phosphate called *Michaelis-Gutmann bodies*.

POLYPOID CYSTITIS. Polypoid cystitis is characterised by papillary projections on the bladder mucosa due to submucosal oedema and can be confused with transitional cell carcinoma.

Urethritis *(p. 724)*

Urethritis may be *gonococcal* or *non-gonococcal*.

■ **Gonococcal (gonorrhoeal) urethritis** is an acute suppurative condition caused by gonococci *(Neisseria gonorrhoeae)*. The mucosa and submucosa are eventually converted into granulation tissue.

■ **Non-gonococcal urethritis** is more common and is most frequently caused by *E. coli*. The infection of urethra often accompanies cystitis in females and prostatitis in males. Urethritis is one of the components in the triad of Reiter's syndrome which comprises arthritis, conjunctivitis and urethritis.

TUMOURS OF THE BLADDER *(p. 724)*

Epithelial (Urothelial) Bladder Tumours *(p. 724)*

More than 90% of bladder tumours arise from transitional epithelial (urothelium) lining of the bladder in continuity with the epithelial lining of the renal pelvis, ureters, and the major part of the urethra. Though many workers consider all transitional cell tumours as transitional cell carcinoma, others distinguish true transitional cell papilloma from grade I transitional cell carcinoma.

Bladder cancer comprises about 3% of all cancers. Most of the cases appear beyond 5th decade of life with preponderance in males.

ETIOPATHOGENESIS. Urothelial tumours in the urinary tract are typically multifocal and the pattern of disease becomes apparent over a period of years. A number of environmental and host factors are associated with increased risk of bladder cancer. These are as under:

1. Industrial occupations. Workers in industries that produce aniline dyes, rubber, plastic, textiles, and cable have high incidence of bladder cancer. Bladder cancer may occur in workers in these factories after a prolonged exposure of about 20 years. The carcinogenic substances responsible for bladder cancer in these cases are the metabolites of β-naphthylamine and benzene.

2. Schistosomiasis. There is increased risk of bladder cancer, particularly squamous cell carcinoma, in patients having bilharzial infestation *(Schistosoma haematobium)* of the bladder. Schistosomiasis is common in Egypt and accounts for high incidence of bladder cancer in that country.

3. Dietary factors. Certain carcinogenic metabolites of tryptophan are excreted in urine of patients with bladder cancer. These metabolites have been shown to induce bladder cancer in experimental animals.

4. Local lesions. A number of local lesions in the bladder predispose to the development of bladder cancer. These include ectopia vesicae (extrophied bladder), vesical diverticulum, leukoplakia of the bladder mucosa and urinary diversion in defunctionalised bladder.

5. Smoking. Tobacco smoking is associated with 2 to 3 fold increased risk of developing bladder cancer.

6. Drugs. Immunosuppressive therapy with cyclophosphamide and patients having analgesic-abuse (phenacetin-) nephropathy have high risk of developing bladder cancer.

Multicentric nature of urothelial cancer and high rate of recurrence has led to the hypothesis that a *field effect* in the urothelium is responsible for this form of cancer.

G/A Urothelial tumours may be single or multiple. About 90% of the tumours are papillary (non-invasive or invasive), whereas the remaining 10% are flat indurated (non-invasive or invasive). The papillary tumours have free floating fern-like arrangement with a broad or narrow pedicle. The non-papillary tumours are bulkier with ulcerated surface. More common locations for either of the two types are the trigone, the region of ureteral orifices and on the lateral walls.

M/E Urothelial tumours are of 3 cell types—transitional cell, squamous cell, and glandular.

A. TRANSITIONAL CELL TUMOURS. Approximately 90% of all epithelial tumours of the bladder are transitional cell tumours. As stated before, transitional cell papilloma is distinguished by some workers from grade I transitional cell carcinoma (TCC), whereas others do not consider this as a distinct entity. Here, we follow the widely accepted classification of Mostofi (1960) adopted by the American Bladder Tumour Registry that divides TCC into 3 grades.

1. Transitional cell papilloma. Papillomas may occur singly or may be multiple. They are generally small, less than 2 cm in diameter, papillary with branching pattern. Each papilla is composed of fibrovascular stromal core covered by normal-looking transitional cells having normal number of layers (not more than six) in thickness. The individual cells resemble the normal transitional cells and do not vary in size and shape. Mitoses are absent and basal polarity is retained.

2. Transitional cell carcinoma. This is the commonest cancer of the bladder and is divided into 3 grades depending upon 2 features: the *degree of anaplasia* and the *extent of invasion*.

■ The *criteria for anaplasia* are: increased cellularity, nuclear crowding, deranged cellular polarity, failure of normal orientation from base to the surface, variation in cell size and shape, variation in nuclear chromatin pattern, mitotic figures and giant cells.

■ The *criteria for invasion* in papillary as well as non-papillary tumours are: penetration of the basement membrane of bladder mucosa.

Based on these salient features, the characteristics of three grades of transitional cell carcinoma are as under (Table 20.18):

TABLE 20.18: Histologic Classification of Epithelial (Urothelial) Tumours (Mostofi, 1960).

A.	**Transitional cell tumours (90%)**
	1. Transitional cell papilloma
	2. Transitional cell carcinoma (grade I, II and III)
B.	**Carcinoma *in situ***
C.	**Squamous cell carcinoma (5%)**
D.	**Adenocarcinoma (Rare)**
E.	**Mixed carcinoma (5%)**

Grade I: The tumour cells are clearly transitional type but show increased number of layers of cells *(c.f.* transitional cell papilloma). The individual cells are generally regular but are slightly larger and show mild hyperchromatism.

Grade II: The tumour cells are still recognisable as of transitional cell origin and the number of layers of cells is increased. The individual tumour cells are less regular, larger in size, and show pronounced nuclear hyperchromatism, mitotic activity and loss of polarity. The tumour may or may not be invasive.

Grade III: This is the anaplastic or undifferentiated grade of the tumour which is always invasive extending into the bladder wall to variable depth depending upon the clinical stage (described later). The tumour cells are no longer recognisable as of transitional origin. The individual tumour cells show pronounced features of anaplasia such as marked pleomorphism, hyperchromatism, total loss of polarity with loosened surface cells exfoliated in the bladder lumen.

B. CARCINOMA *IN SITU*. Foci of epithelial hyperplasia, dysplasia and carcinoma in situ are seen in other parts of the bladder in non-invasive as well as in invasive carcinomas. Similar foci may be present in the ureters and renal pelvis. The malignant potential of epithelial hyperplasia and dysplasia is uncertain but carcinoma *in situ* is certainly precancerous and is currently included as grade 0 transitional cell carcinoma.

C. SQUAMOUS CELL CARCINOMA. Squamous cell carcinoma comprises about 5% of the bladder carcinomas. Unlike transitional cell carcinomas which are mostly papillary and non-ulcerating, most squamous carcinomas of the bladder are sessile, nodular, infiltrating and ulcerating. Association of squamous carcinoma and schistosomiasis has already been highlighted. The carcinoma may be well-differentiated with keratin pearl formation, or may be anaplastic.

D. ADENOCARCINOMA. Adenocarcinoma of the bladder is rare. Adenocarcinoma has association with exostrophy of the bladder with glandular metaplasia, or may arise from urachal rests, periurethral and periprostatic glands, or from cystitis cystica. The tumour is characterised by glandular and tubular pattern with or without mucus production.

STAGING OF BLADDER CANCER. The clinical behaviour and prognosis of bladder cancer can be assessed by the following simple staging system:
Stage 0: Carcinoma confined to the mucosa.
Stage A: Carcinoma invades the lamina propria but not the muscularis.
Stage B1: Carcinoma invades the superficial muscle layer.
Stage B2: Carcinoma invades the deep muscle layer.
Stage C: Carcinoma invades the perivesical tissues.
Stage D1: Carcinoma shows regional metastases.
Stage D2: Carcinoma shows distant metastases.

Non-epithelial Bladder Tumours *(p. 726)*

MALIGNANT. Rhabdomyosarcoma is the most frequent malignant mesenchymal tumour. It exists in 2 forms:
Adult form occurring in adults over 40 years of age and resembles the rhabdomyosarcoma of skeletal muscle.
Childhood form occurring in infancy and childhood and appears as large polypoid, soft, fleshy, grapelike mass and is also called *sarcoma botryoides* or *embryonal rhabdomyosarcoma*. It is morphologically characterised by masses of embryonic mesenchyme consisting of masses of highly pleomorphic stellate cells in myxomatous background. Similar tumours occur in the female genital tract.

URETHRAL CARUNCLE. Urethral caruncle is not uncommon. It is an inflammatory lesion present on external urethral meatus in elderly females.

G/A The caruncle appears as a solitary, 1 to 2 cm in diameter, pink or red mass, protruding from urethral meatus.

M/E The mass may be covered by squamous or transitional epithelium or there may be ulcerated surface. The underlying tissues show proliferating blood vessels, fibroblastic connective tissue and intense acute and chronic inflammatory infiltrate.

■ SELF ASSESSMENT

1. **Glomerular tuft contains capillaries forming following number of lobules:**
   A. Four B. Six
   C. Eight D. Ten
2. **Azotaemia results from elevation of following waste-products of protein metabolism *except:***
   A. Blood urea B. Blood urea nitrogen
   C. Serum uric acid D. Serum creatinine
3. **In end-stage kidney disease, GFR is:**
   A. 5% of normal B. 10% of normal
   C. 15% of normal D. 20% of normal

4. **Infantile polycystic kidney disease has the following features** *except:*
   A. It has autosomal recessive inheritance
   B. It is invariably bilateral
   C. The condition often manifests in adults
   D. The condition is frequently associated with multiple hepatic cysts

5. **The most common features of nephritic syndrome include the following** *except:*
   A. Heavy proteinuria   B. Hypertension
   C. Microscopic haematuria   D. Oliguria

6. **The most common form of glomerulonephritis (GN) in adults is:**
   A. Minimal change disease   B. Membranous GN
   C. Membranoproliferative GN   D. Focal segmental GN

7. **The most frequent form of primary glomerular disease in children is:**
   A. Minimal change disease   B. Acute glomerulonephritis
   C. Membranous GN   D. Membranoproliferative GN

8. **Examples of immune complex GN include the following** *except:*
   A. Acute GN
   B. Membranous GN
   C. Membranoproliferative GN
   D. RPGN in Goodpasture's disease

9. **Classic example of anti-GBM disease is:**
   A. Minimal change disease   B. Acute GN
   C. Membranous GN   D. Goodpasture's disease

10. **Alternate pathway disease occurs in following forms of glomerular disease** *except:*
    A. Membranous GN
    B. Membranoproliferative GN
    C. Rapidly progressive GN
    D. IgA nephropathy

11. **Acute post-streptococcal GN is characterised by proteinuria of:**
    A. Non-selective   B. Selective
    C. Albuminuria only   D. Low molecular weight only

12. **The serum markers for RPGN are as follows** *except:*
    A. Serum C3 levels
    B. Anti-GBM antibody
    C. Anti-neutrophil cytoplasmic antibody (ANCA)
    D. Anti-endothelial cell antibody (AECA)

13. **In Goodpasture disease, the antigen is:**
    A. Collagen IV of basement membrane   B. DNA
    C. Bacterial products   D. Cationic proteins

14. **Children having minimal change disease have selective proteinuria because of:**
    A. Reduction of negative charge on GBM
    B. Extensive damage to the GBM
    C. Deposits of IgG and C3 on GBM
    D. Increased mesangial matrix in the glomeruli

15. **Majority of cases of membranous glomerulonephritis have following etiology:**
    A. SLE   B. Viral infections
    C. History of drugs   D. Idiopathic

16. **Basement membrane material in membranous glomerulonephritis appears as:**
    A. Dense deposits
    B. Spikes protruding from GBM
    C. Double-contoured
    D. Tram-track

17. **Membranoproliferative glomerulonephritis is characterised by lobular proliferation of:**
    - A. Epithelial cells
    - B. Endothelial cells
    - C. Mesangial cells
    - D. Leucocytes

18. **HIV infection commonly produces the following type of glomerular lesions:**
    - A. Membranous GN
    - B. Membranoproliferative GN
    - C. Focal GN
    - D. Focal segmental glomerulosclerosis

19. **The most common and most severe form of lupus nephritis shows the following lesions:**
    - A. Mesangial lupus nephritis
    - B. Focal segmental lupus nephritis
    - C. Diffuse proliferative lupus nephritis
    - D. Membranous lupus nephritis

20. **In diabetic nephropathy, the following lesions are specific for juvenile-onset diabetes:**
    - A. Diffuse glomerulosclerosis
    - B. Nodular glomerulosclerosis
    - C. Diabetic pyelonephritis
    - D. Armanni-Ebstein lesions

21. **In ischaemic ATN, the following holds true *except*:**
    - A. There is dilatation of proximal and distal convoluted tubules
    - B. There is disruption of tubular basement membrane
    - C. There is diffuse tubular necrosis
    - D. Tubular lumina contain casts

22. **The most common mechanism in pathogenesis of chronic pyelonephritis is:**
    - A. Ascending infection
    - B. Reflux nephropathy
    - C. Obstructive nephropathy
    - D. Haematogenous infection

23. **Nephrocalcinosis is characterised by deposition of calcium salt at the following locations *except*:**
    - A. Basement membrane
    - B. Within mitochondria
    - C. Lysosomes
    - D. Cytoplasm

24. **The causes of renal hypertension include the following *except*:**
    - A. Fibromuscular dysplasia of renal artery
    - B. Polyarteritis nodosa
    - C. Sickle cell nephropathy
    - D. Polycystic kidney disease

25. **Causes of flea-bitten kidney include the following *except*:**
    - A. Acute post-streptococcal GN
    - B. Rapidly progressive GN
    - C. Haemolytic uraemic syndrome
    - D. Benign nephrosclerosis

26. **The following type of renal calculi are radiolucent:**
    - A. Calcium oxalate
    - B. Struvite
    - C. Uric acid
    - D. Calcium phosphate

27. **The following type of renal calculi are infection-induced:**
    - A. Calcium oxalate
    - B. Struvite
    - C. Uric acid
    - D. Cystine

28. **In hereditary renal cell carcinoma (RCC), the following syndrome is implicated in carcinogenesis:**
    - A. von Hippel-Lindau disease
    - B. Polycystic kidney disease
    - C. Alport's syndrome
    - D. Fabry's disease

29. **Out of various histologic types of renal cell carcinoma, the following type has worst prognosis:**
    A. Clear cell type   B. Granular cell type
    C. Sarcomatoid type   D. Papillary type
30. **Malakoplakia of the urinary bladder is a form of:**
    A. Dysplasia   B. Metaplasia
    C. Papillary hyperplasia   D. Chronic inflammation
31. **Schistosomiasis of the urinary bladder is implicated in the following type of bladder tumour:**
    A. Transitional cell carcinoma   B. Squamous cell carcinoma
    C. Adenocarcinoma   D. Adenoacanthoma
32. **Collapsing sclerosis is a feature of following type of primary glomerular disease:**
    A. Membranoproliferative GN
    B. IgA nephropathy
    C. Focal segmental glomerulosclerosis
    D. Focal glomerulonephritis

KEY

1 = C	2 = C	3 = A	4 = C
5 = A	6 = B	7 = A	8 = D
9 = D	10 = A	11 = A	12 = D
13 = A	14 = A	15 = D	16 = B
17 = C	18 = D	19 = C	20 = B
21 = C	22 = B	23 = C	24 = C
25 = D	26 = C	27 = B	28 = A
29 = C	30 = D	31 = B	32 = C

21

The Male Reproductive System and Prostate

TESTIS AND EPIDIDYMIS *(p. 728)*

NORMAL STRUCTURE *(p. 728)*

Contents of the scrotal sac include the testicle and epididymis alongwith lower end of the spermatic cord and the tunica vaginalis that forms the outer serous investing layer. The epididymis is attached to body of the testis posteriorly. Thus, the testicle and epididymis may be regarded as one organ.

Structurally, the main components of the testicle are the seminiferous tubules.

M/E The seminiferous tubules are formed of a lamellar connective tissue membrane and contain several layers of cells. In the adult, the cells lining the seminiferous tubules are of 2 types:

1. *Spermatogonia* or germ cells which produce spermatocytes, spermatids and mature spermatozoa.

2. *Sertoli cells* which are larger and act as supportive cells to germ cells, produce oestrogen and androgen.

The seminiferous tubules drain into collecting ducts which form the rete testis from where the secretions pass into the vasa efferentia. Vasa efferentia opens at the upper end of the epididymis.

The fibrovascular stroma present between the seminiferous tubules contains varying number of *interstitial cells of Leydig.* Leydig cells have abundant cytoplasm containing lipid granules and elongated Reinke's crystals. These cells are the main source of testosterone and other androgenic hormones in males.

Cryptorchidism *(p. 728)*

Cryptorchidism or undescended testis is a condition in which the testicle is arrested at some point in its descent. Its incidence is about 0.2% in adult male population. In 70% of cases, the undescended testis lies in the inguinal ring, in 25% in the abdomen and, in the remaining 5%, it may be present at other sites along its descent from intra-abdominal location to the scrotal sac.

ETIOLOGY. A few apparent causes associated with cryptorchidism are as under:

1. **Mechanical factors** e.g. short spermatic cord, narrow inguinal canal, adhesions to the peritoneum.

2. **Genetic factors** e.g. trisomy 13, maldevelopment of scrotum or cremaster muscles.

3. **Hormonal** factors e.g. deficient androgenic secretions.

Cryptorchidism is unilateral in majority of cases but in 25% of patients, it is bilateral.

G/A The cryptorchid testis is small in size, firm and fibrotic.

M/E Contrary to previous beliefs, the changes of atrophy begin to appear by about 2 years of age.

1. *Seminiferous tubules:* There is progressive loss of germ cell elements so that the tubules may be lined by only spermatogonia and spermatids but foci of spermatogenesis are discernible in 10% of cases. The tubular basement membrane is thickened.

2. *Interstitial stroma:* There is usually increase in the interstitial fibrovascular stroma and conspicuous presence of Leydig cells, seen singly or in small clusters.

CLINICAL FEATURES. As such, cryptorchidism is completely asymptomatic and is discovered only on physical examination. However, if surgical correction by orchiopexy is not undertaken by about 2 years of age, or certainly in the prepubertal period, significant adverse clinical outcome may result:

1. Sterility-infertility. Bilateral cryptorchidism is associated with sterility while unilateral disease may result in infertility.

2. Inguinal hernia. A concomitant inguinal hernia is frequently present alongwith cryptorchidism.

3. Malignancy. Cryptorchid testis is at 35 times increased risk of developing testicular malignancy, most commonly seminoma and embryonal carcinoma, than a normally descended testis.

Male Infertility *(p. 729)*

These causes can be divided into 3 groups:

A. PRE-TESTICULAR CAUSES: 1. Hypopituitarism. 2. Oestrogen excess. 3. Glucocorticoid excess. 4. Other endocrine disorders.

B. TESTICULAR CAUSES: 1. Agonadism 2. Cryptorchidism 3. Maturation arrest 4. Hypospermatogenesis 5. Sertoli cell-only syndrome 6. Klinefelter's syndrome 7. Mumps orchitis 8. Irradiation damage.

C. POST-TESTICULAR CAUSES: 1. Congenital block 2. Acquired 3. Impaired sperm motility.

Non-specific Epididymitis and Orchitis *(p. 730)*

Non-specific epididymitis and orchitis, or their combination, may be acute or chronic. The common routes of spread of infection are via the vas deferens, or via lymphatic and haematogenous routes. Most frequently, the infection is caused by urethritis, cystitis, prostatitis and seminal vesiculitis. Other causes are mumps, smallpox, dengue fever, influenza, pneumonia and filariasis.

G/A In acute stage the testicle is firm, tense, swollen and congested. There may be multiple abscesses, especially in gonorrhoeal infection.

M/E Acute orchitis and epididymitis are characterised by congestion, oedema and diffuse infiltration by neutrophils, lymphocytes, plasma cells and macrophages or formation of neutrophilic abscesses. In chronic epididymo-orchitis, there is focal or diffuse chronic inflammation, disappearance of seminiferous tubules, fibrous scarring and destruction of interstitial Leydig cells.

Granulomatous (Autoimmune) Orchitis *(p. 730)*

Non-tuberculous granulomatous orchitis is a peculiar type of unilateral, painless testicular enlargement in middle-aged men that may resemble a testicular tumour clinically. The exact etiology and pathogenesis of the condition are not known though an autoimmune basis is suspected.

G/A The affected testis is enlarged with thickened tunica. Cut section of the testicle is greyish-white to tan-brown.

M/E There are circumscribed non-caseating granulomas lying within the seminiferous tubules. These granulomas are composed of epithelioid cells, lymphocytes, plasma cells, some neutrophils and multinucleate giant cells. The origin of the epithelioid cells is from Sertoli cells lining the tubules.

Tuberculous Epididymo-orchitis *(p. 730)*

Tuberculosis invariably begins in the epididymis and spreads to involve the testis. Tuberculous epididymo-orchitis is generally secondary tuberculosis from elsewhere in the body.

G/A Discrete, yellowish, caseous necrotic areas are seen.

M/E Numerous tubercles which may coalesce to form large caseous mass are seen. Characteristics of typical tubercles such as epithelioid cells, peripheral mantle of lymphocytes, occasional multinucleate giant cells and central areas of caseation necrosis are seen. Numerous acid-fast bacilli can be demonstrated by Ziehl-Neelsen staining.

Spermatic Granuloma *(p. 731)*

Spermatic granuloma is the term used for development of inflammatory lesions due to invasion of spermatozoa into the stroma.

G/A The sperm granuloma is a small nodule, 3 mm to 3 cm in diameter, firm, white to yellowish-brown.

M/E It consists of a granuloma composed of histiocytes, epithelioid cells, lymphocytes and some neutrophils. Characteristically, the centre of spermatic granuloma contains spermatozoa and necrotic debris.

Elephantiasis *(p. 731)*

Elephantiasis is enormous thickening of the scrotal skin resembling the elephant's hide and results in enlargement of the scrotum. The condition results from filariasis in which the adult worm lives in the lymphatics, while the larvae travel in the blood. The most important variety of filaria is *Wuchereria bancrofti.*

G/A The affected leg and scrotum are enormously thickened with enlargement of regional lymph nodes.

M/E The changes begin with lymphatic obstruction by the adult worms. The worm in alive, dead or calcified form may be found in the dilated lymphatics or in the lymph nodes. Dead or calcified worm in lymphatics is usually followed by lymphangitis with intense infiltration by eosinophils. Chronic lymphoedema with tough subcutaneous fibrosis and epidermal hyperkeratosis develops which is termed elephantiasis.

MISCELLANEOUS LESIONS *(p. 731)*

Torsion of Testis *(p. 731)*

Torsion of the testicle may occur either in a fully-descended testis or in an undescended testis. The latter is more common and more severe. It results from sudden cessation of venous drainage and arterial supply to the testis.

There may be coagulative necrosis of the testis and epididymis, or there may be haemorrhagic infarction.

Varicocele *(p. 731)*

Varicocele is the dilatation, elongation and tortuosity of the veins of the pampiniform plexus in the spermatic cord. It is of 2 types:

■ **Primary or idiopathic form** is more frequent and is common in young unmarried men. It is nearly always on the left side as the loaded rectum presses the left vein.

■ **Secondary form** occurs due to pressure on the spermatic vein by enlarged liver, spleen or kidney.

Hydrocele *(p. 732)*

A hydrocele is abnormal collection of serous fluid in the tunica vaginalis. It may be acute or chronic, congenital or acquired. The usual causes are trauma, systemic oedema such as in cardiac failure and renal disease, and as a complication of gonorrhoea, syphilis and tuberculosis.

Haematocele *(p. 732)*

Haematocele is haemorrhage into the sac of the tunica vaginalis. It may result from direct trauma, from injury to a vein by the needle, or from haemorrhagic diseases.

TESTICULAR TUMOURS *(p. 732)*

Testicular tumours are the cause of about 1% of all cancer deaths. They are more frequent in white male population but are less common in Africans and Asians. They have *trimodal* age distribution—a peak during infancy, another during late adolescence and early adulthood, and a third peak after 60 years of age.

Classification *(p. 732)*

The most widely accepted classification is the histogenetic classification proposed by the World Health Organisation (Table 21.1). Based on this, all testicular tumours are divided into: *germ cell tumours, sex cord-stromal tumours* and *mixed forms*. Vast majority of the testicular tumours (95%) arise from germ cells or their precursors in the seminiferous tubules. From clinical point of view, gem cell tumours of testis are distinguished into 2 main groups— seminomatous and non-seminomatous (Table 21.2).

TABLE 21.1: Classification of Testicular Tumours.

I.	GERM CELL TUMOURS
1.	Seminoma
2.	Spermatocytic seminoma
3.	Embryonal carcinoma
4.	Yolk sac tumour (*Syn.* endodermal sinus tumour, orchio blastoma, infantile type embryonal carcinoma)
5.	Polyembryoma
6.	Choriocarcinoma
7.	Teratomas
	(i) Mature
	(ii) Immature
	(iii) With malignant transformation
8.	Mixed germ cell tumours
II.	**SEX CORD-STROMAL TUMOURS**
1.	Leydig cell tumour
2.	Sertoli cell tumour (Androblastoma)
3.	Granulosa cell tumour
4.	Mixed forms
III.	**COMBINED GERM CELL-SEX CORD-STROMAL TUMOURS**
	Gonadoblastoma
IV.	**OTHER TUMOURS**
1.	Malignant lymphoma (5%)
2.	Rare tumours

Etiologic Factors *(p. 732)*

The cause of testicular germ cell tumours is unknown, but the following factors have been implicated:

1. Cryptorchidism. The probability of a germ cell tumour developing in an undescended testis is 35 times greater than in a normally-descended testis. About 10% of testicular germ cell tumours are associated with cryptorchidism.

TABLE 21.2: Distinguishing Features of Seminomatous (SGCT) and Non-seminomatous (NSGCT) Germ Cell Tumours of Testis.

	FEATURE	SGCT	NSGCT
1.	*Primary tumour*	Larger, confined to testis for sufficient time; testicular contour retained	Smaller, at times indistinct; testicular contour may be distorted
2.	*Metastasis*	Generally to regional lymph nodes	Haematogenous spread early
3.	*Response to radiation*	Radiosensitive	Radioresistant
4.	*Serum markers*	hCG; generally low levels	hCG, AFP, or both; high levels
5.	*Prognosis*	Better	Poor

2. Other developmental disorders. Dysgenetic gonads associated with endocrine abnormalities have higher incidence of development of germ cell tumours.

3. Genetic factors. Genetic factors play a role in the development of germ cell tumours supported by the observation of high incidence in other family members, twins and in white male populations.

4. Other factors. i) Orchitis. ii) Trauma. iii) Carcinogens.

Histogenesis *(p. 733)*

Based on current concepts on histogenesis of testicular tumours, following agreements and disagreements have emerged:

1. Developmental disorders: Disorders such as cryptorchidism, gonadal dysgenesis and androgen insensitivity syndrome are high risk factors for development of testicular germ cell tumours.

2. CIS/ITGCN: A preinvasive stage of carcinoma *in situ* (CIS) termed *intratubular germ cell neoplasia* (ITGCN) generally precedes the development of most of the invasive testicular germ cell tumours in adults. CIS originates from spermatogenic elements.

3. 'Three hit' process: Germ cells in seminiferous tubules undergo activation *('first hit')* before undergoing malignant transformation confined to seminiferous tubules (CIS) *('second hit')* and eventually into invasive stage by some epigenetic phenomena *('third hit')*.

Clinical Features and Diagnosis *(p. 733)*

The usual presenting clinical symptoms of testicular tumours are gradual gonadal enlargement and a dragging sensation in the testis.

SPREAD. Testicular tumours may spread by both lymphatic and haematogenous routes:

■ *Lymphatic spread* occurs to retroperitoneal para-aortic lymph nodes, mediastinal lymph nodes and supraclavicular lymph nodes.

■ *Haematogenous spread* primarily occurs to the lungs, liver, brain and bones.

TUMOUR MARKERS. Germ cell tumours of the testis secrete polypeptide hormones and certain enzymes which can be detected in the blood. Two tumour markers widely used in the diagnosis, staging and monitoring the follow-up of patients with testicular tumours are: human chorionic gonadotropin (hCG) and alpha-foetoprotein (AFP). In addition, carcinoembryonic antigen

Chapter Twenty One

(CEA), human placental lactogen (HPL), placental alkaline phosphatase, testosterone, oestrogen and luteinising hormone may also be elevated.

PROGNOSIS. For selecting post-orchiectomy treatment (radiation, surgery, chemotherapy or all the three) and for monitoring prognosis, 3 clinical stages are defined:

Stage I: tumour confined to the testis.

Stage II: distant spread confined to retroperitoneal lymph nodes below the diaphragm.

Stage III: distant metastases beyond the retroperitoneal lymph nodes.

Seminomas tend to remain localised to the testis (stage I) while non-seminomatous germ cell tumours more often present with advanced clinical disease (stage II and III). Seminomas are extremely radiosensitive while non-seminomatous germ cell tumours are radio-resistant. In general, seminomas have a better prognosis with 90% cure rate while the non-seminomatous tumours behave in a more aggressive manner and have poor prognosis.

GERM CELL TUMOURS *(p. 734)*

Germ cell tumours comprise approximately 95% of all testicular tumours and are more frequent before the age of 45 years. *Testicular germ cell tumours are almost always malignant.*

Intratubular Germ Cell Neoplasia *(p. 735)*

The term intratubular germ cell neoplasia (ITGCN) is used to describe the preinvasive stage of germ cell tumours, notably intratubular seminoma and intratubular embryonal carcinoma. Others have used carcinoma *in situ* (CIS) stage of germ cell tumours as synonymous term.

M/E The malignant atypical tumour cells are restricted to the seminiferous tubules without evident invasion into the interstitium.

Seminoma *(p. 735)*

Seminoma is the commonest malignant tumour of the testis and corresponds to dysgerminoma in the female. It constitutes about 45% of all germ cell tumours, and in another 15% comprises the major component of mixed germ cell tumour. The tumour has a peak incidence in the 4th decade of life and is rare before puberty. Undescended testis harbours seminoma more frequently as compared to other germ cell tumours.

G/A The involved testis is enlarged up to 10 times its normal size but tends to maintain its normal contour since the tumour rarely invades the tunica. Cut section of the affected testis shows homogeneous, grey-white lobulated appearance.

M/E The characteristics are as under:

1. Tumour cells. The seminoma cells generally lie in cords, sheets or columns forming lobules. Typically, in a classic seminoma, the tumour cells are fairly uniform in size with clear cytoplasm and well-defined cell borders. The cytoplasm contains variable amount of glycogen that stains positively with PAS reaction. The nuclei are centrally located, large, hyperchromatic and usually contain 1-2 prominent nucleoli.

2. Stroma. The stroma of seminoma is delicate fibrous tissue which divides the tumour into lobules. The stroma shows a characteristic lymphocytic infiltration, indicative of immunologic response of the host to the tumour. About 20% of the tumours show granulomatous reaction in the stroma.

The *prognosis* of seminoma is better than other germ cell tumours. The tumour is highly radiosensitive.

Spermatocytic Seminoma *(p. 736)*

Spermatocytic seminoma is both clinically and morphologically a distinctive tumour from classic seminoma. It is an uncommon tumour having an incidence of about 5% of all germ cell tumours. Spermatocytic seminoma usually occurs in older patients, generally in 6th decade of life.

G/A Spermatocytic seminoma is homogeneous, larger, softer and more yellowish and gelatinous than the classic seminoma.

M/E The distinctive features are as under:

1. Tumour cells. The tumour cells vary considerably in size from lymphocyte-like to huge mononucleate or multinucleate giant cells. Majority of the tumour cells are, however, of intermediate size. The nuclei of intermediate and large cells have filamentous pattern. Mitoses are often frequent.

2. Stroma. The stroma lacks lymphocytic and granulomatous reaction seen in classic seminoma.

The *prognosis* of spermatocytic seminoma is excellent since the tumour is slow-growing and rarely metastasises.

Embryonal Carcinoma *(p. 736)*

Pure embryonal carcinoma constitutes 30% of germ cell tumours but areas of embryonal carcinoma are present in 40% of germ cell tumours. These tumours are more common in 2nd to 3rd decades of life. About 90% cases are associated with elevation of AFP or hCG or both.

G/A Embryonal carcinoma is usually a small tumour in the testis. It distorts the contour of the testis as it frequently invades the tunica and the epididymis. The cut surface of the tumour is grey-white, soft with areas of haemorrhages and necrosis.

M/E 1. The tumour cells are arranged in a variety of *patterns*—glandular, tubular, papillary and solid.

2. The *tumour cells* are highly anaplastic carcinomatous cells having large size, indistinct cell borders, amphophilic cytoplasm and prominent hyperchromatic nuclei. Mitotic figures and tumour giant cells are frequently present. Haemorrhage and necrosis are common.

3. The *stroma* is not as distinct as in seminoma and may contain variable amount of primitive mesenchyme.

Embryonal carcinoma is more aggressive and less radiosensitive than seminoma. Chemotherapy is considered more effective in treating this tumour.

Yolk Sac Tumour *(Synonyms: Endodermal Sinus Tumour, Orchioblastoma, Infantile Embryonal Carcinoma)* *(p. 736)*

This characteristic tumour is the most common testicular tumour of infants and young children up to the age of 4 years. In adults, however, yolk sac tumour in pure form is rare but may be present as the major component in 40% of germ cell tumours. AFP levels are elevated in 100% cases of yolk sac tumours.

G/A The tumour is generally soft, yellow-white, mucoid with areas of necrosis and haemorrhages.

M/E 1. The tumour cells form a variety of *patterns*—loose reticular network, papillary, tubular and solid arrangement.

2. The *tumour cells* are flattened to cuboid epithelial cells with clear vacuolated cytoplasm.

3. The tumour cells may form distinctive,perivascular structures resembling the yolk sac or endodermal sinuses of the rat placenta called *Schiller-Duval bodies.*

4. There may be presence of both intracellular and extracellular PAS-positive *hyaline globules,* many of which contain AFP.

Polyembryoma *(p. 736)*

Polyembryoma is defined as a tumour composed predominantly of embryoid bodies.

Choriocarcinoma *(p. 737)*

Pure choriocarcinoma is a highly malignant tumour composed of elements consisting of syncytiotrophoblast and cytotrophoblast. However, pure form is extremely rare and occurs more often in combination with other germ cell tumours. The serum and urinary levels of hCG are greatly elevated in 100% cases.

G/A The tumour is usually small and may appear as a soft, haemorrhagic and necrotic mass.

M/E The characteristic feature is the identification of intimately related syncytiotrophoblast and cytotrophoblast without formation of definite placental-type villi.

Teratoma *(p. 737)*

Teratomas are complex tumours composed of tissues derived from more than one of the three germ cell layers—endoderm, mesoderm and ectoderm. Testicular teratomas are more common in infants and children and constitute about 40% of testicular tumours in infants, whereas in adults they comprise 5% of all germ cell tumours.

Testicular teratomas are classified into 3 types: 1. Mature (differentiated) teratoma 2. Immature teratoma 3. Teratoma with malignant transformation.

G/A Most teratomas are large, grey-white masses enlarging the involved testis. Cut surface shows characteristic variegated appearance—grey-white solid areas, cystic and honey-combed areas, and foci of cartilage and bone. Dermoid cysts commonly seen in the ovaries are rare in testicular teratomas.

M/E Three types are recognised:

1. Mature (differentiated) teratoma. Mature teratoma is composed of disorderly mixture of a variety of well-differentiated structures such as cartilage, smooth muscle, intestinal and respiratory epithelium, mucous glands, cysts lined by squamous and transitional epithelium, neural tissue, fat and bone. It is believed that *all testicular teratomas in the adults are malignant.*

As mentioned above, dermoid cysts similar to those of the ovary are rare in the testis.

2. Immature teratoma. Immature teratoma is composed of incompletely differentiated and primitive or embryonic tissues alongwith some mature elements. Primitive or embryonic tissue commonly present are poorly-formed cartilage, mesenchyme, neural tissues.

3. Teratoma with malignant transformation. This is an extremely rare form of teratoma in which one or more of the tissue elements show malignant transformation.

Mixed Germ Cell Tumours *(p. 737)*

About 60% of germ cell tumours have more than one of the above histologic types (except spermatocytic seminoma) and are called mixed germ cell tumours.

The most common combinations of mixed germ cell tumours are:

1. teratoma, embryonal carcinoma, yolk sac tumour and syncytiotrophoblast;
2. embryonal carcinoma and teratoma (teratocarcinoma); and
3. seminoma and embryonal carcinoma.

SEX CORD-STROMAL TUMOURS *(p. 738)*

Tumours arising from specialised gonadal stroma are classified on the basis of histogenesis. The primitive mesenchyme which forms the specialised stroma of gonads in either sex gives rise to theca, granulosa and lutein cells in the female, and Sertoli and interstitial Leydig cells in the male. Since the cell of origin of primitive mesenchyme is identical, Sertoli and interstitial Leydig cell tumours may occur in the ovaries (in addition to theca cell, granulosa cell and lutein cell tumours). Likewise, the latter three tumours may occur in the testis (in addition to Sertoli cell and Leydig cell tumours). All these tumours secrete various hormones. The biologic behaviour of these tumours generally cannot be determined on histological grounds alone.

Malignant Lymphoma *(p. 739)*

Malignant lymphomas comprises 5% of testicular malignancies and is the most common testicular tumour in the elderly. Bilaterality is seen in half the cases. Most common are large cell non-Hodgkin's lymphoma of B cell type.

PENIS *(p. 739)*

NORMAL STRUCTURE *(p. 739)*

The penis is covered by skin, foreskin (prepuce) and stratified squamous mucosa. The structure of penis consists of 3 masses of erectile tissue—the two corpora cavernosa, one on each side dorsally, and the corpus spongiosum ventrally through which the urethra passes. The expanded free end of the corpus spongiosum forms the glans.

The lumen of the urethra in sectioned surface of the penis appears as an irregular cleft in the middle of the corpus spongiosum. In the prostatic part, it is lined by transitional epithelium, but elsewhere it is lined by columnar epithelium except near its orifice where stratified squamous epithelium lines it.

ANOMALIES AND INFLAMMATIONS *(p. 739)*

Phimosis *(p. 739)*

Phimosis is a condition in which the prepuce is too small to permit its normal retraction behind the glans. It may be congenital or acquired. *Congenital phimosis* is a developmental anomaly whereas *acquired phimosis* may result from inflammation, trauma or oedema leading to narrowing of preputial opening.

Hypospadias and Epispadias *(p. 739)*

Hypospadias is a developmental defect of the urethra in which the urethral meatus fails to reach the end of the penis, but instead, opens on the ventral surface of the penis. Similar developmental defect with resultant urethral opening on the dorsal surface of the penis is termed *epispadias.*

Balanoposthitis *(p. 739)*

Balanoposthitis is the term used for non-specific inflammation of the inner surface of the prepuce *(balanitis)* and adjacent surface of the glans *(posthitis).*

Balanitis Xerotica Obliterans *(p. 740)*

Balanitis xerotica obliterans is a white atrophic lesion on the glans penis and the prepuce and is a counterpart of the *lichen sclerosus et atrophicus* in the vulva.

BENIGN TUMOURS *(p. 740)*

Condyloma Acuminatum *(p. 740)*

Condyloma acuminatum or venereal wart is a benign tumour caused by human papilloma virus (HPV) types 6 and 11. The tumour may occur singly, or there may be conglomerated papillomas. A more extensive, solitary, exophytic and cauliflower-like warty mass is termed *giant condyloma or Buschke-Löwenstein tumour or verrucous carcinoma.*

G/A The tumour consists of solitary or multiple, warty, cauliflower-shaped lesions of variable size with exophytic growth pattern.

M/E The lesions are essentially like common warts (verruca vulgaris). The features include formation of papillary villi composed of connective tissue stroma and covered by squamous epithelium which shows hyperkeratosis, parakeratosis, and hyperplasia of prickle cell layer. Many of the prickle cells show clear vacuolisation of the cytoplasm (*koilocytosis*) indicative of HPV infection.

PREMALIGNANT LESIONS (CARCINOMA *IN SITU*) *(p. 740)*

The following three lesions display cytological changes of malignancy confined to epithelial layers only without evidence of invasion.

Bowen's Disease. Bowen's disease is located on the shaft of the penis and the scrotum besides the sun-exposed areas of the skin. A fair proportion of cases of Bowen's disease are associated with internal visceral cancers.

Erythroplasia of Queyrat. The lesions of erythroplasia of Queyrat appear on the penile mucosa.

Bowenoid Papulosis. The lesions of bowenoid papulosis appear on the penile shaft and adjacent genital skin.

SQUAMOUS CELL CARCINOMA *(p. 740)*

The incidence of penile carcinoma shows wide variation in different populations. In the United States, the overall incidence of penile cancer is less than 2% of all cancers but it is 3-4 times more common in blacks than in whites. In India, cancer of the penis is rare in Muslims who practice circumcision as a religious rite in infancy, whereas Hindus who do not normally circumcise have higher incidence. The greatest incidence of penile cancer is between 45 and 60 years.

G/A The tumour is located, in decreasing frequency, on frenum, prepuce, glans and coronal sulcus. The tumour may be cauliflower-like and papillary, or flat and ulcerating.

M/E Squamous cell carcinoma of both fungating and ulcerating type is generally well differentiated to moderately-differentiated type.

PROSTATE *(p. 741)*

NORMAL STRUCTURE *(p. 741)*

The prostate gland in the normal adult weighs approximately 20 gm. It surrounds the commencement of the urethra in the male and is composed of 5 lobes during embryonic development—anterior, middle, posterior and two lateral lobes. But at birth, the five lobes fuse to form 3 distinct lobes—two major lateral lobes and a small median lobe.

M/E The prostate is composed of tubular alveoli (acini) embedded in fibromuscular tissue mass. The glandular epithelium forms infoldings and consists of 2 layers—a basal layer of low cuboidal cells and an inner layer of mucus-secreting tall columnar cells. The alveoli are separated by thick fibromuscular septa containing abundant smooth muscle fibres.

Based on hormonal responsiveness, the prostate is divided into 2 separate parts:

- *the inner periurethral female part* which is sensitive to oestrogen and androgen; and
- *outer subcapsular true male part* which is sensitive to androgen.

While benign nodular hyperplasia occurs in the periurethral part distorting and compressing the centrally located urethral lumen, the prostatic carcinoma usually arises from the outer subcapsular part in which case it does not compress the urethra.

PROSTATITIS *(p. 741)*

Inflammation of the prostate i.e. prostatitis, may be acute, chronic and granulomatous types.

Acute Prostatitis *(p. 742)*

Acute focal or diffuse suppurative inflammation of the prostate is not uncommon. It occurs most commonly due to ascent of bacteria from the urethra, less often by descent from the upper urinary tract or bladder, and occasionally by lymphogenous or haematogenous spread from a distant focus of infection. The diagnosis is made by culture of urine specimen.

G/A The prostate is enlarged, swollen and tense. Cut section shows multiple abscesses and foci of necrosis.

M/E The prostatic acini are dilated and filled with neutrophilic exudate. There may be diffuse acute inflammatory infiltrate.

Chronic Prostatitis *(p. 742)*

Chronic prostatitis is more common and foci of chronic inflammation are frequently present in the prostate of men above 40 years of age.

Chronic prostatitis is of 2 types—bacterial and abacterial.

- **Chronic bacterial prostatitis** is caused in much the same way and by the same organisms as the acute prostatitis. It is generally a consequence of recurrent UTI. Diagnosis is made by detection of more than 10-12 leucocytes per high power field in expressed prostatic secretions.

- **Chronic abacterial prostatitis** is more common these days. There is no history of recurrent UTI and culture of urine and prostatic secretions is always negative.

G/A The prostate may be enlarged, fibrosed and shrunken.

M/E The diagnosis of chronic prostatitis is made by foci of lymphocytes, plasma cells, macrophages and neutrophils within the prostatic substance. Corpora amylacea, prostatic calculi and foci of squamous metaplasia in the prostatic acini may accompany inflammatory changes.

Granulomatous Prostatitis *(p. 742)*

Granulomatous prostatitis is a variety of chronic prostatitis, probably caused by leakage of prostatic secretions into the tissue, or could be of autoimmune origin.

NODULAR HYPERPLASIA *(p. 743)*

Non-neoplastic tumour-like enlargement of the prostate, commonly termed benign nodular hyperplasia (BNH) or benign enlargement of prostate (BEP), is a very common condition in men and considered by some as normal ageing process. It becomes increasingly more frequent above the age of 50 years and its incidence approaches 75-80% in men above 80 years.

ETIOLOGY. The cause of BEP has not been fully established. However, a few etiologic factors such as *endocrinologic, racial, inflammation* and *arteriosclerosis* have been implicated but endocrine basis for hyperplasia has been more fully investigated and considered a strong possibility in its genesis. A plausible hypothesis suggested is that there is synergistic stimulation of the prostate by both hormones—the *oestrogen* acting to sensitise the prostatic tissue to the growth promoting effect of *dihydroxy-testosterone* derived from plasma testosterone.

G/A The enlarged prostate is nodular, smooth and firm and weighs 2-4 times its normal weight i.e. may weigh up to 40-80 gm. The appearance on cut section varies depending upon whether the hyperplasia is predominantly of the glandular or fibromuscular tissue.

M/E In every case, there is hyperplasia of all three tissue elements in varying proportions—glandular, fibrous and muscular.

■ *Glandular hyperplasia* predominates in most cases and is identified by exaggerated intra-acinar papillary infoldings with delicate fibrovascular cores.

■ *Fibromuscular hyperplasia* when present as dominant component appears as aggregates of spindle cells forming an appearance akin to fibromyoma of the uterus.

CLINICAL FEATURES. Clinically, the symptomatic cases develop symptoms due to complications such as urethral obstruction and secondary effects on the bladder (e.g. hypertrophy, cystitis), ureter (e.g. hydroureter) and kidneys (e.g. hydronephrosis). The presenting features include frequency, nocturia, difficulty in micturition, pain, haematuria and sometimes, the patients present with acute retention of urine requiring immediate catheterisation.

CARCINOMA OF PROSTATE *(p. 744)*

Cancer of the prostate is the second most common form of cancer in males, followed in frequency by lung cancer. It is a disease of men above the age of 50 years and its prevalence increases with increasing age so that more than 50% of men 80 years old have asymptomatic (latent) carcinoma of the prostate. It is common to classify carcinoma of the prostate into the following 4 types:

1. Latent carcinoma. This is found unexpectedly as a small focus of carcinoma in the prostate during autopsy studies in men dying of other causes.

2. Incidental carcinoma. About 15-20% of prostatectomies done for BEP reveal incidental carcinoma of the prostate.

3. Occult carcinoma. This is the type in which the patient has no symptoms of prostatic carcinoma but shows evidence of metastases on clinical examination and investigations.

4. Clinical carcinoma. Clinical prostatic carcinoma is the type detected by rectal examination and other investigations and confirmed by pathologic examination of biopsy of the prostate.

ETIOLOGY. A few factors have been suspected. These are as under:

1. Endocrinologic factors. Androgens are considered essential for development and maintenance of prostatic epithelium. The etiologic role of androgens is supported by the following indirect evidences:

i) Orchiectomy causes arrest of metastatic prostatic cancer disease (testis being the main source of testosterone).

ii) Administration of oestrogen causes regression of prostatic carcinoma.

iii) Cancer of the prostate is extremely rare in eunuchs and in patients with Klinefelter's syndrome.

iv) Cancer of the prostate begins at the stage of life when androgen levels are high. However, the cancer may remain latent with decline in androgen level with advancing age.

2. Racial and geographic influences. It is uncommon in Japanese and Chinese, while the prevalence is high in Americans. American blacks have a markedly higher incidence as compared to whites.

3. Environmental influences. It is possible that some common, as yet unidentified, environmental factors and carcinogens may play a role in the evolution of prostatic cancer.

4. Nodular hyperplasia. Though nodular prostatic hyperplasia has been suggested by some as precursor for development of prostatic cancer, it is considered unlikely. Most prostatic cancers develop in the periphery of the gland while BEP occurs in the periurethral part of the gland.

5. Genetic factors. The possibility of genetic basis of prostatic cancer has been suggested by the observations of familial clustering and in first degree relatives.

HISTOGENESIS. Histogenesis of prostatic adenocarcinoma has been documented recently as arising from premalignant stage of *prostatic intraepithelial neoplasia (PIN).* PIN refers to multiple foci of cytologically atypical luminal cells overlying diminished number of basal cells in prostatic ducts and is a forerunner of invasive prostatic carcinoma.

G/A The prostate may be enlarged, normal in size or smaller than normal. In 95% of cases, prostatic carcinoma is located in the peripheral zone, especially in the posterior lobe. The malignant prostate is firm and fibrous. Cut section is homogeneous and contains irregular yellowish areas.

M/E Four histologic types are described—adenocarcinoma, transitional cell carcinoma, squamous cell carcinoma and undifferentiated carcinoma. However, *adenocarcinoma* is the most common type found in 96% of cases and is the one generally referred to as carcinoma of the prostate. The other three histologic types are rare and resemble in morphology with similar malignant tumours elsewhere in the body. The histologic characteristics of adenocarcinoma of the prostate are as under:

1.   **Architectural disturbance:** In contrast to convoluted appearance of the glands seen in normal and hyperplastic prostate, there is loss of intra-acinar papillary convolutions. The groups of acini are either closely packed in back-to-back arrangement without intervening stroma or are haphazardly distributed.

2.   **Stroma:** Normally, fibromuscular sling surrounds the acini, whereas malignant acini have little or no stroma between them.

3.   **Gland pattern:** Most frequently, the glands in well-differentiated prostatic adenocarcinoma are small or medium-sized, lined by a single layer of cuboidal or low columnar cells. Moderately-differentiated tumours have cribriform or fenestrated glandular appearance. Poorly-differentiated tumours have little or no glandular arrangement.

4.   **Tumour cells:** In many cases, the individual tumour cells in prostatic carcinoma do not show usual morphologic features of malignancy. The tumour cells may be clear, dark and eosinophilic cells. *Clear cells* have foamy cytoplasm, *dark cells* have homogeneous basophilic cytoplasm, and *eosinophilic cells* have granular cytoplasm.

Chapter Twenty One

5.   Invasion: One of the important diagnostic features of malignancy in prostate is the early and frequent occurrence of invasion of intra-prostatic *perineural spaces*.

SPREAD. The tumour may spread directly and by distant routes.

Direct spread. Direct extension of the tumour occurs into the prostatic capsule and beyond.

Metastases. Distant spread occurs by both lymphatic and haematogenous routes. The rich lymphatic network surrounding the prostate is the main mode of spread to the sacral, iliac and para-aortic lymph nodes. The earliest metastases occur to the obturator lymph node. Haematogenous spread leads most often to osteoblastic *osseous metastases,* especially to pelvis, and lumbar spine; other sites are lungs, kidneys, breast and brain.

CLINICAL FEATURES. By the time symptoms appear, the carcinoma of prostate is usually palpable on rectal examination. In such symptomatic cases, clinical features are: urinary obstruction with dysuria, frequency, retention of urine, haematuria, and in 10% of cases pain in the back due to skeletal metastases. Per-rectal examination shows a hard and nodular gland fixed to the surrounding tissues.

Clinical staging of carcinoma prostate takes into account the following:

■   The tumour found incidentally or a clinically unsuspected cancer in prostate removed for benign disorder *(Stage A).*

■   The tumour palpable by rectal digital examination but confined to the prostate *(Stage B).*

■   The tumour has extended locally beyond the prostate into the surrounding tissues *(Stage C).*

■   The tumour is associated with distant metastases *(Stage D).*

Such clinical staging has good correlation with histologic grading and, thus, has a prognostic significance. *Mostofi's (WHO) histologic grading* categorising prostate cancer into grade I (well-differentiated), grade II (moderately differentiated) and grade III (poorly differentiated) has largely been replaced with *Gleason's microscopic grading system* which is based on two features:

i)   the degree of glandular differentiation; and

ii)   the growth pattern of the tumour in relation to the stroma.

The diagnosis of prostatic carcinoma is made by cytologic, biochemical, radiologic, ultrasonographic and pathologic methods. Two **tumour markers** employed commonly for diagnosis and monitoring the prognosis of prostatic carcinoma are as under:

■   **Prostatic acid phosphatase (PAP)** is secreted by prostatic epithelium. Elevation of serum level of PAP is found in cases of prostatic cancer which have extended beyond the capsule or have metastasised. A reading of 3-5 KA units (normal 1-3 KA units) is highly suspicious but above 5 KA units is diagnostic of prostatic carcinoma.

■   **Prostate-specific antigen (PSA)** can be detected by immunohistochemical method in the malignant prostatic epithelium as well as in the serum. PSA assay is also useful in deciding whether the metastasis originated from the prostate or not. PSA assay is also helpful in distinguishing high-grade prostatic cancer from urothelial carcinoma.

Treatment of prostatic carcinoma consists of surgery, radiotherapy and hormonal therapy. The hormonal dependence of cancer of prostate consists of depriving the tumour cells of growth-promoting influence of testosterone. This can be achieved by orchiectomy and by administration of oestrogen.

■ SELF ASSESSMENT

1. **In an undescended testis the risk of developing a testicular malignancy is increased to average of:**
   A. 20 fold
   B. 25 fold
   C. 30 fold
   D. 35 fold

2. **In an undescended testis, the following tumour develops most often:**
   A. Seminoma
   B. Teratoma
   C. Choriocarcinoma
   D. Yolk sac tumour

3. **Granulomatous orchitis is the term used for inflammation of testis due to following etiology:**
   A. Tuberculosis
   B. Sarcoidosis
   C. Autoimmune
   D. Leprosy

4. **The origin of epithelioid cells in autoimmune orchitis is from:**
   A. Macrophages
   B. Sertoli cells
   C. Leydig cells
   D. Spermatogenic cells

5. **Seminoma is a:**
   A. Benign tumour
   B. Borderline tumour
   C. Malignant tumour
   D. Locally aggressive tumour

6. **Peak incidence of seminoma is in:**
   A. Infancy
   B. Adolescence
   C. Adults
   D. Old age

7. **Spermatocytic seminoma differs from classic seminoma in the following respects** *except:*
   A. It occurs in older age (past 6th decade)
   B. Tumour cells are pleomorphic
   C. The stroma lacks lymphocytic infiltrate
   D. The tumour has worse prognosis

8. **AFP levels are elevated in 100% cases of following type of germ cell tumour:**
   A. Seminoma
   B. Embryonal carcinoma
   C. Yolk sac tumour
   D. Choriocarcinoma

9. **All types of testicular teratomas in adults are:**
   A. Benign tumours
   B. Borderline tumours
   C. Locally aggressive tumours
   D. Malignant tumours

10. **The most common testicular tumour in the elderly is:**
    A. Seminoma
    B. Teratoma
    C. Malignant lymphoma
    D. Leydig cell tumour

11. **The following penile lesions are considered as** *in situ* **carcinoma** *except:*
    A. Condyloma acuminatum
    B. Bowen's disease
    C. Erythroplasia of Queyrat
    D. Bowenoid papulosis

12. **Prostatic hyperplasia affects most often:**
    A. Peripheral prostate
    B. Periurethral prostate
    C. Capsule of prostate
    D. Entire prostate

13. **Normally prostatic tissue responds to hormones as under:**
    A. Periurethral prostate responds to oestrogen as well as androgen
    B. Outer prostate responds to androgen as well as oestrogen
    C. Periurethral prostate responds to rising level of oestrogen
    D. Outer prostate responds to rising level of oestrogen

14. **Prostatic acid phosphatase (PAP) levels given below are diagnostic of prostatic carcinoma:**
    A. 1-2 KA units
    B. 2-3 KA units
    C. 3-5 KA units
    D. 5-7 KA units

15. **Metastasis to the following tissues occur early in prostatic carcinoma:**
    - A. Vertebrae
    - B. Obturator lymph node
    - C. Lungs
    - D. Brain

16. **Areas of intratubular germ cell neoplasia (ITGCN) are frequently found in seminiferous tubules adjacent to the following tumours:**
    - A. Seminoma
    - B. Spermatocytic seminoma
    - C. Embryonal carcinoma
    - D. Immature teratoma

KEY

1 = D	2 = A	3 = C	4 = B
5 = C	6 = C	7 = D	8 = C
9 = D	10 = C	11 = A	12 = B
13 = A	14 = D	15 = B	16 = B

22

The Female Genital Tract

VULVA (p. 747)

The vulva consists of structures of ectodermal origin—labia majora, labia minora, mons pubis, clitoris, vestibule, hymen, Bartholin's glands and minor vestibular glands. The mons pubis and labia majora are covered externally by skin with hair follicles, sebaceous glands and sweat glands including apocrine glands. The inner surface of labia majora, labia minora and vestibule are covered by stratified squamous epithelium.

BARTHOLIN'S CYST AND ABSCESS (p. 747)

Inflammation of Bartholin's vulvovaginal glands (Bartholin's adenitis) may occur due to bacterial infection, notably gonorrhoeal infection. Infection may be *acute* or *chronic*.

■ **Acute Bartholin's adenitis** occurs from obstruction and dilatation of the duct by infection resulting in formation of a Bartholin's abscess.

M/E shows the usual appearance of acute suppurative inflammation with neutrophilic infiltration, hyperaemia, oedema and epithelial degeneration.

■ **Chronic Bartholin's adenitis** results from a less virulent infection so that the process is slow and prolonged. In either case, the chronic inflammatory process terminates into fluid-filled Bartholin's cyst.

M/E shows variable lining of the cyst varying from the transitional epithelium of the normal duct to a flattened lining because of increased intracystic pressure. The cyst wall may show chronic inflammatory infiltrate and a few mucus-secreting acini.

NON-NEOPLASTIC EPITHELIAL DISORDERS (p. 748)

The older term vulvar dystrophy has been replaced by non-neoplastic epithelial disorders of skin and mucosa of vulva. The term is applied to chronic lesions of the vulva characterised clinically by white, plaque-like, pruritic mucosal thickenings and pathologically by disorders of epithelial growth. Clinicians often use the term *'leukoplakia'* for such white lesions. Currently, non-neoplastic epithelial disorders of skin of vulva includes 2 lesions:

1. Lichen sclerosus (older term: atrophic dystrophy).
2. Squamous hyperplasia (older term: hyperplastic dystrophy).

Lichen Sclerosus (p. 748)

Lichen sclerosus may occur anywhere in the skin but is more common and more extensive in the vulva in post-menopausal women. The lesions may extend from vulva onto the perianal and perineal area. Clinically, the patient, usually a post-menopausal woman, complains of intense pruritus which may produce excoriation of the affected skin. Eventually, there is progressive shrinkage and atrophy resulting in narrowing of the introitus, clinically referred to as *kraurosis vulvae*.

M/E 1. Hyperkeratosis of the surface layer.
2. Thinning of the epidermis with disappearance of rete ridges.
3. Amorphous homogeneous degenerative change in the dermal collagen.
4. Chronic inflammatory infiltrate in the mid-dermis.

Lichen sclerosus is *not* a premalignant lesion and responds favourably to topical treatment with androgens.

Squamous Hyperplasia *(p. 748)*

Squamous hyperplasia is characterised by white, thickened vulvar lesions which are usually itchy. The cause is unknown but symptomatic relief results from use of topical treatment with corticosteroids.

M/E 1. Hyperkeratosis.

2. Hyperplasia of squamous epithelium with elongation of rete ridges.
3. Increased mitotic activity of squamous layers but cytologically no atypia.
4. Chronic inflammatory infiltrate in the underlying dermis.

A small proportion of cases of hyperplastic dystrophy (1-4%) may show cytologic atypia and produce vulvar dysplasia which may progress to vulvar carcinoma *in situ* and invasive carcinoma.

VULVAL TUMOURS *(p. 748)*

Stromal Polyps *(p. 749)*

Stromal (fibroepithelial) polyps or acrochordons may form in the vulva or vagina. There may be single or multiple polypoid masses.

M/E They are covered by an orderly stratified squamous epithelium. The stroma consists of loose fibrous and myxomatous connective tissue with some adipose tissue and blood vessels.

Papillary Hidradenoma (Hidradenoma Papilliferum) *(p. 749)*

This is a benign tumour arising from apocrine sweat glands of the vulva.

M/E The tumour lies in the dermis under a normal epidermis. The tumour consists of papillary structures composed of fibrovascular stalk and covered by double layer of epithelial cells.

Condyloma Acuminatum *(p. 749)*

Condyloma acuminata or venereal warts are benign papillary lesions of squamous epithelium which can be transmitted venereally to male sex partner. They may be solitary but more frequently are multiple forming soft warty masses. The common locations are the anus, perineum, vaginal wall, vulva and vagina. They are induced by human papilloma virus (HPV), particularly type 6 and 11.

M/E They are identical to their counterparts on male external genitalia. The features consist of a tree-like proliferation of stratified squamous epithelium, showing marked acanthosis, hyperkeratosis, parakeratosis, papillomatosis and perinuclear vacuolisation of epithelium called *koilocytosis,* indicative of HPV infection.

Condylomas are benign lesions and regress spontaneously except in immunosuppressed individuals.

Extra-Mammary Paget's Disease *(p. 749)*

Paget's disease of the vulva is a rare condition which has skin manifestations like those of Paget's disease of the nipple. The affected skin appears as map-like, red, scaly, elevated and indurated area, most frequently on the labia majora.

M/E Extra-mammary Paget's disease is identified by the presence of large, pale, carcinoma cells lying singly or in small clusters within the epidermis and adnexal structures. These cells characteristically have halo which stains positively with PAS, alcian blue and mucicarmine and are thus believed to be of apocrine epithelial origin.

Unlike Paget's disease of the breast in which case there is always an underlying ductal carcinoma, extra-mammary Paget's disease is confined to epidermis in most cases and only a small proportion of cases have an underlying adenocarcinoma.

Carcinoma and Vulval Intraepithelial Neoplasia *(p. 749)*

Squamous cell carcinoma and vulval intraepithelial neoplasia (VIN) are morphologically similar to those in the cervix and vagina. The etiologic role of certain viruses in carcinogenesis, particularly HPV types 16 and 18, in these sites is well known (high risk types). Vulval carcinoma constitutes 3% of all female genital tract cancers. The usual age for development of cancer or VIN is the 4th to 6th decade.

G/A VIN and vulval carcinoma in early stage is a 'white' lesion (leukoplakia) while later the area develops an exophytic or endophytic (ulcerative) growth pattern.

M/E These lesions are squamous cell type with varying anaplasia and depth of invasion depending upon the stage. HPV-positive tumours are more often poorly-differentiated squamous cell carcinoma while HPV-negative are well-differentiated keratinising type. *Verrucous carcinoma* is a rare variant which is a fungating tumour but is locally malignant.

VAGINA *(p. 750)*

NORMAL STRUCTURE *(p. 750)*

The vagina consists of a collapsed cylinder extending between vestibule externally and the cervix internally.

M/E The vaginal wall consists of 3 layers: an *outer* fibrous, a *middle* muscular and an *inner* epithelial. The muscular coat has a double layer of smooth muscle. The epithelial layer consists of stratified squamous epithelium which undergoes cytologic changes under hormonal stimuli.

VAGINITIS *(p. 750)*

The adult vaginal mucosa is relatively resistant to gonococcal infection because of its histology. However, certain other infections are quite common in the vagina. These are:

■ Bacterial e.g. streptococci, staphylococci, *Escherichia coli, Haemophilus vaginalis.*
■ Fungal e.g. *Candida albicans.*
■ Protozoal e.g. *Trichomonas vaginalis.*
■ Viral e.g. Herpes simplex.

The most common causes of vaginitis are *Candida* (moniliasis) and *Trichomonas* (trichomoniasis). The hyphae of *Candida* can be seen in the vaginal smears. Similarly, the protozoa, *Trichomonas,* can be identified in smears.

TUMOURS *(p. 750)*

Vaginal cysts such as Gartner's duct (Wolffian) cyst lined by glandular epithelium and vaginal inclusion cyst arising from inclusion of vaginal epithelium are more common benign vaginal neoplasms.

Chapter Twenty Two

Carcinoma of Vagina *(p. 750)*

Primary carcinoma of the vagina is an uncommon tumour. Squamous cell dysplasia or vaginal intraepithelial neoplasia occur less frequently as compared to the cervix or vulva and can be detected by Pap smears. Invasive carcinoma of the vagina includes two types:
1. Squamous cell carcinoma
2. Adenocarcinoma of the vagina

Embryonal Rhabdomyosarcoma (Sarcoma Botyroides) *(p. 751)*

This is an unusual and rare malignant tumour occurring in infants and children under 5 years of age. The common location is anterior vaginal wall. Similar tumours may occur in the urinary bladder, orbit, external auditory canal and biliary tract.

G/A The tumour is characterised by bulky and polypoid grape-like mass *(botyroides* = grape) that fills and projects out of the vagina.

M/E 1. Groups of round to fusiform tumour cells are characteristically lying underneath the vaginal epithelium, called *cambium layer* of tumour cells.

2. The central core of polypoid masses is composed of loose and myxoid stroma with many inflammatory cells.

The tumour invades extensively in the pelvis and metastasises to regional lymph nodes and distant sites such as to lungs and liver.

CERVIX *(p. 751)*

The cervix consists of an *internal os* communicating with the endometrial cavity above, and an *external os* opening into the vagina below. *Ectocervix* (exocervix) or *portio vaginalis* is the part of the cervix exposed to the vagina and is lined by stratified squamous epithelium, whereas the endocervix is continuous with the endocervical canal and is lined by a single layer of tall columnar mucus-secreting epithelium. The junction of the ectocervix and endocervix—*junctional mucosa,* consists of gradual transition between squamous and columnar epithelia (squamo-columnar junction) and is clinically and pathologically significant landmark.

CERVICITIS *(p. 751)*

Some degree of cervical inflammation is present in virtually all multiparous women and some nulliparous women.

Cervicitis may be specific or nonspecific, acute or chronic. *Specific cervicitis* may be caused by tuberculosis, syphilis, granuloma inguinale, lymphogranuloma venereum, chlamydia and chancroid. *Nonspecific cervicitis* is more frequent and is generally divided into acute and chronic forms, the latter being quite common.

ACUTE CERVICITIS. Acute cervicitis is usually associated with puerperium or gonococcal infection.

G/A The cervix shows everted endocervical mucosa which is red and oedematous.

M/E There is infiltration of the subepithelial and periglandular tissue with neutrophils, and there is oedema and congestion.

CHRONIC CERVICITIS. Chronic nonspecific cervicitis is encountered quite frequently and is the common cause of leukorrhoea. The most common organisms responsible for chronic cervicitis are the normal mixed vaginal flora that includes streptococci, enterococci (e.g. *E. coli*) and staphylococci. Other infecting organisms include gonococci, *Trichomonas vaginalis, Candida albicans* and herpes simplex.

G/A There is eversion of ectocervix with hyperaemia, oedema and granular surface. Nabothian (retention) cysts may be grossly visible from the surface as pearly grey vesicles.

M/E Chronic cervicitis is characterised by extensive subepithelial inflammatory infiltrate of lymphocytes, plasma cells, large mononuclear cells and a few neutrophils. There may be formation of lymphoid follicles termed *follicular cervicitis.* The surface epithelium may be normal, or may show squamous metaplasia. The squamous epithelium of the ectocervix in cases of uterine prolapse may develop surface keratinisation and hyperkeratosis, so called *epidermidisation.*

TUMOURS *(p. 752)*

Cervical Polyps *(p. 752)*

Cervical polyps are localised benign proliferations of endocervical mucosa though they may protrude through the external os.

G/A Cervical polyp is a small (upto 5 cm in size), bright red, fragile growth which is frequently pedunculated but may be sessile.

M/E Most cervical polyps are endocervical polyps and are covered with endocervical epithelium which may show squamous metaplasia.

Microglandular Hyperplasia *(p. 752)*

Microglandular hyperplasia is a benign condition of the cervix in which there is closely packed proliferation of endocervical glands without intervening stroma. The condition is caused by progestrin stimulation such as during pregnancy, postpartum period and in women taking oral contraceptives.

Squamous Intraepithelial Lesion (SIL)
(Cervical Intraepithelial Neoplasia, CIN) *(p. 752)*

TERMINOLOGY. Presently, the terms dysplasia, CIN, carcinoma *in situ,* and SIL are used synonymously.

DYSPLASIA. The term 'dysplasia' (meaning 'bad moulding') is commonly used for atypical cytologic changes in the layers of squamous epithelium, the changes being progressive. Depending upon the thickness of squamous epithelium involved by atypical cells, dysplasia is conventionally graded as *mild, moderate* and *severe.* Carcinoma *in situ* is the full-thickness involvement by atypical cells, or in other words carcinoma confined to layers above the basement membrane.

CIN. An alternative classification is to group various grades of dysplasia and carcinoma *in situ* together into cervical intraepithelial neoplasia (CIN) which is similarly graded from grade I to III:

■ *CIN-1* represents less than one-third involvement of the thickness of epithelium (mild dysplasia);

■ *CIN-2* is one-third to two-third involvement (moderate dysplasia); and

■ *CIN-3* is full-thickness involvement or equivalent to carcinoma *in situ* (severe dysplasia and carcinoma *in situ*).

SIL. More recently, the National Cancer Institute (NCI) of the US has proposed the *Bethesda System* for reporting cervical and vaginal cytopathology. According to the Bethesda system, the three grades of CIN are readjusted to two grades of squamous intraepithelial lesions (SIL) termed as under:

■ *L-SIL* corresponds to CIN-1 and is a flat condyloma, having koilocytic atypia, usually related to HPV 6 and 11 infection (i.e. includes mild dysplasia and HPV infection).

■ *H-SIL* corresponds to CIN-2 and 3 and has abnormal pleomorphic atypical squamous cells. HPV 16 and 18 are implicated in the etiology of H-SIL (i.e. includes moderate dysplasia, severe dysplasia, and carcinoma *in situ*).

A comparison of these classifications is shown in Table 22.1.

TABLE 22.1: Classification of Cervical Intraepithelial Neoplasia/Squamous Intraepithelial Lesion (CIN/SIL).

BETHESDA SYSTEM	HPV TYPES	MORPHOLOGY	CIN	DYSPLASIA
L-SIL	6, 11	Koilocytic atypia, flat condyloma	CIN-1	Mild
H-SIL	16, 18	Progressive cellular atypia, loss of maturation	CIN-2, CIN-3	Moderate, severe, carcinoma *in situ*

L-SIL = low-grade squamous intraepithelial lesions; H-SIL = high-grade squamous intraepithelial lesion; CIN= cervical intraepithelial neoplasia.

CIN/SIL is a classical example of progression of malignancy through stepwise epithelial changes and that it can be detected early by simple Papanicolaou cytologic test ('Pap smear'). The use of Pap smear followed by colposcopy and biopsy confirms the diagnosis which has helped greatly in instituting early effective therapy and thus has reduced the incidence of cervical cancer in the West.

ETIOPATHOGENESIS. The biology of CIN/SIL and its relationship to invasive carcinoma of the cervix is well understood by epidemiologic, virologic, cytogenetic, immunologic and ultrastructural studies.

1. Epidemiologic studies. Based on epidemiology of large population of women with cervical cancer, several risk factors have been identified which include the following 4 most important factors:

i) Women having *early age of sexual activity.*

ii) Women having *multiple sexual partners.*

iii) Women with *persistent HPV infection* with high risk types of oncogenic virus.

iv) *Potential role of high risk male* sexual partner such as promiscuous male having previous multiple sexual partners, having history of penile condyloma, or male who had previous spouse with cervical cancer.

2. Virologic studies. Human papilloma virus (HPV) infection is strongly implicated in the etiology of cervical cancer:

■ HPV, most commonly of types 16 and 18, and less often types 31, 33 and 35, together termed *high risk types,* are present in cases of cervical cancer in 75-100% cases.

■ HPV types 6 and 11 called *low risk types* are found most frequently in condylomas.

■ Mixed high and low risk types of HPV may be found in dysplasias.

3. Cytogenetic studies. Cytogenetic studies have shown that low risk HPV types do not integrate in the host cell genome. On the other hand, high risk HPV types are integrated into cervical epithelial cells where they activate cell cycle gene, *cyclin E,* and inactivate tumour suppressor genes, *TP53* and *RB-1 gene,* thus permitting uncontrolled cellular proliferation. Women who have persistence of this infection or those who have another cofactor such as cigarette smoking or immunodeficiency, are at greater risk to develop progression of lesions.

4. Immunologic studies. Circulating tumour specific antigens and antibodies are detected in patients of cervical cancer.

5. Ultrastructural studies. The changes observed on ultrastructural studies of cells in CIN/SIL reveal increased mitochondria and free ribosomes, and depletion of normally accumulated glycogen in the surface cells. The latter change forms the basis of *Schiller's test* in which the suspected cervix is painted with solution of iodine and potassium iodide.

G/A No specific picture is associated with cellular atypia found in dysplasias or carcinoma *in situ* except that the changes begin at the squamo-columnar junction or transitional zone.

M/E Distinction between various grades of CIN is quite subjective, but, in general dysplastic cells are distributed in the layers of squamous epithelium for varying thickness, and accordingly graded as mild, moderate and severe dysplasia, and carcinoma *in situ*.

■ In *mild dysplasia (CIN-1)*, the abnormal cells extend upto one-third thickness from the basal to the surface layer;

■ In *moderate dysplasia (CIN-2)* upto two-thirds;

■ In *severe dysplasia (CIN-3)*, these cells extend from 75-90% thickness of epithelium; and

■ In *carcinoma in situ (again CIN-3)*, the entire thickness from the basement membrane to the surface shows dysplastic cells.

The atypical cells migrate to the surface layers from where they are shed off (exfoliated) into vaginal secretions in Pap smear. The individual dysplastic or abnormal cells in these grades of atypia show various cytologic changes such as: crowding of cells, pleomorphism, high nucleocytoplasmic ratio, coarse and irregular nuclear chromatin, numerous mitoses and scattered dyskaryotic cells.

The diagnosis of dysplasia and carcinoma *in situ* or CIN/SIL is best made by *exfoliative cytologic studies*. The degree of atypicality in the exfoliated surface epithelial cells can be objectively graded on the basis of 3 principal features:

1. More severe nuclear dyskaryotic changes such as increased hyperchromasia and nuclear membrane folding.

2. Decreased cytoplasmic maturation i.e. less cytoplasm as the surface cells show less maturation.

3. In lower grades of dysplasia (CIN-1/L-SIL) predominantly superficial and intermediate cells are shed off whereas in severe dysplasia and in carcinoma *in situ* (CIN-3/H-SIL) the desquamated cells are mainly small, dark basal cells.

CERVICAL SCREENING AND BETHESDA SYSTEM OF CYTOLOGIC EXAMINATION. With introduction of effective Pap screening programme in the Western countries, incidence of invasive cervical cancer has declined greatly. However, worldwide cervical cancer remains second most common cancer in women, next to breast cancer. Although accurate statistics are not available from India, but it is perhaps the leading cause of death in women.

The broad principles of *Bethesda system* of cytologic evaluation are as under:

■ Pap smears are evaluated as regards *adequacy of specimen* i.e. satisfactory for evaluation, satisfactory but limited, or unsatisfactory for evaluation giving reason.

■ General diagnosis is given in the form of *normal or abnormal smear*.

■ *Descriptive diagnosis* is given in abnormal smears that includes: benign cellular changes, reactive cellular changes, and abnormalities of epithelial cells.

■ Cellular abnormalities include: *ASCUS* (atypical squamous cells of undetermined significance), *L-SIL* (mentioning HPV infection and CIN-1 present or not), *H-SIL* (stating CIN-2 or CIN-3) and *squamous cell carcinoma*.

Invasive Cervical Cancer *(p. 754)*

Invasive cervical cancer in about 80% of cases is epidermoid (squamous cell carcinoma). The incidence of invasive carcinoma of the cervix has shown a declining trend in developed countries due to increased use of Pap smear technique for early detection and diagnosis but the incidence remains high in countries with low living standards. The risk factors and etiologic factors are the same as for CIN discussed above. The peak incidence of invasive cervical cancer is in 4th to 6th decades of life.

G/A Invasive cervical carcinoma may present 3 types of patterns: fungating, ulcerating and infiltrating. The fungating or exophytic pattern appearing as cauliflower-like growth infiltrating the adjacent vaginal wall is the most common type. Characteristically, cervical carcinoma arises from the squamo-columnar junction.

M/E The following patterns are seen:
1. **Epidermoid (Squamous cell) carcinoma.** This type comprises vast majority of invasive cervical carcinomas (about 80%).
■ The most common pattern (70%) is moderately-differentiated non-keratinising large cell type and has better prognosis.
■ Next in frequency (25%) is well-differentiated keratinising epidermoid carcinoma.
■ Small cell undifferentiated carcinoma (neuroendocrine or oat cell carcinoma) is less common (5%) and has a poor prognosis.
2. **Adenocarcinoma.** Adenocarcinomas comprise about 10% of cases. These may be well-differentiated mucus-secreting adenocarcinoma, or clear cell type containing glycogen but no mucin.
3. **Others.** The remaining 5% cases are a variety of other patterns such as adenosquamous carcinoma, verrucous carcinoma and undifferentiated carcinoma.

MYOMETRIUM AND ENDOMETRIUM *(p. 756)*

The *myometrium* is the thick muscular wall of the uterus which is covered internally by uterine mucosa called the *endometrium*. The endometrium extends above the level of the internal os where it joins the endocervical epithelium. The myometrium is capable of marked alterations in its size, capacity and contractility during pregnancy and labour. The endometrium responds in a cyclic fashion to the ovarian hormones with resultant monthly menstruation.

EFFECTS OF HORMONES *(p. 757)*

In addition to the changes that take place during the normal menstrual cycle, the endometrium undergoes morphologic changes when hormonal preparations are administered, or during pregnancy and menopause.

Oestrogen and Progesterone *(p. 757)*

Oestrogen produces the characteristic changes of proliferative phase at the time of menopause and in young women with anovulatory cycles as occurs in Stein-Leventhal syndrome. The therapeutic addition of progesterone produces secretory pattern in an oestrogen-primed endometrium. Oestrogen-proges-terone combination hormonal therapy is employed for control of conception. The sequential type of oestrogen-progesterone oral contraceptives act by producing prolonged oestrogenic effect past the time of ovulation and implantation so that the secretion is delayed until about 25th day, followed by progestational effect and shedding.

Pregnancy *(p. 757)*

The implantation of a fertilised ovum results in interruption of the endometrial cycle. The endometrial glands are enlarged with abundant glandular secretions and the stromal cells become more plump, polygonal with increased cytoplasm termed *decidual reaction*. About 25% cases of uterine or extrauterine pregnancy show hyperactive secretory state called *Arias-Stella reaction*. It is characterised by hyperchromatic, atypical, tall cells lining the glands and the glandular epithelium may show multilayering and budding which may be mistaken for an adenocarcinoma.

Menopause *(p. 757)*

The onset of menopause is heralded with hormonal transition and consequent varying morphologic changes in the endometrium. Most commonly, the *senile endometrium*, as it is generally called, is thin and atrophic with inactive glands and fibrous stroma. However, some of the glands may show cystic dilatation.

DYSFUNCTIONAL UTERINE BLEEDING (DUB) *(p. 758)*

Dysfunctional uterine bleeding (DUB) may be defined as excessive bleeding occurring during or between menstrual periods without a causative uterine lesion such as tumour, polyp, infection, hyperplasia, trauma, blood dyscrasia or pregnancy. DUB occurs most commonly in association with anovulatory cycles which are most frequent at the two extremes of menstrual life i.e. either when the ovarian function is just beginning (menarche) or when it is waning off (menopause). The causes for *anovulation* at different ages are as follows:

1. In *prepuberty:* precocious puberty of hypothalamic, pituitary or ovarian origin.
2. In *adolescence:* anovulatory cycles at the onset of menstruation.
3. In *reproductive age:* complications of pregnancy, endometrial hyperplasia, carcinoma, polyps, leiomyomas and adenomyosis.
4. At *premenopause:* anovulatory cycles, irregular shedding, endometrial hyperplasia, carcinoma and polyps.
5. At *perimenopause:* endometrial hyperplasia, carcinoma, polyps and senile atrophy.

ENDOMETRITIS AND MYOMETRITIS *(p. 758)*

Inflammatory involvement of the endometrium and myometrium are uncommon clinical problems; myometritis is seen less frequently than endometritis and occurs in continuation with endometrial infections. Endometritis and myometritis may be acute or chronic.

■ The **acute form** generally results from 3 types of causes—puerperal (following full-term delivery, abortion and retained products of conception), intrauterine contraceptive device (IUCD), and extension of gonorrheal infection from the cervix and vagina.

■ The **chronic form** is more common and occurs by the same causes which result in acute phase. In addition, *tuberculous endometritis* is an example of specific chronic inflammation, uncommon in the Western countries but not so uncommon in developing countries. Its incidence in India is reported to be approximately in 5% of women.

ADENOMYOSIS *(p. 758)*

Adenomyosis is defined as abnormal distribution of histologically benign endometrial tissue within the myometrium alongwith myometrial hypertrophy.

The term *adenomyoma* is used for actually circumscribed mass made up of endometrium and smooth muscle tissue. The possible underlying cause of the invasiveness and increased proliferation of the endometrium into the myometrium appears to be either a metaplasia or oestrogenic stimulation due to endocrine dysfunction of the ovary.

G/A The uterus may be slightly or markedly enlarged. On cut section, there is diffuse thickness of the uterine wall with presence of coarsely trabecular, ill-defined areas of haemorrhages.

M/E The diagnosis is based on the finding of normal, benign endometrial islands composed of glands as well as stroma deep within the muscular layer. The minimum distance between the endometrial islands within the myometrium and the basal endometrium should be one low-power microscopic field (2-3 mm) for making the diagnosis.

ENDOMETRIOSIS *(p. 759)*

Endometriosis refers to the presence of endometrial glands and stroma in abnormal locations outside the uterus.

The chief locations where the abnormal endometrial development may occur are as follows (in descending order of frequency): ovaries, uterine ligaments, rectovaginal septum, pelvic peritoneum, laparotomy scars, and infrequently in the umbilicus, vagina, vulva, appendix and hernial sacs.

The **histogenesis** of endometriosis has been a debatable matter for years. Currently, however, the following 3 theories of its histogenesis are described:

1. *Transplantation or regurgitation theory* is based on the assumption that ectopic endometrial tissue is transplanted from the uterus to an abnormal location by way of fallopian tubes due to regurgitation of menstrual blood.

2. *Metaplastic theory* suggests that ectopic endometrium develops *in situ* from local tissues by metaplasia of the coelomic epithelium.

3. *Vascular or lymphatic dissemination* explains the development of endometrial tissue at extrapelvic sites by these routes.

G/A The appearance of endometriosis varies widely depending upon the location and extent of the disease. Often, these foci are surrounded by fibrous tissue resulting in adherence to adjacent structures. The ovary is the most common site of endometriosis and shows numerous cysts varying in diameter from 0.1 to 2.5 cm.

M/E The diagnosis is simple and rests on identification of foci of endometrial glands and stroma, old or new haemorrhages, haemosiderin-laden macrophages and surrounding zone of inflammation and fibrosis.

ENDOMETRIAL HYPERPLASIAS *(p. 759)*

Endometrial hyperplasia is a condition characterised by proliferative patterns of glandular and stromal tissues and commonly associated with prolonged, profuse and irregular uterine bleeding in a menopausal or postmenopausal woman. Hyperplasia results from prolonged oestrogenic stimulation with absence of progestational activity. Endometrial hyperplasia is clinically significant due to the presence of cytologic atypia which is closely linked to endometrial carcinoma.

The following classification of endometrial hyperplasias is widely employed by most gynaecologic pathologists:

SIMPLE HYPERPLASIA (CYSTIC HYPERPLASIA). Commonly termed cystic glandular hyperplasia (CGH), this form of endometrial hyperplasia is characterised by the presence of varying-sized glands, many of which are large and cystically dilated and are lined by atrophic epithelium. Mitoses are scanty. The stroma between the glands is sparsely cellular and oedematous.

There is minimal risk (1%) of adenocarcinoma developing in cystic hyperplasia.

COMPLEX HYPERPLASIA (ADENOMATOUS HYPERPLASIA). This type of hyperplasia shows distinct proliferative pattern. The glands are increased in number, exhibit variation in size and are irregular in shape. The glands are lined by multiple layers of tall columnar epithelial cells with large nuclei which have not lost basal polarity and there is no significant atypia. The glandular epithelium at places is thrown into papillary infolds or out-pouchings into adjacent stroma i.e. there is crowding and complexity of glands without cytologic atypia. The stroma is generally dense, cellular and compact.

The malignant potential of adenomatous hyperplasia in the absence of cytologic atypia is 3%.

ATYPICAL HYPERPLASIA. Some authors have suggested the terms such as anaplasia or carcinoma *in situ* for this form of endometrial hyperplasia but these terms are generally not favoured. Atypical hyperplasia is distinguished from adenomatous hyperplasia by the presence of 'atypical cells' in the hyperplastic epithelium. The extent of cytologic atypia may be mild, moderate or severe. The cytologic features present in these cells include loss of polarity, large size, irregular and hyperchromatic nuclei, prominent nucleoli, and altered nucleocytoplasmic ratio.

Atypical hyperplasia is a precancerous condition and its malignant transformation is related to the degree of cytologic atypia. About 20-25% cases of untreated atypical hyperplasia progress to carcinoma.

TUMOURS OF ENDOMETRIUM AND MYOMETRIUM *(p. 760)*

Endometrial Polyps *(p. 760)*

'Uterine polyp' is clinical term used for a polypoid growth projecting into the uterine lumen and may be composed of benign lesions (e.g. endometrial or mucous polyp, leiomyomatous polyp and placental polyp), or malignant polypoid tumours (e.g. endometrial carcinoma, choriocarcinoma and sarcoma). The most common variety, however, is the one having the structure like that of endometrium and is termed *endometrial or mucous polyp*. They are more common in the perimenopausal age group.

G/A Endometrial polyps may be single or multiple, usually sessile and small (0.5 to 3 cm in diameter) but occasionally they are large and pedunculated.

M/E They are essentially made up of mixture of endometrial glands and stroma. The histologic pattern of the endometrial tissue in the polyp may resemble either functioning endometrium or hyperplastic endometrium of cystic hyperplasia type; the latter being more common.

Endometrial Carcinoma *(p. 761)*

Carcinoma of the endometrium has become more common than the invasive carcinoma of the cervix in women in the United States. Whereas the decline in the incidence of cervical cancer is due to early detection and cure of *in situ* stage, increased frequency of endometrial carcinoma may be due to longevity of women's life to develop this cancer of older females. The peak incidence at onset is 6th to 7th decades of life and is rare below the age of 40 years.

ETIOPATHOGENESIS. The exact etiology of endometrial cancer remains unknown. However, a few factors associated with increased frequency of its development are oestrogen excess, obesity, diabetes, hypertension and nulliparous state. There is irrefutable evidence of *relationship of endometrial carcinoma with prolonged oestrogenic stimulation.*

Papillary serous variant of endometrial carcinoma is associated with mutation in *TP53* tumour suppressor gene while endometrioid carcinoma has mutation in *PTEN* gene located on chromosome 10.

G/A Endometrial carcinoma may have 2 patterns—localised *polypoid tumour,* or a *diffuse tumour;* the latter being more common. The tumour protrudes into the endometrial cavity as irregular, friable and grey-tan mass. In advanced disease, the involvement may extend beyond the physiologic limits—into the cervical canal, into the peritoneum, besides lymphatic metastases and haematogenous metastases to distant sites such as lungs, liver, bones and other organs.

M/E Most endometrial carcinomas are adenocarcinomas. Depending upon the pattern of glands and individual cell changes, these may be well-differentiated, moderately-differentiated or poorly-differentiated.

Cases can also be categorised as regards histologic grade as follows:
G1: Well-differentiated (predominantly glandular).
G2: Moderately-differentiated (glandular and partly solid areas).
G3: Poorly-differentiated (predominantly solid).

Leiomyoma *(p. 762)*

Leiomyomas or fibromyomas, commonly called *fibroids* by the gynaecologists, are the most common uterine tumours of smooth muscle origin, often admixed with variable amount of fibrous tissue component. About 20% of women above the age of 30 years harbour uterine myomas of varying size. Vast majority of them are benign and cause no symptoms. Malignant transformation occurs in less than 0.5% of leiomyomas. Symptomatic cases may produce abnormal uterine bleeding, pain, symptoms due to compression of surrounding structures and infertility.

The cause of leiomyomas is unknown but the possible stimulus to their proliferation is oestrogen.

Leiomyomas are most frequently located in the uterus where they may occur within the myometrium *(intramural or interstitial),* the serosa *(subserosal),* or just underneath the endometrium *(submucosal).*

G/A Irrespective of their location, leiomyomas are often multiple, circumscribed, firm, nodular, grey-white masses of variable size. On cut section, they exhibit characteristic whorled pattern.

M/E They are essentially composed of 2 tissue elements—whorled bundles of smooth muscle cells admixed with variable amount of connective tissue. The smooth muscle cells are uniform in size and shape with abundant cytoplasm and central oval nuclei.

The pathologic appearance may be altered by secondary changes in the leiomyomas. These include: hyaline degeneration, cystic degeneration, infarction, calcification, infection and suppuration, necrosis, fatty change, and rarely, sarcomatous change.

Leiomyosarcoma *(p. 763)*

Leiomyosarcoma is an uncommon malignant tumour as compared to its rather common benign counterpart. The incidence of malignancy in pre-existing leiomyoma is less than 0.5% but primary uterine sarcoma is less common than that which arises in the leiomyoma. The peak age incidence is seen in 4th to 6th decades of life.

G/A The tumour may form a diffuse, bulky, soft and fleshy mass, or a polypoid mass projecting into lumen.

M/E Though there are usually some areas showing whorled arrangement of spindle-shaped smooth muscle cells having large and hyperchromatic nuclei, the hallmark of diagnosis and prognosis is the number of mitoses per high power field (HPF). The essential diagnostic criteria are: more than 10 mitoses per 10 HPF with or without cellular atypia, or 5-10 mitoses per 10 HPF with cellular atypia.

FALLOPIAN TUBES *(p. 763)*

The fallopian tube or oviducts are paired structures, each extending from superior angle of the uterus laterally to the region of the ovaries and running in the superior border of the broad ligaments forming mesosalpinx. Each tube is 7-14 cm long and is divided into 4 parts—*interstitial portion* in the uterine cornual wall; narrow *isthmic portion;* wider *ampullary region;* and funnel-like distal *infundibulum.* The infundibulum is fringed by fimbriae, the longest of which called fimbria ovarica is attached to the ovary.

M/E The wall of tube has 4 coats—*serous* forming the peritoneal covering, *subserous* consisting of fibrovascular tissue, *muscular* composed of longitudinal and circular smooth muscle layers, and *tubal mucosa* having 3 types of cells namely: ciliated, columnar and dark intercalated cells.

SALPINGITIS AND PELVIC INFLAMMATORY DISEASE *(p. 764)*

Pelvic inflammatory disease (PID) by definition is a clinical syndrome characterised by signs and symptoms of ascending infection beginning in the vulva or vagina and spreading through the entire genital tract. Although ascending route of infection is the most common mode of spread, PID may occur following abortion and puerperium, with use of intrauterine contraceptive devices, or from local intra-abdominal infections such as appendicitis with peritonitis.

Most commonly, PID occurs as a venereally-transmitted infection, chiefly caused by *Chlamydia trachomatis* and *Neisseria gonorrhoeae.* Post-abortal and postpartum infections are mainly caused by staphylococci, streptococci, coliform bacteria, clostridia and pneumococci.

Patients generally complain of lower abdominal and pelvic pain which is often bilateral, dysmenorrhoea, menstrual abnormalities and fever with tachycardia. Long-standing chronic PID may lead to infertility and adhesions between small intestine and pelvic organs.

G/A The fallopian tubes are invariably involved bilaterally. The distal end is blocked by inflammatory exudate and the lumina are dilated.

M/E The appearance varies with the duration of inflammatory process.
■ The process begins with *acute salpingitis* characterised by oedema and intense acute inflammatory infiltrate of neutrophils involving the tubal mucosa as well as wall.
■ The purulent process may extend to involve tube as well as ovary causing salpingo-oophoritis and forming *tubo-ovarian abscess.*
■ The escape of purulent exudate into the peritoneal cavity produces *pelvic peritonitis* and *pelvic abscess.*
■ *Pyosalpinx* is distension of the fallopian tube with pus due to occluded fimbrial end.
■ Acute salpingitis may resolve with treatment but some cases pass into *chronic salpingitis* with infiltrate of polymorphs, lymphocytes and plasma cells and fibrosis.
■ *Salpingitis isthmica nodosa* used to be considered another manifestation of chronic salpingitis but currently accepted pathogenesis of this lesion appears to be similar to that of adenomyosis.

TUBERCULOUS SALPINGITIS *(p. 764)*

Tuberculous salpingitis is almost always secondary to focus elsewhere in the body. The tubercle bacilli reach the tube, most commonly by haematogenous route, generally from the lungs, but occasionally from the urinary tract or abdominal cavity. Though infrequent in developed countries of the world, the incidence of tubal tuberculosis in developing countries like India is estimated to be about 5%. It affects more commonly young women in their active reproductive life and the most common complaint is infertility.

G/A The tube is dilated and contains purulent exudate though the fimbrial end is generally patent.

M/E Typical caseating granulomas and chronic inflammation are identified in the tubal serosa, muscularis and mucosa.

ECTOPIC TUBAL PREGNANCY *(p. 764)*

The term ectopic tubal pregnancy is used for implantation of a fertilised ovum in the tube. Though ectopic pregnancy may rarely occur in the uterine horn, cornu, ovary and abdominal cavity, tubal pregnancy is by far the most common form of ectopic gestation. Several factors which predispose to ectopic tubal pregnancy are: PID, previous tubal surgery, use of IUCD and congenital anomalies of the female genital tract. The most frequent site of tubal pregnancy is the ampullary portion.

TUMOURS AND TUMOUR-LIKE LESIONS *(p. 765)*

Tumours in the fallopian tubes are rare. Relatively more common are hydatids of Morgagni or parovarian cysts which are unilocular, thin-walled cysts hanging from the tubal fimbriae. Rare tumours include adenomatoid tumours, leiomyomas, teratomas, adenocarcinomas and choriocarcinoma.

OVARIES *(p. 765)*

The ovaries are paired bean-shaped organs hanging from either tube by a mesentery called the mesovarium, the lateral suspensory ligament and the ovarian ligament. The lateral suspensory ligament of the ovary contains blood vessels, lymphatics and plexuses of nerves.

M/E The ovarian structure consists of covering by coelomic epithelium, outer cortex and inner medulla.

Coelomic epithelium. The surface of the ovary is covered by a single layer of cuboidal epithelial cells.

Cortex. During active reproductive life, the cortex is broad and constitutes the predominant component of the ovary. The cortex contains numerous ovarian follicles and their derivative structures. Each follicle consists of a central *germ cell ovum* surrounded by specialised gonadal stroma. This stroma consists of *granulosa cells* encircling the ovum, and concentrically-arranged plump spindle-shaped *theca cells.*

Medulla. The ovarian medulla is primarily made up of connective tissue fibres, smooth muscle cells and numerous blood vessels, lymphatics and nerves.

NON-NEOPLASTIC CYSTS *(p. 765)*

Follicular and Luteal Cysts *(p. 765)*

Normally follicles and corpus luteum do not exceed a diameter of 2 cm. When their diameter is greater than 3 cm, they are termed as cysts.

■ **Follicular cysts** are frequently multiple, filled with clear serous fluid and may attain a diameter upto 8 cm. When large, they produce clinical symptoms.

M/E They are lined by granulosa cells.

■ **Luteal cysts** are formed by rupture and sealing of corpus haemorrhagicum. The wall of these cysts is composed of yellowish luteal tissue.

Polycystic Ovary Disease (Stein-Leventhal Syndrome) *(p. 766)*

This is a syndrome characterised by oligomenorrhoea, anovulation, infertility, hirsutism and obesity in young women having bilaterally enlarged and cystic ovaries. The principal biochemical abnormalities in most patients are excessive production of androgens, and low levels of pituitary follicle stimulating hormone (FSH). These endocrinologic abnormalities were previously attributed to primary ovarian dysfunction as evidenced by excellent results from wedge resection of the ovary. But current concept of pathogenesis is the unbalanced release of FSH and LH by the pituitary.

G/A The ovaries are usually involved bilaterally and are at least twice the size of the normal ovary. They are grey-white in colour and studded with multiple small (0.5-1.5 cm in diameter) bluish cysts just beneath the cortex.

M/E The outer cortex is thick and fibrous. The subcortical cysts are lined by prominent luteinised theca cells and represent follicles in various stages of maturation but there is no evidence of corpus luteum.

OVARIAN TUMOURS *(p. 766)*

The ovary is third most common site of primary malignancy in the female genital tract, preceded only by endometrial and cervical cancer.

Etiopathogenesis *(p. 766)*

Unlike the other two female genital cancers (cervix and endometrium), not much is known about the etiology of ovarian tumours. However, a few risk factors have been identified which include the following:

1. *Nulliparity.*
2. *Heredity.*
3. *Complex genetic syndromes. e.g.*
i) Peutz-Jeghers syndrome
ii) Gonadal dysgenesis
iii) Nevoid basal cell carcinoma.

Clinical Features and Classification *(p. 767)*

Most benign and malignant ovarian tumours are discovered when they grow sufficiently to cause abdominal discomfort and distension. Urinary tract and gastrointestinal tract symptoms are frequently associated due to compression by the tumour. Ascites is common in both benign and malignant ovarian tumours. Menstrual irregularities may or may not be present. Some ovarian tumours are bilateral.

A simplified classification proposed by the WHO with minor modifications has been widely adopted (Table 22.2). Five major groups have been described:
I. Tumours of surface epithelium (common epithelial tumours)
II. Germ cell tumours
III. Sex cord-stromal tumours
IV. Miscellaneous tumours
V. Metastatic tumours

I. TUMOURS OF SURFACE EPITHELIUM (COMMON EPITHELIAL TUMOURS) *(p. 767)*

This group constitutes about 60-70% of all ovarian neoplasms and 90% of malignant ovarian tumours. The common epithelial tumours are of 3 major

TABLE 22.2: Classification of Ovarian Tumours.

1. TUMOURS OF SURFACE EPITHELIUM (COMMON EPITHELIAL TUMOURS) (60-70%)

A. Serous tumours
   1. Serous cystadenoma
   2. Borderline serous tumour
   3. Serous cystadenocarcinoma
B. Mucinous tumours
   1. Mucinous cystadenoma
   2. Borderline mucinous tumour
   3. Mucinous cystadenocarcinoma
C. Endometrioid tumours
D. Clear cell (mesonephroid) tumours
E. Brenner tumours

II. GERM CELL TUMOURS (15-20%)

A. Teratomas
   1. Benign (mature, adult) teratoma
      ■ Benign cystic teratoma (dermoid cyst)
      ■ Benign solid teratoma
   2. Malignant (immature) teratoma
   3. Monodermal or specialised teratoma
      ■ Struma ovarii
      ■ Carcinoid tumour
B. Dysgerminoma
C. Endodermal sinus (yolk sac) tumour
D. Choriocarcinoma
E. Others (embryonal carcinoma, polyembryoma, mixed germ cell tumours)

III. SEX CORD-STROMAL TUMOURS (5-10%)

A. Granulosa-theca cell tumours
   1. Granulosa cell tumour
   2. Thecoma
   3. Fibroma
B. Sertoli-Leydig cell tumours (Androblastoma, arrhenoblastoma)
C. Gynandroblastoma

IV. MISCELLANEOUS TUMOURS

A. Lipid cell tumours
B. Gonadoblastoma

V. METASTATIC TUMOURS (5%)

A. Krukenberg tumour
B. Others

types—*serous, mucinous* and *endometrioid,* though mixtures of these epithelia may occur in the same tumour. These tumours frequently have prominent cystic component which may have a single or multiple loculations and hence the descriptive prefix *cystadeno-* in these tumours. In addition, surface epithe-lial tumours may differentiate along urothelium to form *Brenner tumour,* and along mesonephroid pattern forming *clear cell (mesonephroid) adenocarcinoma.*

Depending upon the aggressiveness, the surface epithelial tumours are divided into 3 groups: *clearly benign, clearly malignant,* and *borderline* or *low-grade malignant tumours.* In general, the criteria for diagnosis of these 3 grades of aggressiveness are as follows:

■ **Clearly benign tumours** are lined by a single layer of well-oriented columnar epithelium.

■ **Clearly malignant tumours** have anaplastic epithelial component, multilayering, loss of basal polarity and unquestionable stromal invasion.

■ **Borderline tumours** or tumours with low malignant potential have some morphological features of malignancy, apparent detachment of cellular clusters from their site of origin and essential absence of stromal invasion.

Serous Tumours *(p. 768)*

Serous tumours comprise the largest group constituting about 20% of all ovarian tumours and 40% of malignant ovarian tumours. About 60% of serous tumours are benign, 15% borderline and 25% malignant. Only 20% of benign tumours occur bilaterally, whereas 65% of both borderline and malignant serous tumours have bilateral ovarian involvement. Serous tumours occur most commonly in 2nd to 5th decades of life, the malignant forms being more frequent in later life.

Histogenesis of the serous tumours is from the surface (coelomic) epithelium or mesothelium which differentiates along tubal-type of epithelium.

G/A The benign, borderline and malignant serous tumours are large (above 5 cm in diameter) and spherical masses. Small masses are generally unilocular while the larger serous cysts are multiloculated similar to the mucinous variety, but differ from the latter in containing serous fluid rather than the viscid fluid of mucinous tumours. *Malignant serous tumours* may have solid areas in the cystic mass. Exophytic as well as intra-cystic papillary projections may be present in all grades of serous tumours but are more frequent in malignant tumours.

M/E The features are as under:

1. Serous cystadenoma is characteristically lined by properly-oriented low columnar epithelium which is sometimes ciliated and resembles tubal epithelium. Microscopic papillae may be found.

2. Borderline serous tumour usually has stratification (2-3 layers) of benign serous type of epithelium. There is detachment of cell clusters from their site of origin and moderate features of malignancy but there is absence of stromal invasion.

3. Serous cystadenocarcinoma has multilayered malignant cells which show loss of polarity, presence of solid sheets of anaplastic epithelial cells and definite evidence of stromal invasion. Papillae formations are more frequent in malignant variety and may be associated with psammoma bodies.

Mucinous Tumours *(p. 769)*

Mucinous tumours are somewhat less common than serous tumours and constitute about 20% of all ovarian tumours and 10% of all ovarian cancers. Over 80% are benign, 10-15% are borderline and 5-10% are malignant. These predominantly cystic tumours contain mucin which was previously described as pseudomucin. Well-differentiated borderline mucinous tumours are associated with mucinous ascites termed *pseudomyxoma peritonei*. Mucinous tumours as compared with serous tumours are more commonly unilateral. Benign mucinous tumours occur bilaterally in 5% of cases while borderline and malignant are bilateral in 20%. Mucinous tumours occur principally between 2nd and 5th decades of life. Mucinous carcinoma usually develops in women above the age of 40 years.

Histogenesis of mucinous tumours, in line with that of serous tumours, is from the coelomic epithelium that differentiates along endocervical type or intestinal type of mucosa.

G/A Mucinous tumours are larger than serous tumours. They are smooth-surfaced cysts with characteristic multiloculations containing thick and viscid gelatinous fluid. Benign tumours generally have thin wall and septa dividing the loculi are also thin and often translucent, but malignant varieties usually have thickened areas.

M/E The features are as under:

1. **Mucinous cystadenoma** is lined by a single layer of these cells having basal nuclei and apical mucinous vacuoles.

2. **Borderline mucinous tumour** is identified by the same histologic criteria as for borderline serous tumour i.e. stratification (usually 2-3 cell thick) of typical epithelium without stromal invasion.

3. **Mucinous cystadenocarcinoma** likewise is characterised by piling up of malignant epithelium, at places forming solid sheets, papillary formation, adenomatous pattern and infiltration into stroma with or without pools of mucin.

Endometrioid Tumours *(p. 770)*

Endometrioid tumours comprise about 5% of all ovarian tumours. Most of them are malignant accounting for about 20% of all ovarian cancers. Benign and borderline forms are very rare. They are called endometrioid carcinomas because of the close resemblance of histologic pattern to that of uterine endometrial adenocarcinoma. About 40% of endometrioid carcinomas have bilateral ovarian involvement. About 15-30% of cases of endometrioid carcinoma have coexistent endometrial adenocarcinoma.

Histogenesis of these tumours in majority of cases is believed to be from ovarian coelomic epithelium differentiating towards endometrial type of epithelium.

G/A These tumours are partly solid and partly cystic and may have foci of haemorrhages, especially in benign variety.

M/E The endometrioid adenocarcinoma is distinguished from serous and mucinous carcinomas by typical glandular pattern that closely resembles that of uterine endometrial adenocarcinoma. There may be foci of squamous metaplasia justifying the diagnosis of adenoacanthoma.

Clear Cell (Mesonephroid)Tumours *(p. 770)*

Clear cell (mesonephroid) tumours are almost always malignant and comprise about 5% of all ovarian cancers. Rare benign variety is called *clear cell adenofibroma*. They are termed clear cell or mesonephroid carcinomas because of the close histologic resemblance to renal adenocarcinoma.

G/A These tumours are large, usually unilateral, partly solid and partly cystic. Less than 10% are bilateral.

M/E Clear cell or mesonephroid carcinoma is characterised by tubules, glands, papillae, cysts and solid sheets of tumour cells resembling cells of renal adenocarcinoma i.e. clear cells having abundant eosinophilic cytoplasm rich in glycogen.

Brenner Tumour *(p. 771)*

Brenner tumours are uncommon and comprise about 2% of all ovarian tumours. They are characteristically solid ovarian tumours. Less than 10% of Brenner tumours are bilateral. Most Brenner tumours are benign. Rarely, borderline form is encountered and is called 'proliferating Brenner tumour' and one with carcinomatous change is termed 'malignant Brenner tumour'.

G/A Brenner tumour is typically solid, yellow-grey, firm mass of variable size.

M/E Brenner tumour consists of nests, masses and columns of epithelial cells, scattered in fibrous stroma of the ovary. These epithelial cells resemble urothelial cells which are ovoid in shape, having clear cytoplasm, vesicular nuclei with characteristic nuclear groove called 'coffee-bean' nuclei.

II. GERM CELL TUMOURS *(p. 771)*

Ovarian germ cell tumours arising from germ cells which produce the female gametes (i.e. ova) account for about 15-20% of all ovarian neoplasms. Nearly 95% of them are benign and vast majority of them are benign cystic teratomas (dermoid cysts) and occur chiefly in young females. The remainder are malignant germ cell tumours comprising a variety of morphologic forms occurring chiefly in children and young adults and are highly aggressive tumours.

Teratomas *(p. 771)*

Teratomas are tumours composed of different types of tissues derived from the three germ cell layers—ectoderm, mesoderm and endoderm, in different combinations. They are divided into 3 types:

MATURE (BENIGN) TERATOMA. The vast majority of ovarian teratomas are benign and cystic and have the predominant ectodermal elements, often termed clinically as *dermoid cyst.* Infrequently, mature teratoma may be solid and benign and has to be distinguished from immature or malignant teratoma. Benign cystic teratomas are more frequent in young women during their active reproductive life. The tumour is bilateral in 10% of cases. More recently, cytogenetic studies have revealed that these tumours arise from a single germ cell (ovum) after its first meiotic division.

G/A Benign cystic teratoma or dermoid cyst is characteristically a unilocular cyst, 10-15 cm in diameter, usually lined by skin and hence its name. On sectioning, the cyst is filled with paste-like sebaceous secretions and desquamated keratin admixed with masses of hair. The cyst wall is thin and opaque grey-white. Generally, in one area of the cyst wall, a solid prominence is seen (Rokitansky's protuberance) where tissue elements such as tooth, bone, cartilage and various other odd tissues are present.

M/E The most prominent feature is the lining of the cyst wall by stratified squamous epithelium and its adnexal structures such as sebaceous glands, sweat glands and hair follicles. Though ectodermal derivatives are most prominent features, tissues of mesodermal and endodermal origin are commonly present. Various other tissue components frequently found are bronchus, intestinal epithelium, cartilage, bone, tooth, smooth muscle, neural tissue, salivary gland, retina, pancreas and thyroid tissue.

IMMATURE (MALIGNANT) TERATOMA. Immature or malignant teratomas are rare and account for approximately 0.2% of all ovarian tumours. They are predominantly solid tumours that contain immature or embryonal structures in contrast to the mature or adult structures of the benign teratomas.

G/A Malignant teratoma is a unilateral solid mass which on cut section shows characteristic variegated appearance revealing areas of haemorrhages, necrosis, tiny cysts and heterogeneous admixture of various tissue elements.

M/E Parts of the tumour may show mature tissues, while most of it is composed of immature tissues having an embryonic appearance. Immature tissue elements may differentiate towards cartilage, bone, glandular structures, neural tissue etc, and are distributed in spindle-shaped myxoid or undifferentiated sarcoma cells.

MONODERMAL (SPECIALISED) TERATOMA. Monodermal or highly specialised teratomas are rare and include following important examples:

■ **Struma ovarii.** It is a teratoma composed exclusively of thyroid tissue, recognisable grossly as well as microscopically. Most often, the tumour has the appearance of a follicular adenoma of the thyroid.

■ **Carcinoid tumour.** This is an ovarian teratoma arising from argentaffin cells of intestinal epithelium in the teratoma.

■ **Struma-carcinoid** is a rare combination of struma ovarii and ovarian carcinoid.

Dysgerminoma *(p. 773)*

Dysgerminoma is an ovarian counterpart of seminoma of the testes. Dysgerminomas comprise about 2% of all ovarian cancers. They occur most commonly in 2nd to 3rd decades. About 10% of them are bilateral. About 10% of patients with dysgerminoma have elevated hCG level in the plasma. All dysgerminomas are malignant and are extremely radiosensitive.

G/A Dysgerminoma is a solid mass of variable size. Cut section of the tumour is grey-white to pink, lobulated, soft and fleshy with foci of haemorrhages and necrosis.

M/E Their structure is similar to that of seminoma of the testis. The tumour cells are arranged in diffuse sheets, islands and cords separated by scanty fibrous stroma. The tumour cells are uniform in appearance and large, with vesicular nuclei and clear cytoplasm rich in glycogen. The fibrous stroma generally contains lymphocytic infiltrate and sometimes may have sarcoid granulomas.

Endodermal Sinus (Yolk Sac) Tumour *(p. 773)*

Endodermal sinus tumour or yolk sac tumour is the second most common germ cell tumour occurring most commonly in children and young women. The tumour is rich in alphafetoprotein (AFP) and alpha-1-antitrypsin. The tumour is usually unilateral but may metastasise to the other ovary. It is a highly aggressive and rapidly growing tumour.

G/A The tumour is generally solid with areas of cystic degeneration.

M/E Like its testicular counterpart, the endodermal sinus tumour is characterised by the presence of papillary projections having a central blood vessel with perivascular layer of anaplastic embryonal germ cells. Such structures resemble the endodermal sinuses of the rat placenta (Schiller-Duval body).

Choriocarcinoma *(p. 774)*

Choriocarcinoma in females is of 2 types—*gestational and non-gestational.* Gestational choriocarcinoma of placental origin is more common and considered separately later, while non-gestational choriocarcinoma of ovarian origin is rare. Primary ovarian choriocarcinoma more often occurs in combination with other germ cell tumours than in pure form. The patients are usually young girls under the age of 20 years. Morphologically, ovarian choriocarcinoma is identical to gestational choriocarcinoma. Ovarian choriocarcinoma is more malignant than that of placental origin and disseminates widely via blood stream to the lungs, liver, bone, brain and kidneys. The marker for both types of choriocarcinoma is hCG.

Other Germ Cell Tumours *(p. 774)*

Certain other germ cell tumours occasionally encountered in the ovaries are embryonal carcinoma, polyembryoma and mixed germ cell tumours. All these tumours are morphologically identical to similar tumours occurring in the testes.

III. SEX CORD-STROMAL TUMOURS *(p. 774)*

Sex cord-stromal tumours of the ovaries comprise 5-10% of all ovarian neoplasms. They arise from specialised ovarian stromal cells of the developing gonads. Thus, these include tumours originating from granulosa cells, theca cells and Sertoli-Leydig cells.

Granulosa-Theca Cell Tumours *(p. 774)*

Granulosa-theca cell tumours comprise about 5% of all ovarian tumours.

GRANULOSA CELL TUMOUR. Pure granulosa cell tumours may occur at all ages. These tumours invade locally but occasionally may have more aggressive and malignant behaviour. Recurrences after surgical removal are common. Most granulosa cell tumours secrete oestrogen which may be responsible for precocious puberty in young girls, or in older patients may produce endometrial hyperplasia, endometrial adenocarcinoma and cystic disease of the breast.

G/A Granulosa cell tumour is a small, solid, partly cystic and usually unilateral tumour. Cut section of solid areas is yellowish-brown.

M/E The granulosa cells are arranged in a variety of patterns including micro- and macrofollicular, trabecular, bands and diffuse sheets. The microfollicular pattern is characterised by the presence of characteristic rosette-like structures, Call-Exner bodies, having central rounded pink mass surrounded by a circular row of granulosa cells.

THECOMA. Pure thecomas are almost always benign. They occur more frequently in post-menopausal women. Thecomas are typically oestrogenic. Endometrial hyperplasia, endometrial carcinoma and cystic disease of the breast are some of its adverse effects. Occasionally a thecoma may secrete androgen and cause virilisation.

G/A Thecoma is a solid and firm mass, 5-10 cm in diameter. Cut section is yellowish.

M/E Thecoma consists of spindle-shaped theca cells of the ovary admixed with variable amount of hyalinised collagen.

GRANULOSA-THECA CELL TUMOUR. Mixture of both granulosa and theca cell elements in the same ovarian tumour is seen in some cases with elaboration of oestrogen.

FIBROMA. Fibromas of the ovary are more common and account for about 5% of all ovarian tumours. These tumours are hormonally inert but some of them are associated with pleural effusion and benign ascites termed Meig's syndrome.

G/A These tumours are large, firm and fibrous, usually unilateral masses.

M/E They are composed of spindle-shaped well-differentiated fibroblasts and collagen.

IV. METASTATIC TUMOURS *(p. 775)*

About 10% of ovarian cancers are secondary carcinomas. Metastasis may occur by lymphatic or haematogenous route but direct extension from adjacent organs (e.g. uterus, fallopian tube and sigmoid colon) too occurs frequently. Bilaterality of the tumour is the most helpful clue to diagnosis of metastatic tumour. Most common primary sites from where metastases to the ovaries are encountered are: carcinomas of the breast, genital tract, gastrointestinal tract (e.g. stomach, colon appendix, pancreas, biliary tract) and haematopoietic malignancies.

The **Krukenberg tumour** is a distinctive bilateral tumour metastatic to the ovaries by transcoelomic spread characterised by the presence of mucus-filled signet ring cells accompanied by sarcoma-like proliferation of ovarian stroma. This tumour is generally secondary to a gastric carcinoma but other primary sites where mucinous carcinomas occur (e.g. colon, appendix and breast) may also produce Krukenberg tumour in the ovary. Rarely, a tumour having the pattern of Krukenberg tumour is primary in the ovary.

PLACENTA *(p. 776)*

NORMAL STRUCTURE *(p. 776)*

At term, the normal placenta is blue red, rounded, flattened and discoid organ 15-20 cm in diameter and 2-4 cm thick. It weighs 400-600 gm or about one-sixth the weight of the newborn. The placenta secretes a number of hormones and enzymes into the maternal blood. These include: human chorionic gonadotropin (hCG), human placental lactogen (HPL), chorionic thyrotropin and adrenocorticotropin hormone which partake in oestrogen and progesterone metabolism.

HYDATIDIFORM MOLE *(p. 777)*

Hydatidiform mole is a condition characterised by 2 features—hydropic change of the chorionic villi, and trophoblastic proliferation. Most workers consider hydatidiform mole as a benign tumour of placental tissue with potential for developing into choriocarcinoma, while some authors have described mole as a degenerative lesion though capable of neoplastic change.

Hydatidiform mole may be non-invasive or invasive. Two types of non-invasive moles are distinguished—complete (classic) and partial. The pathogenesis of these 2 forms is different:

■ **Complete (classic) mole** by cytogenetic studies has been shown to be derived from the father (androgenesis) and shows 46, XX or rarely 46, XY chromosomal pattern. Complete mole bears relationship to choriocarcinoma.

■ **The partial mole** is mostly triploid (i.e. 69,XXY or 69,XXX) and rarely tetraploid. Partial mole rarely develops into choriocarcinoma.

Clinically, the condition appears in 4th-5th month of gestation and is characterised by increase in uterine size, vaginal bleeding and often with symptoms of toxaemia. Frequently, there is history of passage of grape-like masses per vaginum.

The single most significant investigation is the serial determination of hCG which is elevated more in both blood and urine as compared with the levels in normal pregnancy. Removal of the mole is accompanied by fall in hCG levels. A more ominous behaviour is associated with no fall in hCG levels after expulsion of the mole. About 10% of patients with complete mole develop into invasive moles and 2.5% into choriocarcinoma.

COMPLETE (CLASSIC) MOLE: *G/A* The uterus is enlarged and characteristically filled with grape-like vesicles upto 3 cm in diameter. The vesicles contain clear watery fluid.

M/E 1. Large, round oedematous villi.
2. Hydropic degeneration and decreased vascularity of villous stroma.
3. Trophoblastic proliferation in the form of masses and sheets of both cytotrophoblast and syncytiotrophoblast.

PARTIAL MOLE: *G/A* The uterus is generally smaller than expected and contains some cystic villi, while part of the placenta appears normal. A foetus with multiple malformations is often present.

M/E Some of the villi show oedematous change while others are normal or even fibrotic. Trophoblastic proliferation is usually slight and focal.

INVASIVE (DESTRUCTIVE) MOLE (CHORIOADENOMA DESTRUENS):
G/A Invasive mole shows invasion of the molar tissue into the uterine wall which may be a source of haemorrhage. Rarely, molar tissue may invade the blood vessels and reach the lungs.

M/E The lesion is benign and identical to classic mole but has potential for haemorrhage. It is always associated with persistent elevation of hCG levels.

CHORIOCARCINOMA *(p. 778)*

Gestational choriocarcinoma is a highly malignant and widely metastasising tumour of trophoblast. Approximately 50% of cases occur following hydatidiform mole, 25% following spontaneous abortion, 20% after an otherwise normal pregnancy, and 5% develop in an ectopic pregnancy.

Clinically, the most common complaint is vaginal bleeding following a normal or abnormal pregnancy. Occasionally, the patients present with metastases in the brain or lungs. The diagnosis is confirmed by demonstration of persistently high levels of hCG in the plasma and urine. Widespread haematogenous metastases are early and frequent in choriocarcinoma if not treated and are found chiefly in the lungs, vagina, brain, liver and kidneys.

G/A The tumour appears as haemorrhagic, soft and fleshy mass. Sometimes, the tumour may be small, often like a blood clot, in the uterus.

M/E 1. Absence of identifiable villi.
2. Masses and columns of highly anaplastic and bizarre cytotrophoblast and syncytiotrophoblast cells which are intermixed.
3. Invariable presence of haemorrhages and necrosis.
4. Invasion of the underlying myometrium and other structures, blood vessels and lymphatics.

Gestational choriocarcinoma and its metastases respond very well to chemotherapy while non-gestational choriocarcinoma is quite resistant to therapy and has worse prognosis. With chemotherapy, the cure rate of choriocarcinoma has remarkably improved from dismal 20 to 70% survival rate and almost total cure in localised tumours. The effectiveness of treatment is also monitored by serial hCG determinations.

The contrasting features of complete mole, partial mole and choriocarcinoma are summed up in Table 22.2.

TABLE 22.2: Comparative Features of Major Forms of Gestational Trophoblastic Disease.

	FEATURE	COMPLETE MOLE	PARTIAL MOLE	CHORIO-CARCINOMA
1.	**Karyotype**	46,XX or rarely 46,XY	Triploid i.e. 69,XXY or 69,XXX	46,XY or variable
2.	**Clinical findings**			
	i) Diagnosis	Mole	Missed abortion	Abortion; molar, ectopic or normal pregnancy
	ii) Vaginal bleeding	Marked	Mild	Marked, abnormal
	iii) Uterus size	Large	Small	Generally not bulky
3.	**hCG levels**			
	i) Serum hCG	High	Low	Persistently high
	ii) hCG in tissues	Marked	Mild	Localised in syncytiotropho-blast only

Contd...

Chapter Twenty Two

Table 22.2 Contd...

FEATURE	COMPLETE MOLE	PARTIAL MOLE	CHORIO-CARCINOMA
4. Embryo	Not present	May be present	Not present
5. Gross appearance			
i) Vesicles	Large and regular	Smaller and irregular	No vesicles
ii) Villi	Present	Present	Always absent
6. Microscopy			
i) Villous size	Uniform	Variable	None present
ii) Hydropic villi	All	Some	None
iii) Trophoblastic proliferation	Diffuse, all three (cytotrophoblast, intermediate trophoblast and syncytiotrophoblast)	Focal, syncytiotrophoblast only	Both cytotrophoblast and syncytiotrophoblast
iv) Atypia	Diffuse	Minimal	Marked
v) Blood vessels	Generally absent	Present	Present and abnormal
7. Persistence after initial therapy	20%	7%	May metastasise rapidly if not treated
8. Behaviour	2% may develop choriocarcinoma	Choriocarcinoma almost never develops	Survival rate with chemotherapy 70%

■ **SELF ASSESSMENT**

1. **The following vulval lesion can progress to vulval carcinoma:**
   A. Stromal polyp
   B. Papillary hidradenoma
   C. Squamous hyperplasia
   D. Lichen sclerosus

2. **High risk HPV types implicated in cervical intraepithelial lesions are:**
   A. 6 and 11
   B. 5 and 8
   C. 16 and 18
   D. 19 and 22

3. **The most common histologic type of cervical cancer is:**
   A. Well-differentiated keratinising squamous cell carcinoma
   B. Moderately-differentiated non-keratinising squamous cell carcinoma
   C. Small cell undifferentiated carcinoma
   D. Adenocarcinoma

4. **Arias-Stella reaction occurs in:**
   A. Ectopic tubal gestation only
   B. All ectopic gestations
   C. Uterine gestation
   D. Uterine as well as ectopic gestations

5. **Chocolate cyst of the ovary is:**
   A. Haemorrhagic corpus luteum
   B. Ruptured luteal cyst
   C. Endometriotic cyst
   D. Ruptured follicular cyst

6. **The malignant potential of atypical hyperplasia is:**
   A. About 5%
   B. About 25%
   C. About 50%
   D. About 75%

7. **Peak incidence of endometrial adenocarcinoma is in:**
   A. Reproductive years
   B. Premenopausal years
   C. Perimenopausal years
   D. Postmenopausal years

8. **The commonest site for endometriosis is:**
   A. Hernial sacs
   B. Vulva
   C. Ovaries
   D. Vagina

9. **Bilaterality of following ovarian tumours is most common:**
   A. Benign serous tumours
   B. Malignant serous tumours
   C. Benign mucinous tumours
   D. Brenner tumour

10. **The most common germ cell tumour of the ovary is:**
    A. Dysgerminoma
    B. Benign teratoma
    C. Immature teratoma
    D. Endodermal sinus tumour

11. **The most aggressive ovarian germ cell tumour is:**
    A. Malignant teratoma
    B. Embryonal carcinoma
    C. Endodermal sinus tumour
    D. Dysgerminoma

12. **Granulosa cell tumour is associated with following *except:***
    A. Endometrial hyperplasia
    B. Endometrial adenocarcinoma
    C. Endometrioid tumour
    D. Fibrocystic change in breast

13. **Krukenberg tumour is bilateral metastatic tumour from the following primary sites *except:***
    A. Stomach
    B. Colon
    C. Breast
    D. Endometrium

14. **The following trophoblastic tumour does not respond to chemotherapy:**
    A. Complete mole
    B. Invasive mole
    C. Gestational choriocarcinoma
    D. Ovarian choriocarcinoma

15. **Identifiable chorionic villi are present in the following tumours *except:***
    A. Complete mole
    B. Partial mole
    C. Invasive mole
    D. Gestational choriocarcinoma

16. **According to the Bethesda system, the squamous intraepithelial lesions for the grades of cervical cytology are:**
    A. Two
    B. Three
    C. Four
    D. Five

17. **In the etiology of condyloma acuminatum, the most commonly implicated HPV types are:**
    A. Types 1,2
    B. Types 6, 11
    C. Types 2,3,9
    D. Types 16,18

KEY

1 = C	2 = C	3 = B	4 = D
5 = C	6 = B	7 = D	8 = C
9 = B	10 = B	11 = B	12 = C
13 = D	14 = D	15 = D	16 = A
17 = B			

23

The Breast

NORMAL STRUCTURE *(p. 780)*

The breast is a modified skin appendage which is functional in the females during lactation but is rudimentary in the males. Microanatomy of the breast reveals 2 types of tissue components: *epithelial* and *stromal*. In a fully-developed non-lactating female breast, the epithelial component comprises less than 10% of the total volume but is more significant pathologically since majority of lesions pertain to this portion of the breast.

EPITHELIAL COMPONENT. The epithelial component of the breast consists of the breast lobules and the collecting duct system. The breast is divided into about 20 *lobes.* Each lobe consists of *breast lobules* which drain their secretions through its *collecting duct system* and opens into the nipple through its own main excretory duct, *lactiferous duct.* The segment of lactiferous duct subjacent to the nipple shows a small dilatation called *lactiferous sinus.* Each lactiferous duct has its own collecting duct system which has branches of smaller diameter, ultimately terminating peripherally as *terminal ducts* in the breast lobules which are the main secretory functional units of the mammary tissue during lactation. The breast lobules are composed of *acini* or *ductules* which are lined by cuboidal epithelium during resting mammary gland but develop secretory vacuoles in the last trimester of pregnancy.

STROMAL COMPONENT. The stromal tissue of the breast is present at 2 locations: intralobular and interlobular stroma. *Intralobular stroma* encloses each lobule, and its acini and ducts, and is chiefly made of loose connective tissue, myxomatous stroma and a few scattered lymphocytes. *Interlobular stroma* separates one lobule from the other and is composed mainly of adipose tissue and some loose connective tissue.

INFLAMMATIONS *(p. 780)*

Acute Mastitis and Breast Abscess *(p. 780)*

Acute pyogenic infection of the breast occurs chiefly during the first few weeks of lactation and sometimes by eczema of the nipples. Bacteria such as staphylococci and streptococci gain entry into the breast by development of cracks and fissures in the nipple. Extensive necrosis and replacement by fibrous scarring of the breast with retraction of the nipple may result.

Granulomatous Mastitis *(p. 781)*

Although chronic non-specific mastitis is uncommon, chronic granulomatous inflammation in the breast may occur as a result of the following:
1. *Systemic granulomatous disease* e.g. as part of systemic sarcoidosis, Wegener's granulomatosis.
2. *Infections* e.g. tuberculosis which is not so uncommon in developing countries like India and may be misdiagnosed clinically as breast cancer owing to axillary nodal involvement.
3. *Silicone breast implants* implanted on either breast cancer patients after mastectomy or as breast augmentation cosmetic surgery may rupture or silicone may slowly leak into surrounding breast tissue. This incites chronic inflammatory reaction of lymphocytes, macrophages and foreign body giant cells.
4. *Idiopathic granulomatous mastitis* is an uncommon form of reaction around lobules and ducts in the absence of any known etiology. Exact

pathogenesis is not known but probably it is a form of hypersensitivity reaction to luminal secretion of the breast epithelium during lactation.

Mammary Duct Ectasia (Plasma Cell Mastitis) *(p. 781)*

Mammary duct ectasia is a condition in which one or more of the larger ducts of the breast are dilated and filled with inspissated secretions. These are associated with periductal and interstitial chronic inflammatory changes. Duct ectasia affects women in their 4th to 7th decades of life. The etiology of the condition remains unknown but it appears to begin with periductal inflammation followed by destruction of the elastic tissue to cause ectasia and periductal fibrosis.

G/A The condition appears as a single, poorly-defined indurated area in the breast with ropiness on the surface. Cut section shows dilated ducts containing cheesy inspissated secretions.

M/E 1. Dilated ducts with either necrotic or atrophic lining by flattened epithelium and lumen containing granular, amorphous, pink debris and foam cells.
2. Periductal and interstitial chronic inflammation, chiefly lymphocytes, histiocytes with multinucleate histiocytic giant cells. Sometimes, plasma cells are present in impressive numbers and the condition is then termed *plasma cell mastitis.*
3. Occasionally, there may be obliteration of the ducts by fibrous tissue and varying amount of inflammation and is termed *obliterative mastitis.*

Fat Necrosis *(p. 781)*

Focal fat necrosis of an obese and pendulous breast followed by an inflammatory reaction is generally initiated by trauma. The condition presents as a well defined mass with indurated appearance.

G/A The excised lump has central pale cystic area of necrosis.

M/E There is disruption of the regular pattern of lipocytes with formation of lipid-filled spaces surrounded by neutrophils, lymphocytes, plasma cells and histiocytes having foamy cytoplasm and frequent foreign body giant cell formation.

Galactocele *(p. 782)*

A galactocele is cystic dilatation of one or more ducts occurring during lactation. The mammary duct is obstructed and dilated to form a thin-walled cyst filled with milky fluid.

FIBROCYSTIC CHANGE *(p. 782)*

The term fibrocystic change of the female breast is a histologic entity characterised by:

i)   cystic dilatation of terminal ducts;

ii) relative increase in inter- and intralobular fibrous tissue; and

iii) variable degree of epithelial proliferation in the terminal ducts.

It was previously termed *fibrocystic disease* but is currently considered as an exaggerated physiologic phenomena and not a disease, or was called as *benign mammary dysplasia* under the mistaken belief that all forms are dysplastic or precancerous condition, and hence has attracted considerable interest.

Its incidence has been reported to range from 10-20% in adult women. Most of the patients with fibrocystic change are between 3rd and 5th decades of life.

Chapter Twenty Three

It is important to identify the spectrum of histology or cytology findings by FNAC in fibrocystic changes since only some subset of changes have an increased risk of development of breast cancer. Presently, the spectrum of histologic changes are divided into two clinicopathologically relevant groups:

A. Nonproliferative changes (or cyst formation and fibrosis, or simple fibrocystic change);

B. Proliferative changes (includes epithelial hyperplasia and sclerosing adenosis).

A. Nonproliferative Fibrocystic Changes (Cyst Formation and Fibrosis, Simple Fibrocystic Change) *(p. 782)*

Formation of cysts of varying size and increase in fibrous stroma are the most common features of fibrocystic disease. Cysts are formed by dilatation of obstructed collecting ducts.

G/A The cysts are rarely solitary but are usually multifocal and bilateral. They vary from microcysts to 5-6 cm in diameter. The usual large cyst is rounded, translucent with bluish colour prior to opening (blue-dome cyst).

M/E 1. The cyst lining shows a variety of appearances. Often, the epithelium is flattened or atrophic. Frequently, there is apocrine change or apocrine metaplasia in the lining of the cyst resembling the cells of apocrine sweat glands.

2. There is increased fibrous stroma surrounding the cysts and variable degree of stromal lymphocytic infiltrate.

B. Proliferative Fibrocystic Changes (Epithelial Hyperplasia and Sclerosing Adenosis) *(p. 783)*

EPITHELIAL HYPERPLASIA. Epithelial hyperplasia is defined as increase in the layers of epithelial cells over the basement membrane to three or more layers in the ducts *(ductal hyperplasia)* or lobules *(lobular hyperplasia)*. The latter condition, lobular hyperplasia, must be distinguished from adenosis (discussed separately) in which there is increase in the number of ductules or acini without any change in the number or type of cells lining them.

M/E Epithelial hyperplasia is characterised by epithelial proliferation to more than its normal double layer. In general, ductal hyperplasia is termed as *epithelial hyperplasia of usual type* and may show various grades of epithelial proliferations, while *lobular hyperplasia* involving the ductules or acini is always atypical.

1. **Mild hyperplasia** of ductal epithelium consists of at least three layers of cells above the basement membrane, present focally or evenly throughout the duct.

2. **Moderate and florid hyperplasia** of ductal type is associated with tendency to fill the ductal lumen with proliferated epithelium. Such epithelial proliferations into the lumina of ducts may be focal, forming papillary epithelial projections called *ductal papillomatosis,* or may be more extensive, termed *florid papillomatosis.*

3. Of all the ductal hyperplasias, **atypical ductal hyperplasia** is more ominous and has to be distinguished from intraductal carcinoma. The proliferated epithelial cells in the atypical ductal hyperplasia partially fill the duct lumen and produce irregular microglandular spaces or *cribriform pattern.* The individual cells are uniform in shape but show loss of polarity with indistinct cytoplasmic margin and slightly elongated nuclei.

4. **Atypical lobular hyperplasia** is closely related to lobular carcinoma *in situ* but differs from the latter in having cytologically atypical cells only in half of the ductules or acini.

SCLEROSING ADENOSIS. Sclerosing adenosis is benign proliferation of small ductules or acini and intralobular fibrosis. The lesion may be present as diffusely scattered microscopic foci in the breast parenchyma, or may form an isolated palpable mass.

G/A The lesion may be coexistent with other components of fibrocystic disease, or may form an isolated mass.

M/E There is proliferation of ductules or acini and fibrous stromal overgrowth. The histologic appearance may superficially resemble infiltrating carcinoma but differs from the latter in having maintained lobular pattern and lack of infiltration into the surrounding fat.

Prognostic Significance *(p. 783)*

Since there is a variable degree of involvement of epithelial and mesenchymal elements in fibrocystic change, following prognostic derivations can be made:
1. *Nonproliferative fibrocystic changes* of fibrosis and cyst formation donot carry any increased risk of developing invasive breast cancer.
2. Identification of *general proliferative fibrocystic changes* are associated with 1.5 to 2 times increased risk for development of invasive breast cancer.
3. *Multifocal and bilateral proliferative changes* in the breast pose increased risk to both the breasts equally.
4. Within the group of proliferative fibrocystic changes, *atypical hyperplasia*, in partilcular, carries 4 to 5 times increased risk to develop invasive breast cancer later.

GYNAECOMASTIA (HYPERTROPHY OF MALE BREAST) *(p. 783)*

Unilateral or bilateral enlargement of the male breast is known as gynaecomastia. Since the male breast does not contain secretory lobules, the enlargement is mainly due to proliferation of ducts and increased periductal stroma. Gynaecomastia occurs in response to hormonal stimulation, mainly oestrogen. Such excessive oestrogenic activity in males is seen in young boys between 13 and 17 years of age *(pubertal gynaecomastia)*, in men over 50 years *(senescent gynaecomastia)*, in endocrine diseases associated with increased oestrogenic or decreased androgenic activity e.g. in hepatic cirrhosis, testicular tumours, pituitary tumours, carcinoma of the lung, exogenous oestrogen therapy as in carcinoma of the prostate and testicular atrophy.

G/A One or both the male breasts are enlarged having smooth glistening white tissue.

M/E 1. Proliferation of branching ducts.
2. Increased fibrous stroma with, myxoid appearance.

BREAST TUMOURS *(p. 784)*

FIBROADENOMA *(p. 784)*

Fibroadenoma or adenofibroma is a benign tumour of fibrous and epithelial elements. It is the most common benign tumour of the female breast. Though it can occur at any age during reproductive life, most patients are between 15 to 30 years of age. Clinically, fibroadenoma generally appears as a solitary, discrete, freely mobile nodule within the breast.

G/A Typical fibroadenoma is a small (2-4 cm diameter), solitary, well-encapsu-lated, spherical or discoid mass. The cut surface is firm, grey-white, slightly myxoid and may show slit-like spaces formed by compressed ducts.

M/E Fibrous tissue comprises most of a fibroadenoma. The arrangements between fibrous overgrowth and ducts may produce two types of patterns which may coexist in the same tumour:

■ **Intracanalicular pattern** is one in which the stroma compresses the ducts so that they are reduced to slit-like clefts lined by ductal epithelium.

■ **Pericanalicular pattern** is characterised by encircling masses of fibrous stroma around the patent or dilated ducts.

The fibrous stroma may be quite cellular, or there may be areas of hyalinised collagen. Sometimes, the stroma is loose and myxomatous.

PHYLLODES TUMOUR (CYSTOSARCOMA PHYLLODES) *(p. 785)*

Cystosarcoma phyllodes was the nomenclature given by Müller in 1838 to an uncommon bulky breast tumour with leaf-like gross appearance (*phyllodes*=leaf-like) having an aggressive clinical behaviour. Most patients are between 30 to 70 years of age. Phyllodes tumour can be classified into *benign, borderline* and *malignant* on the basis of histologic features. Local recurrences are much more frequent than metastases.

G/A The tumour is generally large, 10-15 cm in diameter, round to oval, bosselated, and less fully encapsulated than a fibroadenoma. The cut surface is grey-white with cystic cavities, areas of haemorrhages, necrosis and degenerative changes.

M/E The phyllodes tumour is composed of an extremely hypercellular stroma, accompanied by proliferation of benign ductal structures. Thus, phyllodes tumour resembles fibroadenoma except for enhanced stromal cellularity. The histologic criteria used to distinguish benign, borderline and malignant categories of phyllodes tumour are as under:

■ frequency of mitoses;

■ cellular atypia;

■ cellularity; and

■ infiltrative margins.

INTRADUCTAL PAPILLOMA *(p. 785)*

Intraductal papilloma is a benign papillary tumour occurring most commonly in a lactiferous duct or lactiferous sinus near the nipple.

G/A Intraductal papilloma is usually solitary, small, less than 1 cm in diameter, commonly located in the major mammary ducts close to the nipple.

M/E An intraductal papilloma is characterised by multiple papillae having well-developed fibrovascular stalks attached to the ductal wall and covered by benign cuboidal epithelial cells supported by myoepithelial cells.

CARCINOMA OF THE BREAST *(p. 785)*

Cancer of the breast is among the commonest of human cancers throughout the world. Its incidence and mortality are particularly high in developed countries. In the United States, carcinoma of the breast constitutes about 25% of all cancers in females and causes approximately 20% of cancer deaths among females. The incidence of breast cancer is highest in the perimenopausal age group and is uncommon before the age of 25 years.

Currently, emphasis is on early diagnosis by mammography, xero-radiography and thermography. Techniques like fine needle aspiration cytology (FNAC), stereotactic biopsy and frozen section are immensely valuable to the surgeon for immediate pathological diagnosis.

Etiology *(p. 785)*

The following risk factors are considered significant in its etiology:

1. Geography. The incidence of breast cancer is about six times higher in developed countries than the developing countries, with the notable exception of Japan.

2. Genetic factors. Recently, much work has been done on the influence of family history and inherited mutations in breast cancer:

i) *Family history:* First-degree relatives (mother, sister, daughter) of women with breast cancer have 2 to 6-fold higher risk of development of breast cancer. The risk is proportionate to a few factors:

■ number of blood relatives with breast cancer;

■ younger age at the time of development of breast cancer;

■ bilateral cancers; and

■ high risk cancer families having breast and ovarian carcinomas.

ii) *Genetic mutations:* About 10% breast cancers have been found to have inherited mutations. Most important of which is *breast cancer (BRCA)* susceptibility gene in inherited breast cancer:

■ *Mutation in TP53 tumour suppressor gene* on chromosome 17 as an acquired defect accounts for 40% cases of sporadic breast cancer in women but rarely in women with family history of breast cancer.

■ *Other mutations* seen less commonly in breast cancer include ataxia telangiectasia gene, *PTEN* (*phosphate and tensin*) tumour suppressor gene.

3. Oestrogen excess. There is sufficient evidence to suggest that excess endogenous oestrogen or exogenously administered oestrogen for prolonged duration is an important factor in the development of breast cancer.

4. Environmental and dietary factors. Among the environmental influences associated with increased risk of breast cancer are consumption of large amounts of animal fats, high calorie foods, cigarette smoking and alcohol.

5. Fibrocystic change. Fibrocystic change, particularly when associated with atypical epithelial hyperplasia, has about 5-fold higher risk of developing breast cancer subsequently.

General Features and Classification *(p. 787)*

Cancer of the breast occurs more often in left breast than the right and is bilateral in about 4% cases. Anatomically, upper outer quadrant is the site of tumour in half the breast cancers; followed in frequency by central portion, and equally in the remaining both lower and the upper inner quadrant.

Carcinoma of the breast arises from the ductal epithelium in 90% cases while the remaining 10% originate from the lobular epithelium. Table 23.1 presents different types of carcinoma of the breast as proposed in the WHO classification with some modifications.

TABLE 23.1: Classification of Carcinoma of the Breast.

A. NON-INVASIVE (IN SITU) CARCINOMA

  1. Intraductal carcinoma
  2. Lobular carcinoma *in situ*

B. INVASIVE CARCINOMA

  1. Infiltrating (invasive) duct carcinoma-NOS (not otherwise specified)
  2. Infiltrating (invasive) lobular carcinoma
  3. Medullary carcinoma
  4. Colloid (mucinous) carcinoma
  5. Papillary carcinoma
  6. Tubular carcinoma
  7. Adenoid cystic (invasive cribriform) carcinoma
  8. Secretory (juvenile) carcinoma
  9. Inflammatory carcinoma
  10. Carcinoma with metaplasia

C. PAGET'S DISEASE OF THE NIPPLE

A. NON-INVASIVE *(IN SITU)* CARCINOMA *(p. 787)*

In general, non-invasive or *in situ* carcinoma is characterised histologically by presence of tumour cells within the ducts or lobules without evidence of invasion.

1. Intraductal Carcinoma *(p. 787)*

Carcinoma *in situ* confined within the larger mammary ducts is called intraductal carcinoma. The tumour initially begins with atypical hyperplasia of ductal epithelium followed by filling of the duct with tumour cells. Clinically, it produces a palpable mass in 30-75% of cases and presence of nipple discharge in about 30% patients.

G/A The tumour may vary from a small poorly-defined focus to 3-5 cm diameter mass. On cut section, the involved area shows cystically dilated ducts containing cheesy necrotic material *(comedo pattern)*, or the intraductal tumour may be polypoid and friable resembling intraductal papilloma *(papillary pattern)*.

M/E The proliferating tumour cells within the ductal lumina may have 4 types of patterns in different combinations:

i) *Solid pattern* is characterised by filling and plugging of the ductal lumina with tumour cells.

ii) *Comedo pattern* is centrally placed necrotic debris surrounded by neoplastic cells in the duct.

iii) *Papillary pattern* has formation of intraductal papillary projections of tumour cells which lack a fibrovascular stalk.

iv) *Cribriform pattern* is recognised by neat punched out fenestrations in the intraductal tumour.

2. Lobular Carcinoma *in Situ* *(p. 788)*

Lobular carcinoma *in situ* is not a palpable or grossly visible tumour. Patients of *in situ* lobular carcinoma treated with excisional biopsy alone develop invasive cancer of the ipsilateral breast in about 25% cases in 10 years as in intraductal carcinoma but, in addition, have a much higher incidence of developing a contralateral breast cancer (30%).

G/A No visible tumour is identified.

M/E *In situ* lobular carcinoma is characterised by filling up of terminal ducts and ductules or acini by rather uniform cells which are loosely cohesive and have small, rounded nuclei with indistinct cytoplasmic margins.

B. INVASIVE CARCINOMA *(p. 788)*

The invasive breast cancer has various morphologic types which have clinical and prognostic correlates.

1. Infiltrating (Invasive) Duct Carcinoma-NOS *(p. 788)*

Infiltrating duct carcinoma-NOS *(not otherwise specified)* is the classic breast cancer and is the most common histologic pattern accounting for 70% cases of breast cancer. Clinically, majority of infiltrating duct carcinomas have a hard consistency due to dense collagenous stroma (scirrhous carcinoma). Retraction of the nipple and attachment of the tumour to underlying chest wall may be present.

G/A The tumour is irregular, 1-5 cm in diameter, hard cartilage-like mass that cuts with a grating sound. The sectioned surface of the tumour is grey-white to yellowish with chalky streaks and often extends irregularly into the surrounding fat.

M/E i) Anaplastic tumour cells forming solid nests, cords, poorly-formed glandular structures and some intraductal foci.

ii) Infiltration by these patterns of tumour cells into diffuse fibrous stroma and fat.

iii) Invasion into perivascular and perineural spaces as well as lymphatic and vascular invasion.

2. Infiltrating (Invasive) Lobular Carcinoma *(p. 788)*

Invasive lobular carcinoma comprises about 5% of all breast cancers. This peculiar morphologic form differs from other invasive cancers in being more frequently bilateral.

G/A The appearance varies from a well-defined scirrhous mass to a poorly-defined area of induration that may remain undetected by inspection as well as palpation.

M/E Two distinct features are seen:

i) Pattern—A characteristic single file (Indian file) linear arrangement of stromal infiltration by the tumour cells with very little tendency to gland formation is seen.

ii) Tumour cytology—Individual tumour cells resemble cells of *in situ* lobular carcinoma. They are round and regular with very little pleomorphism and infrequent mitoses.

3. Medullary Carcinoma *(p. 789)*

Medullary carcinoma is a variant of ductal carcinoma and comprises about 1% of all breast cancers. The tumour has a significantly better prognosis than the usual infiltrating duct carcinoma, probably due to good host immune response.

G/A The tumour is characterised by a large, well-circumscribed, rounded mass that is typically soft and fleshy or brain-like.

M/E It has 2 distinct features:

i) Tumour cells—Sheets of large, pleomorphic tumour cells with abundant cytoplasm, large vesicular nuclei and many bizarre and atypical mitoses are diffusely spread in the scanty stroma.

ii) Stroma—The loose connective tissue stroma is scanty and usually has a prominent lymphoid infiltrate.

4. Colloid (Mucinous) Carcinoma *(p. 789)*

This is an uncommon pattern of breast cancer occurring more frequently in older women and is slow-growing.

G/A The tumour is usually a soft and gelatinous mass with well-demarcated borders.

M/E Colloid carcinoma contains large amount of extracellular epithelial mucin and acini filled with mucin.

5. Papillary Carcinoma *(p. 790)*

Papillary carcinoma is a rare variety of infiltrating duct carcinoma in which the stromal invasion is in the form of papillary structures.

6. Tubular Carcinoma *(p. 790)*

Tubular carcinoma is another uncommon variant of invasive ductal carcinoma which has more favourable prognosis.

M/E The tumour is highly well-differentiated and has an orderly pattern. The tumour cells are regular and form a single layer in well-defined tubules. The tubules are quite even and distributed in dense fibrous stroma.

7. Adenoid Cystic (Invasive Cribriform) Carcinoma *(p. 790)*

Adenoid cystic or invasive cribriform carcinoma is a unique histologic pattern of breast cancer with excellent prognosis.

8. Secretory (Juvenile) Carcinoma *(p. 790)*

This pattern is found more frequently in children and has a better prognosis. The tumour is generally circumscribed which on histologic examination shows abundant intra- and extracellular PAS-positive clear spaces due to secretory activity of tumour cells.

9. Inflammatory Carcinoma *(p. 790)*

Inflammatory carcinoma of the breast is a clinical entity and does not constitute a histological type. The term has been used for breast cancers in which there is redness, oedema, tenderness and rapid enlargement.

10. Carcinoma with Metaplasia *(p. 790)*

Rarely, invasive ductal carcinomas may have various types of metaplastic alterations such as squamous metaplasia, cartilagenous and osseous metaplasia, or their combinations.

C. PAGET'S DISEASE OF THE NIPPLE *(p. 790)*

Paget's disease of the nipple is an eczematoid lesion of the nipple, often associated with an invasive or non-invasive ductal carcinoma of the underlying breast. The nipple bears a crusted, scaly and eczematoid lesion with a palpable subareolar mass in about half the cases. Most of the patients with palpable mass are found to have infiltrating duct carcinoma, while those with no palpable breast lump are usually subsequently found to have intraductal carcinoma.

G/A The skin of the nipple and areola is crusted, fissured and ulcerated with oozing of serosanguineous fluid from the erosions.

M/E The skin lesion is characterised by the presence of Paget's cells singly or in small clusters in the epidermis. These cells are larger than the epidermal cells, spherical, having hyperchromatic nuclei with cytoplasmic halo that stains positively with mucicarmine. In these respects, Paget's cells are adeno-carcinoma-type cells.

GRADING, STAGING AND PROGNOSIS *(p. 790)*

Histologic grading and clinical staging of breast cancer determines the management and clinical course in these patients.

HISTOLOGIC GRADING. The breast cancers are subdivided into various histologic grades depending upon the following parameters:

1. Histologic type of tumour. Breast cancer can be subdivided into 3 histologic grades:

i) *Non-metastasising*—Intraductal and lobular carcinoma *in situ*.

ii) *Less commonly metastasising*—Medullary, colloid, papillary, tubular, adenoid cystic (invasive cribriform), and secretory (juvenile) carcinomas.

iii) *Commonly metastasising*—Infiltrating duct, invasive lobular, and inflammatory carcinomas.

2. Microscopic grade. Widely used system for microscopic grading of breast carcinoma is that of Nottingham modification of the Bloom-Richardson system. It is based on 3 features: i) Tubule formation ii) Nuclear pleomorphism iii) Mitotic count.

3. Tumour size. There is generally an inverse relationship between diameter of primary breast cancer at the time of mastectomy and long-term survival.

4. Axillary lymph node metastasis. Survival rate is based on the number and level of lymph nodes involved by metastasis. More the number of regional lymph nodes involved, worse is the survival rate. Involvement of the lymph nodes from proximal to distal axilla (i.e. *level I*—superficial axilla, to *level III*—deep axilla) is directly correlated with the survival rate. In this regards, identification and dissection of sentinel lymph node followed by histopathologic examination has attained immense prognostic value (*Sentinel lymph node* is the first node in the vicinity to receive drainage from primary cancer i.e. it stands 'sentinel' over the tumour).

5. Oestrogen and progesterone receptors. Oestrogen is known to promote the breast cancer. Presence or absence of oestrogen receptors on the tumour cells can help in predicting the response of breast cancer to endocrine therapy. Accordingly, patients with high levels of oestrogen receptors on breast tumour cells have a better prognosis.

6. DNA content. Tumour cell subpopulations with aneuploid DNA content as evaluated by flow cytometry have a worse prognosis than purely diploid tumours.

CLINICAL STAGING. The American Joint Committee (AJC) on cancer staging has modified the TNM (primary *T*umour, *N*odal, and distant *M*etastasis) staging proposed by UICC (Union International for Control of Cancer).

Spread of breast cancer to axillary lymph nodes occurs early. Later, however, distant spread by lymphatic route to internal mammary lymphatics, mediastinal lymph nodes, supraclavicular lymph nodes, pleural lymph nodes and pleural lymphatics may occur. Common sites for haematogenous metastatic spread from breast cancer are the lungs, liver, bones, adrenals, brain and ovaries. Breast is one of the most suspect source of inapparent primary carcinoma in women presenting with metastatic carcinoma.

PROGNOSTIC FACTORS IN BREAST CANCER. Based on current knowledge gained by breast cancer screening programmes in the West employing mammography and stereotactic biopsy, various breast cancer risk factors and prognostic factors have been described. These prognostic factors are divided into following 3 groups:

1. Potentially pre-malignant lesions. These conditions are as under:

i) *Atypical ductal hyperplasia* is associated with 4-5 times increased risk than women of the same age. Such lesions are commonest in the age group of 45-55 years.

ii) *Clinging carcinoma* is a related lesion in the duct but different from carcinoma *in situ* and has lower risk of progression to invasive cancer than *in situ* carcinoma.

iii) *Fibroadenoma* is a long-term risk factor (after over 20 years) for invasive breast cancer, the risk being about twice compared to controls.

2. Breast carcinoma *in situ*. Following factors act as determinants:

i) *Ductal carcinoma in situ* (comedo and non-comedo subtypes) is diagnosed on the basis of three histologic features—nuclear grade, nuclear morphology and necrosis, while *lobular neoplasia* includes full spectrum of changes of lobular carcinoma *in situ* and atypical lobular hyperplasia. Ductal carcinoma *in situ* is more important and demands most attention. Comedo type of *in situ* carcinoma has higher recurrence rate.

ii) *Breast conservative therapy* is used more frequently nowadays in carcinoma *in situ* which requires consideration of three factors for management: *margins*, *extent of disease*, and *biological markers*. The biological markers such as *TP53* and *BCL 2* have low positivity in high-grade *in situ* ductal carcinoma and likelihood of recurrences after conservative surgery.

3. Invasive breast cancer. Prognostic and predictive factors for invasive breast cancer have been extensively studied by univariate analysis (examining single factor separately) as well as by multivariate analysis (comparing the value of various factors included in a study). These can be broadly divided into 3 groups: 1. routine histopathology criteria; 2. hormone receptor status; and 3. biological indicators.

■ SELF ASSESSMENT

1. **Mammary duct ectasia is characterised by the following features except:**
   A. It affects women in 2nd to 3rd decade of life
   B. There are dilated ducts containing inspissated secretions
   C. There is periductal chronic inflammation
   D. There may be presence of multinucleate giant cells

2. **Out of the various epithelial hyperplasias in breast the most ominous is:**
   A. Papillary ductal hyperplasia
   B. Florid ductal papillomatosis
   C. Lobular hyperplasia
   D. Epithelial hyperplasia of usual type

3. **Tubular adenoma of breast is mainly composed of:**
   A. Closely-packed ductules
   B. Ductal epithelial hyperplasia
   C. Lobular hyperplasia
   D. Lactational hyperplasia

4. **Phyllodes tumour is distinguished from fibroadenoma by having:**
   A. More ductal hyperplasia
   B. Compressed ducts
   C. More cellular stroma
   D. More lobular hyperplasia

5. **Intraductal papilloma occurs most often in the following region:**
   A. Collecting ducts
   B. Lactiferous ducts
   C. Terminal ducts
   D. Acini

6. **Lobular carcinoma *in situ* has the following features except:**
   A. A palpable lump is generally present
   B. After excision, about 25% cases develop ipsilateral invasive cancer in 10 years
   C. There is a higher incidence of bilaterality
   D. The tumour cells are rather uniform and cohesive

7. **The following type of carcinoma of the breast is characterised by 'Indian file' pattern of tumour cells:**
   A. Infiltrating duct carcinoma
   B. Invasive lobular carcinoma
   C. Medullary carcinoma
   D. Tubular carcinoma

8. **The following type of breast carcinoma is seen in children:**
   A. Papillary carcinoma
   B. Adenoid cystic carcinoma
   C. Secretory carcinoma
   D. Metaplastic carcinoma

9. **Paget's cells in Paget's disease of the breast are malignant cells of following type:**
   A. Squamous cell carcinoma
   B. Basal cell carcinoma
   C. Melanoma
   D. Adenocarcinoma

10. **Patients of breast cancer having high levels of oestrogen receptors imply:**
    A. Patient has an anaplastic breast cancer
    B. Anti-oestrogen therapy will be helpful
    C. Patient has an oestrogen-secreting ovarian tumour
    D. Patient is likely to have poor prognosis

11. **Men who have mutated *BRCA 1* have increased risk of following cancer:**
    A. Male breast
    B. Germ cell tumours of testis
    C. Sex-cord -stromal tumour of testis
    D. Carcinoma of prostate

KEY

1 = A	2 = C	3 = A	4 = C
5 = B	6 = A	7 = B	8 = C
9 = D	10 = B	11 = D	

24

The Skin

NORMAL STRUCTURE *(p. 793)*

In general, the skin is composed of 2 layers, the epidermis and the dermis. Cone-shaped dermal papillae extend upward into the epidermis forming peg-like *rete ridges* of the epidermis.

EPIDERMIS. The epidermis has the following 5 layers from base to the surface:
1. Basal cell layer (stratum germinatum).
2. Prickle cell layer (Stratum spinosum, Stratum malpighii).
3. Granular cell layer (stratum granulosum).
4. Stratum lucidum.
5. Horny layer (Stratum corneum).

DERMIS. The dermis consists of 2 parts—the superficial *pars papillaris* or *papillary dermis,* and the deeper *pars reticularis* or *reticular dermis.* The dermis is composed of fibrocollagenic tissue containing blood vessels, lymphatics and nerves.

Besides these structures, the dermis contains cutaneous appendages or adnexal structures.

1. SWEAT GLANDS. These are of 2 types—eccrine and apocrine.

i) Eccrine glands. They are present all over the skin but are most numerous on the palms, soles and axillae.

ii) Apocrine glands. Apocrine glands are encountered in some areas only—in the axillae, in the anogenital region, in the external ear as modified glands called ceruminous glands, in the eyelids as Moll's glands, and in the breast as mammary glands.

2. SEBACEOUS (HOLOCRINE) GLANDS. Sebaceous glands are found everywhere on the skin except on the palms and soles. They are often found in association with hair but can be seen in a few areas devoid of hair as modified sebaceous glands.

3. HAIR. The hair grows from the bottom of the follicle. It has, therefore, an intracutaneous portion present in the hair follicle and the shaft.

4. ARRECTORES PILORUM. These are small bundles of smooth muscle attached to each hair follicle. When the muscle contracts, the hair becomes more erect.

5. NAILS. The nails are thickenings of the deeper part of the stratum corneum that develop at specially modified portion of the skin called nail bed.

DERMATOSES *(p. 795)*

I. GENETIC DERMATOSES

XERODERMA PIGMENTOSUM. This is an autosomal recessive disorder in which sun-exposed skin is more vulnerable to damage. The condition results from decreased ability to repair the sunlight-induced damage to DNA. Patients of xeroderma pigmentosum are more prone to develop various skin cancers like squamous cell carcinoma, basal cell carcinoma and melanocarcinoma.

M/E The changes include hyperkeratosis, thinning and atrophy of stratum malpighii, chronic inflammatory cell infiltrate in the dermis and irregular accumulation of melanin in the basal cell layer.

URTICARIA PIGMENTOSA. Urticaria pigmentosa may occur as congenital form or may appear without any family history in the adolescents. Clinically, the condition presents as extensive pigmented macules.

M/E The epidermis is normal except for an increase in melanin pigmentation in the basal cell layer. The characteristic feature is the presence of numerous mast cells in the dermis.

ATAXIA TELANGIECTASIA. An autosomal recessive disorder, ataxia appears in infancy, while telangiectasia appears in childhood. The lesions are located on the conjunctivae, cheeks, ears and neck. These children are more prone to develop infections, especially of lungs, and lymphoma-leukaemia.

M/E The papillary dermis shows numerous dilated blood vessels.

II. NON-INFECTIOUS INFLAMMATORY DERMATOSES *(p. 796)*

1. DERMATITIS (ECZEMA). The pathologic term dermatitis is synonymous with the clinical term eczema. Both refer to inflammatory response to a variety of agents acting on the skin from outside or from within the body such as chemicals and drugs, hypersensitivity to various antigens and haptens etc. Accordingly, clinical types such as contact dermatitis, atopic dermatitis, drug-induced dermatitis, photo-eczematous dermatitis and primary irritant dermatitis are described.

M/E Dermatitis reaction may be acute, subacute or chronic:

■ **Acute dermatitis** is characterised by considerable spongiosis (intercellular oedema) that may lead to formation of intraepidermal vesicles or bullae. The vesicles and bullae as well as the oedematous epidermis are permeated by acute inflammatory cells.

■ **Subacute dermatitis** may follow acute dermatitis. Spongiosis and vesicles are smaller than in acute dermatitis. The dermis contains perivascular mononuclear infiltrate. The classical example of subacute dermatitis is *nummular dermatitis*.

■ **Chronic dermatitis** shows hyperkeratosis, parakeratosis and acanthosis with elongation of the rete ridges and broadened dermal papillae.

2. URTICARIA. Urticaria or hives is the presence of transient, recurrent, pruritic wheals (i.e. raised erythematous areas of oedema). Hereditary angioneurotic oedema is an uncommon variant of urticaria in which there is recurrent oedema not only on the skin but also on the oral, laryngeal and gastrointestinal mucosa.

M/E There is dermal oedema and a perivascular mononuclear infiltrate. There is localised mast cell degranulation by sensitisation with specific IgE antibodies but no increase in dermal mast cells.

3. MILIARIA. Miliaria is a condition in which there is cutaneous retention of sweat due to obstruction of sweat ducts. There are 2 types of miliaria.

■ **Miliaria crystallina** occurs when there is obstruction of sweat duct within the stratum corneum. It occurs in areas of skin exposed to sun or may occur during a febrile illness.

■ **Miliaria rubra** occurs when there is obstruction of sweat ducts within the deeper layers of the epidermis. It is seen more often in areas of skin covered by clothes following profuse sweating and the lesions are itchy.

4. PANNICULITIS (ERYTHEMA NODOSUM AND ERYTHEMA INDURA-TUM). Panniculitis is inflammation of the subcutaneous fat. Panniculitis may be acute or chronic. Generally, panniculitis appears as nodular lesions, predominantly on the lower legs. The following types of panniculitis are described:

■ **Erythema nodosum,** acute or chronic, is the most common form. The lesions consist of tender red nodules, 1-5 cm in diameter, seen more often on the anterior surface of the lower legs.

■ **Erythema induratum** is a less common variety. The lesions are chronic, painless, slightly tender, recurrent and found on the calves of lower legs.

M/E The early lesions show necrotising vasculitis involving the blood vessels in the deep dermis and subcutis. In chronic stage, there is inflammatory infiltrate consisting of lymphocytes, histiocytes and multinucleate giant cells.

5. ACNE VULGARIS. Acne vulgaris is a very common chronic inflammatory dermatosis found predominantly in adolescents in both sexes. The lesions are seen more commonly on the face, upper chest and upper back. The appearance of lesions around puberty is related to physiologic hormonal variations.

M/E A comedone consists of keratinised cells, sebum and bacteria. The hair follicle containing a comedone is surrounded by lymphocytic infiltrate in papular acne, and neutrophilic infiltrate in pustular acne.

III. INFECTIOUS DERMATOSES *(p. 797)*

1. IMPETIGO. Impetigo is a common superficial bacterial infection caused by staphylococci and streptococci. The condition may occur in children or in adults and more commonly involves hands and face.

M/E The characteristic feature is the subcorneal pustule which is a collection of neutrophils under the stratum corneum. Often, a few acantholytic cells and gram-positive bacteria are found within the pustule.

2. VERRUCAE (WARTS). Verrucae or warts are common viral lesions of the skin. They are caused by human papillomaviruses (HPV) that belong to papovavirus group, a type of DNA oncogenic virus. More than 80 HPV types have been identified. But it must be appreciated that various types of HPVs produce not only different morphologic lesions but also have variable oncogenic potential. The infection with HPV is acquired by direct contact or by auto-inoculation. Depending upon the clinical appearance and location, they are classified into different types described below.

i) Verruca vulgaris is the most common human wart. The lesions are often multiple, less than 1 cm in size, circumscribed, firm, elevated papules occurring more commonly on the dorsal surfaces of hands and fingers.

ii) Verruca plana on the other hand, is flat or slightly elevated wart, common on the face and dorsal surface of hands.

iii) Palmoplantar warts occur on the palms and soles. They are covered with a thick callus. They may, therefore, resemble calluses or a verrucous carcinoma.

iv) Epidermodysplasia verruciformis resembles verruca plana but differs by having familial occurrence with autosomal recessive inheritance. The genome of HPV types 5 and 8 has been found in some of these tumours. Epidermodysplasia verruciformis is of special clinical significance as it may undergo malignant change, usually into Bowen's disease, and occasionally into squamous cell carcinoma.

v) Condyloma acuminatum (or venereal wart or anogenital wart) occurs on the penis, on the vulva and around the anus. The lesions appear as soft, papillary, cauliflower-like mass that may grow fairly large in size (giant condyloma acuminata). In rare cases, transformation into verrucous carcinoma may occur.

M/E i) Papillomatosis (papillary folds).

ii) Acanthosis (hyperplasia of stratum malpighii containing foci of vacuolated cells in the upper stratum malpighii.

iii) Hyperkaratosis with parakeratosis.

iv) Clumped keratohyaline granules in the granular cells in the valleys between adjacent papillae.

v) Elongation of rete ridges with their lower tips bent inwards.

vi) Virus-infected epidermal cells contain prominent vacuolation (koilocytosis) and keratohyaline granules of intracytoplasmic keratin aggregates due to viral cytopathic effects. These cells on electron microscopy reveal numerous intranuclear viral particles.

3. MOLLUSCUM CONTAGIOSUM. Molluscum contagiosum is a common self-limiting contagious lesion caused by a poxvirus which is a DNA virus. It is more common in children and young adults. Infection is acquired by direct contact. Clinically, the lesions are often multiple, discrete, waxy, papules, about 5 mm in diameter and are seen more frequently on the face and trunk.

M/E Typical lesion consists of sharply circumscribed cup-like epidermal lesion growing down into the dermis. The proliferating epidermal cells contain the pathognomonic intracytoplasmic eosinophilic inclusion bodies called *molluscum bodies.*

4. VIRAL EXANTHEMATA. Viral exanthemata are a group of contagious conditions in which the epidermal cells are destroyed by replicating viruses causing eruption or rash. There are predominantly two groups of viruses which may cause exanthem. These are: the *poxvirus group* (e.g. smallpox or variola, cowpox or vaccinia), and the *herpesvirus group* (e.g. chickenpox or varicella, herpes zoster or shingles, herpes simplex).

Variola (smallpox) has been globally eradicated since 1978. The route of infection is via upper respiratory tract or mouth followed by viraemia and characteristic skin lesions. **Vaccinia (cowpox)** is primarily a disease of the teats and udders of cows but humans are infected by milking the infected animals. **Varicella (chickenpox)** and **herpes zoster (shingles)** are both caused by a common virus, varicella-zoster virus. Chickenpox is transmitted by the respiratory route followed by viraemia and successive crops of lesions. Herpes zoster is different manifestation of infection with the same viral agent after years of latency. It is a disease of the nerves and the tissues supplied by the nerves. **Herpes simplex,** caused by HSV-1, and another related herpetic infection, **herpes genitalis,** caused by HSV-2, are characterised by transmission by direct physical contact and prolonged latency.

M/E The characteristic feature of viral exanthemata is the formation of intra-epidermal vesicles or bullae due to cytopathic effects of viruses. In the early stage, there is proliferation of epidermal cells and formation of multinucleate giant cells. This is followed by intracellular oedema and ballooning degeneration.

5. SUPERFICIAL MYCOSES. Superficial fungal infections of the skin are localised to stratum corneum. These include some of the common dermatophytes such as: *Trichophyton rubrum* and *Pityrosporum.* Clinically, these fungal infections are labelled according to the region involved.

i) *Tinea capitis* occurring on the scalp, especially in children.

ii) *Tinea barbae* affecting the region of beard in adult males.

iii) *Tinea corporis* involving the body surface at all ages.

iv) *Tinea cruris* occurs most frequently in the region of groin in obese men, especially in hot weather.

v) *Tinea pedis* or 'athlete's foot' is located in the web spaces between the toes.

vi) *Onychomycosis* shows disintegration of the nail substance.

vii) *Tinea versicolor* caused by *Malassezia furfur* generally affects the upper trunk.

IV. GRANULOMATOUS DISEASES *(p. 799)*

1. LUPUS VULGARIS. The lesions of lupus vulgaris, the prototype of skin tuberculosis, are found most commonly on the head and neck, especially skin of the nose. They are yellowish-brown to reddish-brown tiny nodules (apple-jelly nodules).

M/E The nodules consist of well-defined tubercles lying in the upper dermis. They consist of accumulation of epithelioid cells surrounded by lymphoid cells. Caseation necrosis may be slight or absent. Langhans' and foreign body type of giant cells are often present.

2. GRANULOMA ANNULARE. The lesions of granuloma annulare are often numerous. Dermal nodules are arranged in a ring-like fashion, commonly on the hands and feet.

M/E The centre of the lesion shows a well demarcated focus of complete collagen degeneration. These foci are surrounded by an infiltrate composed largely of histiocytes and some mononuclear inflammatory cells forming a palisade arrangement and are therefore also referred to as palisading granulomas.

V. CONNECTIVE TISSUE DISEASES *(p. 799)*

1. LUPUS ERYTHEMATOSUS. Two types of lupus erythematosus are recognised—a chronic form, *discoid lupus erythematosus (DLE)* which is confined to the skin; and a systemic form, *systemic lupus erythematosus (SLE)* that has widespread visceral vascular lesions. The discoid variety is more common which is generally benign, while systemic form may be fatal, usually from renal involvement. The characteristic cutaneous lesions in DLE consist of well-defined erythematous discoid patches associated with scaling and atrophy and often limited to the face. In contrast, cutaneous lesions in SLE are present only in a small proportion of cases.

M/E Cutaneous lesion in DLE and SLE may not be distinguishable in all cases. The important features are:
i) Hyperkeratosis with keratotic plugging.
ii) Thinning and flattening of rete malpighii.
iii) Hydropic degeneration of basal layer.
iv) Patchy lymphoid infiltrate around cutaneous adnexal structures.
v) Upper dermis showing oedema, vasodilatation and extravasation of red cells.

High serum titres of antinuclear antibodies and demonstration of LE cells are other notable features, especially in SLE.

2. SYSTEMIC SCLEROSIS (SCLERODERMA). Two types of systemic sclerosis or scleroderma are identified: a localised form called *morphea,* and a generalised form called *progressive systemic sclerosis.* A variant of progressive systemic sclerosis is *CREST syndrome.* (C=calcinosis, R=Raynaud's phenomenon, E=esophageal dismotility, S=sclerodactyly and T=telangiectasia). Morphea consists of lesions limited to the skin and subcutaneous tissue, while progressive systemic sclerosis consists of extensive involvement of the skin and the subcutaneous tissue and has visceral lesions too.

M/E There is thickening of the dermal collagen extending into the subcutaneous tissue. There is pronounced chronic inflammatory infiltrate in the affected area. The epidermis is often thin, devoid of rete ridges and adnexal structures, and there is hyalinised thickening of the walls of dermal arterioles and capillaries. Subcutaneous calcification may develop.

3. LICHEN SCLEROSUS ET ATROPHICUS. This condition involves genital skin most frequently and is often the only site of involvement. It occurs in both sexes, more commonly in women than in men. It is termed *kraurosis vulvae* in women while the counterpart in men is referred to as *balanitis xerotica obliterans.*

M/E i) Hyperkeratosis with follicular plugging.

ii) Thinning and atrophy of the epidermis.

iii) Hydropic degeneration of the basal layer.

iv) Upper dermis showing oedema and hyaline appearance of collagen.

v) Inflammatory infiltrate in mid-dermis.

VI. NON-INFECTIOUS BULLOUS DERMATOSES *(p. 800)*

1. PEMPHIGUS. Pemphigus is an autoimmune bullous disease of skin and mucosa which has 4 clinical and pathologic variants: pemphigus vulgaris, pemphigus vegetans, pemphigus foliaceous and pemphigus erythematosus.

All forms of pemphigus have acantholysis as common histologic feature. Sera from these patients contain IgG antibodies to cement substance of skin and mucosa.

i) Pemphigus vulgaris is the most common type characerised by the development of flaccid bullae on the skin and oral mucosa. These bullae break easily leaving behind denuded surface.

M/E The bullae are suprabasal in location so that the basal layer remains attached to dermis like a row of tombstones.

ii) Pemphigus vegetans is an uncommon variant consisting of early lesions resembling pemphigus vulgaris.

M/E There is considerable acanthosis and papillomatosis. Intraepidermal abscesses composed almost entirely of eosinophils are diagnostic of pemphigus vegetans.

iii) Pemphigus foliaceous is characterised by quite superficial bullae which leave shallow zones of erythema and crust.

M/E Superficial subcorneal bullae are found which contain acantholytic epidermal cells.

iv) Pemphigus erythematosus is an early form of pemphigus foliaceous. The distribution of clinical lesions is similar to lupus erythematosus involving face.

M/E The picture is identical to that of pemphigus foliaceous.

2. PEMPHIGOID. This is a form of bullous disease affecting skin or the mucous membranes. Three variants have been described—*localised form* occurring on the lower extremities; *vesicular form* consisting of small tense blisters; and *vegetating form* having verrucous vegetations found mainly in the axillae and groins.

M/E The characteristic distinguishing feature from pemphigus is the subepidermal location of the non-acantholytic bullae. With passage of time, there is some epidermal regeneration from the periphery at the floor of the bulla. The bullous cavity contains fibrin network and many mononuclear inflammatory cells and some eosinophils. Dermal changes seen in inflammatory bullae consist of infiltrate of mononuclear cells, a few eosinophils and neutrophils.

3. DERMATITIS HERPETIFORMIS. Dermatitis herpetiformis is a form of chronic, pruritic, vesicular dermatosis. The lesions are found more commonly in males in 3rd to 4th decades of life. The disease has an association with gluten-sensitive enteropathy (coeliac disease).

M/E The early lesions of dermatitis herpetiformis consist of neutrophilic micro-abscesses at the tips of papillae, producing separation or blister between the papillary dermis and the epidermis. The older blisters contain fair number of eosinophils causing confusion with bullous pemphigoid.

4. ERYTHEMA MULTIFORME. This is an acute, self-limiting but recurrent dermatosis. The condition occurs due to hypersensitivity to certain infections and drugs, and in many cases, it is idiopathic. As the name suggests, the lesions are *multiform* such as macular, papular, vesicular and bullous. *Stevens-Johnson syndrome* is a severe, at times fatal, form of involvement of skin and mucous membranes of the mouth, conjunctivae, genital and perianal area.

M/E i) *Early lesions* show oedema and lymphocytic infiltrate at the dermo-epidermal junction. The superfical dermis shows perivascular lymphocytic infiltrate.

ii) *Later stage* is associated with migration of lymphocytes upwards into the epidermis resulting in epidermal necrosis and blister formation.

VII. SCALING DERMATOSES *(p. 802)*

The skin surface in some chronic inflammatory dermatoses is roughened due to excessive and abnormal scale formation and desquamation.

1. PSORIASIS. Psoriasis is a chronic inflammatory dermatosis that affects about 2% of the population. It usually appears first between the age of 15 and 30 years. The lesions are characterised by brownish-red papules and plaques which are sharply demarcated and are covered with fine, silvery white scales. As the scales are removed by gentle scrapping, fine bleeding points appear termed *Auspitz sign.*

M/E i) Acanthosis with regular downgrowth of rete ridges to almost the same dermal level with thickening of their lower portion.

ii) Elongation and oedema of the dermal papillae with broadening of their tips.

iii) Suprapapillary thinning of stratum malpighii.

iv) Absence of granular cell layer.

v) Prominent parakeratosis.

vi) Presence of Munro microabscesses in the parakeratotic horny layer is diagnostic of psoriasis.

2. LICHEN PLANUS. Lichen planus is a chronic dermatosis characterised clinically by irregular, violaceous, shining, flat-topped, pruritic papules. The lesions are distributed symmetrically with sites of predilection being flexor surfaces of the wrists, forearms, legs and external genitalia. Buccal mucosa is also involved in many cases of lichen planus.

M/E i) Marked hyperkeratosis.

ii) Focal hypergranulosis.

iii) Irregular acanthosis with elongated saw-toothed rete ridges.

iv) Liquefactive degeneration of the basal layer.

v) A band-like dermal infiltrate of mononuclear cells, sharply demarcated at its lower border and closely hugging the basal layer.

VIII. METABOLIC DISEASES OF SKIN *(p. 803)*

CALCINOSIS CUTIS. There are four types of calcification in the skin: i) Metastatic calcinosis cutis. ii) Dystrophic calcinosis cutis. iii) Idiopathic calcinosis cutis. iv) Subepidermal calcified nodule.

i) Metastatic calcinosis cutis develops due to hypercalcaemia or hyperphosphataemia.

ii) Dystrophic calcinosis cutis results when there is deposition of calcium salts at damaged tissue.

iii) Idiopathic calcinosis cutis resembles dystrophic type but is not associated with any underlying disease. A special manifestation of idiopathic calcinosis cutis is *tumoral calcinosis* in which there are large subcutaneous calcified masses, often accompanied by foreign body giant cell reaction. Calcium may discharge from the surface of the lesion. *Idiopathic calcinosis of the scrotum* consists of multiple asymptomatic nodules of the scrotal skin.

iv) Subepidermal calcified nodule or *cutaneous calculus* is a single raised hard calcified nodule in the upper dermis.

TUMOURS AND TUMOUR-LIKE LESIONS *(p. 803)*

A comprehensive list of tumours and tumour-like lesions of the skin is presented in Table 24.1.

I. TUMOURS AND CYSTS OF THE EPIDERMIS *(p. 804)*

A. Benign Tumours *(p. 804)*

1. SQUAMOUS PAPILLOMA. Squamous papilloma is a benign epithelial tumour of the skin. Though considered by many authors to include common viral warts (verrucae) and condyloma acuminata, true squamous papillomas differ from these viral lesions.

M/E Squamous papillomas are characterised by hyperkeratosis, acanthosis with elongation of rete ridges and papillomatosis. The *verrucae,* in addition to these features, have foci of vacuolated cells in the acanthotic stratum malpighii, vertical tiers of parakeratosis between the adjacent papillae and irregular clumps of keratohyaline granules in the virus-infected granular cells.

2. SEBORRHEIC KERATOSIS. Seborrheic keratosis is a very common lesion in middle-aged adults. There may be only one lesion, but more often these are many. The common locations are trunk and face. They are sharply-demarcated, brownish, smooth-surfaced, measuring a few millimetres in diameter.

M/E The pathognomonic feature is a sharply-demarcated exophytic tumour overlying a straight line from the normal epidermis at one end of the tumour to the normal epidermis at the other end. The other features are hyperkeratosis, acanthosis and papillomatosis as seen in squamous cell papillomas.

3. FIBROEPITHELIAL POLYPS. Also known by other names such as 'skin tags', 'acrochordons' and 'soft fibromas', these are the most common cutaneous lesions. They are often multiple, soft, small (a few mm in size), bag-like tumours commonly seen on the neck, trunk and axillae.

M/E The tumours are composed of loosely-arranged fibrovascular cores with overlying hyperplastic epidermis.

B. Epithelial Cysts *(p. 805)*

1. EPIDERMAL CYST. These intradermal or subcutaneous cysts may occur spontaneously or due to implantation of the epidermis into the dermis or subcutis (implantation cysts).

M/E Epidermal cysts have a cyst wall composed of true epidermis with laminated layers of keratin. Rupture of the cyst may incite foreign body giant cell inflammatory reaction in the wall.

2. PILAR (TRICHILEMMAL, SEBACEOUS) CYST. These cysts clinically resemble epidermal cysts but occur more frequently on the scalp and are more common than the epidermal cysts.

M/E The cyst wall is composed of palisading squamous epithelial cells. These cells undergo degeneration towards the cyst cavity. Rupture of the cyst wall is common and leads to foreign body giant cell inflammatory reaction.

TABLE 24.1: Tumours and Tumour-like Lesions of the Skin.

I. EPIDERMAL TUMOURS

A. Benign tumours
1. Squamous papilloma
2. Seborrhoeic keratosis
3. Fibroepithelial polyps
4. Keratoacanthoma

B. Epithelial cysts
1. Epidermal cyst
2. Pilar (trichilemmal, sebaceous) cyst
3. Dermoid cyst
4. Steatocystoma multiplex

C. Pre-malignant lesions
1. Solar keratosis (actinic keratosis, senile keratosis)
2. Bowen's disease
3. Xeroderma pigmentosum
4. Erythroplasia of Queyrat

D. Malignant tumours
1. Squamous cell carcinoma
2. Basal cell carcinoma (Rodent ulcer)
3. Metatypical (Basosquamous) carcinoma

II. ADNEXAL (APPENDAGEAL) TUMOURS

A. Tumours of hair follicles
1. Trichoepithelioma (Brooke's tumour)
2. Pilomatricoma (Calcifying epithelioma of Malherbe)
3. Trichofolliculoma
4. Trichilemmoma

B. Tumours of sebaceous glands
1. Naevus sebaceus
2. Sebaceous adenoma
3. Sebaceous carcinoma

C. Tumours of sweat glands
1. Eccrine tumours
   i) Eccrine poroma
   ii) Eccrine hidradenoma
   iii) Eccrine spiradenoma
2. Apocrine tumours
   i) Papillary hidradenoma
   ii) Cylindroma (Turban tumour)
3. Sweat gland carcinoma

III. MELANOCYTIC TUMOURS
1. Naevocellular naevi
2. Malignant melanoma

IV. DERMAL TUMOURS
1. Dermatofibroma and malignant fibrous histiocytoma
2. Dermatofibrosarcoma protuberans
3. Xanthoma
4. Lipoma and liposarcoma
5. Leiomyoma and leiomyosarcoma
6. Haemangiomas, lymphangiomas and angiosarcoma
7. Glomangioma
8. Kaposi's sarcoma

V. CELLULAR MIGRANT TUMOURS
1. Mycosis fungoides
2. Langerhans' cell histiocytosis
3. Mastocytosis
4. Lymphomas and leukaemias
5. Plasmacytoma

3. DERMOID CYST. These are subcutaneous cysts often present at birth. Dermoid cysts are more common on the face.

M/E The cyst wall contains epidermis as well as appendages such as hair follicles, sebaceous glands and sweat glands.

4. STEATOCYSTOMA MULTIPLEX. This is an inherited autosomal dominant disorder having multiple cystic nodules, 1-3 cm in size. They are more common in the axillae, sternum and arms.

M/E The cyst walls are composed of several layers of epithelial cells and contain lobules of sebaceous glands in the cyst wall.

C. Pre-malignant Lesions (p. 805)

1. SOLAR KERATOSIS (ACTINIC KERATOSIS, SENILE KERATOSIS). Solar (sun-induced) or actinic (induced by a variety of rays) keratoses are the multiple lesions occurring in sun-exposed areas of the skin in fair-skinned elderly people. Similar lesions may be induced by exposure to ionising radiation, hydrocarbons and arsenicals. The condition is considered to be a fore-runner of invasive squamous cell and/or basal cell carcinoma.

M/E Solar keratoses are squamous cell carcinoma *in situ* with the following characteristic features:

i) Considerable hyperkeratosis. ii) Marked acanthosis. iii) Dyskeratosis and dysplasia of the epidermal cells showing features such as hyperchromatism, loss of polarity, pleomorphism and increased number of mitotic figures. iv) Non-specific chronic inflammatory cell infiltrate in the upper dermis encroaching upon the basement membrane of the epidermis.

2. BOWEN'S DISEASE. Bowen's disease is also a carcinoma *in situ* of the entire epidermis but differs from solar keratosis in having often solitary lesion that may occur on sun-exposed as well as sun-unexposed skin. The condition may occur anywhere on the skin but is found more often on the trunk, buttocks and extremities.

M/E i) Marked hyperkeratosis.
ii) Pronounced parakeratosis.
iii) Marked epidermal hyperplasia with disappearance of dermal papillae.
iv) Scattered bizarre dyskeratotic cells distributed throughout the epidermis.

D. Malignant Tumours (p. 806)

1. SQUAMOUS CELL CARCINOMA. Squamous cell carcinoma may arise on any part of the skin and mucous membranes lined by squamous epithelium but is more likely to occur on sun-exposed parts in older people. Various predisposing conditions include: i) xeroderma pigmentosum; ii) solar keratosis; iii) chronic inflammatory conditions such as chronic ulcers and draining osteomyelitis; iv) old burn scars (Marjolin's ulcers); v) chemical burns; vi) psoriasis; vii) HIV infection; viii) ionising radiation; ix) industrial carcinogens (coal tars, oils etc); and x) in the case of cancer of oral cavity, chewing betel nuts and tobacco.

Cancer of scrotal skin in chimney-sweeps was the first cancer in which an occupational carcinogen (soot) was implicated. *'Kangari cancer'* of the skin of inner side of thigh and lower abdomen common in natives of Kashmir is another example of skin cancer due to chronic irritation.

Although squamous carcinomas can occur anywhere on the skin, most common locations are the face, pinna of the ears, back of hands and mucocutaneous junctions such as on the lips, anal canal and glans penis.

G/A Squamous carcinoma of the skin and squamous-lined mucosa can have one of the following two patterns:

i) More commonly, an *ulcerated growth* with elevated and indurated margin.

ii) Less often, a raised *fungating or polypoid verrucous* lesion without ulceration.

M/E i) There is irregular downward proliferation of epidermal cells into the dermis.

ii) Depending upon the grade of malignancy, the masses of epidermal cells show atypical features such as variation in cell size and shape, nuclear hyperchromatism, absence of intercellular bridges, individual cell keratinisation and occurrence of atypical mitotic figures.

iii) Better-differentiated squamous carcinomas have whorled arrangement of malignant squamous cells forming horn pearls. The centres of these horn pearls may contain laminated, keratin material.

iv) Higher grades of squamous carcinomas, however, have fewer or no horn pearls and may instead have highly atypical cells.

v) An uncommon variant of squamous carcinoma may have spindle-shaped tumour cells *(spindle cell carcinoma)*.

vi) Adenoid changes may be seen in a portion of squamous cell carcinoma *(adenoid squamous cell carcinoma)*.

vii) *Verrucous carcinoma* is a low grade squamous cell carcinoma in which the superficial portion of the tumour resembles verruca.

viii) All variants of squamous cell carcinoma show inflammatory reaction between the collections of tumour cells, while in *pseudocarcinomatous hyperplasia* there is permeation of the epithelial proliferations by inflammatory cells.

A system of grading of squamous cell carcinoma called **Broders' grading** has been proposed that depends upon the percentage of anaplastic cells present in a tumour. Accordingly, following 4 grades are recognised:

Grade I: Less than 25% anaplastic cells

Grade II :   25-50% anaplastic cells

Grade III :   50-75% anaplastic cells

Grade IV: More than 75% anaplastic cells.

However, it is important to take into account other factors for grading the tumour such as: the degree of atypicality of the tumour cells, presence or absence of keratinisation and the depth of penetration of the lesion. Therefore, based on combination of these factors, it is customary with pathologists to label squamous cell carcinomas with descriptive terms such as: well-differentiated, moderately-differentiated, undifferentiated, keratinising, non-keratinising, spindle cell type etc.

2. BASAL CELL CARCINOMA (RODENT ULCER). Typically, the basal cell carcinoma is a locally invasive, slow-growing tumour of middle-aged that rarely metastasises. It occurs exclusively on hairy skin, the most common location (90%) being the face, usually above a line from the lobe of the ear to the corner of the mouth. Basal cell carcinoma is seen more frequently in white-skinned people and in those who have prolonged exposure to strong sunlight like in those living in Australia and New Zealand.

G/A The most common pattern is a nodulo-ulcerative basal cell carcinoma in which a slow-growing small nodule undergoes central ulceration with pearly, rolled margins. The tumour enlarges in size by burrowing and by destroying the tissues locally like a rodent and hence the name 'rodent ulcer'.

M/E The most characteristic feature is the proliferation of basaloid cells (resembling basal layer of epidermis). A variety of patterns of these cells may be seen: solid masses, masses of pigmented cells, strands and nests of tumour cells in morphea pattern, keratotic masses, cystic change with sebaceous differentiation, and adenoid pattern with apocrine or eccrine differentiation. The most common pattern is *solid basal cell carcinoma* in which the dermis contains irregular masses of basaloid cells having characteristic peripheral palisaded appearance of the nuclei.

II. ADNEXAL (APPENDAGEAL) TUMOURS *(p. 808)*

A. Tumours of Hair Follicle *(p. 808)*

1. TRICHOEPITHELIOMA (BROOKE'S TUMOUR). This tumour may occur as a solitary lesion or as multiple inherited lesions, predominantly on the face, scalp and neck.

2. PILOMATRICOMA (CALCIFYING EPITHELIOMA OF MALHERBE). Pilomatricoma usually occurs as a solitary lesion, more often on the face and upper extremities. It may be seen at any age. The lesions vary in size from 0.5-5 cm and appear as well-demarcated dark red nodules.

B. Tumours of Sebaceous Glands *(p. 808)*

1. NAEVUS SEBACEUS. Naevus sebaceus of Jadassohn occurs mainly on the scalp or face as a solitary lesion that may be present at birth.

2. SEBACEOUS ADENOMA. Sebaceous adenoma occurs in middle-aged persons, most commonly on the face.

3. SEBACEOUS CARCINOMA. Sebaceous carcinoma is a rare tumour that may occur anywhere in the body except the palms and soles. Variants of sebaceous carcinoma are carcinoma of the Meibomian glands of the eyelids and carcinoma of the ceruminous glands in the external meatus.

M/E The tumour is composed of variable-sized lobules of poorly-differentiated cells containing some sebaceous cells. The tumour cells show marked cytologic atypia such as pleomorphism and hyperchromasia.

C. Tumours of Sweat Glands *(p. 809)*

1. ECCRINE TUMOURS. Depending upon the portion of eccrine sweat gland from which the tumour takes origin, the eccrine tumours are of 3 types:
i) *arising from intraepidermal portion of the duct* e.g. eccrine poroma;
ii) *arising from intradermal portion of the duct* e.g. hidradenoma; and
iii) *arising from secretory coils* e.g. eccrine spiradenoma.

2. APOCRINE TUMOURS. Apocrine sweat glands may give rise to tumours; the two common examples being papillary hidradenoma and cylindroma.

■ **Papillary hidradenoma.** Papillary hidradenoma or hidradenoma papilliferum is usually located as a small lesion commonly in women in the skin of the anogenital area.

■ **Cylindroma.** Also called as 'turban tumour' due to its common location on the scalp, cylindroma may occur as both solitary and multiple lesions.

3. SWEAT GLAND CARCINOMA. Rarely, the eccrine and apocrine gland tumours described above may turn malignant. All these carcinomas are adenocarcinomas.

III. MELANOCYTIC TUMOURS *(p. 810)*

Melanocytic tumours may arise from one of the three cell types: naevus cells, epidermal melanocytes and dermal melanocytes.

■ Benign tumours originating from *naevus cells* are called naevocellular naevi.

- The examples of benign tumours *arising from epidermal melanocytes* are lentigo, freckles, pigmentation associated with Albright's syndrome and *cafe-au-lait* spots of neurofibromatosis.

- Benign tumours *derived from dermal melanocytes* are Mongolian spots, naevi of Ota and of Ito and the blue naevus.

- *Malignant melanoma* is the malignant counterpart of melanocytic tumours.

1. NAEVOCELLULAR NAEVI. Pigmented naevi or moles are extremely common lesions on the skin of most individuals. They are often flat or slightly elevated lesions; rarely they may be papillomatous or pedunculated.

M/E Irrespective of the histologic types, all naevocellular naevi are composed of 'naevus cells' which are actually identical to melanocytes but differ from melanocytes in being arranged in clusters or nests. Naevus cells are cuboidal or oval in shape with homogeneous cytoplasm and contain large round or oval nucleus. Melanin pigment is abundant in the naevus cells present in the lower epidermis and upper dermis, but the cells in the mid-dermis and lower dermis hardly contain any melanin.

The important *histological variants* of naevi are as under:

i) **Lentigo** is the replacement of the basal layer of the epidermis by melanocytes.

ii) **Junctional naevus** is the one in which the naevus cells lie at the epidermal-dermal junction. The naevus cells form well-circumscribed nests.

iii) **Compound naevus** is the commonest type of pigmented naevus. These lesions, in addition to the junctional activity as in junctional naevi, show nests of naevus cells in the dermis to a variable depth.

iv) **Intradermal naevus** shows slight or no junctional activity. The lesion is mainly located in the upper dermis as nests and cords of naevus cells. Multinucleate naevus cells are common.

v) **Spindle cell (epithelioid) naevus or juvenile melanoma** is a compound naevus with junctional activity. The naevus cells are, however, elongated and epithelioid in appearance which may or may not contain melanin.

vi) **Blue naevus** is characterised by dendritic spindle naevus cells rather than the usual rounded or cuboidal naevus cells.

vii) **Dysplastic naevi** are certain atypical naevi which have increased risk of progression to malignant melanoma.

2. MALIGNANT MELANOMA. Malignant melanoma or melanocarcinoma arising from melanocytes is one of the most rapidly spreading malignant tumour of the skin that can occur at all ages but is rare before puberty. The tumour spreads locally as well as to distant sites by lymphatics and by blood. The etiology is unknown but there is role of excessive exposure of white skin to sunlight. Besides the skin, melanomas may occur at various other sites such as oral and anogenital mucosa, oesophagus, conjunctiva, orbit and lepto-meninges.

Some high risk factors associated with increased incidence of malignant melanoma are:

i) persistent change in appearance of a mole;

ii) presence of pre-existing naevus (especially dysplastic naevus);

iii) family history of melanoma in a patient of atypical mole;

iii) higher age of the patient; and

iv) more than 50 moles 2 mm or more in diameter.

Clinically, melanoma often appears as a flat or slightly elevated naevus which has variegated pigmentation, irregular borders and, of late, has undergone secondary changes of ulceration, bleeding and increase in size. Many of the malignant melanomas, however, arise *de novo* rather than from a pre-existing naevus. Malignant melanoma can be differentiated from benign pigmented lesions by subtle features which dermatologists term as ABCD of melanoma; these are summed up in Table 24.2.

TABLE 24.2: Distinguishing Features of Benign Mole and Malignant Melanoma.

	FEATURE	BENIGN MOLE	MALIGNANT MELANOMA
1.	**Clinical features**		
	i) Symmetry	Symmetrical	A = Asymmetry
	ii) Border	well-demarkated	B = Border irregularity
	iii) Colour	Uniformly pigmented	C = Colour change
	iv) Diameter	Small, less than 6 mm	D = Diameter more than 6 mm
2.	**Common locations**	Skin of face, mucosa	Skin; mucosa of nose, bowel, anal region
3.	**Histopathology**		
	i) Architecture	Nests of cells	Various paterns: solid sheets, alveoli, nests, islands
	ii) Cell morphology	Uniform looking naevus cells	Malignant cells, atypia, mitoses, nucleoli
	iii) Melanin pigment	Irregular, coarse clumps	Fine granules, uniformly distributed
	iv) Inflammation	May or may not be present	Often present
4.	**Spread**	Remains confined, poses cosmetic problem only	Haematogenous and/or lymphatic spread early

Depending upon the clinical course and prognosis, cutaneous malignant melanomas are of the following 4 types:

i) Lentigo maligna melanoma. This often develops from a pre-existing lentigo (a flat naevus characterised by replacement of basal layer of epidermis by naevus cells). It is essentially a malignant melanoma *in situ*. It is slow-growing and has good prognosis.

ii) Superficial spreading melanoma. This is a slightly elevated lesion with variegated colour and ulcerated surface. It often develops from a superficial spreading melanoma *in situ* (pagetoid melanoma) in 5 to 7 years. The prognosis is worse than for lentigo maligna melanoma.

iii) Acral lentigenous melanoma. This occurs more commonly on the soles, palms and mucosal surfaces.

iv) Nodular melanoma. This often appears as an elevated and deeply pigmented nodule that grows rapidly and undergoes ulceration. This variant carries the worst prognosis.

M/E The following characteristics are observed:

i) Origin. The malignant melanoma, whether arising from a pre-existing naevus or starting *de novo*, has marked junctional activity at the epidermo-dermal junction and grows downward into the dermis.

ii) Tumour cells. The malignant melanoma cells are usually larger than the naevus cells. They may be epithelioid or spindle-shaped, the former being more common. The tumour cells have amphophilic cytoplasm and large, pleomorphic nuclei with conspicuous nucleoli. Mitotic figures are often present and multinucleate giant cells may occur.

iii) Melanin. Melanin pigment may be present (melanotic) or absent (amelanotic melanoma) without any prognostic influence. The pigment, if present, tends to be in the form of uniform fine granules.

iv) Inflammatory infiltrate. Some amount of inflammatory infiltrate is present in the invasive melanomas.

The prognosis for patients with malignant melanoma is related to the depth of invasion of the tumour in the dermis.

Metastatic spread of malignant melanoma is very common and takes place via lymphatics to the regional lymph nodes, and through blood to distant sites like lungs, liver, brain, spinal cord, and adrenals.

IV. TUMOURS OF THE DERMIS (p. 812)

1. DERMATOFIBROMA AND MALIGNANT FIBROUS HISTIOCYTOMA. These soft tissue tumours are composed of cells having mixed features of fibroblasts, myofibroblasts, histiocytes and primitive mesenchymal cells. The histogenesis of these tumours is not quite clear but probably they arise from multi-directional differentiation of the primitive mesenchymal cells. The commonest sites are the lower and upper extremities. The benign variant is also known by various synonyms like dermatofibroma, histiocytoma, sclerosing haemangioma, fibroxanthoma and xanthogranuloma.

M/E The tumours are composed of spindle-shaped fibrohistiocytoid cells which are characteristically arranged in cartwheel or storiform pattern. The benign variety contains uniform spindle-shaped cells with admixture of numerous foamy histiocytes. The malignant fibrous histiocytoma shows pleomorphic tumour cells and some multinucleate giant cells in a stroma that may show myxoid change and inflammatory infiltrate.

2. DERMATOFIBROSARCOMA PROTUBERANS. This is a low grade fibrosarcoma that rarely metastasises but is locally recurrent. The tumour usually forms a solid nodule, within the dermis and subcutaneous fat, protruding the epidermis outwards. Sometimes multiple nodules may form.

M/E The tumour is very cellular and is composed of uniform fibroblasts arranged in a cartwheel or storiform pattern. The overlying epidermis is generally thinned and may be ulcerated.

3. XANTHOMAS. These are solitary or multiple tumour-like lesions, often associated with high levels of serum cholesterol and phospholipids. Many of the cases result from familial hyperlipidaemia. They may occur at different sites such as buttocks, knees, elbows, tendo-achilles, palmar creases and on the eyelids (referred to as xanthelasma).

V. CELLULAR MIGRANT TUMOURS (p. 813)

MYCOSIS FUNGOIDES (CUTANEOUS T CELL LYMPHOMA). Mycosis fungoides or cutaneous T cell lymphoma (CTCL) is the commonest form of lymphoma in the skin but in advanced stage, mycosis fungoides may disseminate to the lymph nodes and other organs. Clinically, mycosis fungoides may manifest in 3 stages:

i) **Premycotic stage** in which the lesions are erythematous, red-brown, scaly and pruritic, resembling eczema or psoriasis.

ii) **Infiltrative stage** has slightly elevated, bluish-red, firm plaques.

iii) **Fungoid (Tumour) stage** is characterised by red-brown nodules of tumour which often undergo ulceration.

Lesions may affect different body surfaces but more often involve the trunk, extremities, face and scalp.

M/E It has the following characteristics:
i) Initially, lower portion of the epidermis contains hyperchromatic enlarged lymphocytes. In about half the cases, there is formation of intraepidermal clusters of atypical lymphoid cells forming *Darier-Pautrier's microabscesses.*
ii) Later, there are band-like sharply demarcated aggregates of polymorphous cellular infiltrate in the dermis including atypical lymphoid cells (Sézary-Lutzner cells) and multinucleated cells.

iii) The individual mycosis cells are malignant T lymphocytes which have hyperchromatic and cerebriform nuclei and express CD4 and HLA-DR antigen.

The etiology of mycosis fungoides or cutaneous T cell-lymphoma has been found to be the same as for adult T cell lymphoma-leukaemia syndrome which is human T cell-leukaemia virus-I (HTLV-I).

Sézary syndrome is a variant of CTCL, often due to dissemination of underlying CTCL to the blood and infiltration into the skin causing generalised erythroderma, lymphadenopathy and hepatosplenomegaly.

■ SELF ASSESSMENT

1. **Molluscum contagiosum is caused by:**
   A. Papilloma virus
   B. Herpes virus
   C. Pox virus
   D. EB virus

2. **Xeroderma pigmentosum is characterised by the following features *except*:**
   A. Autosomal recessive inheritance
   B. Inability to repair sunlight-induced damage to DNA
   C. Proneness to develop various skin cancers
   D. Irregular accumulation of melanin in the basal layer

3. **The etiologic agent implicated in epidermodysplasia verruciformis is:**
   A. Herpes virus (HSV)
   B. Pox virus
   C. EB virus
   D. Papilloma virus (HPV)

4. **Herpesviruses cause the following exanthemata *except*:**
   A. Herpes simplex
   B. Herpes zoster
   C. Vaccinia
   D. Varicella

5. **The following bullous dermatosis is associated with coeliac disease:**
   A. Pemphigus vulgaris
   B. Pemphigoid
   C. Erythema multiforme
   D. Dermatitis herpetiformis

6. **Psoriasis has the following features *except*:**
   A. Acanthosis with thickened lower portion
   B. Suprapapillary thinning of epidermis
   C. Prominent granular cell layer
   D. Munro abscesses in parakeratotic layer

7. **Lichen planus is characterised by the following features *except*:**
   A. Marked hyperkeratosis
   B. Acanthosis with elongated saw-toothed lower border
   C. Band-like dermal infiltrate of inflammatory cells
   D. Intact basal cell layer

8. **The following conditions are premalignant *except*:**
   A. Solar keratosis
   B. Seborrheic keratosis
   C. Bowen's disease
   D. Xeroderma pigmentosum

9. **The following tumour is commonly non-metastasising:**
   A. Squamous cells carcinoma
   B. Basal cell carcinoma
   C. Melanoma
   D. Sweat gland carcinoma

10. **Papillary hidradenoma occurs most commonly in the following region:**
    A. Scalp
    B. Back
    C. Anogenital region
    D. Extremities

11. **The following type of naevi most often progress to malignant melanoma:**
    A. Compound naevus
    B. Blue naevus
    C. Dysplastic naevus
    D. Epithelioid naevus

12. **The following type of malignant melanoma has worse prognosis:**
    A. Nodular melanoma
    B. Superficial spreading melanoma
    C. Acral lentigenous melanoma
    D. Lentigo maligna melanoma

13. **Darier-Pautrier's abscess is composed of the following cells:**
    A. Neutrophils
    B. Macrophages
    C. Plasma cells
    D. Atypical lymphoid cells

14. **The following HPV types are implicated in the etiology of verruca vulgaris:**
    A. Types 1, 2
    B. Types 6, 11
    C. Types 2, 3
    D. Types 16, 18

15. **High risk factor for malignant melanoma include the following except:**
    A. Change in appearance
    B. Higher age of the patient
    C. More than 50 or more moles 2 mm or more in diameter
    D. Uniform pigmentation

KEY

1 = C	2 = D	3 = D	4 = C
5 = D	6 = C	7 = D	8 = B
9 = B	10 = C	11 = C	12 = A
13 = D	14 = A	15 = D	

25

The Endocrine System

GENERAL PRINCIPLES *(p. 814)*

The development, structure and functions of human body are governed and maintained by 2 mutually interlinked systems—*the endocrine system* and *the nervous system,* a third system combining features of both these systems is appropriately called *neuroendocrine system.*

NEUROENDOCRINE SYSTEM *(p. 814)*

This system forms a link between the endocrine and nervous systems. The cells of this system elaborates polypeptide hormones; owing to these biochemical properties, it has also been called as *APUD cell system* (for Amine Precursor Uptake and Decarboxylation properties).

1. Neuroendocrine cells are present in the gastric and intestinal mucosa and elaborate peptide hormones.

2. Neuroganglia cells lie in the ganglia cells in the sympathetic chain and elaborate amines.

3. Adrenal medulla elaborates epinephrine and norepinephrine.

4. Parafollicular C cells of the thyroid secrete calcitonin.

5. Islets of Langerhans in the pancreas (included in both endocrine and neuroendocrine systems) secrete insulin.

6. Isolated cells in the left atrium of the heart secrete atrial natriuretic (salt-losing) peptide hormone.

THE ENDOCRINE SYSTEM *(p. 814)*

Anatomically, the endocrine system consists of 6 distinct organs: pituitary, adrenals, thyroid, parathyroids, gonads, and pancreatic islets (also included in neuroendocrine system). Understanding the pathology of these endocrine organs requires the knowledge of overall framework of hormone secretions, their actions and broad principles of feedback mechanisms.

Broadly speaking, human hormones are divided into 5 major classes which are further grouped under two headings depending upon their site of interactions on the target cell receptors (whether cell membrane or nuclear):

Group I: Those interacting with cell-surface membrane receptors:

1. *Amino acid derivatives:* thyroid hormone, catecholamines.

2. *Small neuropeptides:* gonadotropin-releasing hormone (GnRH), thyrotropin-releasing hormone (TRH), somatostatin, vasopressin.

Group II: Those interacting with intracellular nuclear receptors:

3. *Large proteins:* insulin, luteinising hormone (LH), parathormone hormone.

4. *Steroid hormones:* cortisol, estrogen.

5. *Vitamin derivatives:* retinol (vitamin A) and vitamin D.

The *synthesis* of these hormones and their precursors takes place through a prescribed genetic pathway that involves: transcription → mRNA → protein synthesis → post-translational protein processing → intracellular sorting/ membrane integration → secretion.

Major functions of hormones are as under:

i) Growth and differentiation of cells

ii) Maintenance of homeostasis

iii) Reproduction

A basic feature of all endocrine glands is the existence of both negative and positive **feedback control system** that stimulates or regulates hormone production in a way that levels remain within the normal range (abbreviated as S or R respectively with the corresponding hormone e.g. TSH-TRH pathway, GnRH-LH/FSH pathway etc). This system is commonly termed *hypothalamic-pituitary hormone axis* for different hormones

In general, pathologic processes affecting endocrine glands with resultant hormonal abnormalities may occur from following processes:

■ **Hyperfunction:** This results from excess of hormone secreting tissues e.g. hyperplasia, tumours (adenoma, carcinoma), ectopic hormone production, excessive stimulation from inflammation (often autoimmune), infections, iatrogenic (drugs-induced, hormonal administration).

■ **Hypofunction:** Deficiency of hormones occurs from destruction of hormone-forming tissues from inflammations (often autoimmune), infections, iatrogenic (e.g. surgical removal, radiation damage), developmental defects (e.g. Turner's syndrome, hypoplasia), enzyme deficiency, haemorrhage and infarction (e.g. Sheehan's syndrome), nutritional deficiency (e.g. iodine deficiency).

■ **Hormone resistance:** There may be adequate or excessive production of a hormone but there is peripheral resistance, often from inherited mutations in receptors (e.g. defect in membrane receptors, nuclear receptors or receptor for signal transduction).

PITUITARY GLAND *(p. 816)*

NORMAL STRUCTURE *(p. 816)*

The pituitary gland or hypophysis in an adult weighs about 500 mg and is slightly heavier in females. It is situated at the base of the brain in a hollow called *sella turcica* formed out of the sphenoid bone. The gland is composed of 2 major anatomic divisions:

A. ANTERIOR LOBE (ADENOHYPOPHYSIS). It is composed of round to polygonal epithelial cells arranged in cords and islands having fibrovascular stroma. These epithelial cells, depending upon their staining characteristics and functions, are divided into 3 types, each of which performs separate functions:

1. Chromophil cells with acidophilic granules: The acidophils are further of 2 types:

i) *Somatotrophs (GH cells)* which produce growth hormone (GH); and

ii) *Lactotrophs (PRL cells)* which produce prolactin (PRL).

Cells containing both GH and PRL called *mammosomatotrophs* are also present.

2. Chromophil cells with basophilic granules: The basophils include 3 types of cells:

i) *Gonadotrophs (FSH-LH cells)* which are the source of the FSH and LH or interstitial cell stimulating hormone (ICSH).

ii) *Thyrotrophs (TSH cells)* are the cells producing TSH.

iii) *Corticotrophs (ACTH-MSH cells)* produce ACTH, melanocyte stimulating hormone (MSH), β-lipoprotein and β-endorphin.

3. Chromophobe cells without visible granules: These include sparsely granulated corticotrophs, thyrotrophs and gonadotrophs.

B. POSTERIOR LOBE (NEUROHYPOPHYSIS). The neurohypophysis is composed mainly of interlacing nerve fibres in which are scattered specialised glial cells called *pituicytes*. These nerve fibres on electron microscopy contain granules of neurosecretory material made up of 2 octapeptides.

1. **ADH** causes reabsorption of water from the renal tubules and is essential for maintenance of osmolality of the plasma. Its deficiency results in diabetes insipidus.

2. **Oxytocin** causes contraction of mammary myoepithelial cells resulting in ejection of milk from the lactating breast and causes contraction of myometrium of the uterus at term.

HYPERPITUITARISM (p. 817)

Hyperpituitarism is characterised by oversecretion of one or more of the pituitary hormones. Such hypersecretion may be due to diseases of the anterior pituitary, posterior pituitary or hypothalamus. For all practical purposes, however, hyperfunction of the anterior pituitary is due to the development of a hormone-secreting pituitary adenoma

A. Hyperfunction of Anterior Pituitary (p. 817)

Three common syndromes of adenohypophyseal hyperfunction are: gigantism and acromegaly, hyperprolactinaemia and Cushing's syndrome.

Gigantism. When GH excess occurs prior to epiphyseal closure, gigantism is produced. Gigantism, therefore, occurs in prepubertal boys and girls and is much less frequent than acromegaly.

Acromegaly. Acromegaly results when there is overproduction of GH in adults following cessation of bone growth and is more common than gigantism. The term 'acromegaly' means increased growth of extremities.

2. HYPERPROLACTINAEMIA. Hyperprolactinaemia is the excessive production of prolactin (PRL), most commonly by lactotroph (PRL-secreting) adenoma, also called prolactinoma.

3. CUSHING'S SYNDROME. Pituitary-dependent Cushing's syndrome results from ACTH excess. Most frequently, it is caused by corticotroph (ACTH-secreting) adenoma.

B. Hyperfunction of Posterior Pituitary and Hypothalamus (p. 817)

Two of the syndromes associated with hyperfunction of the posterior pituitary and hypothalamus are: inappropriate release of ADH and precocious puberty.

1. INAPPROPRIATE RELEASE OF ADH. Inappropriate release of ADH occurs most often in paraneoplastic syndrome e.g. in oat cell carcinoma of the lung, carcinoma of the pancreas, lymphoma and thymoma.

2. PRECOCIOUS PUBERTY. A tumour in the region of hypothalamus or the pineal gland may result in premature release of gonadotropins causing the onset of pubertal changes prior to the age of 9 years.

HYPOPITUITARISM (p. 818)

A. Hypofunction of Anterior Pituitary (p. 818)

Adenohypophyseal hypofunction is invariably due to destruction of the anterior lobe of more than 75% because the anterior pituitary possesses a large functional reserve. This may result from anterior pituitary lesions or pressure and destruction from adjacent lesions. Lesions of the anterior pituitary include nonsecretory (chromophobe) adenoma, metastatic carcinoma, craniopharyngioma, trauma, postpartum ischaemic necrosis (Sheehan's syndrome), empty-sella syndrome, and rarely, tuberculosis.

1. PANHYPOPITUITARISM. Three most common causes of panhypopituitarism are: non-secretory (chromophobe) adenoma, Sheehan's syndrome and Simmond's disease, and empty-sella syndrome.

Sheehan's syndrome and Simmond's disease. Pituitary insufficiency occurring due to postpartum pituitary (Sheehan's) necrosis is called Sheehan's syndrome, whereas occurrence of similar process without preceding pregnancy as well as its occurrence in males is termed Simmond's disease.

Empty-sella syndrome. Most commonly, it results from herniation of subarachnoid space into the sella turcica due to an incomplete diaphragma sella creating an empty sella.

2. PITUITARY DWARFISM. Severe deficiency of GH in children before growth is completed results in retarded growth and pituitary dwarfism. Most commonly, isolated GH deficiency is the result of an inherited autosomal recessive disorder. Less often it may be due to a pituitary adenoma or craniopharyngioma, infarction and trauma to the pituitary.

B. Hypofunction of Posterior Pituitary and Hypothalamus (p. 818)

Insufficiency of the posterior pituitary and hypothalamus is uncommon. The only significant clinical syndrome due to hypofunction of the neurohypophysis and hypothalamus is diabetes insipidus.

DIABETES INSIPIDUS. Deficient secretion of ADH causes diabetes insipidus. The causes of ADH deficiency are: inflammatory and neoplastic lesions of the hypothalamo-hypophyseal axis, destruction of neurohypophysis due to surgery, radiation, head injury, and lastly, are those cases where no definite cause is known and are labelled as idiopathic. The main features of diabetes insipidus are excretion of a very large volume of dilute urine of low specific gravity (below 1.010), polyuria and polydipsia.

PITUITARY TUMOURS (p. 819)

Tumours of the anterior pituitary are more common than those of the posterior pituitary and hypothalamus. The most common of the anterior pituitary tumours are adenomas.

All pituitary tumours, whether benign or malignant, cause symptoms in 2 ways: by pressure effects, and by hormonal effects.

Pituitary Adenomas (p. 819)

Adenomas are the most common pituitary tumours. They are conventionally classified according to their haematoxylin-eosin staining characteristics of granules into acidophil, basophil and chromophobe adenomas. A recent classification of pituitary adenomas based on functional features as correlated with morphologic features of older classification is given in Table 25.1.

G/A Pituitary adenomas range in size from small foci of less than 10 mm in size (termed microadenoma) to large adenomas several centimeters in diameter.

M/E By light microscopy of H & E stained sections, an adenoma is composed predominantly of one of the normal cell types of the anterior pituitary i.e. acidophil, basophil or chromophobe cells. These cells may have 3 types of patterns: diffuse, sinusoidal and papillary.

Pituitary adenocarcinoma is rare and is demonstrated by metastasis only.

Craniopharyngioma (p. 820)

Craniopharyngioma is a benign tumour arising from remnants of Rathke's pouch. It is more common in children and young adults. The tumour, though benign, compresses as well as invades the adjacent structures extensively.

G/A The tumour is encapsulated, adherent to surrounding structures and is typically cystic, reddish-grey mass.

TABLE 25.1: Morphologic and Functional Classification of Pituitary Adenomas.

	FUNCTIONAL TYPE	FREQUENCY	HORMONES PRODUCED	CLINICAL SYNDROME
1.	*Lactotroph adenoma (Prolactinoma)*	20-30%	PRL	Hypogonadism, galactorrhoea
2.	*Somatotroph adenoma*	5%	GH	Acromegaly/gigantism
3.	*Mixed somatotroph-lactotroph adenoma*	5%	PRL, GH	Acromegaly, hypogonadism, galactorrhoea
4.	*Corticotroph adenoma*	10-15%	ACTH	Cushing's syndrome
5.	*Gonadotroph adenoma*	10-15%	FSH-LH	Inactive or hypogonadism
6.	*Thyrotroph adenoma*	1%	TSH	Thyrotoxicosis
7.	*Null cell adenoma/ oncocytoma*	20%	Nil	Pituitary failure
8.	*Pleurihormonal adenoma*	15%	Multiple hormones	Mixed

M/E Craniopharyngioma closely resembles ameloblastoma of the jaw. There are 2 distinct histologic features:
1. Stratified squamous epithelium frequently lining, a cyst and containing loose stellate cells in the centre; and
2. Solid ameloblastous areas.

Granular Cell Tumour (Choristoma) *(p. 820)*

Though tumours of the posterior pituitary are rare, granular cell tumour or choristoma is the most common tumour of the neurohypophysis. It is composed of a mass of cells having granular eosinophilic cytoplasm similar to the cells of the posterior pituitary.

ADRENAL GLAND *(p. 820)*

NORMAL STRUCTURE *(p. 820)*

The adrenal glands lie at the upper pole of each kidney. Each gland weighs approximately 4 gm in the adult but in children the adrenals are proportionately larger. On sectioning, the adrenal is composed of 2 distinct parts: an outer yellow-brown *cortex* and an inner grey *medulla*.

ADRENAL CORTEX. It is composed of 3 layers:

1. **Zona glomerulosa** is the outer layer and comprises about 10% of the cortex. This layer is responsible for the synthesis of *mineralocorticoids*.

2. **Zona fasciculata** is the middle layer and constitutes approximately 70% of the cortex. Various *steroid hormones* are manufactured in the adrenal cortex such as glucocorticoids (e.g. cortisol) and sex steroids (e.g. testosterone).

3. **Zona reticularis** is the inner layer which makes up the remainder of the adrenal cortex. It has similar functional characteristics of synthesis and secretion of *glucocorticoids* and *androgens*.

The synthesis of glucocorticoids and adrenal androgens is under the control of ACTH from hypothalamus-anterior pituitary.

ADRENAL MEDULLA. The adrenal medulla is a component of the dispersed neuroendocrine system derived from primitive neuroectoderm; the other components of this system being *paraganglia* distributed in the vagi, paravertebral and visceral autonomic ganglia. The cells comprising this system are neuro-endocrine cells, the major function of which is synthesis and secretion of catecholamines (epinephrine and norepinephrine). Various other peptides such as calcitonin, somatostatin and vasoactive intestinal polypeptide (VIP) are also secreted by these cells. The major metabolites of catecholamines are metanephrine, nor-metanephrine, vanillyl mandelic acid (VMA) and homo-vanillic acid (HVA).

ADRENOCORTICAL HYPERFUNCTION (HYPERADRENALISM) *(p. 821)*

Hypersecretion of each of the three types of corticosteroids elaborated by the adrenal cortex causes distinct corresponding hyperadrenal clinical syndromes:

Cushing's Syndrome (Chronic Hypercortisolism) *(p. 821)*

Cushing's syndrome is caused by excessive production of cortisol of whatever cause.

ETIOPATHOGENESIS. There are 4 major etiologic types of Cushing's syndrome which should be distinguished for effective treatment.

1. Pituitary Cushing's syndrome. About 60-70% cases of Cushing's syndrome are caused by excessive secretion of ACTH due to a lesion in the pituitary gland, most commonly a corticotroph adenoma or multiple corticotroph microadenomas.

2. Adrenal Cushing's syndrome. Approximately 20-25% cases of Cushing's syndrome are caused by disease in one or both the adrenal glands.

3. Ectopic Cushing's syndrome. About 10-15% cases of Cushing's syndrome have an origin in ectopic ACTH elaboration by non-endocrine tumours. Most often, the tumour is an oat cell carcinoma of the lung

4. Iatrogenic Cushing's syndrome. Prolonged therapeutic administration of high doses of glucocorticoids or ACTH may result in Cushing's syndrome.

Conn's Syndrome (Primary Hyperaldosteronism) *(p. 821)*

This is an uncommon syndrome occurring due to overproduction of aldosterone, the potent salt-retaining hormone.

Adrenogenital Syndrome (Adrenal Virilism) *(p. 822)*

Adrenal cortex secretes a smaller amount of sex steroids than the gonads. However, adrenocortical hyperfunction may occasionally cause sexual disturbances.

ADRENOCORTICAL INSUFFICIENCY (HYPOADRENALISM) *(p. 822)*

Adrenocortical insufficiency may result from deficient synthesis of cortical steroids from the adrenal cortex or may be secondary to ACTH deficiency. Three types of adrenocortical hypofunction are distinguished:

1. *Primary adrenocortical insufficiency* caused primarily by the disease of the adrenal glands. Two forms are described: acute or 'adrenal crisis', and chronic or 'Addison's disease'.

2. *Secondary adrenocortical insufficiency* resulting from diminished secretion of ACTH.

3. *Hypoaldosteronism* characterised by deficient secretion of aldosterone.

Primary Adrenocrotical Insufficiency *(p. 822)*

Primary adrenal hypofunction occurs due to defect in the adrenal glands and normal pituitary function. It may develop in 2 ways:

A. Primary Acute Adrenocortical Insufficiency (Adrenal Crisis) *(p. 822)*

Sudden loss of adrenocortical function may result in an acute condition called *adrenal crisis.*

ETIOPATHOGENESIS. Causes of acute insufficiency are: 1. Bilateral adrenalectomy 2. Septicaemia 3. Rapid withdrawal of steroids 4. Acute stress in a case of chronic insufficiency.

B. Primary Chronic Adrenocortical Insufficiency (Addison's Disease) *(p. 823)*

Progressive chronic destruction of more than 90% of adrenal cortex on both sides results in an uncommon clinical condition called Addison's disease.

ETIOPATHOGENESIS. Any condition which causes marked chronic adrenal destruction may produce Addison's disease. These include: tuberculosis, autoimmune or idiopathic adrenalitis, histoplasmosis, amyloidosis, metastatic cancer, sarcoidosis and haemochromatosis. However, currently the first two causes—tuberculosis and autoimmune chronic destruction of adrenal glands, are implicated in majority of cases of Addison's disease.

Secondary Adrenocortical Insufficiency *(p. 823)*

Adrenocortical insufficiency resulting from deficiency of ACTH is called secondary adrenocortical insufficiency.

ETIOPATHOGENESIS. It includes following mechanisms:
1. *Selective ACTH deficiency* due to prolonged administration of high doses of glucocorticoids.
2. *Panhypopituitarism* due to hypothalamus-pituitary diseases.

Hypoaldosteronism *(p. 823)*

Isolated deficiency of aldosterone with normal cortisol level may occur in association with reduced renin secretion.

ETIOPATHOGENESIS. It may be form following factors:
1. Congenital defect due to deficiency of an enzyme required for its synthesis.
2. Prolonged administration of heparin.
3. Certain diseases of the brain.
4. Excision of an aldosterone-secreting tumour.

TUMOURS OF ADRENAL GLANDS *(p. 823)*

Cortical Adenoma *(p. 823)*

Adenomas of adrenal cortex are indistinguishable from hyperplastic nodules except that lesions smaller than 2 cm diameter are labelled *hyperplastic nodules.* A cortical adenoma is a benign and slow-growing tumour. It is usually small and nonfunctional.

G/A An adenoma is usually a small, solitary, spherical and encapsulated tumour which is well-delineated from the surrounding normal adrenal gland. Cut section is typically bright yellow.

M/E The tumour cells are arranged in trabeculae and generally resemble the cells of zona fasciculata.

Cortical Carcinoma *(p. 824)*

Carcinoma of the adrenal cortex is an uncommon tumour occurring mostly in adults. It invades locally as well as spreads to distant sites.

Pheochromocytoma (Chromaffin Tumour) *(p. 824)*

Pheochromocytoma (meaning *dusky brown tumour*) is generally a benign tumour arising from the adrenal medulla. The extra-adrenal pheochromocytomas arising from other paraganglia are preferably called *paragangliomas*.

Pheochromocytoma may occur at any age but most patients are 20-60 years old. Most pheochromocytomas are slow-growing and benign but about 5% of the tumours are malignant, invasive and metastasising.

The *clinical features* of pheochromocytoma are predominantly due to secretion of catecholamines, both epinephrine and norepinephrine. The most common feature is hypertension.

G/A The tumour is soft, spherical, about 5 cm in diameter, and well-demarcated from the adjacent adrenal gland. On cut section, the tumour is grey to dusky brown with areas of haemorrhages, necrosis, calcification and cystic change. On immersing the tumour in dichromate fixative, it turns brown-black due to oxidation of catecholamines in the tumour and hence the name chromaffin tumour.

M/E 1. The tumour cells are arranged in solid columns, sheets, trabeculae or clumps.
2. The tumour cells are large, polyhedral and pleomorphic with abundant granular amphophilic or basophilic cytoplasm and vesicular nuclei.
3. The tumour cells of pheochromocytoma stain positively with neuroendocrine markers such as neuron-specific enolase (NSE) and chromogranin.
4. The tumour has abundant fibrovascular stroma.

Myelolipoma *(p. 824)*

Myelolipoma is an uncommon benign adrenal medullary tumour found incidentally at autopsy. Less often, it may produce symptoms due to excessive hormone elaboration.

Neuroblastoma *(p. 824)*

Neuroblastoma, also called as sympathicoblastoma, is a common malignant tumour of embryonic nerve cells, occurring most commonly in children under 5 years of age. Vast majority of cases occur within the abdomen (in the adrenal medulla and paravertebral autonomic ganglia) and rarely in the cerebral hemisphere. Most cases are sporadic but familial occurrence with autosomal dominant transmission is also seen.

The *clinical manifestations* of neuroblastoma are related to its rapid local growth, metastatic spread or development of hormonal syndrome. Local symptoms include abdominal distension, fever, weight loss and malaise. Foci of calcification may be observed on radiologic examination of the abdomen. Metastatic spread occurs early and widely through haematogenous as well as lymphatic routes and involves bones (especially skull), liver, lungs and regional lymph nodes. Neuroblastoma produces variable amounts of catecholamines and its metabolites such as vanillyl mandelic acid (VMA).

Prognosis of neuroblastoma depends upon a few variables:
1. *Age* of the child below 2 years is associated with better prognosis.
2. Extra-abdominal *location* of the tumour have better outlook than abdominal masses.
3. *Patients in clinical stage* I (confined to the organ of origin) or stage II (tumour extending in continuity beyond the organ of origin but not crossing the midline) have better prognosis than higher stages with distant metastases.
4. Tumours with amplification of *MYC oncogene* and *TP53* are associated with poor prognosis.

G/A The tumour is generally large, soft and lobulated mass with extensive areas of necrosis and haemorrhages. The tumour is usually diffusely infiltrating into the adjacent tissues.

M/E 1. The tumour cells are small, round and oval, slightly larger than lymphocytes, and have scanty and poorly-defined cytoplasm and hyperchromatic nuclei.

2. The tumour cells stain positively with immunohistochemical markers such as neuron-specific enolase (NSE), neurofilaments (NF) and chromogranin.

3. They are generally arranged in irregular sheets separated by fibrovascular stroma.

4. Classical neuroblastomas show Homer-Wright's rosettes (pseudorosettes) which have a central fibrillar eosinophilic material surrounded by radially arranged tumour cells.

Ganglioneuroma *(p. 825)*

A ganglioneuroma is a mature, benign and uncommon tumour occurring in adults. It is derived from ganglion cells, most often in the posterior mediastinum, and uncommonly in other peripheral ganglia and brain.

Extra-adrenal Paraganglioma (Chemodectoma) *(p. 825)*

Parasympathetic paraganglia located in extra-adrenal sites such as the carotid bodies, vagus, jugulotympanic and aorticosympathetic (pre-aortic) paraganglia may produce neoplasms, collectively termed *paragangliomas* with the anatomic site of origin e.g. carotid body paraganglioma, intravagal paraganglioma, jugulotympanic paraganglioma etc. These tumours are also called chemodectomas because of their responsiveness to chemoreceptors.

THYROID GLAND *(p. 826)*

NORMAL STRUCTURE *(p. 826)*

Embryologically, the thyroid gland arises from a midline invagination at the root of the tongue and grows downwards in front of trachea and thyroid cartilage to reach its normal position.

The thyroid gland in an adult weighs 15-40 gm and is composed of two lateral lobes connected in the midline by a broad isthmus which may have a pyramidal lobe extending upwards.

M/E The thyroid is composed of lobules of colloid-filled spherical follicles or acini. The lobules are enclosed by fibrovascular septa. The follicles are the main functional units of the thyroid. They are lined by cuboidal epithelium with numerous fine microvilli extending into the follicular colloid that contains the glycoprotein, *thyroglobulin.*

FUNCTIONS. The major function of the thyroid gland is to maintain a high rate of metabolism which is done by means of iodine-containing thyroid hormones, thyroxine (T_4) and tri-iodothyronine (T_3).

The *synthesis and release* of the two main circulating thyroid hormones, T_3 and T_4 are regulated by hypophyseal thyroid-stimulating hormone (TSH) and involves the following steps: 1. Iodine trapping by thyroidal cells 2. Oxidation of the iodide   3. Iodination 4. Coupling of MIT and DIT.

HYPERTHYROIDISM (THYROTOXICOSIS) *(p. 827)*

Hyperthyroidism, also called thyrotoxicosis, is a hypermetabolic clinical and biochemical state caused by excess production of thyroid hormones. The condition is more frequent in females and is associated with rise in both T_3 and T_4 levels in blood, though the increase in T_3 is generally greater than that of T_4.

ETIOPATHOGENESIS. Hyperthyroidism may be caused by many diseases but three most common causes are: Graves' disease (diffuse toxic goitre), toxic multinodular goitre and a toxic adenoma.

HYPOTHYROIDISM *(p. 827)*

Hypothyroidism is a hypometabolic clinical state resulting from inadequate production of thyroid hormones for prolonged periods, or rarely, from resistance of the peripheral tissues to the effects of thyroid hormones. The clinical manifestations of hypothyroidism, depending upon the age at onset of disorder, are divided into 2 forms:

Cretinism *(p. 827)*

A cretin is a child with severe hypothyroidism present at birth or developing within first two years of postnatal life. This is the period when brain development is taking place so that in the absence of treatment the child is both physically and mentally retarded.

ETIOPATHOGENESIS. 1. *Developmental anomalies* e.g. thyroid agenesis and ectopic thyroid.
2. *Genetic defect* in thyroid hormone synthesis
3. *Foetal exposure* to iodides and antithyroid drugs.
4. *Endemic cretinism* in regions with endemic goitre due to dietary lack of iodine.

Myxoedema *(p. 828)*

The adult-onset severe hypothyroidism causes myxoedema. The term myxoedema connotes non-pitting oedema due to accumulation of hydrophilic mucopolysaccharides in the ground substance of dermis and other tissues.

ETIOPATHOGENESIS. 1. Ablation of the thyroid by surgery or radiation.
2. Autoimmune (lymphocytic) thyroiditis (termed primary idiopathic myxoedema).
3. Endemic or sporadic goitre.
4. Hypothalamic-pituitary lesions.
5. Thyroid cancer.
6. Prolonged administration of antithyroid drugs.
7. Mild developmental anomalies and dyshormonogenesis.

THYROIDITIS *(p. 828)*

Inflammation of the thyroid, thyroiditis, is more often due to non-infectious causes and is classified on the basis of onset and duration of disease into acute, subacute and chronic as under:

I. Acute thyroiditis:
1. Bacterial infection e.g. *Staphylococcus, Streptococcus.*
2. Fungal infection e.g. *Aspergillus, Histoplasma, Pneumocystis.*
3. Radiation injury

II. Subacute thyroiditis:
1. Subacute granulomatous thyroiditis (de Quervain's thyroiditis, giant cell thyroiditis, viral thyroiditis)
2. Subacute lymphocytic (postpartum, silent) thyroiditis
3. Tuberculous thyroiditis

III. Chronic thyroiditis:
1. Autoimmune thyroiditis (Hashimoto's thyroiditis or chronic lymphocytic thyroiditis)
2. Riedel's thyroiditis (or invasive fibrous thyroiditis).

Important examples are considered below.

Hashimoto's (Autoimmune, Chronic Lymphocytic) Thyroiditis *(p. 828)*

Hashimoto's thyroiditis, also called diffuse lymphocytic thyroiditis, struma lymphomatosa or goitrous autoimmune thyroiditis, is characterised by 3 principal features:

■ diffuse goitrous enlargement of the thyroid;

■ lymphocytic infiltration of the thyroid gland; and

■ occurrence of thyroid autoantibodies.

Hashimoto's thyroiditis occurs more frequently between the age of 30 and 50 years and shows an approximately ten-fold preponderance among females. Though rare in children, about half the cases of adolescent goitre are owing to autoimmune thyroiditis. Hashimoto's thyroiditis is the most common cause of *goitrous hypothyroidism* in regions where iodine supplies are *adequate*. Regions where iodine intake is highest have higher incidence of Hashimoto's thyroiditis e.g. in Japan and the United States.

ETIOPATHOGENESIS. Hashimoto's thyroiditis is an autoimmune disease is well established. Autoimmune pathogenesis of Hashimoto's thyroiditis is explained by the following observations:

1. Other autoimmune disease association: Like in other autoimmune diseases, Hashimoto's disease has been found in association with other autoimmune diseases such as Graves' disease, SLE, Sjögren's syndrome, rheumatoid arthritis, pernicious anaemia and Type 1 (juvenile-onset) diabetes mellitus.

2. Immune destruction of thyroid cells: The sequence of immune phenomena is initial activation of CD4+ T helper cells. These cells then induce infiltration of CD8+ T cytotoxic cells in the thyroid parenchyma as well as activate B cells to form autoantibodies, which bring about immune destruction of thyroid parenchyma.

3. Detection of autoantibodies: The following autoantibodies against different thyroid cell antigens are detectable in the sera of most patients with Hashimoto's thyroiditis:

i) Thyroid microsomal autoantibodies (against the microsomes of the follicular cells).

ii) Thyroglobulin autoantibodies.

iii) TSH receptor autoantibodies.

4. Inhibitory TSH-receptor antibodies: TSH-receptor antibody seen on the surface of thyroid cells in Hashimoto's thyroiditis is inhibitory to TSH, producing hypothyroidism.

5. Genetic basis: The disease has higher incidence in first-degree relatives of affected patients. Hashimoto's thyroiditis is seen more often with HLA-DR3 and HLA-DR5 subtypes.

G/A The *classic form* is characterised by diffuse, symmetric, firm and rubbery enlargement of the thyroid which may weigh 100-300 gm. Sectioned surface of the thyroid is fleshly with accentuation of normal lobulations but with retained normal shape of the gland. The *fibrosing variant* has a firm, enlarged thyroid with compression of the surrounding tissues.

M/E The *classic form* shows the following features

1. There is extensive infiltration of the gland by lymphocytes, plasma cells, immunoblasts and macrophages, with formation of lymphoid follicles having germinal centres.

2. There is decreased number of thyroid follicles which are generally atrophic and are often devoid of colloid.

3. The follicular epithelial cells are transformed into their degenerated state termed Hurthle cells (also called Askanazy cells, or oxyphil cells, or oncocytes). These cells have abundant oxyphilic or eosinophilic and granular cytoplasm due to large number of mitochondria and contain large bizarre nuclei.

4. There is slight fibrous thickening of the septa separating the thyroid lobules.

The less common *fibrosing variant* of Hashimoto's thyroiditis shows considerable fibrous replacement of thyroid parenchyma and a less prominent lymphoid infiltrate.

There is no increased risk of developing thyroid carcinoma in Hashimoto's thyroiditis but there is increased frequency of malignant lymphoma in these cases.

Subacute Lymphocytic Thyroiditis *(p. 829)*

Subacute lymphocytic (or painless or silent or postpartum) thyroiditis is another variety of autoimmune thyroiditis. Clinically, it differs from subacute granulomatous in being non-tender thyroid enlargement. It occurs frequently 3-6 months after delivery.

Subacute Granulomatous Thyroiditis *(p. 830)*

Granulomatous thyroiditis, also called de Quervain's or subacute, or giant cell thyroiditis, is a distinctive form of self-limited inflammation of the thyroid gland. Etiology of the condition is not known but clinical features of a prodromal phase and preceding respiratory infection suggest a possible viral etiology. The disease is more common in young and middle-aged women and may present clinically with painful moderate thyroid enlargement with fever.

G/A There is moderate enlargement of the gland which is often asymmetric or focal. The cut surface of the involved area is firm and yellowish-white.

M/E

■ *Initially,* there is acute inflammatory destruction of the thyroid parenchyma and formation of microabscesses.

■ *Later,* the more characteristic feature of granulomatous appearance is produced. These granulomas consist of central colloid material surrounded by histiocytes and scattered multinucleate giant cells.

■ More *advanced* cases may show fibroblastic proliferation.

Riedel's Thyroiditis *(p. 830)*

Riedel's thyroiditis, also called Riedel's struma or invasive fibrous thyroiditis, is a rare chronic disease characterised by stony-hard thyroid that is densely adherent to the adjacent structures in the neck. The condition is clinically significant due to compressive clinical features (e.g. dysphagia, dyspnoea, recurrent laryngeal nerve paralysis and stridor) and resemblance with thyroid cancer. The etiology is unknown but possibly Riedel's thyroiditis is a part of *multifocal idiopathic fibrosclerosis*. This group of disorders includes: idiopathic retroperitoneal, mediastinal and retro-orbital fibrosis, and sclerosing cholangitis, all of which may occur simultaneously with Riedel's thyroiditis.

G/A The thyroid gland is usually contracted, stony-hard, asymmetric and firmly adherent to the adjacent structures. Cut section is hard and devoid of lobulations.

M/E There is extensive fibrocollagenous replacement, marked atrophy of the thyroid parenchyma, focally scattered lymphocytic infiltration and invasion of the adjacent muscle tissue by the process.

GRAVES' DISEASE (DIFFUSE TOXIC GOITRE) *(p. 830)*

Graves' disease, also known as Basedow's disease, primary hyperplasia, exophthalmic goitre, and diffuse toxic goitre, is characterised by a triad of features:

■ hyperthyroidism (thyrotoxicosis);

■ diffuse thyroid enlargement; and

■ ophthalmopathy.

The disease is more frequent between the age of 30 and 40 years and has five-fold increased prevalence among females.

ETIOPATHOGENESIS. Graves' disease is an autoimmune disease, there are many immunologic similarities between this condition and Hashimoto's thyroiditis.

1. HLA association. Like in Hashimoto's thyroiditis. Graves'disease too has genetic predisposition. A familial occurrence has been observed. Graves' disease has been found strongly associated with HLA-DR3.

2. Autoimmune disease association. Graves' disease may be found in association with other organ-specific autoimmune diseases. Hashimoto's thyroiditis and Graves' disease are frequently present in the same families and the two diseases may coexist in the same patient.

3. Other factors. Besides these two factors, other factors observed in Graves' disease are higher prevalence in women (7 to 10 times), association with emotional stress and smoking.

4. Autoantibodies. Autoantibodies against thyroid antigens are detectable in the serum of these patients too but their sites of action are different from that of Hashimoto's thyroiditis.

i) Thyroid-stimulating immunoglobulin (TSI):

ii) Thyroid growth-stimulating immunoglobulins (TGI):

iii) TSH-binding inhibitor immunoglobulins (TBII):

G/A The thyroid is moderately, diffusely and symmetrically enlarged and may weigh up to 70-90 gm. On cut section, the thyroid parenchyma is typically homogeneous, red-brown and meaty and lacks the normal translucency.

M/E 1. There is considerable epithelial hyperplasia and hypertrophy as seen by increased height of the follicular lining cells and formation of papillary infoldings.

2. The colloid is markedly diminished and is lightly staining, watery and finely vacuolated.

3. The stroma shows increased vascularity and accumulation of lymphoid cells.

GOITRE *(p. 831)*

The term goitre is defined as thyroid enlargement caused by compensatory hyperplasia and hypertrophy of the follicular epithelium in response to thyroid hormone deficiency. The end-result of this hyperplasia is generally a *euthyroid state* (in contrast to thyrotoxicosis occurring in diffuse toxic goitre or Graves' disease) though at some stages there may be hypo- or hyperthyroidism. Two morphologic forms of goitre are distinguished:

A. Diffuse goitre (simple nontoxic goitre or colloid goitre).

B. Nodular goitre (multinodular goitre or adenomatous goitre).

Pathogenesis of Goitre *(p. 831)*

The pathogenetic mechanisms of both forms of goitre can be considered together since nodular goitre is generally regarded as the end-stage of long-standing simple goitre (Fig. 25.1). The fundamental defect is deficient production

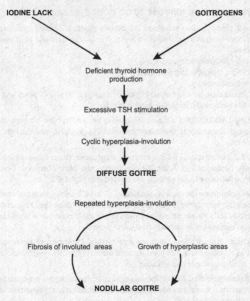

IODINE LACK   **GOITROGENS**

Deficient thyroid hormone
production

↓

Excessive TSH stimulation

↓

Cyclic hyperplasia-involution

↓

DIFFUSE GOITRE

↓

Repeated hyperplasia-involution

Fibrosis of involuted areas   Growth of hyperplastic areas

NODULAR GOITRE

Fig. 25.1: Pathogenesis of simple and nodular goitre

of thyroid hormones due to various etiologic factors described below, but most common is *dietary lack of iodine*. Deficient thyroid hormone production causes excessive TSH stimulation which leads to hyperplasia of follicular epithelium as well as formation of new thyroid follicles.

Diffuse Goitre (Simple Non-toxic Goitre, Colloid Goitre) *(p. 832)*

Diffuse, nontoxic simple or colloid goitre is the name given to diffuse enlargement of the thyroid gland, unaccompanied by hyperthyroidism. Most cases are in a state of euthyroid though they may have passed through preceding stage of hypothyroidism due to inadequate supply of iodine. TSH levels are invariably elevated. In general, goitre is more common in females.

ETIOLOGY. Epidemiologically, goitre occurs in 2 forms:

Endemic goitre. Prevalence of goitre in a geographic area in more than 10% of the population is termed endemic goitre. Such endemic areas are several high mountainous regions far from the sea where iodine content of drinking water and food is low such as in the regions of the Himalayas, the Alps and the Ande.

Sporadic goitre. Non-endemic or sporadic simple goitre is less common than the endemic variety. In most cases, the etiology of sporadic goitre is unknown. A number of causal influences have been attributed:
- Suboptimal iodine intake in conditions of increased demand as in puberty and pregnancy.
- Genetic factors.
- Dietary goitrogenes.
- Hereditary defect in thyroid hormone synthesis and transport.
- Inborn errors of iodine metabolism.

G/A The enlargement of the thyroid gland in simple goitre is moderate (weighing upto 100-150 gm), symmetric and diffuse. Cut surface is gelatinous and translucent brown.

M/E Two stages are distinguished:

1. *Hyperplastic stage* is the early stage and is characterised by tall columnar follicular epithelium showing papillary infoldings and formation of small new follicles.

2. *Involution stage* generally follows hyperplastic stage after variable period of time. This stage is characterised by large follicles distended by colloid and lined by flattened follicular epithelium.

Nodular Goitre (Multinodular Goitre, Adenomatous Goitre) *(p. 833)*

It is characterised by most extreme degree of tumour-like enlargement of the thyroid gland and characteristic nodularity. The enlargement of the gland may be sufficient to cause not only cosmetic disfigurement, but in many cases may cause dysphagia and choking due to compression of oesophagus and trachea.

ETIOLOGY. Etiologic factors implicated in endemic and non-endemic or sporadic variety of simple goitre are involved in the etiology of nodular goitre too.

G/A The thyroid in nodular goitre shows asymmetric and extreme enlargement, weighing 100-500 gm or even more. The *five* cardinal macroscopic features are: 1. nodularity with poor encapsulation; 2. fibrous scarring; 3. haemorrhages; 4. focal calcification; and 5. cystic degeneration.

Cut surface generally shows multinodularity but occasionally there may be only one or two nodules which are poorly-circumscribed.

M/E 1. Partial or incomplete encapsulation of nodules.

2. The follicles varying from small to large and lined by flat to high epithelium. A few may show macropapillary formation.

3. Areas of haemorrhages, haemosiderin-laden macrophages and cholesterol crystals.

4. Fibrous scarring with foci of calcification.

5. Micro-macrocystic change.

The features of diffuse and nodular goitre are summarised in Table 25.2.

FOLLICULAR ADENOMA *(p. 834)*

Follicular adenoma is the most common benign thyroid tumour occurring more frequently in adult women. Clinically, it appears as a solitary nodule which can be found in approximately 1% of the population.

G/A The follicular adenoma is characterised by *four* features so as to distinguish it from a nodule of nodular goitre: 1. solitary nodule; 2. complete encapsulation; 3. clearly distinct architecture inside and outside the capsule; and 4. compression of the thyroid parenchyma outside the capsule.

Usually, an adenoma is small (upto 3 cm in diameter) and spherical. On cut section, the adenoma is grey-white to red-brown, less colloidal than the surrounding thyroid parenchyma and may have degenerative changes.

M/E The tumour shows complete fibrous encapsulation. The tumour cells are benign follicular epithelial cells forming follicles of various sizes or may show trabecular, solid and cord patterns with little follicle formation. Accordingly, the following 6 types of growth patterns are distinguished,

1. *Microfollicular (foetal) adenoma* consists of small follicles containing little or no colloid and separated by abundant loose stroma

2. *Normofollicular (simple) adenoma* has closely packed follicles like that of normal thyroid gland.

TABLE 25.2: Contrasting Features of Simple and Nodular Goitre.

FEATURE	DIFFUSE GOITRE	NODULAR GOITRE
1. *Nomenclature*	Simple goitre, hyperplastic goitre, nontoxic goitre	Multinodular, adenomatous goitre
2. *Etiology*	Graves' disease, thyroiditis, puberty	Endemic thyroiditis, cancer
3. *Pathogenesis*	Hyperplasia-involution	Repeated cycles of hyperplasia with growth and involution with fibrosis
4. *Composition*	Cellular-rich	Colloid-rich
5. *Gross*	Moderate, symmetric, diffuse enlargement, colloid-filled follicles, gelatinous	Nodular asymmetric, haemorrhages, scarring, cystic change, calcification
6. *Microscopy*	Hyperplastic phase: papillary infoldings, Involution stage: large colloid filled follicles with flat epithelium	Incomplete ecapsulation, nodularity, variable-sized follicles, fibrous scarring, haemorrhages, calcification, cyst formation
7. *Functional status*	Hyperthyroidism, euthyroid	Hypothyroidism, euthyroid

3. Macrofollicular (colloid) adenoma contains large follicles of varying size and distended with colloid.

4. Trabecular (embryonal) adenoma resembles embryonal thyroid.

5. Hurthle cell (oxyphilic) adenoma is an uncommon variant composed of solid trabeculae of large cells having abundant granular oxyphilic cytoplasm and vesicular nuclei.

6. Atypical adenoma is the term used for a follicular adenoma which has more pronounced cellular proliferation so that features may be considered indicative of malignancy such as pleomorphism, increased mitoses and nuclear atypia.

THYROID CANCER *(p. 835)*

Approximately 95% of all primary thyroid cancers are carcinomas. Primary lymphomas of the thyroid comprise less than 5% of thyroid cancers and majority of them possibly evolve from autoimmune (lymphocytic) thyroiditis. About 20% of patients dying of metastasising malignancy have metastatic deposits in the thyroid gland, most commonly from malignant melanoma, renal cell carcinoma and bronchogenic carcinoma.

Carcinoma of the thyroid gland has 4 main morphologic types with distinctly different clinical behaviour and variable prevalence. These are: papillary, follicular, medullary and undifferentiated (anaplastic) carcinoma (Table 25.3).

In line with most other thyroid lesions, most carcinomas of the thyroid too have female preponderance. Irrespective of the histologic types, two types of factors are implicated in the pathogenesis of thyroid cancer:

1. Environmental factors: The single most important environmental factor associated with increased risk of developing thyroid carcinoma after many years is exposure to external radiation of high dose.

2. Genetic factors: Familial clustering of thyroid cancer has been observed. Molecular studies reveal a variety of mutations: i) Mutation in RET gene on chromosome 10 ii) Mutation in RAS gene.

TABLE 25.3: Contrasting Features of Main Histologic Types of Thyroid Carcinoma.

FEATURE	PAPILLARY CARCINOMA	FOLLICULAR CARCINOMA	MEDULLARY CARCINOMA	ANAPLASTIC CARCINOMA
1. Frequency	75-80%	10-20%	5%	5%
2. Age	All ages	Middle to old age	Middle to old age; familial too	Old age
3. Female/male ratio	3:1	2.5:1	1:1	1.5:1
4. Cell of origin	Follicular	Follicular	Parafollicular	Follicular
5. Gross	Small, multifocal	Moderate size, nodular	Moderate size	Invasive growth
6. Pathognomonic microscopy	Nuclear features, papillary pattern	Vascular and capsular invasion	Solid nests, amyloid stroma	Undifferentiated, spindle-shaped, giant cells
7. Regional metastases	Common	Rare	Common	Common
8. Distant metastases	Rare	Common	Rare	Common
9. 10-year survival	80-95%	50-70%	60-70%	5-10% (median survival about 2 months)

Papillary Carcinoma (p. 836)

Papillary carcinoma is the most common type of thyroid carcinoma, comprising 75-85% of cases. It can occur at all ages including children and young adults but the incidence is higher with advancing age. The tumour is found about three times more frequently in females than in males. The following associations have been observed to explain the etiology of papillary carcinoma: 1. External radiation. 2. Iodine excess. 3. Genetic factors.

Papillary carcinoma is typically a slow-growing malignant tumour, most often presenting as an asymptomatic solitary nodule. Involvement of the regional lymph nodes is common but distant metastases to organs are rare. *'Lateral aberrant thyroid'* is the term used for occurrence of thyroid tissue in the lateral cervical lymph node, which in most patients represents a well-differentiated metastasis of an occult papillary carcinoma of the thyroid.

G/A Papillary carcinoma may range from microscopic foci to nodules upto 10 cm in diameter and is generally poorly delineated. Cut surface of the tumour is greyish-white, hard and scar-like

M/E 1. **Papillary pattern.** Papillae composed of fibrovascular stalk and covered by single layer of tumour cells is the predominant feature.
2. **Tumour cells.** The tumour cells have characteristic nuclear features due to dispersed nuclear chromatin imparting it *ground glass or optically clear appearance* and clear or oxyphilic cytoplasm.
3. **Invasion.** The tumour cells invade the capsule and intrathyroid lymphatics but invasion of blood vessels is rare.
4. **Psammoma bodies.** Half of papillary carcinomas show typical small, concentric, calcified spherules called psammoma bodies in the stroma.

Follicular Carcinoma (p. 837)

Follicular carcinoma is the other common type of thyroid cancer, next only to papillary carcinoma and comprises about 10-20% of all thyroid carcinomas. It is more common in middle and old age and has preponderance in females (female-male ratio 2.5:1). In contrast to papillary carcinoma, follicular carcinoma has a positive correlation with endemic goitre but the role of external radiation in its etiology is unclear.

G/A Follicular carcinoma may be either in the form of a solitary adenoma-like circumscribed nodule or as an obvious cancerous irregular thyroid enlargement. The cut surface of the tumour is grey-white with areas of haemorrhages, necrosis and cyst formation.

M/E 1. *Follicular pattern:* Follicular carcinoma, like follicular adenoma, is composed of follicles of various sizes and may show trabecular or solid pattern. The tumour cells have hyperchromatic nuclei and the cytoplasm resembles that of normal follicular cells. However, variants like *clear cell type* and *Hurthle cell (oxyphilic) type* of follicular carcinoma may occur. The tumour differs from papillary carcinoma in lacking: papillae, ground-glass nuclei of tumour cells and psammoma bodies.

2. *Vascular invasion and direct extension:* Vascular invasion and direct extension to involve the adjacent structures (e.g. into the capsule) are significant features but lymphatic invasion is rare.

Medullary Carcinoma *(p. 837)*

Medullary carcinoma is a less frequent type derived from parafollicular or C-cells present in the thyroid and comprises about 5% of thyroid carcinomas. It is equally common in men and women. There are 3 distinctive features which distinguish medullary carcinoma from the other thyroid carcinomas:

1. Familial occurrence. Most cases of medullary carcinoma occur sporadically, but about 10% have a genetic background with mutation in chromosome 10. The familial form of medullary carcinoma has association with pheochromocytoma and parathyroid adenoma (multiple endocrine neoplasia, MEN II A), or with pheochromocytoma and multiple mucosal neuromas (MEN II B).

2. Secretion of calcitonin and other peptides. Like normal C-cells, tumour cells of medullary carcinoma secrete calcitonin, the hypocalcaemic hormone. In addition, the tumour may also elaborate prostaglandins, histaminase, somatostatin, vasoactive intestinal peptide (VIP) and ACTH.

3. Amyloid stroma. Most medullary carcinomas have amyloid deposits in the stroma which stains positively with usual amyloid stains such as Congo red.

G/A The tumour may either appear as a unilateral solitary nodule *(sporadic form)*, or have bilateral and multicentric involvement *(familial form)*. Cut surface of tumour in both forms shows well-defined tumour areas which are firm to hard, grey-white to yellow-brown with areas of haemorrhages and necrosis.

M/E 1. *Tumour cells:* Like other neuroendocrine tumours (e.g. carcinoid, islet cell tumour, paraganglioma etc), medullary carcinoma of the thyroid too has a well-defined organoid pattern, forming nests of tumour cells separated by fibrovascular septa.

2. *Amyloid stroma:* The tumour cells are separated by amyloid stroma derived from altered calcitonin which can be demonstrated by immunostain for calcitonin.

3. *C-cell hyperplasia:* Familial cases generally have C-cell hyperplasia as a precursor lesion but not in sporadic cases.

Anaplastic Carcinoma *(p. 839)*

Undifferentiated or anaplastic carcinoma of the thyroid comprises less than 5% of all thyroid cancers and is one of the most malignant tumour in humans.

The tumour is predominantly found in old age (7th-8th decades) and is slightly more common in females than in males (female-male ratio 1.5:1). The tumour is widely aggressive and rapidly growing. The features at presentation are usually those of extensive invasion of adjacent soft tissue, trachea and oesophagus. The tumour metastasises both to regional lymph nodes and to distant organs such as the lungs.

G/A The tumour is generally large and irregular, often invading the adjacent strap muscles of the neck and other structures in the vicinity of the thyroid.

M/E The tumour is too poorly-differentiated to be placed in any other histologic type of thyroid cancer, but usually shows a component of either papillary or follicular carcinoma in better differentiated areas. The tumour is generally composed of 3 types of cells occurring in varying proportions: small cells, spindle cells and giant cells. There are 3 histologic variants:

1. Small cell carcinoma: This type of tumour is composed of closely packed small cells having hyperchromatic nuclei and numerous mitoses. This variant closely resembles malignant lymphoma.

2. Spindle cell carcinoma: These tumours are composed of spindle cells resembling sarcoma. Some tumours may contain obvious sarcomatous component such as areas of osteosarcoma, chondrosarcoma or rhabdomyosarcoma.

3. Giant cell carcinoma: This type is composed of highly anaplastic giant cells showing numerous atypical mitoses, bizarre and lobed nuclei and some assuming spindle shapes.

PARATHYROID GLANDS *(p. 839)*

NORMAL STRUCTURE *(p. 839)*

The parathyroid glands are usually 4 in number: the *superior pair* derived from the 3rd branchial pouch and *inferior pair* from the 4th branchial pouch of primitive foregut. Both pairs are usually embedded in the posterior aspect of the thyroid substance but separated from it by a connective tissue capsule. In the adults, each gland is an oval, yellowish-brown, flattened body, weighing 35-45 mg.

M/E Parathyroid glands are composed of solid sheets and cords of parenchymal cells and variable amount of stromal fat. The parenchymal cells are of 3 types: *chief cells, oxyphil cells* and *water-clear cells.* The chief cells are most numerous and are the major source of parathyroid hormone.

The major *function* of the parathyroid hormone, in conjunction with calcitonin and vitamin D, is to regulate serum calcium levels and metabolism of bone. The role of parathyroid hormone in regulating calcium metabolism in the body is at the following 3 levels:

1. Parathyroid hormone *stimulates osteoclastic activity* and results in resorption of bone and release of calcium.
2. Parathyroid hormone acts *directly on renal tubular epithelial cells* and increases renal reabsorption of calcium and inhibits reabsorption of phosphate.
3. Parathyroid hormone increases renal production of the *most active metabolite of vitamin D*, 1, 25-dihydrocholecalciferol.

HYPERPARATHYROIDISM *(p. 840)*

Primary Hyperparathyroidism *(p. 840)*

Primary hyperparathyroidism is not uncommon and occurs more commonly with increasing age. It is especially likely to occur in women near the time of menopause.

ETIOLOGY. 1. Most commonly, parathyroid adenomas in approximately 80% cases.
2. Carcinoma of the parathyroid glands in 2-3% patients.

3. Primary hyperplasia in about 15% cases (usually chief cell hyperplasia).

Clinical presentation of individuals with primary hyperparathyroidism may be in a variety of ways:

1. Most commonly, nephrolithiasis and or/nephrocalcinosis.
2. Metastatic calcification.
3. Generalised osteitis fibrosa cystica.
4. Neuropsychiatric disturbances.
5. Hypertension.
6. Other changes such as pancreatitis, cholelithiasis and peptic ulcers.

Secondary Hyperparathyroidism *(p. 840)*

Secondary hyperparathyroidism occurs due to increased parathyroid hormone elaboration secondary to a disease elsewhere in the body. Hypocalcaemia stimulates compensatory hyperplasia of the parathyroid glands and causes secondary hyperparathyroidism.

ETIOLOGY. 1. Chronic renal insufficiency

2. Vitamin D deficiency and consequent rickets and osteomalacia.

3. Intestinal malabsorption syndromes causing deficiency of calcium and vitamin D.

Tertiary Hyperparathyroidism *(p. 841)*

Tertiary hyperparathyroidism is a complication of secondary hyperparathyroidism in which the hyperfunction persists in spite of removal of the cause of secondary hyperplasia. Possibly, a hyperplastic nodule in the parathyroid gland develops which becomes partially autonomous and continues to secrete large quantities of parathyroid hormone.

HYPOPARATHYROIDISM *(p. 841)*

Primary Hypoparathyroidism *(p. 841)*

Primary hypoparathyroidism is caused by disease of the parathyroid glands. Most common causes of primary hypoparathyroidism are: surgical procedures involving thyroid, parathyroid, or radical neck dissection for cancer.

Pseudo-hypoparathyroidism *(p. 841)*

In pseudo-hypoparathyroidism, the tissues fail to respond to parathyroid hormone though parathyroid glands are usually normal.

Pseudopseudo-hypoparathyroidism *(p. 841)*

Pseudopseudo-hypoparathyroidism is another rare familial disorder in which all the clinical features of pseudo-hypoparathyroidism are present except that these patients have no hypocalcaemia or hyperphosphataemia and the tissues respond normally to parathyroid hormone.

PARATHYROID ADENOMA *(p. 841)*

The commonest tumour of the parathyroid glands is an adenoma. It may occur at any age and in either sex but is found more frequently in adult life. Most adenomas are first brought to attention because of excessive secretion of parathyroid hormone causing features of hyperparathyroidism.

G/A A parathyroid adenoma is small (less than 5 cm diameter) encapsulated, yellowish-brown, ovoid nodule and weighing up to 5 gm or more.

M/E Majority of adenomas are predominantly composed of chief cells arranged in sheets or cords. Oxyphil cells and water-clear cells may be found intermingled in varying proportions.

PARATHYROID CARCINOMA *(p. 842)*

Carcinoma of the parathyroid is rare and produces manifestations of hyperparathyroidism which is often more pronounced.

ENDOCRINE PANCREAS *(p. 842)*

NORMAL STRUCTURE *(p. 842)*

The endocrine pancreas consists of microscopic collections of cells called islets of Langerhans found scattered within the pancreatic lobules, as well as individual endocrine cells found in duct epithelium and among the acini. The total weight of endocrine pancreas in the adult, however, does not exceed 1-1.5 gm (total weight of pancreas 60-100 gm). The islet cell tissue is greatly concentrated in the tail than in the head or body of the pancreas.

A. Major cell types:

1. *Beta (B) cells* comprise about 70% of islet cells and secrete insulin, the defective response or deficient synthesis of which causes diabetes mellitus.

2. *Alpha (A) cells* comprise 20% of islet cells and secrete glucagon which induces hyperglycaemia.

3. *Delta (D) cells* comprise 5-10% of islet cells and secrete somatostatin which suppresses both insulin and glucagon release.

4. *Pancreatic polypeptide (PP) cells or F cells* comprise 1-2% of islet cells and secrete pancreatic polypeptide having some gastrointestinal effects.

B. Minor cell types:

1. *D1 cells* elaborate vasoactive intestinal peptide (VIP) which induces glycogenolysis and hyperglycaemia and causes secretory diarrhoea by stimulation of gastrointestinal fluid secretion.

2. *Enterochromaffin cells* synthesise serotonin which in pancreatic tumours may induce carcinoid syndrome.

DIABETES MELLITUS *(p. 842)*

Definition and Epidemiology *(p. 842)*

As per the WHO, diabetes mellitus (DM) is a hetrogeneous metabolic disorder characterised by common feature of chronic hyperglycaemia with disturbance of carbohydrate, fat and protein metabolism.

DM is a leading cause of morbidity and mortality the world over. It is estimated that approximately 1% of population suffers from DM. The incidence is rising in the developed countries of the world, especially of type 2 DM, due to rising incidence of obesity and reduced activity levels.

Classification and Etiology *(p. 842)*

The older classification systems dividing DM into primary (idiopathic) and secondary types, juvenile-onset and maturity onset types, and insulin-dependent (IDDM) and non-insulin independent (NIDDM) types, have become obsolete and undergone major revision due to extensive understanding of etiology and pathogenesis of DM in recent times.

As outlined in Table 25.4 based on etiology, currently DM is classified into two broad categories (type 1 and type 2), a few uncommon specific etiologic types, and gestational DM.

The contrasting features of the two main forms of diabetes mellitus are presented in Table 25.5.

Pathogenesis *(p. 843)*

Depending upon etiology of DM, hyperglycaemia may result from:

■ reduced insulin secretion;

TABLE 25.4: Etiologic Classification of Diabetes Mellitus
(as per American Diabetes Association, 2000).

I. **Type 1 diabetes mellitus (10%)** (earlier called Insulin-dependent, or juvenile-onset diabetes)

Type IA DM: Immune-mediated
Type IB DM: Idiopathic

II. **Type 2 diabetes mellitus (80%)** (earlier called non-insulin-dependent, or maturity-onset diabetes)

III. **Other specific types of diabetes (10%)**

A. Genetic defect of β-cell function due to mutations in various enzymes (earlier called maturity-onset diabetes of the young or MODY) (e.g. hepatocyte nuclear transcription factor HNF, glucokinase)

B. Genetic defect in insulin action (e.g. type A insulin resistance)

C. Diseases of exocrine pancreas (e.g. chronic pancreatitis, pancreatic tumours, post-pancreatectomy)

D. Endocrinopathies (e.g. acromegaly, Cushing's syndrome, pheochromocytoma)

E. Drug- or chemical-induced (e.g. steroids, thyroid hormone, thiazides, β-blockers etc)

F. Infections (e.g. congenital rubella, cytomegalovirus)

G. Uncommon forms of immune-mediated DM (stiff man syndrome, anti-insulin receptor antibodies)

H. Other genetic syndromes (e.g. Down's syndrome, Klinefelter's syndrome, Turner's syndrome)

IV. **Gestational diabetes mellitus**

TABLE 25.5: Contrasting Features of Type 1 and Type 2 Diabetes Mellitus.

	FEATURE	TYPE 1 DM	TYPE 2 DM
1.	*Frequency*	10-20%	80-90%
2.	*Age at onset*	Early (below 35 years)	Late (after 40 years)
3.	*Type of onset*	Abrupt and severe	Gradual and insidious
4.	*Weight*	Normal	Obese/non-obese
5.	*HLA*	Linked to HLA DR3, HLA DR4, HLA DQ	No HLA association
6.	*Family history*	< 20%	About 60%
7.	*Genetic locus*	Unknown	Chromosome 6
8.	*Diabetes in identical twins*	50% concordance	80% concordance
9.	*Pathogenesis*	Autoimmune destruction of β-cells	Insulin resistance, impaired insulin secretion
10.	*Islet cell antibodies*	Yes	No
11.	*Blood insulin level*	Decreased insulin	Normal or increased insulin
12.	*Islet cell changes*	Insulitis, β-cell depletion	No insulitis, later fibrosis of islets
13.	*Amyloidosis*	Infrequent	Common in chronic cases
14.	*Clinical management*	Insulin and diet	Diet, exercise, oral drugs, insulin
15.	*Acute complications*	Ketoacidosis	Hyperosmolar coma

■ decreased glucose use by the body; and
■ increased glucose production.

Pathogenesis of two main types of DM and its complications is distinct. In order to understand it properly, it is essential to relearn physiology of normal insulin synthesis and secretion.

NORMAL INSULIN METABOLISM. *The major stimulus for both synthesis and release of insulin is glucose.* The steps involved in biosynthesis, release and actions of insulin are as follows:

Synthesis. Insulin is synthesised in the β-cells of pancreatic islets of Langerhans:

i) It is initially formed as *pre-proinsulin* which is single-chain 86-amino acid precursor polypeptide.

ii) Subsequent proteolysis removes the amino terminal signal peptide, forming *proinsulin*.

iii) Further cleavage of proinsulin gives rise to *A (21 amino acids) and B (30 amino acids) chains* of insulin, linked together by connecting segment called *C-peptide*, all of which are stored in the secretory granules in the β-cells.

iv) For therapeutic use, *human insulin* is now produced by recombinant DNA technology.

Release. Glucose is the key regulator of insulin secretion from β-cells by a series of steps:

i) Hypoglycaemia (glucose level below 70 mg/dL or below 3.9 mmol/L) stimulates transport into β-cells of a *glu*cose transporter, *GLUT2.*

ii) An islet transcription factor, *glucokinase,* causes glucose phosphorylation.

iii) Metabolism of glucose to glucose-6-phosphate by glycolysis generates *ATP.*

iv) Generation of ATP *alters the ion channel activity* on the membrane. It causes inhibition of ATP-sensitive K^+ channel on the cell membrane and opening up of calcium channel with resultant influx of calcium, which stimulates insulin release.

Action. Half of insulin secreted from β-cells into portal vein is degraded in the liver while the remaining half enters the systemic circulation for action on the target cells:

i) Insulin from circulation binds to its receptor on the target cells. This *insulin receptor* has intrinsic tyrosine kinase activity.

ii) This, in turn, activates post-receptor intracellular signalling pathway molecules, *insulin receptor substrates (IRS) 1 and 2 proteins.*

iii) These reactions on the target cells are responsible for the main *mitogenic and anabolic actions of insulin*—glycogen synthesis, glucose transport, protein synthesis, lipogenesis.

iv) Besides the role of glucose in maintaining equilibrium of insulin release, *low insulin level in the fasting state* promotes hepatic gluconeogenesis and glycogenolysis.

PATHOGENESIS OF TYPE 1 DM. *The basic phenomena in type 1 DM is destruction of β-cell mass, usually leading to absolute insulin deficiency.* While type 1B DM remains idiopathic, pathogenesis of type 1A DM is immune-mediated and has been extensively studied. Currently, pathogenesis of type 1A DM is explained on the basis of 3 mutually-interlinked mechanisms: genetic susceptibility, autoimmune factors, and certain environmental factors.

Pathogenesis of type 1A DM can be summed up by interlinking the above three factors as under:

1. At birth, individuals with *genetic susceptibility* to this disorder have normal β-cell mass.

2. Destruction of β–cell mass occurs by *autoimmune phenomena* and takes months to years. Clinical features of diabetes manifest after more than 80% of β-cell mass has been destroyed.

3. The trigger for autoimmune process appears to be some *infectious or environmental factor* which specifically targets β-cells.

PATHOGENESIS OF TYPE 2 DM. The basic metabolic defect in type 2 DM is either a delayed insulin secretion relative to glucose load *(impaired insulin secretion)*, or the peripheral tissues are unable to respond to insulin *(insulin resistance)*.

Type 2 DM is a heterogeneous disorder with a more complex etiology and is far more common than type 1, but much less is known about its pathogenesis. A number of factors have been implicated though, but HLA association and autoimmune phenomena are not implicated. These factors are as under.

1. Genetic factors. 2. Constitutional factors. 3. Insulin resistance. 4. Impaired insulin secretion. 5. Increased hepatic glucose synthesis.

In essence, hyperglycaemia in type 2 DM is not due to destruction of β-cells but is instead a failure of β-cells to meet the requirement of insulin in the body. Its pathogenesis can be summed up by interlinking the above factors as under:

1. Type 2 DM is a more *complex multifactorial disease*.

2. There is greater role of *genetic defect and heredity*.

3. The two main mechanisms for hyperglycaemia in type 2 DM—*insulin resistance and impaired insulin secretion*, are interlinked.

4. While *obesity* plays a role in pathogenesis of insulin resistance, impaired insulin secretion may be from many constitutional factors.

5. *Increased hepatic synthesis of glucose* in initial period of disease contributes to hyperglycaemia.

Pathologic Changes in Pancreatic Islets *(p. 847)*

Pathologic changes in islets have been demonstrated in both types of diabetes, though the changes are more distinctive in type 1 DM.

1. INSULITIS: In type 1 DM, characteristically, in early stage there is lymphocytic infiltrate, mainly by T cells, in the islets which may be accompanied by a few macrophages and polymorphs. Diabetic infants born to diabetic mothers, however, have eosinophilic infiltrate in the islets.

In type 2 DM, there is no significant leucocytic infiltrate in the islets but there is variable degree of fibrous tissue in the islets.

2. ISLET CELL MASS: In type 1 DM, as the disease becomes chronic there is progressive depletion of β–cell mass, eventually resulting in total loss of pancreatic β–cells.

In type 2 DM, β-cell mass is either normal or mildly reduced. Infants of diabetic mothers, however, have hyperplasia and hypertrophy of islets as a compensatory response to maternal hyperglycaemia.

3. β-CELL DEGRANULATION: In type 1 DM, EM shows degranulation of remaining β-cells of islets.

In type 2 DM, no such change is observed.

4. AMYLOIDOSIS: In type 1 DM, deposits of amyloid around islets are absent.

In type 2 DM, characteristically chronic long-standing cases show deposition of amyloid material around the capillaries of the islets causing compression and atrophy of islet tissue.

Clinical Features *(p. 848)*

It can be appreciated that hyperglycaemia in DM does not cause a single disease but is associated with numerous diseases and symptoms, especially due to complications. Two main types of DM can be distinguished clinically to the extent shown in Table 25.5. However, overlapping of clinical features occurs as regards the age of onset, duration of symptoms and family history.

Type 1 DM: i) Patients of type 1 DM usually manifest at early age, generally below the age of 35.

ii) The onset of symptoms is often abrupt.

iii) At presentation, these patients have polyuria, polydipsia and polyphagia.

iv) The patients are not obese but have generally progressive loss of weight.

v) These patients are prone to develop metabolic complications such as ketoacidosis and hypoglycaemic episodes.

Type 2 DM: i) This form of diabetes generally manifests in middle life or beyond, usually above the age of 40.

ii) The onset of symptoms in type 2 DM is slow and insidious.

iii) Generally, the patient is asymptomatic when the diagnosis is made on the basis of glucosuria or hyperglycaemia during physical examination, or may present with polyuria and polydipsia.

iv) The patients are frequently obese and have unexplained weakness and loss of weight.

v) Metabolic complications such as ketoacidosis are infrequent.

Pathogenesis of Complications *(p. 849)*

It is now known that in both type 1 and 2 DM, *severity and chronicity of hyperglycaemia* forms the main pathogenetic mechanism for 'microvascular complications' (e.g. retinopathy, nephropathy, neuropathy); therefore control of blood glucose level constitutes the mainstay of treatment for minimising development of these complications. Longstanding cases of type 2 DM, however, in addition, frequently develop 'macrovascular complications' (e.g. atherosclerosis, coronary artery disease, peripheral vascular disease, cerebrovascular disease) which are more difficult to explain on the basis of hyperglycaemia alone.

The following biochemical mechanisms have been proposed to explain the development of complications of diabetes mellitus:

1. Non-enzymatic protein glycosylation: The free amino group of various body proteins binds by non-enzymatic mechanism to glucose; this process is called *glycosylation* and is directly proportionate to the severity of hyperglycaemia. Various body proteins undergoing chemical alterations in this way include haemoglobin, lens crystalline protein, and basement membrane of body cells. An example is the measurement of a fraction of haemoglobin called glycosylated haemoglobin (HbA_{1C}) as a test for monitoring glycaemic control in a diabetic patient during the preceding 100 to 120 days which is lifespan of red cells.

2. Polyol pathway mechanism: This mechanism is responsible for producing lesions in the aorta, lens of the eye, kidney and peripheral nerves. These tissues have an enzyme, aldose reductase, that reacts with glucose to form sorbitol and fructose in the cells of the hyperglycaemic patient.

Intracellular accumulation of sorbitol and fructose so produced results in entry of water inside the cell and consequent cellular swelling and cell damage.

3. Excessive oxygen free radicals. In hyperglycaemia, there is increased production of reactive oxygen free radicals from mitochondrial oxidative phosphorylation which may damage various target cells in diabetes.

Complications of Diabetes *(p. 850)*

As a consequence of hyperglycaemia of diabetes, every tissue and organ of the body undergoes biochemical and structural alterations which account for the major complications in diabetics which may be *acute metabolic* or *chronic systemic.*

Both types of diabetes mellitus may develop complications which are broadly divided into 2 major groups:

I. ACUTE METABOLIC COMPLICATIONS. Metabolic complications develop acutely. While ketoacidosis and hypoglycaemic episodes are primarily complications of type 1 DM, hyperosmolar nonketotic coma is chiefly a complication of type 2 DM.

1. Diabetic ketoacidosis. Ketoacidosis is almost exclusively a complication of type 1 DM. It can develop in patients with severe insulin deficiency combined with glucagon excess. Failure to take insulin and exposure to stress are the usual precipitating causes. Severe lack of insulin causes lipolysis in the adipose tissues, resulting in release of free fatty acids into the plasma. These free fatty acids are taken up by the liver where they are oxidised through acetyl coenzyme-A to ketone bodies, principally acetoacetic acid and β-hydroxy-butyric acid. Such free fatty acid oxidation to ketone bodies is accelerated in the presence of elevated level of glucagon.

2. Hyperosmolar nonketotic coma. Hyperosmolar nonketotic coma is usually a complication of type 2 DM. It is caused by severe dehydration resulting from sustained hyperglycaemic diuresis. The loss of glucose in urine is so intense that the patient is unable to drink sufficient water to maintain urinary fluid loss.

3. Hypoglycaemia. Hypoglycaemic episode may develop in patients of type 1 DM. It may result from excessive administration of insulin, missing a meal, or due to stress.

II. LATE SYSTEMIC COMPLICATIONS. A number of systemic complications may develop after a period of 15-20 years in either type of diabetes.

1. Atherosclerosis. Diabetes mellitus of both type 1 and type 2 accelerates the development of atherosclerosis so that consequent atherosclerotic lesions appear earlier than in the general population, are more extensive, and are more often associated with complicated plaques such as ulceration, calcification and thrombosis

The possible ill-effects of accelerated atherosclerosis in diabetes are early onset of coronary artery disease, silent myocardial infarction, cerebral stroke and gangrene of the toes and feet. Gangrene of the lower extremities is 100 times more common in diabetics than in non-diabetics.

2. Diabetic microangiopathy. Microangiopathy of diabetes is characterised by basement membrane thickening of small blood vessels and capillaries of different organs and tissues such as the skin, skeletal muscle, eye and kidney. Similar type of basement membrane-like material is also deposited in nonvascular tissues such as peripheral nerves, renal tubules and Bowman's capsule.

3. Diabetic nephropathy. Renal involvement is a common complication and a leading cause of death in diabetes. Four types of lesions are described in diabetic nephropathy:

i) *Diabetic glomerulosclerosis* which includes diffuse and nodular lesions of glomerulosclerosis.

ii) *Vascular lesions* that include hyaline arteriolosclerosis of afferent and efferent arterioles and atheromas of renal arteries.

iii) *Diabetic pyelonephritis* and *necrotising renal papillitis.*

iv) *Tubular lesions or Armanni-Ebstein lesion.*

4. Diabetic neuropathy. Diabetic neuropathy may affect all parts of the nervous system but symmetric peripheral neuropathy is most characteristic. The basic pathologic changes are segmental demyelination, Schwann cell injury and axonal damage.

5. Diabetic retinopathy. Diabetic retinopathy is a leading cause of blindness. There are 2 types of lesions involving retinal vessels: *background* and *proliferative*. Besides retinopathy, diabetes also predisposes the patients to early development of cataract and glaucoma.

6. Infections. Diabetics have enhanced susceptibility to various infections such as tuberculosis, pneumonias, pyelonephritis, otitis, carbuncles and diabetic ulcers. This could be due to various factors such as impaired leucocyte functions, reduced cellular immunity, poor blood supply due to vascular involvement and hyperglycaemia *per se.*

Diagnosis of Diabetes *(p. 851)*

Hyperglycaemia remains the fundamental basis for the diagnosis of diabetes mellitus. In *symptomatic cases,* the diagnosis is not a problem and can be confirmed by finding glucosuria and a random plasma glucose concentration above 200 mg/dl.

■ The severity of clinical symptoms of polyuria and polydipsia is directly related to the degree of hyperglycaemia.

■ In *asymptomatic cases,* when there is persistently elevated fasting plasma glucose level, diagnosis again poses no difficulty.

■ The problem arises in asymptomatic patients who have normal fasting glucose level in the plasma but are suspected to have diabetes on other grounds and are thus subjected to oral glucose tolerance test (GTT). If abnormal GTT values are found, these subjects are said to have *'chemical diabetes'.* The WHO-American Diabetes Association (2000) have suggested definite diagnostic criteria for early diagnosis of diabetes mellitus (Table 25.6).

TABLE 25.6: Revised Criteria for Diagnosis of Diabetes by Oral GTT (as per WHO-American Diabetes Association, 2000).

	PATIENT STATUS	PLASMA GLUCOSE VALUE*	DIAGNOSIS
1.	Fasting value	below 110 mg/dl (6.1 mmol/L)	Normal fasting value
2.	Fasting value	110-126 mg/dl (6.1-7.0 mmol/L)	Impaired fasting glucose (IFG)**
3.	Fasting value	126 mg/dl (7.0 mmol/L) or more	Diabetes mellitus
4.	Two-hour after 75 g oral glucose load	140-200 mg/dl (7.8-11.1 mmol/L)	Impaired glucose tolerance (IGT)**
5.	Two-hour after 75 g oral glucose load	200 mg/dl (11.1 mmol/L) or more	Diabetes mellitus
6.	Random value	200 mg/dl (11.1 mmol/L) or more in a symptomatic patient	Diabetes mellitus

Note: * Plasma glucose values are 15% higher than whole blood glucose value.
** Individuals with IFG and IGT are at increased risk for development of type 2 DM later.

The following investigations are helpful in establishing the diagnosis of diabetes mellitus:

I. URINE TESTING. Urine tests are cheap and convenient but the diagnosis of diabetes cannot be based on urine testing alone since there may be false-positives and false-negatives. They can be used in population screening surveys. Urine is tested for the presence of glucose and ketones.

Chapter Twenty Five

1. Glucosuria. *Benedict's qualitative test* detects any reducing substance in the urine and is not specific for glucose. More sensitive and glucose specific test is *dipstick* method based on enzyme-coated paper strip.

Besides diabetes mellitus, *glucosuria* may also occur in certain other conditions such as: renal glycosuria, alimentary (lag storage) glucosuria, many metabolic disorders, starvation and intracranial lesions (e.g. cerebral tumour, haemorrhage and head injury).

■ *Renal glucosuria:* After diabetes, the next most common cause of glucosuria is the reduced renal threshold for glucose. In such cases although the blood glucose level is below 180 mg/dl (i.e. below normal renal threshold for glucose) but glucose still appears regularly and consistently in the urine due to lowered renal threshold.

Renal glucosuria is a benign condition unrelated to diabetes and runs in families and may occur temporarily in pregnancy without symptoms of diabetes.

■ *Alimentary (lag storage) glucosuria:* A rapid and transitory rise in blood glucose level above the normal renal threshold may occur in some individuals after a meal. During this period, glucosuria is present. This type of response to meal is called 'lag storage curve' or more appropriately 'alimentary glucosuria'. A characteristic feature is that unusually high blood glucose level returns to normal 2 hours after meal.

2. Ketonuria. Tests for ketone bodies in the urine are required for assessing the severity of diabetes and not for diagnosis of diabetes.

II. SINGLE BLOOD SUGAR ESTIMATION. For diagnosis of diabetes, blood sugar determinations are absolutely necessary. *Whole blood or plasma may be used but whole blood values are 15% lower than plasma values.*

A grossly elevated single determination of plasma glucose may be sufficient to make the diagnosis of diabetes. A *fasting plasma glucose value above 126 mg/dl (7 mmol/L) is certainly indicative of diabetes.* In other cases, oral GTT is performed.

III. ORAL GLUCOSE TOLERANCE TEST. The patient who is scheduled for oral GTT is instructed to eat a high carbohydrate diet for at least 3 days prior to the test and come after an overnight fast on the day of the test (for at least 8 hours). A fasting blood sugar sample is first drawn. Then 75 gm of glucose dissolved in 300 ml of water is given. Blood and urine specimen are collected at half-hourly intervals for at least 2 hours. Blood or plasma glucose content is measured and urine is tested for glucosuria to determine the approximate renal threshold for glucose.

■ Individuals with fasting value of plasma glucose higher than 126 mg/dl and 2-hour value after 75 gm oral glucose higher than 200 mg/dl are labelled as *diabetics.*

■ In a symptomatic case the random blood glucose value above 200 mg/dl is diagnosed as diabetes mellitus.

■ Normal cut off value for fasting blood glucose level is considered as 110 mg/dl. Cases with fasting blood glucose value between 110 and 126 mg/dl are considered as *impaired fasting glucose tolerance (IGT);* these cases are at increased risk of developing diabetes later and therefore kept under observation for repeating the test. During pregnancy, however, a case of IGT is treated as a diabetic.

IV. OTHER TESTS. A few other tests are sometimes performed in specific conditions in diabetics and for research purposes:

1. Glycosylated haemoglobin (HbA_{1C}). Measurement of blood glucose level in diabetics suffers from variation due to dietary intake of the previous day. Long-term objective assessment of degree of diabetic control is better done by measurement of glycosylated haemoglobin (HbA_{1C}), a minor haemoglobin component present in normal persons.

2. Extended GTT. The oral GTT is extended to 3-4 hours for appearance of symptoms of hyperglycaemia.

3. Intravenous GTT. This test is performed in persons who have intestinal malabsorption or in postgastrectomy cases.

4. Cortisone-primed GTT. This provocative test is a useful investigative aid in cases of potential diabetics.

5. Insulin assay. Plasma insulin levels can be measured by radio-immunoassay and ELISA techniques.

6. C-peptide assay. This test is even more sensitive than insulin assay because its levels are not affected by insulin therapy.

ISLET CELL TUMOURS *(p. 853)*

Insulinoma (β-Cell Tumour) *(p. 853)*

Insulinomas or beta (β)-cell tumours are the most common islet cell tumours. The neoplastic β-cells secrete insulin into the blood stream which remains unaffected by normal regulatory mechanisms. This results in characteristic attacks of hypolgycaemia with blood glucose level falling to 50 mg/dl or below, high plasma insulin level (hyperinsulinism) and high insulin-glucose ratio.

Gastrinoma (G-Cell Tumour, Zollinger-Ellison Syndrome) *(p. 853)*

Zollinger and Ellison described diagnostic triad consisting of:
- fulminant peptic ulcer disease;
- gastric acid hypersecretion; and
- presence of non-β pancreatic islet cell tumour.

Such non-β pancreatic islet cell tumour is the source of gastrin, producing hypergastrinaemia and hence named gastrinoma.

MULTIPLE ENDOCRINE NEOPLASIA (MEN) SYNDROMES *(p. 854)*

Multiple adenomas and hyperplasias of different endocrine organs are a group of genetic diorders which produce heterogeneous clinical features called multiple endocrine neoplasia (MEN) syndromes. Presently, 4 distinct types of MEN syndromes are distinguished. These are briefly outlined below along with major disease associations:

1. MEN type 1 syndrome (Wermer's syndrome) includes adenomas of the parathyroid glands, pancreatic islets and pituitary. The syndrome is inherited as an autosomal dominant trait.
1. *Parathyroid:* Hyperplasia or adenoma; hyperparathyroidism is the most common (90%) clinical manifestation.
2. *Pancreatic islet cells:* Hyperplasia or adenoma seen in 80% cases; frequently with Zollinger-Ellison syndrome.
3. *Pituitary:* Hyperplasia or adenoma in 65% cases; manifest as acromegaly or hypopituitarism.
4. *Adrenal cortex:* Uncommonly involved by adenoma or pheochromocytoma.
5. *Thyroid:* Less commonly involved by adenoma or hyperplasia.

2. MEN type 2 syndrome (Sipple's syndrome) is characterised by medullary carcinoma thyroid and pheochromocytoma.

■ **MEN type 2A** is the combination of medullary carcinoma thyroid, pheochromocytoma and hyperparathytroidism.

■ **MEN type 2B** is the combination of medullary carcinoma thyroid, pheo-chromocytoma, mucosal neuromas, intestinal ganglioneuromatosis, and marfanoid features.

3. Mixed syndromes include a variety of endocrine neoplastic combinations which are distinct from those in MEN type 1 and type 2.

POLYGLANDULAR AUTOIMMUNE (PGA) SYNDROMES *(p. 854)*

Immunologic syndromes affecting two or more endocrine glands and some non-endocrine immune disturbances produce syndromic presentation termed polyglandular autoimmune (PGA) syndromes. PGA syndromes are of two types:

☒ PGA type I occurring in children is characterised by mucocutaneous candidiasis, hypoparathyroidism, and adrenal insufficiency.

☒ PGA type II (Schmidt syndrome) presents in adults and commonly comprises of adrenal insufficiency, autoimmune thyroiditis, and type 1 diabetes mellitus.

■ SELF ASSESSMENT

1. **Hyperfunction of anterior pituitary in pre-pubertal children generally results in:**
   A. Acromegaly
   B. Gigantism
   C. Hyperprolactinaemia
   D. Cushing's syndrome

2. **Excessive secretion of ADH from posterior pituitary results from the following conditions** *except:*
   A. Oat cell carcinoma
   B. Carcinoma pancreas
   C. Pituitary adenoma
   D. Thymoma

3. **Hypofunction of anterior pituitary results in the following** *except:*
   A. Sheehan's syndrome
   B. Diabetes insipidus
   C. Pituitary dwarfism
   D. Empty-sella syndrome

4. **The most common form of pituitary adenoma is:**
   A. Somatotroph
   B. Lactotroph
   C. Gonadotroph
   D. Corticotroph

5. **Craniopharyngioma arises from:**
   A. Arachnoid cap cells
   B. Lining epithelium of pharynx
   C. Chromophil cells
   D. Remnants of Rathke's pouch

6. **Cushing's syndrome due to ectopic elaboration of cortisol occurs in the following conditions** *except:*
   A. Oat cell carcinoma lung
   B. Adrenal cortical adenoma
   C. Malignant thymoma
   D. Pancreatic carcinoma

7. **Main causes of Addison's disease include the following** *except:*
   A. Tuberculosis
   B. Amyloidosis
   C. Adrenal cortical adenoma
   D. Autoimmune diseases

8. **Pheochromocytoma has the following features** *except:*
   A. It is generally a benign tumour of adrenal medulla
   B. Hypertension is generally presenting feature
   C. It arises from embryonal nerve cells
   D. 24 hour urinary measurement of catecholamines is diagnostic

9. **Neuroblastoma has the following features** *except:*
   A. It arises from primitive nerve cells
   B. It is a common malignant tumour in children under 5 years of age
   C. The tumour spreads by haematogenous route early
   D. The tumour cells are highly pleomorphic and large

10. **Common causes of myxoedema are as under** *except:*
    A. Follicular adenoma
    B. Ablation of thyroid by surgery
    C. Thyroid cancer
    D. Autoimmune thyroiditis

11. **There is higher incidence of lymphoma of the thyroid in the following condition:**
    A. Graves' disease
    B. Hashimoto's thyroiditis
    C. Nodular goitre
    D. Riedel's thyroiditis

12. **There is considerable depletion of colloid in the follicles in the following thyroid disease:**
    A. Graves' disease
    B. Hashimoto's thyroiditis
    C. Nodular goitre
    D. Follicular adenoma

13. **Nodular goitre is characterised by the following features** *except:*
    A. Iodine deficiency plays role in etiology
    B. There is repeated hyperplasia and involution
    C. There is deficient thyroid hormone production
    D. There is decreased TSH stimulation

14. **Role of external radiation in etiology of thyroid cancer is maximum in:**
    A. Papillary carcinoma
    B. Follicular carcinoma
    C. Medullary carcinoma
    D. Anaplastic carcinoma

15. **Haematogenous spread is rare and exceptional in following thyroid cancer:**
    A. Follicular carcinoma
    B. Medullary carcinoma
    C. Papillary carcinoma
    D. Anaplastic carcinoma

16. **Male: female ratio is equal in the following thyroid cancer:**
    A. Papillary carcinoma
    B. Follicular carcinoma
    C. Medullary carcinoma
    D. Anaplastic carcinoma

17. **The following thyroid cancer is a neuroendocrine tumour:**
    A. Papillary carcinoma
    B. Follicular carcinoma
    C. Medullary carcinoma
    D. Anaplastic carcinoma

18. **Prognosis is best in the following thyroid cancer:**
    A. Anaplastic carcinoma
    B. Medullary carcinoma
    C. Papillary carcinoma
    D. Follicular carcinoma

19. **Secondary hyperparathyroidism secondary to disease elsewhere in the body causes:**
    A. Hypercalcaemia
    B. Hypocalcaemia
    C. Normocalcaemia
    D. Normal parathormone levels

20. **Islets of Langerhans are concentrated in the pancreas in the following zone:**
    A. Head
    B. Body
    C. Tail
    D. Uncinate process

21. **The following holds true for type 1 diabetes** *except:*
    A. There is association with HLA-DR 3 and HLA-DR 4
    B. There is autoimmune disease association
    C. There is more than 90% concordance for monozygotic twins to develop diabetes
    D. Viral infection may precede type I diabetes

22. **The following are correct statements for type 2 diabetes (NIDDM)** *except:*
    A. It is more than common than IDDM
    B. These patients are generally obese
    C. There is role of insulin resistance
    D. There is presence of 'insulitis'

23. **The following complication is almost exclusive for type 1 diabetes mellitus (IDDM):**
    A. Hyperosmolar nonketotic coma
    B. Diabetic ketoacidosis
    C. Atherosclerosis
    D. Diabetic nephropathy

24. **Renal glucosuria is characterised by:**
    A. Elevation of fasting blood glucose level
    B. Elevation of blood glucose at 1 hour after meal
    C. Elevation of blood glucose at 2 hours after meal
    D. Normal blood glucose level during entire GTT

25. **Long term assessment of diabetes is provided by the following investigation:**
    A. Whole blood glucose estimation
    B. Plasma glucose estimation
    C. Capillary method of glucose estimation
    D. Glycosylated haemoglobin

26. **Hypoglycaemia (blood glucose 50 mg/dl or lower) is a characteristic finding in:**

    A. Gastrinoma
    B. Insulinoma
    C. Glucagonoma
    D. VIPoma

27. **Lateral aberrant thyroid is the term used for the following:**
    A. Ectopic normal thyroid tissue in lateral cervical region
    B. Abnormal thyroid tissue at unusual site
    C. Metastatic deposits in cervical lymph node from papillary carcinoma thyroid
    D. Metastatic deposits in cervical lymph node from gastric carcinoma

28. **Following pathologic finding is invariably present in pancreas in type 2 diabetes mellitus:**

    A. Insulitis
    B. Depleted islet cell mass
    C. B-cell degranulation
    D. Amyloidosis of islets

KEY

1 = B	2 = C	3 = B	4 = B
5 = D	6 = B	7 = C	8 = C
9 = D	10 = A	11 = B	12 = A
13 = D	14 = A	15 = C	16 = C
17 = C	18 = C	19 = B	20 = C
21 = C	22 = D	23 = B	24 = D
25 = D	26 = B	27 = C	28 = D

26

The Musculoskeletal System

SKELETAL SYSTEM *(p. 855)*

The skeleton consists of cartilage and bone. Cartilage has a role in growth and repair of bone, and in the adults forms the articular skeleton responsible for movement of joints. Bone is a specialised form of connective tissue which performs the function of providing mechanical support and is also a mineral reservoir for calcium homeostasis. There are 206 bones in the human body, and depending upon their size and shape may be long, flat, tubular etc.

NORMAL STRUCTURE OF BONE *(p. 855)*

Bone is divided into 2 components:
■ **Cortical or compact bone** comprises 80% of the skeleton and is the dense outer shell responsible for structural rigidity.
■ **Trabecular or cancellous bone** composes 20% of the skeleton and has trabeculae traversing the marrow space. Its main role is in mineral homeostasis.

M/E Bone consists of large quantities of extracellular matrix which is loaded with calcium hydroxyapatite and relatively small number of bone cells which are of 3 main types besides osteoid matrix.

1. **Osteoblasts.** Osteoblasts are uninucleate cells found abundantly along the new bone-forming surfaces. They synthesise bone matrix. The serum levels of bone-related *alkaline phosphatase* (other being hepatic alkaline phosphatase) is a marker for osteoblastic activity.

2. **Osteocytes.** Osteocytes are those osteoblasts which get incorporated into bone matrix during its synthesis. Osteocytes are found within small spaces called lacunae lying in the bone matrix.
■ **Woven bone** is immature and rapidly deposited bone containing large number of closely-packed osteocytes and consists of irregular interlacing pattern of collagen fibre bundles in bone matrix.
■ **Lamellar bone** differs from woven bone in having smaller and less numerous osteocytes and fine and parallel or lamellar sheets of collagen fibres.

3. **Osteoclasts.** Osteoclasts are large multinucleate cells of mononuclear-macrophage origin and are responsible for bone resorption. The osteoclastic activity is determined by bone-related serum *acid phosphatase* levels (other being prostatic acid phosphatase).

4. **Osteoid matrix.** The osteoid matrix of bone consists of 90-95% of collagen type I and comprises nearly half of total body's collagen. Virtually whole of body's hydroxyproline and hydroxylysine reside in the bone.

BONE FORMATION AND RESORPTION. Bone is not a static tissue but its formation and resorption are taking place during period of growth as well as in adult life. Bone deposition is the result of osteoblasts while bone resorption is the function of osteoclasts. Bone formation may take place directly from collagen called *membranous ossification* seen in certain flat bones, or may occur through an intermediate stage of cartilage termed *endochondral ossification* found in metaphysis of long bones.

NORMAL STRUCTURE OF CARTILAGE *(p. 856)*

Unlike bone, the cartilage lacks blood vessels, lymphatics and nerves. It may have focal areas of calcification. Cartilage consists of 2 components.

■ **Cartilage matrix.** Like bone, cartilage too consists of organic and inorganic material. Inorganic material of cartilage is calcium hydroxyapatite similar to that in bone matrix but the organic material of cartilage is distinct from bone. High water content of cartilage matrix is responsible for function of articular cartilage and lubrication. Proteoglycans are macromolecules having proteins complexed with polysaccharides termed glycosaminoglycans. Cartilage glyco-saminoglycans consist of chondroitin sulfate and keratan sulfate, the former being most abundant.

■ **Chondrocytes.** Primitive mesenchymal cells which form bone cells form chondroblasts which give rise to chondrocytes. However, calcified cartilage is removed by the osteoclasts.

Depending upon location and structural composition, cartilage is of 3 types:

1. *Hyaline cartilage* is the basic cartilaginous tissue comprising articular cartilage of joints, cartilage in the growth plates of developing bones, costochondral cartilage, cartilage in the trachea, bronchi and larynx and the nasal cartilage.

2. *Fibrocartilage* is a hyaline cartilage that contains more abundant type II collagen fibres. It is found in annulus fibrosus of intervertebral disc, menisci, insertions of joint capsules, ligament and tendons.

3. *Elastic cartilage* is hyaline cartilage that contains abundant elastin.

OSTEOMYELITIS *(p. 857)*

An infection of the bone is termed osteomyelitis. A number of systemic infectious diseases may spread to the bone such as enteric fever, actino-mycosis, mycetoma (madura foot), syphilis, tuberculosis and brucellosis.

Pyogenic Osteomyelitis *(p. 857)*

Suppurative osteomyelitis is usually caused by bacterial infection and rarely by fungi. Haematogenous pyogenic osteomyelitis occurs most commonly in the long bones of infants and young children (5-15 years of age), particularly in the developing countries of the world. Bacterial osteomyelitis may be a complication at all ages in patients with compound fractures, surgical procedures involving prosthesis or implants, gangrene of a limb in diabetics, debilitation and immunosuppression. Though any etiologic agent may cause osteomyelitis, *Staphylococcus aureus* is implicated in a vast majority of cases. Less frequen-tly, other organisms such as streptococci, *Escherichia coli, Pseudomonas, Klebsiella* and anaerobes are involved.

Clinically, the child with acute haematogenous osteomyelitis has painful and tender limb. Fever, malaise and leucocytosis generally accompany the bony lesion.

MORPHOLOGY. Depending upon the duration, osteomyelitis may be *acute, subacute* or *chronic.* The basic pathologic changes in any stage of osteomyelitis are: suppuration, ischaemic necrosis, healing by fibrosis and bony repair. The *sequence of pathologic changes* is as under:

1. The infection begins in the metaphyseal end of the *marrow cavity* which is largely occupied by *pus*.

2. The tension in the marrow cavity is increased due to pus and results in spread of infection along the marrow cavity, causing *periosteitis*.

3. The infection may reach the subperiosteal space forming *subperiosteal abscesses*.

4. Combination of suppuration and impaired blood supply to the cortical bone results in infarction necrosis of the cortex called *sequestrum*.

5. With passage of time, there is formation of new bone beneath the periosteum present over the infected bone. This forms an encasing sheath around the necrosed bone and is known as *involucrum*.

6. Long continued neo-osteogenesis gives rise to dense sclerotic pattern of osteomyelitis called *chronic sclerosing nonsuppurative osteomyelitis of Garré*.

7. Occasionally, acute osteomyelitis may be contained to a localised area and walled off by fibrous tissue and granulation tissue. This is termed *Brodie's abscess*.

8. Occasionally, *vertebral osteomyelitis* may occur in which case infection begins from the disc (discitis) and spreads to involve the vertebral bodies.

COMPLICATIONS. Osteomyelitis may result in the following complications:
1. Septicaemia.
2. Acute bacterial arthritis.
3. Pathologic fractures.
4. Development of squamous cell carcinoma in long-standing cases.
5. Secondary amyloidosis in long-standing cases.
6. Vertebral osteomyelitis may cause vertebral collapse with paravertebral abscess, epidural abscess, cord compression and neurologic deficits.

Tuberculous Osteomyelitis *(p. 858)*

Tuberculous osteomyelitis, though rare in developed countries, continues to be a common condition in under-developed and developing countries of the world. The tubercle bacilli, *M. tuberculosis,* reach the bone marrow and synovium most commonly by haematogenous dissemination from infection elsewhere, usually the lungs, and infrequently by direct extension from the pulmonary or gastrointestinal tuberculosis. The disease affects adolescents and young adults more often. Most frequently involved are the spine and bones of extremities.

M/E The bone lesions in tuberculosis have the same general histological appearance as in tuberculosis elsewhere and consist of central caseation necrosis surrounded by tuberculous granulation tissue. The tuberculous lesions appear as a focus of bone destruction and replacement of the affected tissue by caseous material and formation of multiple discharging sinuses through the soft tissues and skin. Involvement of joint spaces and intervertebral disc are frequent. Tuberculosis of the spine, *Pott's disease,* often commences in the vertebral body and may be associated with compression fractures and destruction of intervertebral discs.

DISORDERS OF BONE GROWTH AND DEVELOPMENT (SKELETAL DYSPLASIAS) *(p. 859)*

Achondroplasia *(p. 859)*

Achondroplasia is an autosomal dominant genetic abnormality. There is selective interference with normal endochondral ossification at the level of epiphyseal cartilaginous growth plates of long bones. Thus, the long bones are abnormally short but the skull grows normally leading to relatively large skull. Achondroplasia is the commonest cause of dwarfism.

Osteogenesis Imperfecta *(p. 859)*

Osteogenesis imperfecta is an autosomal dominant or recessive disorder of synthesis of type I collagen that constitutes 90-95% of bone matrix. The disorder, thus, involves not only the skeleton but other extra-skeletal tissues as well containing type I collagen such as sclera, eyes, joints, ligaments, teeth and skin. The skeletal manifestations of osteogenesis imperfecta are due to defective osteoblasts which normally synthesise type I collagen. This results in thin or non-existent cortices and irregular trabeculae *(too little bone)* so that the bones are very fragile and liable to multiple fractures. The growth plate cartilage is, however, normal.

Osteopetrosis *(p. 860)*

Osteopetrosis, also called *marble bone disease,* is an autosomal dominant or recessive disorder of increased skeletal mass or osteosclerosis caused by a hereditary defect in osteoclast function. The condition may appear in 2 forms: autosomal recessive (malignant infantile form) and autosomal dominant (benign adult form). Failure of normal osteoclast function of bone resorption coupled with continued bone formation and endochondral ossification results in net overgrowth of calcified dense bone *(too much bone)* which occupies most of the available marrow space. Despite increased density of the bone, there is poor structural support so that the skeleton is susceptible to fractures.

METABOLIC AND ENDOCRINE BONE DISEASES *(p. 860)*

Osteoporosis *(p. 860)*

Osteoporosis or osteopenia is a common clinical syndrome involving multiple bones in which there is quantitative reduction of bone tissue mass but the bone tissue mass is otherwise normal. This reduction in bone mass results in fragile skeleton which is associated with increased risk of fractures and consequent pain and deformity. The condition is particularly common in elderly people and more frequent in postmenopausal women. The condition may remain asymptomatic or may cause only backache. Levels of serum calcium, inorganic phosphorus and alkaline phosphatase are usually within normal limits.

PATHOGENESIS. Osteoporosis is conventionally classified into 2 major groups:

■ **Primary osteoporosis** results primarily from osteopenia without an underlying disease or medication. Primary osteoporosis is further subdivided into 2 types: *idiopathic type* found in the young and juveniles and is less frequent, and *involutional type* seen in postmenopausal women and aging individuals and is more common. A number of risk factors have been attributed to cause this imbalance between bone resorption and bone formation:

1. *Genetic factors*—more marked in whites and Asians than blacks.
2. *Sex*—more frequent in females than in males.
3. *Reduced physical activity*—as in old age.
4. *Deficiency of sex hormones*—oestrogen deficiency in women as in postmenopausal osteoporosis and androgen deficiency in men.
5. *Combined deficiency of calcitonin and oestrogen.*
6. *Hyperparathyroidism.*
7. *Deficiency of vitamin D.*
8. *Local factors*—which may stimulate osteoclastic resorption or slow osteoblastic bone formation.

■ **Secondary osteoporosis** is attributed to a number of factors and conditions (e.g. immobilisation, chronic anaemia, acromegaly, hepatic disease, hyperparathyroidism, hypogonadism, thyrotoxicosis and starvation), or as an effect of medication (e.g. hypercortisonism, administration of anticonvulsant drugs and large dose of heparin).

MORPHOLOGY. Except disuse or immobilisation osteoporosis which is localised to the affected limb, other forms of osteoporosis have systemic skeletal distribution. Most commonly encountered osteoporotic fractures are:

vertebral crush fracture, femoral neck fracture and wrist fracture. There is enlargement of the medullary cavity and thinning of the cortex.

M/E Osteoporosis may be active or inactive type.

■ **Active osteoporosis** is characterised by increased bone resorption and formation i.e. *accelerated turnover.*

■ **Inactive osteoporosis** has the features of minimal bone formation and reduced resorptive activity i.e. *reduced turnover.*

Osteitis Fibrosa Cystica *(p. 861)*

Hyperparathyroidism of primary or secondary type results in oversecretion of parathyroid hormone which causes increased osteoclastic resorption of the bone. Severe and prolonged hyperparathyroidism results in osteitis fibrosa cystica. The lesion is generally induced as a manifestation of primary hyperparathyroidism, and less frequently, as a result of secondary hyperparathyroidism such as in chronic renal failure (renal osteodystrophy).

The clinical manifestations of bone disease in hyperparathyroidism are its susceptibility to fracture, skeletal deformities, joint pains and dysfunctions as a result of deranged weight bearing. The chief biochemical abnormality of excessive parathyroid hormone is hypercalcaemia, hypophosphataemia and hypercalciuria.

G/A There are focal areas of erosion of cortical bone and loss of lamina dura at the roots of teeth.

M/E The following features are seen:

■ Earliest change is *demineralisation* and *increased bone resorption* beginning at the subperiosteal and endosteal surface of the cortex and then spreading to the trabecular bone.

■ There is replacement of bone and bone-marrow by fibrosis coupled with increased number of bizarre osteoclasts at the surfaces of moth-eaten trabeculae and cortex *(osteitis fibrosa).*

■ As a result of increased resorption, microfractures and microhaemorrhages occur in the marrow cavity leading to development of cysts *(osteitis fibrosa cystica).*

■ Haemosiderin-laden macrophages and multinucleate giant cells appear at the areas of haemorrhages producing an appearance termed as *'brown tumour'* or *'reparative giant cell granuloma of hyperparathyroidism'.*

Renal Osteodystrophy (Metabolic Bone Disease) *(p. 862)*

Renal osteodystrophy is a loosely used term that encompasses a number of skeletal abnormalities appearing in cases of chronic renal failure and in patients treated by dialysis for several years. Renal osteodystrophy is more common in children than in adults.

PATHOGENESIS. Renal osteodystrophy involves two main events: *hyperphosphataemia* and *hypocalcaemia* which, in turn, leads to parathormone elaboration and resultant osteoclastic activity and major lesions of renal osteodystrophy—osteomalacia (rickets in children), secondary hyperpara-thyroidism, osteitis fibrosa cystica, osteosclerosis and metastatic calcification.

The mechanisms underlying renal osteodystrophy are briefly outlined below:

1. Hyperphosphataemia: In CRF, there is impaired renal excretion of phosphate, causing phosphate retention and hyperphosphataemia. Hyper-phosphataemia, in turn, causes hypocalcaemia which is responsible for secondary hyperparathyroidism.

2. Hypocalcaemia: Hypocalcaemia may also result from the following:

■ Due to renal dysfunction, there is decreased conversion of vitamin D metabolite 25(OH) cholecalciferol to its active form $1,25 \, (OH)_2$ cholecalciferol.

■ Reduced intestinal absorption of calcium.

3. Parathormone secretion: Hypocalcaemia stimulates secretion of parathormone, eventually leading to secondary hyperparathyroidism which, in turn, causes increased osteoclastic activity.

4. Metabolic acidosis: As a result of decreased renal function, acidosis sets in which may cause osteoporosis and bone decalcification.

5. Calcium phosphorus product > 70: When the product of biochemical value of calcium and phosphate is higher than 70, metastatic calcification may occur at extraosseous sites.

6. Dialysis-related metabolic bone disease: Long-term dialysis employing use of aluminium-containing dialysate is currently considered to be a major cause of metabolic bone lesions. Aluminium interferes with deposition of calcium hydroxyapatite in bone and results in osteomalacia, secondary hyperparathyroidism and osteitis fibrosa cystica. In addition, accumulation of β_2-microglobulin amyloid in such cases causes dialysis-related amyloidosis.

MORPHOLOGY. The following skeletal lesions can be identified in renal osteodystrophy:

1. *Mixed osteomalacia-osteitis fibrosa* is the most common manifestation of renal osteodystrophy resulting from disordered vitamin D metabolism and secondary hyperparathyroidism.

2. *Pure osteitis fibrosa* results from metabolic complications of secondary hyperparathyroidism.

3. *Pure osteomalacia* of renal osteodystrophy is attributed to aluminium toxicity.

4. *Renal rickets* resembling the changes seen in children with nutritional rickets with widened osteoid seams may occur.

5. *Osteosclerosis* is characterised by enhanced bone density in the upper and lower margins of vertebrae.

6. *Metastatic calcification* is seen at extraosseous sites such as in medium-sized blood vessels, periarticular tissues, myocardium, eyes, lungs and gastric mucosa.

Skeletal Fluorosis *(p. 863)*

Fluorosis of bones occurs due to high sodium fluoride content in soil and water consumed by people in some geographic areas and is termed endemic fluorosis. Such endemic regions exist in some tropical and subtropical areas; in India it exists in parts of Punjab and Andhra Pradesh. The condition affects farmers who consume drinking water from wells.

PATHOGENESIS. In fluorosis, fluoride replaces calcium as the mineral in the bone and gets deposited without any regulatory control. This results in heavily mineralised bones which are thicker and denser but are otherwise weak and deformed (just as in osteopetrosis).

G/A The long bones and vertebrae develop nodular swellings present both inside the bones and on the surface.

M/E These nodules are composed of heavily mineralised irregular osteoid admixed with fluoride which requires confirmation chemically.

PAGET'S DISEASE OF BONE (OSTEITIS DEFORMANS) *(P. 863)*

Paget's disease of bone is an osteolytic and osteosclerotic bone disease of uncertain etiology involving one (monostotic) or more bones (polyostotic). The condition affects predominantly males over the age of 50 years. Though the etiology remains obscure, recently there has been a suggestion that osteitis deformans is a form of slow-virus infection by paramyxovirus detected in osteoclasts.

Clinically, the *monostotic form* of the disease may remain asymptomatic and the lesion is discovered incidentally or on radiologic examination. *Polyostotic form,* however, is more widespread and may produce pain, fractures, skeletal deformities, and occasionally, sarcomatous transformation.

1. Initial osteolytic stage: This stage is characterised by areas of osteoclastic resorption produced by increased number of large osteoclasts.

2. Mixed osteolytic-osteoblastic stage: In this stage, there is imbalance between osteoblastic laying down of new bone and osteoclastic resorption so that mineralisation of the newly-laid matrix lags behind, resulting in development of characteristic *mosaic pattern* of osteoid seams or cement lines.

3. Quiescent osteosclerotic stage: After many years, excessive bone formation results so that the bone becomes more compact and dense producing osteosclerosis.

TUMOUR-LIKE LESIONS OF BONE *(p. 864)*

Fibrous Dysplasia *(p. 864)*

Fibrous dysplasia is not an uncommon tumour-like lesion of the bone. It is a benign condition, possibly of developmental origin, characterised by the presence of localised area of replacement of bone by fibrous connective tissue with a characteristic whorled pattern and containing trabeculae of woven bone.

Three types of fibrous dysplasia are distinguished:

■ **Monostotic fibrous dysplasia.** Monostotic fibrous dysplasia affects a solitary bone and is the most common type, comprising about 70% of all cases. The condition affects either sex and most patients are between 20 and 30 years of age. The bones most often affected, in descending order of frequency, are: ribs, craniofacial bones (especially maxilla), femur, tibia and humerus.

■ **Polyostotic fibrous dysplasia.** Polyostotic form of fibrous dysplasia affecting several bones constitutes about 25% of all cases. Both sexes are affected equally but the lesions appear at a relatively earlier age than the monostotic form. Most frequently affected bones are: craniofacial, ribs, vertebrae and long bones of the limbs. Approximately a quarter of cases with polyostotic form have more than half of the skeleton involved by disease.

■ **Albright syndrome.** Also called McCune-Albright syndrome, this is a form of polyostotic fibrous dysplasia associated with endocrine dysfunctions and accounts for less than 5% of all cases. Unlike monostotic and polyostotic varieties, Albright syndrome is more common in females. The syndrome is characterised by polyostotic bone lesions, skin pigmentation *(cafe-au-lait* macular spots) and sexual precocity, and infrequently other endocrinopathies.

G/A The lesions appear as sharply-demarcated, localised defects measuring 2-5 cm in diameter, present within the cancellous bone, having thin and smooth overlying cortex.

M/E The lesions of fibrous dysplasia have characteristic benign-looking fibroblastic tissue arranged in a loose, whorled pattern in which there are irregular and curved trabeculae of woven (nonlamellar) bone. There may be numerous osteoclasts in relation to bony trabeculae.

Fibrous Cortical Defect (Metaphyseal Fibrous Defect, Non-ossifying Fibroma) *(p. 864)*

Fibrous cortical defect or metaphyseal fibrous defect is a rather common benign tumour-like lesion occurring in the metaphyseal cortex of long bones in children. Most commonly involved bones are upper or lower end of tibia or lower end of femur. The lesion is generally solitary but rarely there may be multiple and bilaterally symmetrical defects.

G/A The lesion is generally small, less than 4 cm in diameter, granular and brown. Larger lesion (5-10 cm) occurring usually in response to trauma is referred to as non-ossifying fibroma.

M/E Fibrous cortical defect consists of cellular masses of fibrous tissue showing storiform pattern. There are numerous multinucleate osteoclast-like giant cells, haemosiderin-laden macrophages and foamy cells.

Solitary (Simple, Unicameral) Bone Cyst *(p. 865)*

Solitary, simple or unicameral bone cyst is a benign condition occurring in children and adolescents, most frequently located in the metaphyses at the upper end of humerus and femur. The cyst expands the bone causing thinning of the overlying cortex.

G/A The simple cyst of the bone is generally unilocular with smooth inner surface. The cavity is filled with clear fluid.

M/E The cyst wall consists of thin collagenous tissue having scattered osteoclast giant cells and newly formed reactive bony trabeculae.

Aneurysmal Bone Cyst *(p. 865)*

Aneurysmal bone cyst, true to its name, is an expanding osteolytic lesion filled with blood. The condition is seen more commonly in young patients under 30 years of age. Most frequently involved bones are shafts of metaphyses of long bones or the vertebral column.

G/A The lesion consists of a large haemorrhagic mass covered over by thinned out reactive bone.

M/E The cyst consists of blood-filled aneurysmal spaces of variable size, some of which are endothelium-lined. The spaces are separated by connective tissue septa containing osteoid tissue, numerous osteoclast-like multinucleate giant cells and trabeculae of bone.

Ganglion Cyst of Bone *(p. 866)*

Ganglion cyst of bone or intraosseous ganglion is a benign condition occurring in middle-aged patients.

BONE TUMOURS *(p. 866)*

Bone tumours are comparatively infrequent but they are clinically quite significant since some of them are highly malignant. Bone tumours may be primary or metastatic. Since histogenesis of some bone tumours is obscure, the WHO has recommended a widely accepted classification of primary bone tumours based on both histogenesis and histologic criteria. Table 26.1 lists the various types of bone tumours arising from different tissue components—osseous and non-osseous, indigenous to the bone.

BONE-FORMING (OSTEOBLASTIC)TUMOURS *(p. 866)*

Osteoma *(p. 866)*

An osteoma is a rare benign, slow-growing lesion, regarded by some as a hamartoma rather than a true neoplasm. Similar lesions may occur following trauma, subperiosteal haematoma or local inflammation.

The lesion is composed of well-differentiated mature lamellar bony trabeculae separated by fibrovascular tissue.

TABLE 26.1: Classification of Primary Bone Tumours.

HISTOLOGIC DERIVATION	BENIGN	MALIGNANT
A. OSSEOUS TUMOURS		
I. Bone-forming (osteogenic, osteoblastic) tumours	Osteoma (40-50 yrs) Osteoid osteoma (20-30 yrs) Osteoblastoma (20-30 yrs)	Osteosarcoma (10-20 yrs) Parosteal (juxtacortical) osteosarcoma (50-60 yrs)
II. Cartilage-forming (chondrogenic) tumours	Enchondroma (20-50 yrs) Osteochondroma (20-50 yrs) (Osteocartilaginous exostosis) Chondroblastoma (10-20 yrs) Chondromyxoid fibroma (20-30 yrs)	Chondrosarcoma (40-60 yrs)
III. Haematopoietic (marrow) tumours	—	Myeloma (50-60 yrs) Lymphoplasmacytic lymphoma (50-60 yrs)
IV. Unknown	Giant cell tumour (20-40 yrs) (osteoclastoma)	Malignant giant cell tumour (30-50 yrs) Ewing's sarcoma (5-20 yrs) Adamantinoma of long bones
V. Notochordal tumour	—	Chordoma (40-50 yrs)
B. NON-OSSEOUS TUMOURS		
I. Vascular tumours	Haemangioma	Haemangioendothelioma Haemangiopericytoma Angiosarcoma
II. Fibrogenic tumours	Non-ossifying fibroma (metaphyseal fibrous defect)	Fibrosarcoma
III. Neurogenic tumours	Neurilemmoma and neurofibroma	Neurofibrosarcoma
IV. Lipogenic tumours	Lipoma	Liposarcoma
V. Histiocytic tumours	Fibrous histiocytoma	Malignant fibrous histiocytoma

Figures in brackets indicate common age of occurrence.

Osteoid Osteoma and Osteoblastoma (p. 866)

Osteoid osteoma and osteoblastoma (or giant osteoid osteoma) are closely related benign tumours occurring in children and young adults. Osteoid osteoma is more common than osteoblastoma. There are no clear-cut histologic criteria to distinguish the two. The distinction between them is based on clinical features, size and radiographic appearance.

■ **Osteoid osteoma** is generally small (usually less than 1 cm) and painful tumour, located in the cortex of a long bone. The tumour is clearly demarcated having surrounding zone of reactive bone formation.

■ **Osteoblastoma**, on the other hand, is larger in size (usually more than 1 cm), painless, located in the medulla, commonly in the vertebrae, ribs, ilium and long bones, and there is absence of reactive bone formation.

M/E The distinction between osteoid osteoma and osteoblastoma is not obvious. In either case, the lesion consists of trabeculae of osteoid, rimmed by osteoblasts and separated by highly vascularised connective tissue stroma.

Osteosarcoma *(p. 867)*

Osteosarcoma or osteogenic sarcoma is the most common primary malignant tumour of the bone. The tumour is characterised by formation of *osteoid or bone, or both, directly by sarcoma cells*. The tumour is thought to arise from primitive osteoblast-forming mesenchyme. Depending upon their locations within the bone, osteosarcomas are classified into 2 main categories: *medullary* (central) and *parosteal* (juxtacortical).

Medullary or central osteosarcoma is the more common type and is generally referred to as 'osteosarcoma' if not specified. The tumour occurs in young patients between the age of 10 and 20 years. Males are affected more frequently than females. The tumour arises in the metaphysis of long bones. Most common sites, in descending order of frequency, are: the lower end of femur and upper end of tibia (i.e. around knee joint about 60%); the upper end of humerus (10%); pelvis and the upper end of femur (i.e. around hip joint about 15%).

Based upon the pathogenesis, osteosarcoma is divided into 2 types:

■ *Primary osteosarcoma* is more common and occurs in the absence of any known underlying disease. Its etiology is unknown but there is evidence linking this form of osteosarcoma with genetic factors (e.g. hereditary mutation of chromosome 13 in common with retinoblastoma locus), period of active bone growth (occurrence of the tumour in younger age), and certain environmental influences (e.g. radiation and an oncogenic virus).

■ *Secondary osteosarcoma,* on the other hand, develops following pre-existing bone disease e.g. Paget's disease of bone, fibrous dysplasia, multiple osteochondromas, chronic osteomyelitis, infarcts and fractures of bone. The tumour has a more aggressive behaviour than the primary osteosarcoma.

Medullary osteosarcoma is a highly malignant tumour. The tumour arises centrally in the metaphysis, extends longitudinally for variable distance into the medullary cavity, expands laterally on either side breaking through the cortex and lifting the periosteum. The radiographic appearance is quite distinctive: characteristic *'sunburst pattern'* due to osteogenesis within the tumour and presence of *Codman's triangle* formed at the angle between the elevated periosteum and underlying surface of the cortex.

G/A The tumour appears as a grey-white, bulky mass at the metaphyseal end of a long bone of the extremity. The articular end of the bone is generally uninvolved in initial stage. Cut surface of the tumour is grey-white with areas of haemorrhages and necrotic bone.

M/E Following features are seen:

1. Sarcoma cells: The tumour cells of osteosarcomas are undifferentiated mesenchymal stromal cells which show marked pleomorphism and polymorphism i.e. variation in size as well as shape. The tumour cells may have various shapes such as spindled, round, oval and polygonal and bizarre tumour giant cells. The tumour cells have variable size and show hyperchromatism and atypical mitoses.

2. Osteogenesis: The anaplastic sarcoma cells form osteoid matrix and bone directly which are found interspersed in the areas of tumour cells.

A variant of the usual osteosarcoma is *telangiectatic osteosarcoma* in which the tumour has large, cavernous, dilated vascular channels.

Parosteal (Juxtacortical) Osteosarcoma *(p. 868)*

Parosteal or juxtacortical osteosarcoma is an uncommon form of osteosarcoma having its origin from the external surface of the bone (*parosteal* or *juxtacortical* means outer to cortex). The tumour should be distinguished from the more common medullary osteosarcoma because of its better prognosis and different presentation. The tumour occurs in older age group, has no sex predilection and is slow growing.

G/A The tumour is lobulated and circumscribed, calcified mass in the subperiosteal location.

M/E Though the features which characterise the usual osteosarcoma (sarcomatous stroma and production of neoplastic osteoid and bone) are present, the tumour shows a high degree of structural differentiation.

CARTILAGE-FORMING (CHONDROBLASTIC)TUMOURS *(p. 869)*

Osteocartilaginous Exostoses (Osteochondromas) *(p. 869)*

Osteocartilaginous exostoses or osteochondromas are the commonest of benign cartilage-forming lesions. Though designated and discussed with neoplasms, exostosis or osteochondroma is not a true tumour but is regarded as a disorder of growth and development. It may occur as a '*solitary sporadic exostosis*' or there may be '*multiple hereditary exostoses*'.

Exostoses arise from metaphyses of long bones as exophytic lesions, most commonly lower femur and upper tibia (i.e. around knee) and upper humerus. They are discovered most commonly in late childhood or adolescence and are more frequent in males. Both solitary and multiple exostoses may undergo transformation into chondrosarcoma but the risk is much greater with multiple hereditary exostoses.

G/A Osteochondromas have a broad or narrow base (i.e. may be either sessile or pedunculated) which is continuous with the cortical bone. They protrude exophytically as mushroom-shaped, cartilage-capped lesions enclosing well-formed cortical bone and marrow.

M/E They are composed of outer mature cartilage resembling epiphyseal cartilage and the inner mature lamellar bone and bone marrow.

Enchondroma *(p. 869)*

Enchondroma is the term used for the benign cartilage-forming tumour that develops centrally within the interior of the affected bone, while chondroma refers to the peripheral development of lesion similar to osteochondromas. The coexistence of multiple enchondromas with multiple soft tissue haemangiomas constitutes a familial syndrome called *Maffucci's syndrome*. Most common locations for enchondromas are short tubular bones of the hands and feet.

G/A The enchondroma is lobulated, bluish-grey, translucent, cartilaginous mass lying within the medullary cavity.

M/E The tumour has characteristic lobulated appearance. The lobules are composed of normal adult hyaline cartilage separated by vascularised fibrous stroma. Foci of calcification may be evident within the tumour. Enchondroma is distinguished from chondrosarcoma by the absence of invasion into surrounding tissues.

Chondroblastoma *(p. 870)*

Chondroblastoma is a relatively rare benign tumour arising from the epiphysis of long bones adjacent to the epiphyseal cartilage plate. Most commonly affected bones are upper tibia and lower femur (i.e. about knee) and upper humerus. The tumour usually occurs in patients under 20 years of age with male preponderance (male-female ratio 2:1).

G/A Chondroblastoma is a well-defined mass, up to 5 cm in diameter, lying in the epiphysis.

M/E The tumour is highly cellular and is composed of small, round to polygonal mononuclear cells resembling chondroblasts and also contains multinucleate osteoclast-like giant cells.

Chondromyxoid Fibroma *(p. 870)*

Chondromyxoid fibroma is an uncommon benign tumour of cartilaginous origin arising in the metaphysis of long bones. Most common locations are upper end of tibia and lower end of femur i.e. around the knee joint. Majority of tumours appear in 2nd to 3rd decades of life with male preponderance.

G/A Chondromyxoid fibroma is sharply-demarcated, grey-white lobulated mass, not exceeding 5 cm in diameter, lying in the metaphysis. The tumour is often surrounded by a layer of dense sclerotic bone.

M/E The tumour has essentially lobulated pattern. The lobules are separated by fibrous tissue and variable number of osteoclast-like giant cells.

Chondrosarcoma *(p. 871)*

Chondrosarcoma is a malignant tumour of chondroblasts. In frequency, it is next in frequency to osteosarcoma but is relatively slow-growing and thus has a much better prognosis than that of osteosarcoma. Two types of chondrosarcoma are distinguished:

■ **Central chondrosarcoma** is more common and arises within the medullary cavity of diaphysis or metaphysis. This type of chondrosarcoma is generally primary i.e. occurs de novo.

■ **Peripheral chondrosarcoma** arises in the cortex or periosteum of metaphysis. It may be primary or secondary occurring on a pre-existing benign cartilaginous tumour such as osteocartilaginous exostoses (osteochondromas), multiple enchondromatosis.

Both forms of chondrosarcoma usually occur in patients between 3rd and 6th decades of life with slight male preponderance. In contrast to benign cartilaginous tumours, majority of chondrosarcomas are found in the central skeleton (i.e. in the pelvis, ribs and shoulders) and around the knee joint.

G/A Chondrosarcoma may vary in size from a few centimeters to extremely large and lobulated masses of firm consistency. Cut section of the tumour shows translucent, bluish-white, gelatinous or myxoid appearance with foci of ossification.

M/E The hallmarks of chondrosarcoma are invasive character and formation of lobules of anaplastic cartilage cells showing cytologic features of malignancy such as hyperchromatism, pleomorphism, two or more cells in the lacunae and tumour giant cells.

GIANT CELL TUMOUR (OSTEOCLASTOMA) *(p. 871)*

Giant cell tumour or osteoclastoma is a distinctive neoplasm with uncertain histogenesis and hence classified separately. The tumour arises in the epiphysis of long bones close to the articular cartilage. Most common sites of involvement are lower end of femur and upper end of tibia (i.e. about the knee), lower end of radius and upper end of fibula. Giant cell tumour occurs in patients between 20 and 40 years of age with no sex predilection.

G/A Giant cell tumour is eccentrically located in the epiphyseal end of a long bone which is expanded. The tumour is well-circumscribed, dark-tan and covered by a thin shell of subperiosteal bone. Cut surface of the tumour is characteristically haemorrhagic, necrotic, and honey-combed.

M/E The hallmark of giant cell tumour is the presence of large number of multinucleate osteoclast-like giant cells which are regularly scattered throughout the stromal mononuclear cells.

Giant cell tumour of bone has certain peculiarities which deserve further elaboration.

■ **Cell of orign.** Though designated as giant cell tumour or osteoclastoma, the true tumour cells are round to spindled mononuclear cells and not osteoclast-like giant cells. Histogenesis of tumour cells is uncertain but possibly they are of mesenchymal origin. The available evidence suggests that osteoclasts are perhaps derived from fusion of monocytes and are reactive in nature.

■ **Other giant cell lesions.** This peculiar tumour with above description is named 'giant cell tumour' but giant cells are present in several other benign tumours and tumour-like lesions from which the giant cell tumour is to be distinguished. These *benign giant cell lesions* are: chondroblastoma, brown tumour of hyperparathyroidism, reparative giant cell granuloma, aneurysmal bone cyst, simple bone cyst and metaphyseal fibrous defect (non-ossifying fibroma).

■ **Biologic behaviour.** Giant cell tumours are best described as aggressive lesions. About 40% to 60% of them recur after curettage, sometimes after a few decades of initial resection. Approximately 4% cases result in distant metastases, mainly to lungs.

EWING'S SARCOMA AND PRIMITIVE NEUROECTODERMAL TUMOUR (PNET) *(p. 873)*

Ewing's sarcoma is a highly malignant small round cell tumour occurring in patients between the age of 5 and 20 years with predilection for occurrence in females. Currently Ewing's sarcoma includes:

i)   classic (skeletal) Ewing's sarcoma;
ii) soft tissue Ewing's sarcoma; and
iii) primitive neuroectodermal tumour (PNET).

The three are linked together by a common neural origin and by a common cytogenetic translocation abnormality t(11; 22) (q24; q12). This suggests a phenotypic spectrum in these conditions varying from undifferentiated Ewing's sarcoma to PNET positive for rosettes and neural markers.

The skeletal Ewing's sarcoma arises in the medullary canal of diaphysis or metaphysis. The common sites are shafts and metaphysis of long bones, particularly femur, tibia, humerus and fibula.

Clinical features include pain, tenderness and swelling of the affected area accompanied by fever, leucocytosis and elevated ESR.

G/A Ewing's sarcoma is typically located in the medullary cavity and produces expansion of the affected diaphysis (shaft) or metaphysis, often extending into the adjacent soft tissues. The tumour tissue is characteristically grey-white, soft and friable.

M/E Ewing's tumour is a member of *small round cell tumours* which includes other tumours such as: PNET, neuroblastoma, embryonal rhabdomyosarcoma, lymphoma-leukaemias, and metastatic small cell carcinoma. Ewing's tumour shows the following microscopic characteristics:

1. **Pattern.** The tumour is divided by fibrous septa into irregular lobules of closely-packed tumour cells. These tumour cells are characteristically arranged around capillaries termed 'pseudorosette pattern'.

2. Tumour cells. The individual tumour cells comprising the lobules are small and uniform resembling lymphocytes and have ill-defined cytoplasmic outlines, scanty cytoplasm and round nuclei having 'salt and pepper' chromatin and frequent mitoses. Based on these cytological features the tumour is also called *round cell tumour* or *small blue cell tumour.* The cytoplasm contains glycogen that stains with periodic acid-Schiff (PAS) reaction.

Ewing's sarcoma metastasises early by haematogenous route to the lungs, liver, other bones and brain. Involvement of other bones has prompted a suggestion of *multicentric origin* of Ewing's sarcoma. Currently, use of combined regimen consisting of radiotherapy and systemic chemotherapy has improved the outcome greatly (5-year survival rate 40-75%).

CHORDOMA *(p. 873)*

Chordoma is a slow-growing malignant tumour arising from remnants of notochord. Notochord is the primitive axial skeleton which subsequently develops into the spine. Normally, remnants of notochord are represented by notochordal or physaliphorous *(physalis* = bubble, *phorous* = bearing) cells present in the nucleus pulposus. Chordomas thus occur in the axial skeleton, particularly sacral and spheno-occipital region, and infrequently in the vertebrae. Chordoma is usually found in patients over the age of 40 years with no sex predilection.

G/A The tumour is soft, lobulated, translucent and gelatinous with areas of haemorrhages.

M/E Chordoma is composed of highly vacuolated physaliphorous cells surrounded by a sea of intercellular mucoid material.

METASTATIC BONE TUMOURS *(p. 874)*

Metastases to the skeleton are more frequent than the primary bone tumours. Metastatic bone tumours are exceeded in frequency by only 2 other organs—lungs and liver. Most skeletal metastases are derived from haematogenous spread.

Bony metastases of carcinomas predominate over the sarcomas. Some of the common *carcinomas* metastasising to the bones are of: breast, prostate, lung, kidney, stomach, thyroid, cervix, body of uterus, urinary bladder, testis, melanoma and neuroblastoma of adrenal gland. Examples of *sarcomas* which may metastasise to bone are: embryonal and alveolar rhabdomyosarcoma, Ewing's sarcoma and osteosarcoma.

Skeletal metastases may be single or multiple. Most commonly involved bones are: the spine, pelvis, femur, skull, ribs and humerus. Usual radiographic appearance is of an *osteolytic* lesion. *Osteoblastic* bone metastases occur in cancer of the prostate, carcinoid tumour and small cell carcinoma of lung.

JOINTS *(p. 874)*

NORMAL STRUCTURE *(p. 874)*

The joints are of 2 types—*diarthrodial or synovial joints* with a joint cavity, and *synarthrodial or nonsynovial joints* without a joint cavity. Most of the diseases of joints affect diarthrodial or synovial joints. In diarthrodial joints, the ends of two bones are held together by joint capsule with ligaments and tendons inserted at the outer surface of the capsule. The articular surfaces of bones are covered by hyaline cartilage which is thicker in weight-bearing areas than in nonweight-bearing areas. The joint space is lined by synovial membrane or synovium which forms synovial fluid that lubricates the joint during movements.

OSTEOARTHRITIS *(p. 875)*

Osteoarthritis (OA), also called osteoarthrosis or degenerative joint disease, is the most common form of chronic disorder of synovial joints. It is characterised by progressive degenerative changes in the articular cartilages over the years, particularly in weight-bearing joints.

TYPES AND PATHOGENESIS. OA occurs in 2 clinical forms:

■ **Primary OA** occurs in the elderly, more commonly in women than in men. The process begins by the end of 4th decade and then progressively and steadily increases producing clinical symptoms. Probably, wear and tear with repeated minor trauma, heredity, obesity, aging *per se,* all contribute to focal degenerative changes in the articular cartilage of the joints.

■ **Secondary OA** may appear at any age and is the result of any previous wear and tear phenomena involving the joint such as previous injury, fracture, inflammation, loose bodies and congenital dislocation of the hip.

The manifestations of OA are most conspicuous in large joints such as hips, knee and back. However, the pattern of joint involvement may be related to the type of physical activity.

MORPHOLOGY The pathologic changes occur in the articular cartilages, adjacent bones and synovium:

1. Articular cartilages. The regressive changes are most marked in the weight-bearing regions of articular cartilages. Initially, there is loss of cartilaginous matrix (proteoglycans) resulting in progressive loss of normal metachromasia. Radiologically, this progressive loss of cartilage is apparent as narrowed joint space.

The molecular mechanism of damage to cartilage in OA appears to be the breakdown of collagen type II, probably by IL-1, TNF and nitric oxide.

2. Bone. The denuded subchondral bone appears like polished ivory. There is death of superficial osteocytes and increased osteoclastic activity causing rarefaction, microcyst formation and occasionally microfractures of the subjacent bone. The margins of the joints respond to cartilage damage by *osteophyte* or *spur formation.*

3. Synovium. Initially, there are no pathologic changes in the synovium but in advanced cases there is low-grade chronic synovitis and villous hypertrophy.

RHEUMATOID ARTHRITIS *(p. 876)*

Rheumatoid arthritis (RA) is a chronic multisystem disease of unknown cause. Though the most prominent manifestation of RA is inflammatory arthritis of the peripheral joints, usually with a symmetrical distribution, its systemic manifestations include haematologic, pulmonary, neurological and cardiovascular abnormalities.

RA is a common disease having peak incidence in 3rd to 4th decades of life, with 3-5 times higher preponderance in females. The condition has high association with HLA-DR4 and HLA-DR1 and familial aggregation.

About 80% of cases are seropositive for *rheumatoid factor (RF)*. However, RF titres are elevated in certain unrelated diseases too such as in: viral hepatitis, cirrhosis, sarcoidosis and leprosy. Advanced cases show characteristic radiologic abnormalities such as narrowing of joint space and ulnar deviation of the fingers and radial deviation of the wrist.

ETIOPATHOGENESIS. Present concept on etiology and pathogenesis proposes that RA occurs in an *immunogenetically predisposed individual to the effect of microbial agents acting as trigger antigen.* More recently, the role of *superantigens* which are produced by several microorganisms with capacity to bind to HLA-DR molecules (MHC-II region) has been proposed.

Chapter Twenty Six

The proposed events in **immunopathogenesis** of RA consists of the following sequence:

■ In response to antigenic exposure (? infectious agent) in a genetically predisposed individual (HLA-DR), *CD4+ T-cells* are activated.

■ These cells elaborate *cytokines;* the important ones being tumour necrosis factor (TNF)-α, interferon (IF)-γ and interleukin (IL)-1.

■ These cytokines *activate* endothelial cells, B lymphocytes and macrophages.

■ Activation of B-cells releases IgM antibody against IgG (i.e. anti-IgG); this molecule is termed *rheumatoid factor (RF)*.

■ IgG and IgM immune complexes trigger *inflammatory damage* to the synovium, small blood vessels and collagen.

■ Activated endothelial cells express *adhesion molecules* which stimulate collection of inflammatory cells.

■ Activation of macrophages releases more cytokines which cause damage to joint tissues and vascularisation of cartilage termed *pannus formation*.

■ Eventually damage and destruction of bone and cartilage are followed by *fibrosis* and *ankylosis* producing joint deformities.

MORPHOLOGY. The predominant pathologic lesions are found in the joints and tendons, and less often, extra-articular lesions are encountered.

ARTICULAR LESIONS. RA involves first the small joints of hands and feet and then symmetrically affects the joints of wrists, elbows, ankles and knees. The proximal interphalangeal and metacarpophalangeal joints are affected most severely.

M/E 1. Numerous folds of large villi of synovium.
2. Marked thickening of the synovial membrane.
3. Intense inflammatory cell infiltrate in the synovial membrane.
4. Foci of fibrinoid necrosis and fibrin deposition.

The pannus progressively destroys the underlying cartilage and subchondral bone.

EXTRA-ARTICULAR LESIONS. Nonspecific inflammatory changes are seen in the blood vessels (acute vasculitis), lungs, pleura, pericardium, myocardium, lymph nodes, peripheral nerves and eyes. But one of the characteristic extra-articular manifestation of RA is occurrence of rheumatoid nodules in the skin.

There are some *variants* of RA:

1. Juvenile RA found in adolescent patients under 16 years of age is characterised by acute onset of fever and predominant involvement of knees and ankles.

2. Felty's syndrome consists of polyarticular RA associated with splenomegaly and hypersplenism and consequent haematologic derangements.

3. Ankylosing spondylitis or rheumatoid spondylitis is rheumatoid involvement of the spine, particularly sacro-iliac joints, in young male patients.

SUPPURATIVE ARTHRITIS *(p. 878)*

Infectious or suppurative arthritis is invariably an acute inflammatory involvement of the joint. Bacteria usually reach the joint space from the blood stream but other routes of infection by direct contamination of an open wound or lymphatic spread may also occur. Immunocompromised and debilitated patients are increasingly susceptible to suppurative arthritis.

G/A The haematogenous infectious joint involvement is more often monoarticular rather than polyarticular. The large joints of lower extremities such as the knee, hip and ankle, shoulder and sternoclavicular joints are particularly favoured sites.

M/E There may be formation of inflammatory granulation tissue and onset of fibrous adhesions between the opposing articular surfaces resulting in permanent ankylosis.

TUBERCULOUS ARTHRITIS *(p. 878)*

Tuberculous infection of the joints results most commonly from haematogenous dissemination of the organisms from pulmonary or other focus of infection. Another route of infection is direct spread from tuberculous osteomyelitis close to the joint.

G/A The affected articular surface shows deposition of grey-yellow exudate and occasionally tubercles are present.

M/E The synovium is studded with solitary or confluent caseating tubercles. The underlying articular cartilage and bone may be involved by extension of tuberculous granulation tissue and cause necrosis *(caries)*.

GOUT AND GOUTY ARTHRITIS *(p. 878)*

Gout is a disorder of purine metabolism manifested by the following features, occurring singly or in combination:
1. Increased serum uric acid concentration *(hyperuricaemia)*.
2. Recurrent attacks of characteristic type of acute arthritis in which crystals of *monosodium urate monohydrate* may be demonstrable in the leucocytes present in the synovial fluid.
3. Aggregated deposits of monosodium urate monohydrate *(tophi)* in and around the joints of the extremities.
4. *Renal disease* involving interstitial tissue and blood vessels.
5. Uric acid *nephrolithiasis*.
   The disease usually begins in 3rd decade of life and affects men more often than women. A family history of gout is present in a fairly large proportion of cases indicating role of inheritance in hyperuricaemia. Clinically, the natural history of gout comprises 4 stages: asymptomatic hyperuricaemia, acute gouty arthritis, asymptomatic intervals of intercritical periods, and chronic tophaceous stage. In addition, gout nephropathy and urate nephrolithiasis may occur.

TYPES AND PATHOGENESIS. The fundamental biochemical hallmark of gout is *hyperuricaemia*. A serum uric acid level in excess of 7 mg/dl, which represents the upper limit of solubility of monosodium urate in serum at 37°C at blood pH, is associated with increased risk of development of gout. Thus, *pathogenesis of gout is pathogenesis of hyperuricaemia.*
   Hyperuricaemia and gout may be classified into 2 types:

1. Hyperuricaemia of metabolic origin. This group comprises about 10% cases of gout which are characterised by overproduction of uric acid. There is either an accelerated rate of purine biosynthesis *de novo*, or an increased turnover of nucleic acids. The causes of *primary metabolic gout* include a number of specific enzyme defects in purine metabolism. The *secondary metabolic gout* is due to either increased purine biosynthesis or a deficiency of glucose-6-phosphatase.

2. Hyperuricaemia of renal origin. About 90% cases of gout are the result of reduced renal excretion of uric acid.

MORPHOLOGY. The pathologic manifestations of gout include:

1. Acute gouty arthritis. This stage is characterised by acute synovitis triggered by precipitation of sufficient amount of needle-shaped crystals of monosodium urate from serum or synovial fluid. Acute gouty arthritis is predominantly a disease of lower extremities, affecting most commonly *great toe*.

2. Chronic tophaceous arthritis. Recurrent attacks of acute gouty arthritis lead to progressive evolution into chronic arthritis.

3. Tophi in soft tissue. A *tophus* (meaning 'a porous stone') is a mass of urates measuring a few millimeters to a few centimeters in diameter. Tophi may be located in the periarticular tissues as well as subcutaneously such as on the hands and feet.

4. Renal lesions. Chronic gouty arthritis frequently involves the kidneys. Three types of renal lesions are described in the kidneys: acute urate nephropathy, chronic urate nephropathy and uric acid nephrolithiasis.

PSEUDOGOUT (PYROPHOSPHATE ARTHROPATHY) *(p. 880)*

Pseudogout refers to an inflammatory joint involvement due to deposition of calcium pyrophosphate in the joint space. The condition is seen in middle-aged and elderly individuals of either sex. The pain is usually less severe and involvement of big toe is rare.

MORPHOLOGY. The involvement may be monoarticular or polyarticular but large joints such as knees, hips and shoulders are more often affected.

PIGMENTED VILLONODULAR SYNOVITIS AND GIANT CELL TUMOUR OF TENDON SHEATH (NODULAR TENOSYNOVITIS) *(p. 880)*

The terms 'pigmented villonodular synovitis' and 'nodular tenosynovitis' represent diffuse and localised form respectively of the same underlying process. The localised form of lesion is also termed *xanthofibroma* or *benign synovioma*. When the giant cells are numerous in localised tenosynovitis, the condition is called *giant cell tumour of tendon sheath*.

MORPHOLOGY. Though the two conditions have many morphologic similarities, they are best described separately.

■ **Giant cell tumour of tendon sheath (Nodular tenosynovitis).** The localised nodular tenosynovitis is seen most commonly in the tendons of fingers.

G/A It takes the form of a solitary, circumscribed, pedunculated, small and lobulated nodule, measuring less than 2 cm in diameter. It is closely attached to and sometimes grooved by the underlying tendon.

M/E It is well encapsulated and is composed of sheets of small oval to spindle-shaped cells, foamy xanthoma cells, scattered multinucleate giant cells and irregular bundles of collagen.

■ **Pigmented villonodular tenosynovitis.** This is a diffuse form of synovial overgrowth seen most commonly in the knee and hip.

G/A The synovium has characteristic sponge-like reddish-brown or tan appearance with intermingled elongated villous projections and solid nodules.

M/E The changes are modified by recurrent injury. The enlarged villi are covered by hyperplastic synovium and abundant subsynovial infiltrate of lymphocytes, plasma cells and macrophages, many of which are lipid-laden and haemosiderin-laden. Multinucleate giant cells are scattered in these areas.

CYST OF GANGLION *(p. 881)*

A ganglion is a small, round or ovoid, movable, subcutaneous cystic swelling. The most common location is dorsum of wrist but may be found on the dorsal surface of foot near the ankle. It may be the result of herniated synovium.

G/A A ganglion is a small cyst filled with clear mucinous fluid.

M/E The cyst has a wall composed of dense or oedematous connective tissue which is sometimes lined by synovial cells but more often is lined by necrotic cells.

BURSITIS *(p. 881)*

Inflammation of bursa is termed bursitis. Bursae are synovial-lined sacs found over bony prominences. Bursitis occurs following mechanical trauma or inflammation. It may result following single injury such as *olecranon bursitis* and *prepatellar bursitis,* but is more often due to repeated injuries from excessive pressure such as in *housemaid's knee* or *tennis elbow.*

SKELETAL MUSCLES *(p. 881)*

NORMAL STRUCTURE *(p. 881)*

Striated skeletal muscles consist of bundles of fibres called *fascicles,* each of which is surrounded by connective tissue sheath termed *perimysium.* Perimysium contains blood vessels and nerve supply of the muscle fascicles. Each muscle fibre is enveloped by delicate fibrous stroma called *endomysium.*

Myofilaments are of 2 types—*myosin* comprising thick filaments and *actin* constituting thin filaments. These together produce cross-striations in muscle fibres seen in longitudinal sections on light microscopy. *Sarcomeres* are the partitions of myofilaments into equal zones.

NEUROGENIC DISEASES *(p. 882)*

The group of neurogenic diseases affecting skeletal muscles is characterised by a combination of muscular weakness and fatiguability. The most common of these is myasthenia gravis; others are congenital myasthenia, an acquired Eaton-Lambert syndrome associated with carcinoma of the lung, and denervation atrophy.

MYASTHENIA GRAVIS *(p. 882)*

Myasthenia gravis (MG) is a neuromuscular disorder of autoimmune origin in which the acetylcholine receptors (AChR) in the motor end-plates of the muscles are damaged. The term *'myasthenia'* means muscular weakness and *'gravis'* implies serious; thus both together denote the clinical characteristics of the disease. MG may be found at any age but adult women are affected more often than adult men in the ratio of 3:2. The condition presents clinically with muscular weakness and fatiguability, initially in the ocular musculature but later spreads to involve the trunk and limbs.

PATHOGENESIS. The pathogenesis of MG is best understood in the context of normal muscle metabolism.

■ **Normally,** acetylcholine is synthesised in the motor nerve terminal and stored in vesicles that are released spontaneously when an action potential reaches the nerve terminal.

■ **In MG,** the basic defect is reduction in the number of available AChRs at the post-synaptic muscle membrane. In addition, the post-synaptic folds are flattened. About 85-90% patients of MG have anti-AChR-antibodies in their sera. Majority of patients of MG may have either thymoma or thymic hyperplasia; thymectomy is helpful in ameliorating the condition. The thymus possibly sensitises B cells to produce anti-AChR antibodies.

G/A The muscles appear normal until late in the course of disease when they become wasted.

M/E A few clumps of lymphocytes may be found around small blood vessels. Degenerating muscle fibres are present in half the cases.

EM Reveals reduction in synaptic area of the motor axons due to flattening or simplification of post-synaptic folds. The number of AChRs is greatly reduced.

DENERVATION ATROPHY *(P. 883)*

If the muscle or a part of muscle is deprived of its motor nerve supply, the affected muscle undergoes atrophy. In demyelination, on the other hand, there is conduction block in the nerve impulse but no denervation and hence muscle atrophy does not occur.

Denervating diseases are characterised by axonal degeneration and consequent muscle atrophy. These include *amyotrophic lateral sclerosis* as an example of anterior horn cell disease, and *peripheral neuropathy* causing injury to myelinated axon.

M/E Denervation atrophy is pathologically characterised by groups of small angulated muscle fibres alternating with groups of plump, normal or even hypertrophic fibres with intact innervation.

MYOPATHIC DISEASES (MYOPATHIES) *(p. 883)*

Myopathies are primary skeletal muscle diseases resulting in chronic muscle weakness. These are divided into 5 broad groups: hereditary (muscular dystrophies), inflammatory, endocrine, metabolic and toxic myopathies. Only the hereditary myopathies, also termed muscular dystrophies, are briefly considered below.

MUSCULAR DYSTROPHIES *(p. 883)*

Muscular dystrophies are a group of genetically-inherited primary muscle diseases, having in common, progressive and unremitting muscular weakness. Six major forms of muscular dystrophies are described: *Duchenne's, Becker's, myotonic, facio-scapulohumeral, limb-girdle and oculo-pharyngeal type.* Each type of muscular dystrophy is a distinct entity having differences in inheritance pattern, age at onset, clinical features, other organ system involvements and clinical course.

M/E Common to all forms of muscular dystrophies are muscle fibre necrosis, regenerative activity, replacement by interstitial fibrosis and adipose tissue.

■ SELF ASSESSMENT

1. **The serum marker for increased osteoclastic activity is:**
   A. Total acid phosphatase level
   B. Bony acid phosphatase level
   C. Total alkaline phosphatase level
   D. Bony alkaline phosphatase level

2. **The serum marker for increased osteoblastic activity is:**
   A. Total acid phosphatase level
   B. Bony acid phosphatase level
   C. Total alkaline phosphatase level
   D. Bony alkaline phosphatase level

3. **Mineralisation of uncalcified osteoid matrix takes about:**
   A. 3-5 days   B   5-8 days
   C. 8-12 days   D. 12-15 days

4. **Cartilage matrix largely consists of:**
   A. Chondroitin sulfate   B. Keratan sulfate
   C. Heparan sulfate   D. Dermatan sulfate

5. **Long-term complications of chronic osteomyelitis are as follows** *except:*
   A. Secondary amyloidosis
   B. Draining sinus tracts
   C. Development of Ewing's sarcoma
   D. Squamous carcinoma in sinus tract

6. **Osteopetrosis is characterised by the following features** *except:*
   A. Overgrowth of calcified dense bone
   B. Hereditary defect in osteoclast function
   C. There is hypercalcaemia
   D. Skeleton is susceptible to fractures

7. **Osteoporosis is characterised by the following laboratory investigation** *except:*
   A. Normal inorganic phosphate
   B. Raised serum calcium
   C. Normal alkaline phosphatase
   D. Normal acid phosphatase

8. **Renal osteodystrophy has the following biochemical parameters** *except:*
   A. Raised parathormone level
   B. Hyperphosphataemia
   C. Hypercalcaemia
   D. Calcium phosphorus product >70

9. **Paget's disease of the bone has following features** *except:*
   A. Affects older age past 50 years
   B. Elevation of serum alkaline phosphatase
   C. There is generally hypocalcaemia
   D. Role of virus in its etiology

10. **Albright's syndrome has the following features** *except:*
    A. There are monostotic bony lesions
    B. Skin pigmentation
    C. Sexual precocity
    D. More common in females

11. **Osteoblastoma differs from osteoid osteoma by the following features** *except:*
    A. It is larger than osteoid osteoma
    B. It is generally painful
    C. It is commonly located in the medulla of vertebrae, ribs etc.
    D. There is absence of reactive bone formation

12. **Classic osteosarcoma has the following features** *except:*
    A. It occurs in age range of 10-20 years
    B. There is role of mutation in Rb gene in its etiology
    C. It is a highly malignant tumour
    D. Serum alkaline phosphatase levels are generally lowered.

13. **Parosteal osteosarcoma has the following features** *except:*
    A. It occurs at extracortical location
    B. It occurs in older age group
    C. Worse prognosis than classic osteosarcoma
    D. It has no sex predilection

14. **There is a higher possibility of development of chondrosarcoma in the following benign cartilage-forming tumour:**
    A. Solitary enchondroma
    B. Multiple enchondroma
    C. Chondroblastoma
    D. Chondromyxoid fibroma

15. **In giant cell tumour of bone, the tumour cells are:**
    A. Osteoclastic giant cells
    B. Mononuclear stromal cells
    C. Fibroblastic cells
    D. Sinusoidal lining cells

16. **The cell of origin of Ewing's sarcoma is:**
    A. Endothelial cell
    B. Marrow cell
    C. Osteoblast
    D. Primitive neuroectodermal cell

17. **Chordoma is a:**
   A. Benign tumour
   B. Locally recurrent tumour
   C. Intermediate grade tumour
   D. Malignant tumour

18. **Osteoblastic skeletal metastasis are characteristically seen in:**
   A. Thyroid cancer
   B. Breast cancer
   C. Prostatic cancer
   D. Malignant melanoma

19. **Osteoarthritis has the following pathologic changes** *except:*
   A. Progressive loss of cartilaginous matrix
   B. Increased osteoclastic activity
   C. Osteophyte formation at the joint margin
   D. Atrophy of synovium

20. **Most frequently and severely involved joints in rheumatoid arthritis are:**
   A. Knees
   B. Elbows
   C. Interphalangeal
   D. Sacroiliac

21. **Most frequently affected joint in acute gouty arthritis in the beginning is:**
   A. Knee
   B. Elbow
   C. Shoulder
   D. Great toe

22. **The origin of villonodular tenosynovitis and giant cell tumour of tendon sheath is:**
   A. Inflammatory
   B. Neoplastic
   C. Traumatic
   D. Autoimmune

23. **Patients of myasthenia gravis have the following features** *except:*
   A. There is reduction in AChRs
   B. Majority of patients have anti-AChR antibodies in their serum
   C. Thymic hypoplasia has a risk in its etiology
   D. The disease has other autoimmune associations

24. **All the following tumours are benign** *except:*
   A. Osteoma
   B. Chondroma
   C. Chordoma
   D. Osteoblastoma

KEY

1 = B	2 = D	3 = D	4 = A
5 = C	6 = C	7 = B	8 = C
9 = C	10 = A	11 = B	12 = D
13 = C	14 = B	15 = B	16 = D
17 = D	18 = C	19 = D	20 = C
21 = D	22 = B	23 = C	24 = C

27

Soft Tissue Tumours

GENERAL FEATURES *(p. 885)*

INTRODUCTION. For the purpose of classification of this group of tumours, the WHO has defined soft tissues as including all non-epithelial extra-skeletal tissues of the body except the reticuloendothelial system, the glia and the supporting tissues of specific organs and viscera. Thus, tissues included in soft tissues are: fibrous tissue, adipose tissue, muscle tissue, synovial tissue, blood vessels and neuroectodermal tissues of the peripheral and autonomic nervous system.

In general, the benign tumours of soft tissues are designated by a prefix indicating the tissue of origin followed by suffix-*oma* and malignant counterparts by adding the suffix -*sarcoma*. Benign soft tissue tumours are about 100 times more common than sarcomas. Sarcomas rarely arise from malignant transformation of a pre-existing benign tumour. It may be recalled here that soft tissue sarcomas metastasise most frequently by the haematogenous route and disseminate commonly to the lungs, liver, bone and brain. Lymph node metastases are often late.

A few important principles apply to majority of soft tissue tumours:

■ Superficially-located tumours tend to be benign while *deep-seated lesions* are more likely to be malignant.

■ *Large-sized tumours* are generally more malignant than small ones.

■ A *rapidly-growing tumour* often behaves as a malignant tumour than the one that develops slowly.

■ Malignant tumours have frequently *increased vascularity* while benign tumours are selectively avascular.

■ Although soft tissue tumours may arise anywhere in the body but in general *more common locations* are: lower extremity (40%), upper extremity (20%), trunk and retroperitoneum (30%) and head and neck (10%).

■ In general *males* are affected more commonly than females.

■ Approximately 15% of soft tissue tumours occur in *children* and includes some specific examples of soft tissue sarcomas e.g. rhabdomyosarcoma, synovial sarcoma.

ETIOLOGY AND PATHOGENESIS. A few common features characterise many soft tissue tumours:

1. Frequently there is history of antecedent *trauma*.

2. Molecular and cytogenetic studies in many soft tissue tumours reveal *chromosomal abnormalities and mutations* in genes e.g. translocations, various fusion genes etc.

3. Most of the soft tissue tumours occur *sporadically;* however there are a few examples which are components of *genetic syndromes* e.g. neurofibromatosis type 1, Li-Fraumeni syndrome, Osler-Weber-Rendu syndrome etc.

CLASSIFICATION AND DIAGNOSTIC CRITERIA. Soft tissue tumours are generally classified clinically on the basis of tissue produced by the tumour e.g. fibrous, lipogenic etc. However, accurate pathological diagnosis of soft tissue tumours is based on histogenesis which can be made by the following plan:

1. Cell patterns:

i) *Smooth muscle tumours:* interlacing fascicles of pink staining tumour cells.

ii) *Fibrohistiocytic tumours:* characteristically have storiform pattern.

iii) Herringbone pattern: is seen in fibrosarcoma.

iv) Pallisaded arrangement: characteristically is seen in schwannomas.

v) Biphasic pattern: is the term used for a combination arrangement of two types—fascicles and epithelial-like; e.g. in synovial sarcoma.

2. Cell types:

i) Spindle cells: These are the most common cell types in most sarcomas.

ii) Small round cells: Some soft tissue sarcomas are characterised by dominant presence of small round cells or blue cells and are accordingly termed as malignant small round cell tumours, round cell sarcomas, or blue cell tumours (due to presence of lymphocyte-like nuclear size and dense blue chromatin). For example:

a) rhabdomyosarcoma (embryonal and alveolar types);

b) primitive neuroectodermal tumour (PNET),

c) Ewing's sarcoma;

d) neuroblastoma; and

e) malignant lymphomas.

iii) Epithelioid cells: Some soft tissue tumours have either epithelioid cells as the main cells (e.g. epithelioid sarcoma) or have epithelial-like cells as a part of biphasic pattern of the tumour (e.g. synovial sarcoma).

3. Immunohistochemistry: Soft tissue tumours are distinguished by application of immunohistochemical stains. Some common examples are:

i) smooth muscle actin (SMA) for smooth muscle tumours;

ii) vimentin as common marker to distinguish mesenchymal cells from epithelium;

iii) desmin for skeletal muscle cells;

iv) S-100 for nerve fibres;

v) factor VIII antigen for vascular endothelium; and

vi) LCA (leucocyte common antigen) common marker for lymphocytes.

4. Electron microscopy: EM as such is mainly a research tool and does not have much diagnostic value in soft tissue tumours but can be applied sometimes to look for tonofilaments or cell organelles.

5. Cytogenetics: As mentioned above, many soft tissue tumours have specific genetic and chromosomal changes which can be done for determining histogenesis, or for diagnosis and prognosis.

STAGING AND GRADING. Pathological grading of soft tissue tumours based on degree of cytologic atypia is similar to grading for other tumours (grade 0 to 4). However, a different staging system for soft tissue sarcomas *(Enneking's staging)* based on grade and location of tumour is accepted.

■ *Low grade or stage I* (combines histologic grades 1 and 2).

■ *High grade or stage II* (combines histologic grades 3 and 4).

■ *Stage III* is given to any histologic grade of soft tissue tumour having distant metastases.

TUMOURS AND TUMOUR-LIKE LESIONS OF FIBROUS TISSUE *(p. 887)*

FIBROMAS *(p. 887)*

True fibromas are uncommon tumours in soft tissues. Many fibromas are actually examples of hyperplastic fibrous tissue rather than true neoplasms. On the other hand, combinations of fibrous growth with other mesenchymal tissue elements are more frequent e.g. neurofibroma, fibromyoma etc.

1. Fibroma durum is a benign, often pedunculated and well-circumscribed tumour occurring on the body surfaces and mucous membranes. It is composed of fully matured and richly collagenous fibrous connective tissue.

2. Fibroma molle or fibrolipoma, also termed **soft fibroma,** is similar type of benign growth composed of mixture of mature fibrous connective tissue and adult-type fat.

3. **Elastofibroma** is a rare benign fibrous tumour located in the subscapular region. It is characterised by association of collagen bundles and branching elastic fibres.

FIBROMATOSIS (p. 887)

'Fibromatosis' is the term used for tumour-like lesions of fibrous tissue which continue to proliferate actively and may be difficult to differentiate from sarcomas. These lesions may, therefore, be regarded as non-metastasising fibroblastic tumours which tend to invade locally and recur after surgical excision.

A. Infantile or juvenile fibromatoses include: fibrous hamartoma of infancy, fibromatosis colli, diffuse infantile fibromatosis, juvenile aponeurotic fibroma, juvenile nasopharyngeal angiofibroma and congenital (generalised and solitary) fibromatosis.

B. Adult type of fibromatoses are: palmar and plantar fibromatosis, nodular fasciitis, cicatricial fibromatosis, keloid, irradiation fibromatosis, penile fibromatosis (Peyronie's disease), abdominal and extra-abdominal desmoid fibromatosis, and retroperitoneal fibromatosis.

KELOID. A keloid is a progressive fibrous overgrowth in response to cutaneous injury such as burns, incisions, insect bites, vaccinations and others.

G/A The keloid is a firm, smooth, pink, raised patch from which extend claw-like processes (keloid-claw).

M/E It is composed of thick, homogeneous, eosinophilic hyalinised bands of collagen admixed with thin collagenous fibres and large active fibroblasts.

NODULAR FASCIITIS. Nodular fasciitis, also called pseudosarcomatous fibromatosis, is a form of benign and reactive fibroblastic growth extending from superficial fascia into the subcutaneous fat, and sometimes into the subjacent muscle. The most common locations are the upper extremity, trunk and neck region of young adults.

G/A The lesion appears as a solitary well-cirumscribed nodule (true to its name) in the superficial fascia.

M/E Various morphologic patterns may be seen but most common is a whorled or S-shaped pattern of fibroblasts present in oedematous background. The individual cells are spindle-shaped, plump fibroblasts showing mild nuclear atypia.

PALMAR AND PLANTAR FIBROMATOSES. These fibromatoses, also called Dupuytren-like contractures are the most common form of fibromatoses occurring superficially.

■ **Palmar fibromatosis** is more common in the elderly males occurring in the palmar fascia and leading to flexion contractures of the fingers (Dupuytren's contracture).

■ **Plantar fibromatosis** is a similar lesion occurring on the medial aspect of plantar arch. Essentially similar lesions occur in the shaft of the penis *(penile fibromatosis* or *Peyronie's disease)* and in the soft tissues of the knuckles *(knuckle pads).*

M/E All these forms of fibromatoses have similar appearance. The nodules are composed of fibrovascular tissue having plump, tightly-packed fibroblasts which have high mitotic rate.

DESMOID FIBROMATOSES. Desmoid fibromatoses or musculo-aponeurotic fibromatoses, commonly referred to as desmoid tumours, are of 2 types: abdominal and extra-abdominal. Both types are, however, histologically similar. Recurrences are frequent and multiple.

■ **Abdominal desmoids** are locally aggressive infiltrating tumour-like fibroblastic growths, often found in the musculo-aponeurotic structures of the rectus muscle in the anterior abdominal wall in women during or after pregnancy.

■ **Extra-abdominal desmoids,** on the other hand, are more common in men and are widely distributed such as in the upper and lower extremities, chest wall, back, buttocks and head and neck region.

■ **Intra-abdominal desmoids** present at the root of the small bowel mesentery are associated with Gardner's syndrome (consisting of fibromatosis, familial intestinal polyposis, osteomas and epidermal cysts).

G/A Desmoids are solitary, large, grey-white, firm and unencapsulated tumours infiltrating the muscle locally. Cut surface is whorled and trabeculated.

M/E Their appearance is rather misleadingly bland in contrast with aggressive local behaviour. They are composed of uniform-looking fibroblasts arranged in bands and fascicles.

FIBROSARCOMA *(p. 888)*

Fibrosarcoma is a slow-growing tumour, affecting adults between 4th and 7th decades of life. Most common locations are the lower extremity (especially thigh and around the knee), upper extremity, trunk, head and neck, and retroperitoneum.

G/A Fibrosarcoma is a grey-white, firm, lobulated and characteristically circum-scribed mass. Cut surface of the tumour is soft, fishflesh-like, with foci of necrosis and haemorrhages.

M/E The tumour is composed of uniform, spindle-shaped fibroblasts arranged in intersecting fascicles. In well-differentiated tumours, such areas produce *'herring-bone pattern'* (herring-bone is a sea fish).

FIBROHISTIOCYTIC TUMOURS *(p. 889)*

BENIGN FIBROUS HISTIOCYTOMA *(p. 889)*

Depending upon the location and predominant pattern, benign fibrous histiocytomas include a number of diverse entities such as dermatofibroma, sclerosing haemangioma, fibroxanthoma, xanthogranuloma, giant cell tumour of tendon sheath and pigmented villonodular synovitis.

DERMATOFIBROSARCOMA PROTUBERANS *(p. 889)*

Dermatofibrosarcoma protuberans is a low-grade malignant cutaneous tumour of fibrohistiocytic origin. The tumour recurs locally, and in rare instances gives rise to distant metastases.

G/A The tumour forms a firm, solitary or multiple, satellite nodules extending into the subcutaneous fat and having thin and ulcerated skin surface.

M/E The tumour is highly cellular and is composed of fibroblasts arranged in a cart-wheel or storiform pattern.

MALIGNANT FIBROUS HISTIOCYTOMA *(p. 889)*

Malignant fibrous histiocytomas now represent approximately 20-30% of all soft tissue sarcomas. It is the most common soft tissue sarcoma and is the most frequent sarcoma associated with radiotherapy. The tumour occurs more commonly in males and more frequently in the age group of 5th to 7th decades. Most common locations are lower and upper extremities and retroperitoneum.

G/A Malignant fibrous histiocytoma is a multilobulated, well-circumscribed, firm or fleshy mass, 5-10 cm in diameter. Cut surface is grey-white, soft and myxoid.

M/E There is marked variation in appearance from area to area within the same tumour. In general, there is admixture of spindle-shaped *fibroblast-like cells* and mononuclear round to oval *histiocyte-like cells* which may show phagocytic function. There is tendency for the spindle shaped cells to be arranged in characteristic cart-wheel or storiform pattern. The tumour cells show varying degree of pleomorphism, hyperchromatism, mitotic activity and presence of multinucleate bizarre tumour giant cells.

TUMOURS OF ADIPOSE TISSUE *(p. 890)*

LIPOMA *(p. 890)*

Lipoma is the commonest soft tissue tumour. It appears as a solitary, soft, movable and painless mass which may remain stationary or grow slowly. Lipomas occur most often in 4th to 5th decades of life and are frequent in females. They may be found at different locations in the body but most common sites are the subcutaneous tissues in the neck, back and shoulder.

G/A A subcutaneous lipoma is usually small, round to oval and encapsulated mass. The cut surface is soft, lobulated, yellowish-orange and greasy.

M/E The tumour is composed of lobules of mature adipose cells separated by delicate fibrous septa. A thin fibrous capsule surrounds the tumour.

LIPOSARCOMA *(p. 890)*

Liposarcoma is one of the common soft tissue sarcomas, perhaps next in frequency only to malignant fibrous histiocytoma. Unlike lipoma which originates from mature adipose cells, liposarcoma arises from primitive mesenchymal cells, the *lipoblasts*. The peak incidence is in 5th to 7th decades of life. In contrast to lipomas which are more frequently subcutaneous in location, liposarcomas often occur in the deep tissues.

G/A Liposarcoma appears as a nodular mass, 5 cm or more in diameter. The tumour is generally circumscribed but infiltrative. Cut surface is grey-white to yellow, myxoid and gelatinous.

M/E The hallmark of diagnosis of liposarcoma is the identification of variable number of *lipoblasts* which may be univacuolated or multivacuolated. Four major histologic varieties of liposarcomas are distinguished.
1. *Well-differentiated liposarcoma* resembles lipoma but contains uni- or multi-vacuolated lipoblasts.
2. *Myxoid liposarcoma* is the most common histologic type. It is composed of monomorphic, fusiform or stellate cells representing primitive mesenchymal cells, lying dispersed in mucopolysaccharide-rich ground substance.
3. *Round cell liposarcoma* is composed of uniform, round to oval cells having fine multivacuolated cytoplasm with central hyperchromatic nuclei.
4. *Pleomorphic liposarcoma* is highly undifferentiated and the most anaplastic type. There are numerous large tumour giant cells and bizarre lipoblasts.

SKELETAL MUSCLE TUMOURS *(p. 891)*

RHABDOMYOMA *(p. 891)*

Rhabdomyoma is a rare benign soft tissue tumour. Soft tissue rhabdomyomas are predominantly located in the head and neck, most often in the upper neck, tongue, larynx and pharynx.

RHABDOMYOSARCOMA *(p. 892)*

Rhabdomyosarcoma is a much more common soft tissue tumour than rhabdomyoma, and is the commonest soft tissue sarcoma in children and young adults. It is a highly malignant tumour arising from rhabdomyoblasts in varying stages of differentiation with or without demonstrable cross-striations. Depending upon the growth pattern and histology, 4 types are distinguished.

1. EMBRYONAL RHABDOMYOSARCOMA. The embryonal form is the most common of the rhabdomyosarcomas. It occurs predominantly in children under 12 years of age. The common locations are in the head and neck region, most frequently in the orbit, urogenital tract and the retroperitoneum.

G/A The tumour forms a gelatinous mass growing between muscles or in the deep subcutaneous tissues.

M/E There is considerable variation in cell types. Generally, the tumour consists of a mixture of small, round to oval cells and spindle-shaped strap cells having tapering bipolar cytoplasmic processes in which cross-striations may be evident. Mitoses are frequent.

2. BOTRYOID RHABDOMYOSARCOMA. Botryoid variety is regarded as a variant of embryonal rhabdomyosarcoma occurring in children under 10 years of age. It is seen most frequently in the vagina, urinary bladder and nose.

G/A The tumour forms a distinctive grape-like gelatinous mass protruding into the hollow cavity.

M/E The tumour grows underneath the mucosal layer, forming the characteristic *cambium layer* of tumour cells.

3. ALVEOLAR RHABDOMYOSARCOMA. Alveolar type of rhabdomyosarcoma is more common in older children and young adults under the age of 20 years. The most common locations, unlike the embryonal variety, are the extremities.

G/A The tumour differs from embryonal type in arising directly from skeletal muscle and grows rapidly as soft and gelatinous mass.

M/E The tumour shows characteristic alveolar pattern resembling pulmonary alveolar spaces. These spaces are formed by fine fibrocollagenous septa. The tumour cells lying in these spaces and lining the fibrous trabeculae are generally small, lymphocyte-like with frequent mitoses. Cross-striation can be demonstrated in about a quarter of cases.

4. PLEOMORPHIC RHABDOMYOSARCOMA. This less frequent variety of rhabdomyosarcoma occurs predominantly in older adults above the age of 40 years. They are most common in the extremities, most frequently in the lower limbs.

G/A The tumour forms a well-circumscribed, soft, whitish mass with areas of haemorrhages and necrosis.

M/E The tumour cells show considerable variation in size and shape. The tumour is generally composed of highly anaplastic cells having bizarre appearance and numerous multinucleate giant cells. Cross-striations can be demonstrated with PTAH stain in a few tumours.

TUMOURS OF UNCERTAIN HISTOGENESIS (p. 893)

SYNOVIAL SARCOMA (MALIGNANT SYNOVIOMA) (p. 893)

Synovial sarcoma or malignant synovioma, is a distinctive soft tissue sarcoma arising from synovial tissues close to the large joints, tendon sheaths, bursae and joint capsule but almost never arising within joint cavities. Most common locations are the extremities, most frequently the lower extremity. The tumour principally occurs in young adults, usually under 40 years of age. The tumour grows slowly as a painful mass but may metastasise via blood stream, chiefly to the lungs.

G/A The tumour is of variable size and is grey-white, round to multilobulated and encapsulated. Cut surface shows fishflesh-like sarcomatous appearance with foci of calcification, cystic spaces and areas of haemorrhages and necrosis.

M/E Classic *synovial sarcoma* shows a characteristic *biphasic cellular pattern* composed of clefts or gland-like structures lined by cuboidal to columnar epithelial-like cells and plump to oval spindle cells.

An uncommon variant of synovial sarcoma is *monophasic pattern* in which the epithelial component is exceedingly rare.

ALVEOLAR SOFT PART SARCOMA *(p. 893)*

Alveolar soft part sarcoma is a histologically distinct, slow-growing malignant tumour of uncertain histogenesis. The tumour may occur at any age but affects children and young adults more often.

G/A The tumour is well-demarcated, yellowish and firm.

M/E The tumour shows characteristic alveolar pattern. Organoid masses of tumour cells are separated by fibrovascular septa. The tumour cells are large and regular and contain abundant, eosinophilic, granular cytoplasm which contains diastase-resistant PAS-positive material.

GRANULAR CELL MYOBLASTOMA *(p. 894)*

Granular cell tumour is a benign tumour of unknown histogenesis. It may occur at any age but most often affected are young to middle-aged adults. The most frequent locations are the tongue and subcutaneous tissue of the trunk and extremities.

EPITHELIOID SARCOMA *(p. 894)*

This soft tissue sarcoma occurring in young adults is peculiar in that it presents as an ulcer with sinuses, often located on the skin and subcutaneous tissues as a small swelling. The tumour is slow growing but metastasising.

CLEAR CELL SARCOMA *(p. 894)*

Clear cell sarcoma, first described by Enginzer, is seen in skin and subcutaneous tissues, especially of hands and feet.

MYOSITIS OSSIFICANS *(p. 894)*

Myositis ossificans is a benign, tumour-like lesion characterised by osteoid and heterotopic bone formation in the soft tissues. It is a misnomer since the lesion neither occurs exclusively in the skeletal muscle as the name leads one to believe, nor are the inflammation or ossification always essential.

Myositis ossificans is generally preceded by history of antecedent trauma to a skeletal muscle or its tendon. The patient generally complains of pain, tenderness and swelling. Richly vascularised granulation tissue replaces the affected muscle or tendon. Then follows development of osteoid and bone at the periphery, giving characteristic X-ray appearance.

G/A The lesion appears as unencapsulated, gritty mass replacing the muscle.

M/E The central region of the mass shows loosely-arranged fibroblasts having high mitotic activity. Towards the periphery, there is presence of osteoid matrix and formation of woven mineralised bone with trapped skeletal muscle fibres and regenerating muscle (myogenic) giant cells. The appearance is sufficiently atypical to suggest osteosarcoma. This is why the condition is also called *pseudomalignant osseous tumour* of the soft tissues.

■ **SELF ASSESSMENT**

1. **The term soft tissue tumours includes:**
   - A. Mesodermal tissue
   - B. Epithelial tissues
   - C. Reticuloendothelial tissues
   - D. Glial tissue

2. **Nodular fascitis has the following features** *except:*
   - A. It is an inflammatory condition
   - B. Local excision is curative
   - C. There are whorls of fibroblasts
   - D. There is mild nuclear atypia and mitosis

3. **Desmoid tumour has the following characteristics** *except:*
   - A. It has an aggressive behaviour
   - B. The lesion is generally solitary and unencapsulated
   - C. It has pleomorphic fibroblasts having moderate mitotic activity
   - D. It may be abdominal or extra-abdominal

4. **The following lesions generally do not metastasise** *except:*
   - A. Dermatofibrosarcoma protuberans
   - B. Fibrosarcoma
   - C. Granular cell myoblastoma
   - D. Fibromatosis

5. **The most common soft tissue sarcoma is:**
   - A. Fibrosarcoma
   - B. Rhabdomyosarcoma
   - C. Liposarcoma
   - D. Malignant fibrous histiocytoma

6. **The commonest soft tissue sarcoma in children is:**
   - A. Liposarcoma
   - B. Rhabdomyosarcoma
   - C. Malignant fibrous histiocytoma
   - D. Synovial sarcoma

7. **Synovial sarcoma has the following characteristics** *except:*
   - A. It generally arises from synovial tissues
   - B. It has a biphasic growth pattern
   - C. It always grows within joint cavities
   - D. Most common locations are extremities

8. **Granular cell myoblastoma is seen most frequently in:**
   - A. Extremities
   - B. Trunk
   - C. Tongue
   - D. Visceral organs

9. **The term pseudomalignant osseous tumour is used for the following condition:**
   - A. Myositis ossificans
   - B. Osteochondroma
   - C. Osteoid osteoma
   - D. Osteoblastoma

10. **The following tumour is characterised by biphasic pattern of growth:**
    - A. Osteosarcoma
    - B. Osteochondroma
    - C. Synovial sarcoma
    - D. Malignant fibrous histiocytoma

KEY

1 = A	2 = A	3 = C	4 = B
5 = D	6 = B	7 = C	8 = C
9 = A	10 = C		

28

The Nervous System

NORMAL STRUCTURE (p. 895)

The average weight of the brain is about 1400 gm in men and 1250 gm in women. The two main divisions of the brain, the cerebrum and the cerebellum, are quite distinct in structure. There is absence of lymphatic drainage in the brain. There are 2 types of tissues in the nervous system:

1. *Neuroectodermal tissues* which include neurons (nerve cells) and neuroglia, and together form the predominant constituent of the CNS.

2. *Mesodermal tissues* are microglia, dura mater, the leptomeninges (pia-arachnoid), blood vessels and their accompanying mesenchymal cells.

1. NEURONS. The neurons are highly specialised cells of the body which are incapable of dividing after the first few weeks of birth. Thus, brain damage involving the neurons is irreversible. A neuron consists of 3 main parts: the cell body, an axon and numerous dendrites. Lipofuscin may be present due to ageing. Neuromelanin is found in neurons in the substantia nigra and pigmented nucleus of the pons.

Neurons respond to injury in a variety of ways depending upon the etiologic agent and the pathologic processes. These include central chromatolysis, atrophy and degeneration of neurons and axons, and intraneuronal storage of substances.

2. NEUROGLIA. The neuroglia provides supportive matrix and maintenance to the neurons. It includes 3 types of cells: astrocytes, oligodendrocytes and ependymal cells. Neuroglia is generally referred to as *glia;* the tumours originating from it are termed *gliomas,* and reactive proliferation of the astrocytes being called *gliosis.*

i) Astrocytes. The astrocytes are stellate cells with numerous fine branching processes. In routine haematoxylin and eosin stains, an astrocyte has round or oval vesicular nucleus, but unlike neuron, lacks a prominent nucleolus. Depending upon the type of processes, two types of astrocytes are distinguished:

■ *Protoplasmic astrocytes* have branched processes and are found mostly in the grey matter.

■ *Fibrous astrocytes* have long, thin processes and are present mainly in the white matter.

The astrocytic processes may not be visible by routine stains but can be demonstrated by phosphotungstic acid haematoxylin (PTAH) stain.

The astrocytes in respond to injury undergo hyperplasia and hypertrophy termed 'gliosis' which is an equivalent of scar elsewhere in the body. *Gemistocytic astrocytes* are early reactive astrocytes having prominent pink cytoplasm. Long-standing progressive gliosis results in the development of *Rosenthal fibres* which are eosinophilic, elongated or globular bodies present on the astrocytic processes. *Corpora amylacea* are basophilic, rounded, sometimes laminated bodies, present in elderly people in the white matter.

ii) Oligodendrocytes. Oligodendrocytes are so named because of their short and fewer processes when examined by light microscopy with special stains. In grey matter, they are clustered around the neurons and are called *satellite cells.* In white matter, they are present along the myelinated nerve fibres and are termed *interfascicular oligodendroglia.*

Chapter Twenty Eight

The major function of oligodendrocytes is formation and maintenance of myelin.

iii) Ependymal cells. The ependymal cells are epithelium-like and form a single layer of cells lining the ventricular system, the aqueduct, the central canal of the spinal cord and cover the choroid plexus. They are cuboidal to columnar cells and have ciliated luminal surface, just beneath which are present small bodies termed *blepharoplasts*. The ependymal cells influence the formation and composition of the cerebrospinal fluid (CSF) by processes of active secretion, diffusion, absorption and exchange.

3. MICROGLIA. The microglia is the nervous system counterpart of the monocyte-macrophage system. The commonly used term 'microglia' is inappropriate since these cells, unlike neuroglia, are not of neuroectodermal origin. Microglial cells (or Hortega cells) are not fixed but are mobile cells. Microglial cells may actually assume the shape and phagocytic function of macrophages and form *gitter cells*.

Neuropil is the term used for the fibrillar network formed by processess of all the neuronal cells.

4. THE DURA MATER. The dura mater is a tough fibrous covering of the brain which is closely attached to the skull on its inner layer of endocranial periosteum. In the region of spinal canal, it encloses a potential space, the *epidural space,* between the bone and the dura.

5. THE PIA-ARACHNOID (LEPTOMENINGES). The leptomeninges (*lepto* = thin, slender) consisting of the pia and arachnoid mater form the delicate vascular membranous covering of the central nervous system. The pia mater is closely applied to the brain and its convolutions, while the arachnoid mater lies between the pia mater and the dura mater without dipping into sulci. Thus, a space is left between the two layers of leptomeninges, known as *subarachnoid space,* which contains the CSF. Extension of the subarachnoid space between the wall of blood vessels entering the brain and their pial sheaths form a circumvascular space called *Virchow-Robin space.*

DEVELOPMENTAL ANOMALIES *(p. 897)*

Spinal Cord Defects *(p. 897)*

Spina bifida is the term applied to the malformations of the vertebral column involving incomplete embryologic closure of one or more of the vertebral arches (rachischisis), most frequently in the lumbosacral region. The least serious form is **spina bifida occulta** in which there is only vertebral defect but no abnormality of the spinal cord and its meninges. The larger bony defect, however, appears as a distinct cystic swelling over the affected site called **spina bifida cystica.**

Herniation of the meninges alone through the bony defect, **meningocele,** is a less common variety. The herniated sac in meningocele consists of dura and arachnoid. The commonest and more serious form is, however, **meningomyelocele** in which spinal cord or its roots also herniate through the defect and are attached to the posterior wall of the sac. A more serious variant of meningomyelocele is associated with hydrocephalus and Arnold-Chiari malformation. A rare form of the defect is **myelocele** or **syringomyelocele.**

The existence of defect in bony closure in the region of occipital bone or fronto-ethmoid junction may result in **cranial meningocele** and **encephalocele.**

Syringomyelia and Syringobulbia *(p. 898)*

These are probably congenital malformations since they manifest clinically later in life and often develop in association with certain acquired lesions involving the CNS. Syringomyelia and syringobulbia are characterised by development of a *syrinx* or a tubular cavity in the spinal cord and medulla respectively.

Arnold-Chiari Malformations *(p. 898)*

Arnold-Chiari malformation is the term used for a group of malformations of the brain involving the brainstem and cerebellum. Approximately 50% of children with hydrocephalus have the Arnold-Chiari malformation. Four types are described, of which type II malformation is the most common and is most frequently associated with congenital hydrocephalus:

1. elongation of the medulla with part of fourth ventricle in the cervical canal;
2. distortion of the medulla forming a characteristic S-shaped bend at the junction with the cervical spinal cord; and
3. lengthening and herniation of the cerebellar vermis and cerebellar tonsils through the foramen magnum resulting in formation of a mass over the upper cervical cord.

Combination of these abnormalities results in stenosis of the aqueduct or obstruction of the foramina of Luschka and Magendie causing internal hydrocephalus.

HYDROCEPHALUS *(p. 898)*

Hydrocephalus is the term used for increased volume of CSF within the skull, accompanied by dilatation of the ventricles. In majority of cases of hydrocephalus, there is increased intracranial pressure. This type of hydrocephalus involving ventricular dilatation is termed *internal hydrocephalus*. A localised collection of CSF in the subarachnoid space is called *external hydrocephalus.*

Source and Circulation of CSF *(p. 898)*

CSF is mainly produced by choroid plexus in the lateral, third and fourth ventricle, and a small part is formed on the surface of the brain and spinal cord. The total volume of CSF is about 120-150 ml. It is absorbed into the blood by the arachnoid villi present along the dural venous sinuses.

Types and Etiopathogenesis *(p. 898)*

Hydrocephalus is classified into primary and secondary types, the former being much more common.

PRIMARY HYDROCEPHALUS. Primary hydrocephalus is defined as actual increase in the volume of CSF within the skull along with elevated intracranial pressure. There are 3 possible mechanisms of primary hydrocephalus:

1. Obstruction to the flow of CSF.
2. Overproduction of CSF.
3. Deficient reabsorption of CSF.

Obstruction to the flow of CSF is by far the commonest cause and is termed *obstructive hydrocephalus.* The terms *non-communicating* and *communicating hydrocephalus* are used to denote the site of obstruction.

Non-communicating hydrocephalus. When the site of obstruction of CSF pathway is in the third ventricle or at the exit foramina in the fourth ventricle, the ventricular system enlarges and CSF cannot pass into the subarachnoid space. This is termed as non-communicating hydrocephalus. Among the common causes are the following:

i) Congenital non-communicating hydrocephalus
ii) Acquired non-communicating hydrocephalus

Communicating hydrocephalus. When obstruction to the flow of CSF is in the subarachnoid space at the base of the brain, it results in enlargement of the ventricular system but CSF flows freely between dilated ventricles and the spinal canal. The causes of communicating hydrocephalus are:

i) Overproduction of CSF

ii) Deficient reabsorption of CSF

SECONDARY HYDROCEPHALUS. Secondary hydrocephalus is much less common and is defined as compensatory increase of CSF due to loss of neural tissue e.g. from cerebral atrophy and infarction.

INFECTIONS *(p. 899)*

The micro-organisms may gain entry into the nervous system by one of the following routes:

1. Via bloodstream. Spread of infection by the arterial route from another focus is the most common mode of spread of infection in the nervous system.

2. Direct implantation. Spread of infection by direct implantation occurs following skull fractures or through defects in the bony and meningeal coverings of the nervous system.

3. Local extension. Extension of infection from contiguous focus such as otitis media and frontal or mastoid sinusitis may occur.

4. Along nerve. Certain viruses such as herpes simplex, herpes zoster and rabies spread along cranial and peripheral nerves and ascend to the CNS.

MENINGITIS *(p. 899)*

Meningitis is inflammatory involvement of the meninges. Meningitis may involve the dura called *pachymeningitis,* or the leptomeninges (pia-arachnoid) termed *leptomeningitis.*

An *extradural abscess* may form by suppuration between the bone and dura. Further spread of infection may penetrate the dura and form a *subdural abscess.* Other effects of pachymeningitis are localised or generalised leptomeningitis and *cerebral abscess.*

Infectious meningitis is broadly classified into 3 types: acute pyogenic, acute lymphocytic (viral, aseptic) and chronic (bacterial or fungal).

Acute Pyogenic Meningitis *(p. 900)*

Acute pyogenic or acute purulent meningitis is acute infection of the pia-arachnoid and of the CSF enclosed in the subarachnoid space. Since the subarachnoid space is continuous around the brain, spinal cord and the optic nerves, infection spreads immediately to whole of the cerebrospinal meninges as well as to the ventricles.

ETIOPATHOGENESIS. The causative organisms are:

1. *Escherichia coli* infection is common in neonates with neural tube defects.

2. *Haemophilus influenzae* is commonly responsible for infection in infants and children.

3. *Neisseria meningitidis* causes meningitis in adolescent and young adults and is causative for epidemic meningitis.

4. *Streptococcus pneumoniae* is causative for infection at extremes of age and following trauma.

The **routes** of infection are as follows:

1. Most commonly by the bloodstream.

2. From an adjacent focus of infection.

3. By iatrogenic infection such as introduction of micro-organisms at operation or during lumbar puncture.

G/A Pus accumulates in the subarachnoid space so that normally clear CSF becomes turbid or frankly purulent. The turbid fluid is particularly seen in the sulci and at the base of the brain where the space is wide.

M/E There is presence of numerous polymorphonuclear neutrophils in the subarachnoid space as well as in the meninges. Gram-staining reveals varying number of causative bacteria.

Acute Lymphocytic (Viral, Aseptic) Meningitis *(p. 900)*

Acute lymphocytic meningitis is a viral or aseptic meningitis, especially common in children and young adults. Among the etiologic agents are numerous viruses such as enteroviruses, mumps, ECHO viruses, coxsackie virus, Epstein-Barr virus and herpes simplex II.

G/A Some cases show swelling of the brain while others show no distinctive change.

M/E There is mild lymphocytic infiltrate in the leptomeninges.

Chronic (Tuberculous and Cryptococcal) Meningitis *(p. 901)*

There are two principal types of chronic meningitis—one bacterial (tuberculous meningitis) and the other fungal (cryptococcal meningitis). Both types cause chronic granulomatous reaction and may produce parenchymal lesions.

■ *Tuberculous meningitis* occurs in children and adults through haematogenous spread of infection from tuberculosis elsewhere in the body, or it may simply be a manifestation of miliary tuberculosis. Less commonly, the spread may occur directly from tuberculosis of a vertebral body.

■ *Cryptococcal meningitis* develops particularly in debilitated or immunocompromised persons, usually as a result of haematogenous dissemination from a pulmonary lesion. Cryptococcal meningitis is especially an important cause of meningitis in patients with AIDS.

G/A In tuberculous meningitis, the subarachnoid space contains thick exudate, particularly abundant in the sulci and the base of the brain. Tubercles, 1-2 mm in diameter, may be visible, especially adjacent to the blood vessels. The exudate in cryptococcal meningitis is scanty, translucent and gelatinous.

M/E Tuberculous meningitis shows exudate of acute and chronic inflammatory cells, and granulomas with or without caseation necrosis and giant cells. Acid-fast bacilli may be demonstrated. Cryptococcal meningitis is characterised by infiltration by lymphocytes, plasma cells, an occasional granuloma and abundant characteristic capsulated cryptococci.

Table 28.1 summarises the CSF findings in the three important types of meningitis in comparison with those in health.

ENCEPHALITIS *(p. 901)*

Parenchymal infection of brain is termed encephalitis. Encephalitis may be the result of bacterial, viral, fungal and protozoal infections.

Bacterial Encephalitis *(p. 901)*

Bacterial infection of the brain substance is usually secondary to involvement of the meninges rather than a primary bacterial parenchymal infection. This results in bacterial cerebritis that progresses to form *brain abscess*. However, *tuberculosis* and *neurosyphilis* are the two primary bacterial involvements of the brain parenchyma.

BRAIN ABSCESS. Brain abscesses may arise by one of the following routes:

1. By direct implantation of organisms e.g. following compound fractures of the skull.

TABLE 28.1: CSF Findings in Health and Various Types of Meningitis.

FEATURE	NORMAL	ACUTE PYOGENIC (BACTERIAL) MENINGITIS	ACUTE LYMPHO-CYTIC (VIRAL) MENINGITIS	CHRONIC (TUBERCULOUS) MENINGITIS
1. Naked eye appearance	Clear and colourless	Cloudy or frankly purulent	Clear or slightly turbid	Clear or slightly turbid, forms fibrin coagulum on standing
2. CSF pressure	60-150 mm water	Elevated (above 180 mm water)	Elevated (above 250 mm water)	Elevated (above 300 mm water)
3. Cells	0-4 lymphocytes/µl	10-10,000 neutrophils/µl	10-100 lymphocytes/µl	100-1000 lymphocytes/µl
4. Proteins	15-45 mg/dl	Markedly raised	Raised	Raised
5. Glucose	50-80 mg/dl	Markedly reduced	Normal	Reduced
6. Bacteriology	Sterile	Causative organisms present	Sterile	Tubercle bacilli present

2. By local extension of infection e.g. chronic suppurative otitis media, mastoiditis and sinusitis.

3. By haematogenous spread e.g. from primary infection in the heart such as acute bacterial endocarditis, and from lungs such as in bronchiectasis.

G/A It appears as a localised area of inflammatory necrosis and oedema surrounded by fibrous capsule.

M/E The changes consist of liquefactive necrosis in the centre of the abscess containing pus. It is surrounded by acute and chronic inflammatory cells, neovascularisation, oedema, septic thrombosis of vessels, fibrous encapsulation and zone of gliosis.

TUBERCULOMA. Tuberculoma is an intracranial mass occurring secondary to dissemination of tuberculosis elsewhere in the body. Tuberculomas may be solitary or multiple.

G/A It has a central area of caseation necrosis surrounded by fibrous capsule.
M/E There is typical tuberculous granulomatous reaction around the central caseation necrosis. A zone of gliosis generally surrounds the tuberculoma. Advanced cases may show areas of calcification.

NEUROSYPHILIS. Syphilitic lesions of the CNS used to be common and serious, but more recently there is evidence of atypical neurosyphilis in cases of AIDS. The lesions in syphilis may be in the form of *syphilitic meningitis* found in secondary syphilis, and *neurosyphilis* consisting of tabes dorsalis and generalised paralysis of the insane occurring in tertiary stage.

■ **Syphilitic meningitis.** This is a form of chronic meningitis characterised by distinctive perivascular inflammatory reaction of plasma cells and endarteritis obliterans.

■ **Tabes dorsalis (Locomotor ataxia).** There is slowly progressive degeneration of the posterior roots of the spinal nerves and the posterior columns of the spinal cord by the spirochaetes.

■ **General paralysis of the insane.** This is the result of diffuse parenchymal involvement by the spirochaetes with widespread lesions in the nervous system.

Viral Encephalitis *(p. 902)*

A number of viruses can infect the CNS and produce either aseptic meningitis (described already) or viral encephalitis, but sometimes combination of both termed meningoencephalitis, is present. Most viral infections of the CNS are the end-result of preceding infection in other tissues and organs.

Most of the viruses reach the nervous system via bloodstream before which they enter the body by various routes e.g. infection of the skin and mucous membrane (in herpes simplex and herpes zoster-varicella), by the alimentary tract (in enteroviruses including polio virus), by arthropod bite (in arbovirus), by transplacental infection (in cytomegalovirus), and through body fluids in AIDS (in HIV infection). Rabies virus travels along the peripheral nerves to reach the CNS. Herpes zoster-varicella is a distinct primary disease (chickenpox) but the virus remains latent for a long time before it gets reactivated to cause severe hyperalgesia and pain along the distribution of nerve related to acutely inflamed posterior root ganglia (herpes zoster). All these viral infections enumerated so far cause *acute viral encephalitis. Slow virus diseases* are another group of CNS infections in which the agents have not only a long latent period but the disease also develops slowly.

M/E 1. Parenchymal infiltrate, chiefly in perivascular location, of mononuclear cells consisting of lymphocytes, plasma cells and macrophages.
2. Microscopic clusters of microglial cells and presence of neuronophagia.

3. Intranuclear inclusion bodies in most viral diseases and specific cytoplasmic inclusions of Negri bodies in rabies.

HIV Encephalopathy (AIDS-Dementia Complex) *(p. 903)*

Late in the course of AIDS, a group of signs and symptoms of CNS disease appear termed HIV encephalopathy or AIDS-dementia complex. One major clinical feature of this entity is the occurrence of *dementia* i.e. fall in the cognitive ability of the individual compared to previous level. The condition is believed to be the result of direct effect of HIV on the CNS. Clinically, the disease develops in about 25% cases of AIDS while autopsy studies reveal presence of HIV encephalopathy in 80-90% cases of AIDS.

M/E The changes are more in subcortical area of the brain and consist of gliosis, multinucleate giant cell encephalitis, and vacuolar myelopathy.

Table 28.2 lists important forms of CNS diseases in patients with AIDS.

TABLE 28.2: Major Forms of CNS Diseases in AIDS.

	DISEASE	INCIDENCE
1.	HIV encephalopathy (AIDS-dementia complex)	25%
2.	Toxoplasmosis	15%
3.	Cryptococcal meningitis	9%
4.	Progressive multifocal leucoencephalopathy	4%
5.	Neurosyphilis	1%
6.	CNS lymphoma	1%
7.	Tuberculous meningitis	1%

Progressive Multifocal Leucoencephalopathy *(p. 903)*

Progressive multifocal leucoencephalopathy (PML) is a slow viral infection of the CNS caused by a papovavirus called *JC virus* (not to be confused with CJ disease or mad-cow disease; JC virus here stands for the initials of the patient first infected). PML develops in immunocompromised individual like CMV and Toxoplasma encephalitis.

G/A The lesions consist of focal, irregular gelatinous areas most prominent at the junction of grey and white matter.

M/E The changes are:

■ focal areas of demyelination;

■ many lipid-laden macrophages in the centre of foci; and

■ enlarged oligodendroglial nuclei containing purple viral inclusions at the periphery of the lesion.

Spongiform Encephalopathy (Creutzfeldt-Jakob Disease) *(p. 903)*

Spongiform encephalopathy, also called Creutzfeldt-Jakob disease (CJD) or mad-cow disease, though included under the group of viral encephalitis but is caused by accumulation of prion proteins. *Prion proteins* are a modified form of normal structural proteins present in the mammalian CNS and are peculiar in two respects: they lack nucleic acid (DNA or RNA), and they can be transmitted as an infectious proteinaceous particles.

Majority of cases occur sporadically though familial predisposition with autosomal dominant inheritance has also been reported in 5-15% cases. Other methods of transmission are by iatrogenic route (e.g. by tissue transplantation from an infected individual) and by human consumption of BSE (bovine spongiform encephalopathy)-infected beef; the last-named route came to be called as mad-cow disease.

G/A The changes are too rapid to become noticeable but brain atrophy may be seen in long-standing cases.

M/E The hallmark is spongiform change i.e. there are small round vacuoles in the neuronal cells. These changes are predominantly seen in the cortex and other grey matter areas.

Fungal and Protozoal Encephalitis *(p. 904)*

Mycotic diseases of the CNS usually develop by bloodstream from systemic deep mycoses elsewhere in the body. They are particularly more common in immunosuppressed individuals such as in AIDS, patients of lymphomas and other cancers. Some of the fungi which may disseminate to the CNS are *Candida albicans, Mucor, Aspergillus fumigatus, Cryptococcus neoformans, Histoplasma capsulatum* and *Blastomyces dermatitidis.* These fungal infections may produce one of the three patterns: fungal chronic meningitis, vasculitis and encephalitis.

CEREBROVASCULAR DISEASES *(p. 904)*

Various pathologic processes commonly implicated in cerebrovascular diseases are: thrombosis, embolism, rupture of a vessel, hypoxia, hypertensive arteriolosclerosis, atherosclerosis, arteritis, trauma, aneurysm and developmental malformations. These processes can result in 2 main types of parenchymal diseases of the brain:

A. Ischaemic brain damage:

a) Generalised reduction in blood flow resulting in *global hypoxic-ischaemic encephalopathy*

b) Local vascular obstruction causing *infarcts.*

B. Intracranial haemorrhage:

a) Haemorrhage in the brain parenchyma *(intracerebral haemorrhage)*

b) Haemorrhage in the subarachnoid space *(subarachnoid haemorrhage).*

The *stroke syndrome* is the cardinal feature of cerebrovascular disease. The term stroke is used for sudden and dramatic development of focal neurologic deficit, varying from trivial neurologic disorder to hemiplegia and coma. Other less common effects of vascular disease include: transient ischaemic attacks (TIA), vascular headache (e.g. in migraine, hypertension and arteritis), local pressure of an aneurysm and increased intracranial pressure (e.g. in hypertensive encephalopathy and venous thrombosis).

A. ISCHAEMIC BRAIN DAMAGE *(p. 904)*

Ischaemic necrosis in the brain results from ischaemia caused by considerable reduction or complete interruption of blood supply to neural tissue which is insufficient to meet its metabolic needs. The brain requires sufficient quantities of oxygen and glucose so as to sustain its aerobic metabolism, mainly by citric acid (Krebs') cycle which requires oxygen. Moreover, neural tissue has limited stores of energy reserves so that cessation of continuous supply of oxygen and glucose for more than 3-4 minutes results in permanent damage to neurons and neuroglial cells.

Deprivation of oxygen (anoxia) to the brain may occur in 4 different ways:

1. *Anoxic anoxia,* in which there is low inspired pO_2.
2. *Anaemic anoxia,* in which the oxygen-carrying haemoglobin is reduced.

3. *Histotoxic anoxia,* in which there is direct toxic injury as occurs in cyanide poisoning.

4. *Stagnant (ischaemia) anoxia,* in which the damage is caused by cessation of blood with resultant local accumulation of metabolites and changes in pH.

In all these different forms of anoxia, the end-result is ischaemic brain damage which may have one of the following two patterns:

1. *Global hypoxic-ischaemic encephalopathy,* resulting from generalised cerebral hypoperfusion.

2. *Cerebral infarction,* resulting from severe localised reduction or cessation of blood supply.

Global Hypoxic-Ischaemic Encephalopathy *(p. 904)*

The brain receives 20% of cardiac output for maintaining its vital aerobic metabolism. A number of factors determine the maximum length of time the CNS can *survive irreversible ischaemic damage.* These include:

i) severity of the hypoxic episode;

ii) presence of pre-existing cerebrovascular disease;

iii) age of the patient; and

iv) body temperature.

In normal individuals, the brain continues to be perfused adequately up to systolic arterial pressure of 50 mmHg by an auto-regulatory vascular control mechanism. However, fall of systemic arterial systolic pressure below this critical value results in rapid fall in cerebral perfusion pressure and eventual ischaemic encephalopathy. Such types of medical emergencies occur at the time of cardiac arrest followed by relatively delayed resuscitation, severe episode of hypotension, carbon monoxide intoxication and status epilepticus.

Depending upon the proneness of different cells of the brain to the effects of ischaemia-hypoxia, three types of lesion may occur:

1. Selective neuronal damage: Neurons are most vulnerable to damaging effect of ischaemia-hypoxia and irreversible injury. In particular, oligodendroglial cells are most susceptible, followed by astrocytes while microglial cells and vascular endothelium survive the longest.

2. Laminar necrosis: Global ischaemia of cerebral cortex results in uneven damage because of different cerebral vasculature which is termed laminar or pseudolaminar necrosis.

3. Watershed infarcts: Circulatory flow in the brain by anterior, middle and posterior cerebral arteries has overlapping circulations. In ischaemia-hypoxia, perfusion of overlapping zones, being farthest from the blood supply, suffers maximum damage. This results in wedge-shaped areas of coagulative necrosis called watershed or border zone infarcts.

G/A The features are as under:

■ **Survival for a few hours:** No pathologic changes are visible.

■ **Survival 12-24 hours:** No macroscopic change is discernible but microscopic examination reveals early neuronal damage in the form of eosinophilic cytoplasm and pyknotic nuclei, so called red neurons.

■ **After 2-7 days:** There is focal softening. The area supplied by distal branches of the cerebral arteries suffers from the most severe ischaemic damage and may develop *border zone* or *watershed infarcts* in the junctional zones between the territories supplied by major arteries.

M/E The nerve cells die and disappear and are replaced by reactive fibrillary gliosis. There are minor variations in the distribution of neuronal damage to the cortex.

Cerebral Infarction *(p. 905)*

Cerebral infarction is a localised area of tissue necrosis caused by local vascular occlusion—arterial or venous. Occasionally, it may be the result of non-occlusive causes such as compression on the cerebral arteries from outside and from hypoxic encephalopathy. In general, the focal neurologic deficit termed stroke, is present. However, significant atherosclerotic cerebrovascular disease may produce transient ischaemic attacks (TIA).

1. Arterial occlusion. Occlusion of the cerebral arteries by either thrombi or emboli is the most common cause of cerebral infarction. Thrombotic occlusion of the cerebral arteries is most frequently the result of atherosclerosis, and rarely, from arteritis of the cranial arteries.

2. Venous occlusion. Venous infarction in the brain is an infrequent phenomenon due to good communications of the cerebral venous drainage.

3. Non-occlusive causes. Compression of the cerebral arteries from outside such as occurs during herniation may cause cerebral infarction. Mechanism of watershed (border zone) cerebral infarction in hypoxic encephalopathy has already been explained above.

In any case, the extent of damage produced by any of the above causes depends upon:
i) rate of reduction of blood flow;
ii) type of blood vessel involved; and
iii) extent of collateral circulation.

G/A An *anaemic infarct* becomes evident 6-12 hours after its occurrence. The affected area is soft and swollen and there is blurring of junction between grey and white matter. Within 2-3 days, the infarct undergoes softening and disintegration. Eventually, there is central liquefaction with peripheral firm glial reaction and thickened leptomeninges, forming a cystic infarct. A *haemorrhagic infarct* is red and superficially resembles a haematoma. It is usually the result of fragmentation of occlusive arterial emboli or venous thrombosis.

M/E The features are as under:
1. Initially, there is eosinophilic neuronal necrosis and lipid vacuolisation produced by breakdown of myelin.
2. After the first 2-3 days, there is progressive invasion by macrophages and there is astrocytic and vascular proliferation.
3. In the following weeks to months, the macrophages clear away the necrotic debris by phagocytosis followed by reactive astrocytosis, often with little fine fibrosis.
4. Ultimately, after 3-4 months an old cystic infarct is formed which shows a cyst traversed by small blood vessels and has peripheral fibrillary gliosis.

B. INTRACRANIAL HAEMORRHAGE *(p. 906)*

Haemorrhage into the brain may be traumatic, non-traumatic, or spontaneous. There are two main types of spontaneous intracranial haemorrhage:
1. Intracerebral haemorrhage, which is usually of hypertensive origin.
2. Subarachnoid haemorrhage, which is commonly aneurysmal in origin.

In addition to hypertension and rupture of an aneurysm, other causes of spontaneous intracranial haemorrhage include vascular malformations which produce mixed intracerebral and subarachnoid haemorrhage, haemorrhagic diathesis and haemorrhage into tumours.

Intracerebral Haemorrhage *(p. 907)*

Spontaneous intracerebral haemorrhage occurs mostly in patients of hypertension. Most hypertensives over middle age have microaneurysms in very small cerebral arteries in the brain tissue. Rupture of one of the numerous microaneurysms is believed to be the cause of intracerebral haemorrhage.

M/E The haemorrhage consists of dark mass of clotted blood replacing brain parenchyma. The borders of the lesion are sharply defined and have a narrow rim of partially necrotic parenchyma. Small ring haemorrhages in the Virchow-Robin space in the border zone are commonly present. Ipsilateral ventricles are distorted and compressed and may contain blood in their lumina. After a few weeks to months, the haematoma undergoes resolution with formation of a slit-like space called *apoplectic cyst* and containing yellowish fluid.

Subarachnoid Haemorrhage *(p. 907)*

Haemorrhage into the subarachnoid space is most commonly caused by rupture of an aneurysm, and rarely, rupture of a vascular malformation.

Of the three types of aneurysms affecting the larger intracranial arteries, namely berry, mycotic and fusiform, *berry aneurysms* are most important and most common. Berry aneurysms are saccular in appearance with rounded or lobulated bulge arising at the bifurcation of intracranial arteries and varying in size from 2 mm to 2 cm or more. They account for 95% of aneurysms which are liable to rupture.

In more than 85% cases of subarachnoid haemorrhage, the cause is massive and sudden bleeding from a berry aneurysm on or near the circle of Willis.

The remaining 15% cases of subarachnoid haemorrhage are the result of rupture in the posterior circulation, vascular malformations and rupture of mycotic aneurysms that occurs in the setting of bacterial endocarditis.

M/E An intracerebral haematoma may develop if the blood tracks into the brain parenchyma. The region of the brain supplied by the affected artery frequently shows infarction, partly attributed to vasospasm.

TRAUMA TO THE CNS *(p. 908)*

Trauma to the CNS constitutes an important cause of death and permanent disability in the modern world. Important causes of head injuries are: motor vehicle accidents, accidental falls and violence. Traumatic injuries to the CNS may result in three consequences which may occur in isolation or in combination:
- epidural haematoma;
- subdural haematoma; and
- parenchymal brain damage.

A. Epidural Haematoma *(p. 908)*

Epidural haematoma is accumulation of blood between the dura and the skull following fracture of the skull, most commonly from rupture of middle meningeal artery.

B. Subdural Haematoma *(p. 908)*

Subdural haematoma is accumulation of blood between the dura and subarachnoid and develops most often from rupture of veins which cross the surface convexities of the cerebral hemispheres. Subdural haematoma may be acute or chronic.

- **Acute subdural haematoma.** Acute subdural haematoma develops following trauma and consists of clotted blood, often in the frontoparietal region. There is no significant compression of gyri. Since the accumulated blood is of venous origin, symptoms appear slowly and may become chronic with passage of time if not fatal.

■ **Chronic subdural haematoma.** Chronic subdural haematoma occurs often with brain atrophy and less commonly following trauma. Chronic subdural haematoma is composed of liquid blood. Separating the haematoma from underlying brain is a membrane composed of granulation tissue.

C. Parenchymal Brain Damage (p. 908)

Trauma to the CNS may result in damage to brain parenchyma and includes the following forms:

1. Concussion. Concussion is caused by closed head injury and is characterised by transient neurologic dysfunction and loss of consciousness. Invariably, there is complete neurologic recovery after some hours to days.

2. Diffuse axonal injury. Diffuse axonal injury is the most common cause of persistent coma or vegetative state following head injury. The underlying cause is sudden angular acceleration or deceleration resulting in widespread axonal shearing in the deep white matter of both the hemispheres.

3. Contusions and lacerations. Contusions and lacerations are the result of direct damage to the brain parenchyma, particularly cerebral hemispheres, as occurs in the soft tissues. Most often, they are the result of blunt trauma. The overlying skull may or may not be fractured. Traumatic subarachnoid haemorrhage invariably accompanies cerebral contusions.

4. Traumatic intracerebral haemorrhage. On trauma to the CNS, the parenchymal vessels of the hemispheres may get torn and cause multiple intracerebral haemorrhages.

5. Brain swelling. Head injury may be accompanied by localised or diffuse brain swelling.

DEMYELINATING DISEASES (p. 909)

Demyelinating diseases are an important group of neurological disorders which have, in common, the pathologic features of focal or patchy destruction of myelin sheaths in the CNS accompanied by an inflammatory response. Demyelination may affect peripheral nervous system as well. Some degree of axonal damage may also occur but demyelination is the predominant feature.

Loss of myelin may occur in certain other conditions as well, but without an inflammatory response. These conditions have known etiologies such as: genetically-determined defects in the myelin metabolism (leucodystrophies), slow virus diseases of oligodendrocytes (progressive multifocal leuco-encephalopathy), and exposure to toxins (central pontine myelinolysis). All these entities are currently not classified as demyelinating diseases. Only those conditions in which the myelin sheath or the myelin-forming cells (i.e. oligo-dendrocytes and Schwann cells) are primarily injured and are associated with considerable inflammatory exudate are included under the term 'demyelinating diseases'. Pathologically and clinically, two demyelinating diseases are distinguished:

Multiple (Disseminated) Sclerosis (p. 909)

Multiple or disseminated sclerosis is the most common of the CNS demyelinating diseases. The usual age at onset is 20 to 40 years. The disease presents as recurrent attacks of focal neurologic disorder with predilection for involvement of the spinal cord, optic nerve and brain. The etiology of multiple sclerosis remains unknown but a role for genetic susceptibility, infectious agent and immunologic mechanism has been proposed.

Perivenous Encephalomyelitis *(p. 910)*

Perivenous encephalomyelitis includes two uncommon diseases: *acute disseminated encephalomyelitis* and *acute necrotising haemorrhagic leucoencephalitis*. Both are monophasic diseases characterised by perivenous mononuclear inflammatory cell infiltration. Both diseases occur following a viral infection, vaccination or a respiratory illness.

Degenerative Diseases *(p. 910)*

Degenerative diseases are disorders of unknown etiology and pathogenesis, characterised pathologically by progressive loss of CNS neurons and their processes accompanied by fibrillary astrocytosis. The identification of these diseases depends upon exclusion of diseases with known etiologies such as metabolic disturbances, vascular diseases, nutritional deficiencies or infection. A considerable proportion of degenerative disorders are genetic in origin, with either dominant or recessive inheritance; others occur sporadically. Family history is, of course, of great importance.

Some of the more common degenerative diseases are listed in Table 28.3. Two of the important examples—Alzheimer's disease and parkinsonism are discussed below.

ALZHEIMER'S DISEASE. Alzheimer's disease is the most common cause of dementia in the elderly. The condition occurs after 5th decade of life and incidence progressively increases with advancing age. The exact cause is not known but a few factors are implicated in its etiology which include positive family history and deposition of Aβ amyloid derived from amyloid precursor protein (APP) forming *neuritic 'senile' plaques* and *neurofibrillary tangles.*

G/A The brain is often reduced in weight and bilaterally atrophic.

M/E The features are as under:

i)   *Senile neuritic plaque* is the most conspicuous lesion and consists of focal area which has a central core containing Aβ amyloid.

ii)   *Neurofibrillary tangle* is a filamentous collection of neurofilaments and neurotubules within the cytoplasm of neurons.

iii)   *Amyloid angiopathy* is deposition of the same amyloid in the vessel wall which is deposited in the amyloid core of the plaque.

iv)   *Granulovacular degeneration* is presence of multiple, small intraneuronal cytoplasmic vacuoles, some of which contain one or more dark granules called *Hirano bodies.*

PARKINSONISM. Parkinsonism is a syndrome of chronic progressive disorder of motor function and is clinically characterised by tremors which are most conspicuous at rest and worsen with emotional stress.

G/A The brain is atrophic or may be normal externally.

M/E The hallmark is depigmentation of substantia nigra and locus ceruleus due to loss of neuromelanin pigment from neurons and accumulation of neuromelanin pigment in the glial cells.

Metabolic Diseases *(p. 911)*

Metabolic diseases of the CNS result from neurochemical disturbances which are either inherited or acquired. *Hereditary metabolic disorders* predominantly manifest in infancy or childhood and include genetically-determined disorders of carbohydrate, lipid, amino acid and mineral metabolism. *Acquired or secondary metabolic diseases* are the disturbances of cerebral function due to disease in some other organ system such as the heart and circulation, lungs and respiratory function, kidneys, liver, endocrine glands and pancreas.

TABLE 28.3: Common Degenerative Diseases.

REGION AFFECTED	DISEASE	MAIN FEATURES	PREDOMINANT PATHOLOGY
I. **Cerebral cortex**	Alzheimer's disease	Progressive senile dementia	Cortical atrophy, senile plaques (neurites), neurofibrillary tangles, amyloid angiopathy
	Pick's disease	Pre-senile dementia	Lobar cortical atrophy, ballooning degeneration of neurons (Pick's cells)
II. **Basal ganglia and brainstem**	Huntington's disease	Progressive dementia with choreiform movements	Atrophy of frontal lobes, fibrillary astrocytosis
	Parkinson's disease	Abnormalities of posture and movement	Aggregates of melanin-containing nerve cells in brainstem, intracytoplasmic neuronal inclusions (Lewy bodies)
III. **Spinal cord and cerebellum**	Cerebellar cortical degeneration	Progressive cerebellar ataxia	Loss of Purkinje cells in cerebellar cortex
	Olivopontocerebellar atrophy	Cerebellar ataxia	Combination of atrophy of cerebellar cortex, inferior olivary nuclei and pontine nuclei
	Spinocerebellar atrophy (Friedreich's ataxia)	Gait ataxia, dysarthria	Degeneration of spinocerebellar tracts, peripheral axons and myelin sheaths
IV. **Motor neurons (UMN and LMN)**	Motor neuron disease (Amyotrophic lateral sclerosis)	Syndromes of muscular weakness and wasting without sensory loss	Progressive loss of motor neurons, both in the cerebellar cortex (UMN) and in the anterior horn of spinal cord (LMN)
	Werdnig-Hoffmann's disease	Spinal muscular atrophy in infants	Loss of lower motor neurons, denervation atrophy of muscles

The predominant types of hereditary and acquired metabolic disorders are as under:

A. Hereditary Metabolic Diseases:

1. Neuronal storage diseases—characterised by storage of a metabolic product in the neurons due to specific enzyme deficiency. Common examples are: gangliosidoses (e.g. Tay-Sachs disease or GM2 gangliosidosis), mucopolysaccharidoses, Gaucher's disease and Niemann-Pick disease).

2. Leucodystrophies—are diseases of white matter characterised by diffuse demyelination and gliosis. They are caused by deficiency of one of the enzymes required for formation and maintenance of myelin.

3. Other inborn errors of metabolism—e.g. Wilson's disease (hepato-lenticular degeneration), glycogen storage diseases, phenylketonuria and galactosaemia.

B. Acquired Metabolic Diseases:

1. Anoxic-ischaemic encephalopathy
2. Hypoglycaemic encephalopathy
3. Hyperglycaemic coma
4. Acute hepatic encephalopathy (Reye's syndrome)
5. Chronic hepatic encephalopathy
6. Kernicterus
7. Uraemic encephalopathy
8. Encephalopathy due to electrolyte and endocrine disturbances.

Nutritional Diseases *(p. 912)*

Neurologic disorders may be caused by malnutrition from lack of adequate diet in many underdeveloped countries and many poor socio-economic groups. In the United States and Europe, however, nutritionally-induced disease is chiefly found in association with chronic alcoholism or due to defect in absorption, transport or metabolism of dietary nutrients.

Some of the common neurologic diseases included in the category of deficiency diseases are:
1. Wernicke's encephalopathy and Korsakoff's psychosis (vitamin B_1 or thiamine deficiency).
2. Subacute combined degeneration of the spinal cord (vitamin B_{12} deficiency).
3. Folic acid deficiency.
4. Spinocerebellar syndrome (vitamin E deficiency).
5. Pellagra (niacin deficiency).
6. Alcoholic cerebellar degeneration.

TUMOURS OF THE CNS *(p. 912)*

Tumours of the CNS may originate in the brain or spinal cord (primary tumours), or may spread from another primary site of cancer (metastatic tumours). More than one-quarter of the CNS tumours are secondary meta-stases arising in patients undergoing treatment for systemic cancer. Primary CNS tumours are the second commonest form of cancer in infants and children under the age of 15 years, exceeded in frequency only by leukaemia. Both benign and malignant CNS tumours are capable of producing neurologic impairment depending upon their site.

Primary CNS tumours or intracranial tumours include: tumours arising from *constituent cells of the brain* (with the sole exception of microglial cells) and from *the supporting tissues*. In childhood, tumours arise from more primitive cells (e.g. neuroblastoma, medulloblastoma).

A classification of intracranial tumours abbreviated from the WHO classification is given in Table 28.4.

TABLE 28.4: Classification of Intracranial Tumours.

I.	**TUMOURS OF NEUROGLIA (GLIOMAS)**
1.	Astrocytoma
2.	Oligodendroglioma
3.	Ependymoma
4.	Choroid plexus papilloma
II.	**TUMOURS OF NEURONS**
1.	Neuroblastoma
2.	Ganglioneuroblastoma
3.	Ganglioneuroma
III.	**TUMOURS OF NEURONS AND NEUROGLIA**
	Ganglioglioma
IV.	**POORLY-DIFFERENTIATED AND EMBRYONAL TUMOURS**
1.	Medulloblastoma
2.	Neuroblastoma
3.	PNET
V.	**TUMOURS OF MENINGES**
1.	Meningioma
2.	Meningeal sarcoma
VI.	**NERVE SHEATH TUMOURS**
1.	Schwannoma (neurilemmoma)
2.	Neurofibroma
3.	Malignant nerve sheath tumour
VII.	**OTHER PRIMARY INTRAPARENCHYMAL TUMOURS**
1.	Haemangioblastoma
2.	Primary CNS lymphoma
3.	Germ cell tumours
VIII.	**MISCELLANEOUS TUMOURS**
1.	Malignant melanoma
2.	Craniopharyngioma
3.	Pineal cell tumours
4.	Pituitary tumours
IX.	**TUMOUR-LIKE LESIONS**
	(epidermal cyst, dermoid cyst, colloid cyst)
X.	**METASTATIC TUMOURS**

GLIOMAS *(p. 912)*

The term glioma is used for all tumours arising from neuroglia, or more precisely, from neuroectodermal epithelial tissue. Gliomas are the most common of the primary CNS tumours and collectively account for 40% of all intracranial tumours. They include: tumours arising *from astrocytes* (astrocytomas and glioblastoma multiforme); *from oligodendrocytes* (oligodendroglioma); *from ependyma* (ependymoma); and *from choroid plexus* (choroid plexus papilloma). Gliomas may be well-differentiated or poorly-differentiated.

Astrocytoma and Glioblastoma Multiforme *(p. 913)*

Astrocytomas are the most common type of gliomas. In general, they are found in the late middle life with a peak in 6th decade of life. They occur predominantly in the cerebral hemispheres, and occasionally in the spinal cord. In children and young adults, pilocytic astrocytomas arise in the optic nerves, cerebellum and brainstem. Astrocytomas have tendency to progress from low grade to higher grades of anaplasia.

PATHOLOGIC CHANGES. Pathologically, astrocytomas are divided into 3 progressive histologic grades:

1. LOW-GRADE ASTROCYTOMA. *G/A* It is a poorly defined, grey-white tumour of variable size.

M/E It is composed of well-differentiated astrocytes separated by variable amount of fibrillary background of astrocytic processes. Based on the type of astrocytes, three subtypes are distinguished: *fibrillary, protoplastic* and *gemistocytic astrocytoma.*

PILOCYTIC ASTROCYTOMA. It is a distinctly benign astrocytoma occurring in children and young adults.

G/A It is usually cystic or solid and circumscribed.

M/E It is predominantly composed of fusiform pilocytic astrocytes having unusually long, wavy fibrillary processes.

2. ANAPLASTIC ASTROCYTOMA. *G/A* It may not be distinguishable from the low-grade astrocytoma.

M/E It contains features of anaplasia such as hypercellularity, pleomorphism, nuclear hyperchromatism and mitoses. Another characteristic feature of anaplastic variety of astrocytoma is the proliferation of vascular endothelium.

3. GLIOBLASTOMA MULTIFORME. *G/A* It shows variegated appearance, with some areas showing grey-white appearance while others are yellow and soft with foci of haemorrhages and necrosis. The surrounding normal brain tissue is distorted and infiltrated by yellow tumour tissue.

M/E i) Highly anaplastic and cellular appearance.

ii) Areas of tumour necrosis around which tumour cells may form pseudo-palisading.

iii) Microvascular endothelial proliferation is marked.

Oligodendroglioma *(p. 914)*

Oligodendroglioma is an uncommon glioma of oligodendroglial origin and may develop in isolation or may be mixed with other glial cells. The tumour commonly presents in 3rd to 4th decades of life.

G/A Oligodendroglioma is well-circumscribed, grey-white and gelatinous mass having cystic areas, foci of haemorrhages and calcification.

M/E The tumour is characterised by uniform cells with round to oval nuclei surrounded by a clear halo of cytoplasm and well-defined cell membranes. Tumour cells tend to cluster around the native neurons forming *satellitosis.* Typically, there are varying degree of endothelial cell hyperplasia and foci of calcification.

Ependymoma *(p. 914)*

Ependymoma is not an uncommon tumour, derived from the layer of epithelium that lines the ventricles and the central canal of the spinal cord. It occurs chiefly in childhood and young adulthood (below 20 years of age). Typically, it is encountered in the fourth ventricle (posterior fossa tumour).

G/A Ependymoma is a well-demarcated tumour but complete surgical removal may not be possible due to close proximity to vital structures in the medulla and pons.

M/E The tumour is composed of uniform epithelial (ependymal) cells forming rosettes, canals and perivascular pseudorosettes. By light microscopy under high magnification, PTAH-positive structures, blepharoplasts, representing basal bodies of cilia may be demonstrated in the cytoplasm of tumour cells.

Two variants of ependymoma deserve special mention:

1. Myxopapillary ependymoma. Characteristically, it occurs in the region of cauda equina and originates from the filum terminale in adults. True to its name, it contains myxoid and papillary structures interspersed in the typical ependymal cells. It is a slow-growing tumour.

2. Subependymoma. It occurs as a small, asymptomatic, incidental solid nodule in the fourth and lateral ventricle of middle-aged or elderly patients. Areas of microcysts and calcification may be encountered.

Choroid Plexus Papilloma *(p. 914)*

Tumours derived from choroid plexus epithelium are uncommon intracranial tumours. They are found in the distribution of the choroid plexus. In children, they occur most frequently in the lateral ventricles, whereas in adults fourth ventricle is the most common site.

G/A The tumour projects as rounded, papillary mass into one of the ventricles.

M/E Choroid plexus papilloma is a papillary tumour resembling normal choroid plexus with a vascular connective tissue core covered by a single layer of cuboidal epithelium which lies upon a basement membrane.

Medulloblastoma *(p. 915)*

Medulloblastoma is the most common variety of primitive neuroectodermal tumour. It comprises 25% of all childhood brain tumours but a quarter of cases occur in patients over the age of 20 years. The most common location is the cerebellum in the region of roof of fourth ventricle, in the midline of cerebellum, in the vermis, and in the cerebellar hemispheres. Medulloblastoma is a highly malignant tumour and spreads to local as well as to distant sites.

G/A The tumour typically protrudes into the fourth ventricle as a soft, grey-white mass or invades the surface of the cerebellum.

M/E Medulloblastoma is composed of small, poorly-differentiated cells with ill-defined cytoplasmic processes and a tendency to be arranged around blood vessels and occasionally forms pseudorosettes (Homer-Wright rosettes).

OTHER PRIMARY INTRAPARENCHYMAL TUMOURS *(p. 915)*

Haemangioblastoma *(p. 915)*

Haemangioblastoma is a tumour of uncertain origin and constitutes about 2% of all intracranial tumours. It is seen more commonly in young adults and is commoner in males. It may occur sporadically or be a part of von Hippel-Lindau syndrome (along with cysts in the liver, kidney, and benign/malignant renal tumour).

G/A The tumour is usually a circumscribed cystic mass with a mural nodule. The cyst contains haemorrhagic fluid.

M/E i) Large number of thin-walled blood vessels lined by plump endothelium. ii) Vascular spaces are separated by groups of polygonal lipid-laden foamy stromal cells.

Primary CNS Lymphoma *(p. 915)*

Lymphomas in the brain may occur as a part of disseminated non-Hodgkin's lymphoma or may be a primary CNS lymphoma. The incidence of the primary CNS lymphoma has shown a rising trend in patients of AIDS and other immunosuppressed conditions. They occur in men above 5th decade of life. Primary CNS lymphoma has a poor prognosis.

G/A The tumour is frequently periventricular in location and may appear nodular or diffuse.

M/E i) Characteristically, the tumour grows around blood vessels i.e. has an angiocentric growth pattern. Reticulin stain highlights this feature well.

ii) Typically, CNS lymphomas are diffuse, large cell type with high mitotic activity.

iii) They are generally B-cell type.

Germ Cell Tumours *(p. 915)*

Rarely, germ cell tumours may occur in the brain, especially in children. Common locations are suprasellar region and pineal area. Some common examples of such tumours are germinoma (seminoma/dysgerminoma), teratoma and embryonal carcinoma. Morphologically, they are similar to their counterparts elsewhere.

Meningioma *(p. 916)*

Meningiomas arise from the cap cell layer of the arachnoid. Their most common sites are in the front half of the head and include: lateral cerebral convexities, midline along the falx cerebri adjacent to the major venous sinuses parasagittally, and olfactory groove. Less frequent sites are: within the cerebral ventricles, foramen magnum, cerebellopontine angle and the spinal cord. Meningiomas are generally solitary. They have an increased frequency in patients with neurofibromatosis 2 and are often multiple in them. They are usually found in 2nd to 6th decades of life, with slight female preponderance. Most are benign and can be removed successfully.

G/A Meningioma is well-circumscribed, solid, spherical or hemispherical mass of varying size (1-10 cm in diameter). The tumour is generally firmly attached to the dura and indents the surface of the brain but rarely ever invades it. Cut surface of the tumour is firm and fibrous, sometimes with foci of calcification.

M/E Meningiomas are divided into 5 subtypes:

1. Meningotheliomatous (syncytial) meningioma. This pattern of meningioma resembles the normal arachnoid cap cells. The tumour consists of solid masses of polygonal cells with poorly-defined cell membranes (i.e. syncytial appearance).

2. Fibrous (fibroblastic) meningioma. A less frequent pattern is of a spindle-shaped fibroblastic tumour in which the tumour cells form parallel or interlacing bundles.

3. Transitional (mixed) meningioma. This pattern is characterised by a combination of cells with syncytial and fibroblastic features with conspicuous whorled pattern of tumour cells, often around central capillary-sized blood vessels. Some of the whorls contain psammoma bodies due to calcification of the central core of whorls.

4. Angioblastic meningioma. An angioblastic meningioma includes 2 patterns: *haemangioblastic pattern* resembling haemangioblastoma of the cerebellum, and *haemangiopericytic pattern* which is indistinguishable from haemangiopericytoma elsewhere in the body.

5. Anaplastic (malignant) meningioma. Rarely, a meningioma may display features of anaplasia and invade the underlying brain or spinal cord.

METASTATIC TUMOURS *(p. 917)*

Approximately a quarter of intracranial tumours are metastatic tumours. The clinical features are like those of a primary brain tumour. Most common primary tumours metastasising to the brain are: carcinomas of the lung, breast, skin (malignant melanoma), kidney and the gastrointestinal tract and choriocarcinoma. Infiltration from lymphoma and leukaemias may also occur.

PERIPHERAL NERVOUS SYSTEM *(p. 917)*

NORMAL STRUCTURE *(p. 917)*

The peripheral nervous system (PNS) consists of cranial and spinal nerves, sympathetic and parasympathetic autonomic nervous system and the peripheral ganglia. The PNS is involved in electric transmission of sensory and motor impulses to and from the CNS. A peripheral nerve is surrounded by an outer layer of fibrous tissue, the *epineurium.* Each nerve is made of several fascicles enclosed in multilayered membrane of flattened cells, the *perineurium.* Each fascicle is composed of bundles of connective tissue, the *endoneurium.* There are 2 main types of nerve fibres or axons comprising a peripheral nerve—myelinated and non-myelinated. *Myelinated axons* are thicker (diameter greater than 2 *µm*) and are surrounded by a chain of Schwann cells which produce myelin sheath. *Non-myelinated axons* have diameter of 0.2-3 µm and about ten non-myelinated fibres may be enclosed by a Schwann cell. *Nodes of Ranvier* on myelinated fibres are the boundaries between each Schwann cell surrounding the fibre.

PATHOLOGIC REACTIONS TO INJURY *(p. 917)*

The pathologic reactions of the PNS in response to injury may be in the form of one of the types of degenerations causing *peripheral neuropathy* or formation of a *traumatic neuroma.* There are 3 main types of degenerative processes in the PNS.

WALLERIAN DEGENERATION. Wallerian degeneration occurs after transection of the axon which may be as a result of knife wounds, compression, traction and ischaemia. Following transection, initially there is accumulation of organelles in the proximal and distal ends of the transection sites. The process of regeneration occurs by sprouting of axons and proliferation of Schwann cells from the proximal end.

AXONAL DEGENERATION. In axonal degeneration, degeneration of the axon begins at the peripheral terminal and proceeds backward towards the nerve cell body. The cell body often undergoes chromatolysis. There is Schwann cell proliferation in the region of axonal degeneration.

SEGMENTAL DEMYELINATION. Segmental demyelination is similar to demyelination within the brain. Segmental demyelination is demyelination of the segment between two consecutive nodes of Ranvier, leaving a denuded axon segment. Repeated episodes of demyelination and remyelination are associated with concentric proliferation of Schwann cells around axons producing *'onion bulbs'* found in hypertrophic neuropathy.

TRAUMATIC NEUROMA. Normally, the injured axon of a peripheral nerve regenerates at the rate of approximately 1 mm per day. However, if the process of regeneration is hampered due to an interposed haematoma or fibrous scar, the axonal sprouts together with Schwann cells and fibroblasts form a peripheral mass called as traumatic or stump neuroma.

PERIPHERAL NEUROPATHY *(p. 918)*

Peripheral neuropathy is the term used for disorders of the peripheral nerves of any cause. It may be polyneuropathy, mononeuropathy multiplex, and mononeuropathy.

■ **Polyneuropathy** is characteristically symmetrical with noticeable sensory features such as tingling, pricking, burning sensation or dysaesthesia in feet and toes.

M/E Polyneuropathy may be the result of axonal degeneration (axonopathy) or segmental demyelination (demyelinating polyneuropathy). In each type, acute, subacute and chronic forms are distinguished. *Guillain-Barré syndrome* is the classical example of acute demyelinating polyneuropathy which has probably an autoimmune etiology.

■ **Mononeuropathy multiplex or multifocal neuropathy** is defined as simultaneous or sequential multifocal involvement of nerve trunks which are not in continuity. The involvement may be partial or complete and may evolve over days or years.

■ **Mononeuropathy,** on the other hand, is focal involvement of a single nerve. It is generally the result of local causes such as direct trauma, compression and entrapment.

NERVE SHEATH TUMOURS *(p. 919)*

Schwannoma (Neurilemmoma) *(p. 919)*

Schwannomas or neurilemmomas arise from cranial and spinal nerve roots. An *acoustic schwannoma* or *acoustic neuroma* is an intracranial schwannoma located within the internal auditory canal originating from vestibular portion of the acoustic nerve. *Intraspinal schwannomas* are found as intradural tumours in the thoracic region.

G/A A schwannoma is an encapsulated, solid, sometimes cystic, tumour that produces eccentric enlargement of the nerve root from where it arises.

M/E The tumour is composed of fibrocellular bundles forming whorled pattern. There are areas of dense and compact cellularity *(Antoni A pattern)* alternating with loose acellular areas *(Antoni B pattern)*. Areas of Antoni A pattern show palisaded nuclei called *Verocay bodies*. Nerve fibres are usually found stretched over the capsule but not within the tumour. Areas of degeneration contain haemosiderin and lipid-laden macrophages. Schwann cells characteristically express S-100 protein. A schwannoma rarely ever becomes malignant.

Neurofibroma and von Recklinghausen's Disease *(p. 919)*

Neurofibromas may occur as solitary, fusiform cutaneous tumour of a single nerve, but more often are multiple associated with von Recklinghausen's disease. Solitary neurofibroma is a tumour of adults but multiple neurofibromas or neurofibromatosis is a hereditary disorder with autosomal dominant inheritance. Solitary neurofibroma is generally asymptomatic but patients with von Recklinghausen's disease have a triad of features;

■ multiple cutaneous neurofibromas

■ numerous pigmented skin lesions (*'cafe au lait'* spots); and

■ pigmented iris hamartomas.

Neurofibromatosis type 1 is a genetic disorder having mutation in chromosome 17 while type 2 has mutation in chromosome 22.

G/A Neurofibroma is an unencapsulated tumour producing fusiform enlargement of the affected nerve. Neurofibromatosis in von Recklinghausen's disease is characterised by numerous nodules of varying size, seen along the small cutaneous nerves but may also be found in visceral branches of sympathetic nerves.

M/E A neurofibroma is composed of bundles and interlacing fascicles of delicate and elongated spindle-shaped cells having wavy nuclei. The cellular area is separated by loose collagen and mucoid material. Residual nerve fibres (neurites) may be demonstrable.

It is estimated that about 3% of patients with von Recklinghausen's neurofibromatosis develop malignant transformation of one of the nodules.

Malignant Peripheral Nerve Sheath Tumour (p. 920)

Malignant peripheral nerve sheath tumour (MPNST) is a poorly differentiated spindle cell sarcoma of the peripheral nerves occurring most often in adults. The tumour may arise *de novo* or from malignant transformation of a pre-existing neurofibroma than a schwannoma, generally at an early age (20-40 years). About 50% of the tumours are seen in patients with neurofibromatosis type 1, while some develop at sites of previous irradiation.

G/A The tumour appears as an unencapsulated fusiform enlargement of a nerve.

M/E The tumour has the appearance of a fibrosarcoma. The tumour has frequent mitosis and areas of necrosis. *Triton tumour* is the name use for MPNST which has areas of poorly-differentiated rhabdomyosarcoma, cartilage and bone.

■ SELF ASSESSMENT

1. **Astrocytic processes can be demonstrated by:**
   A. Reticulin stain
   B. Phosphotungstic acid haematoxylin (PTAH)
   C. Periodic acid Schiff (PAS)
   D. van Gieson

2. **Normally, the most numerous of the cells in the central nervous system are:**
   A. Astrocytes   B. Neurons
   C. Oligodendrocytes   D. Microglia

3. **Arnold-Chiari malformation consists of the following *except:***
   A. Elongation of the medulla with part of 4th ventricle
   B. S-shaped bend in the medulla
   C. Encephalocele
   D. Lengthening and herniation of cerebellar vermix

4. **Secondary hydrocephalus has the following features *except:***
   A. There is compensatory increase of CSF
   B. It occurs due to loss of neural tissue
   C. There is increased intracranial pressure
   D. Common causes are cerebral atrophy and infarction

5. **The most common route of spread of infection to the brain is:**
   A. Via venous route   B. Via arterial route
   C. Via lymphatics   D. Along nerves

6. **Glucose content of CSF is unaltered in the following type of meningitis:**
   A. Acute pyogenic meningitis   B. Acute viral meningitis
   C. Cryptococcal meningitis   D. Tuberculous meningitis

7. **The following viral infection of the brain produces intra-cytoplasmic inclusions:**
   A. Herpes simplex virus   B. Cytomegalovirus
   C. Rabies virus   D. Enteroviruses

8. **The etiologic agent for Creutzfeldt-Jakob disease (CJD) is as under:**
   A. HIV   B. JC virus
   C. Prions   D. Zoster-varicella virus

9. **The lowest limit of critical level of systolic pressure upto which the brain continues to be perfused is:**
   A. 70 mm Hg   B. 60 mm Hg
   C. 50 mm Hg   D. 40 mm Hg

10. **Subarachnoid haemorrhage results most often from the following:**
    - A. Hypertension
    - B. Aneurysm
    - C. Vascular malformation
    - D. Bleeding diathesis

11. **Acute subdural haematoma has the following features *except*:**
    - A. Blood is of venous origin
    - B. Accumulated blood is in liquid form
    - C. No significant compression of gyri
    - D. Symptoms develop slowly

12. **Neuritic plaques are seen in the brain in:**
    - A. Multiple sclerosis
    - B. Alzheimer's disease
    - C. Parkinsonism
    - D. Perivenous encephalomyelitis

13. **Primary CNS tumours may arise from the following constituent cells *except*:**
    - A. Neuroglia
    - B. Microglia
    - C. Neurons
    - D. Meninges

14. **Out of the following, the most common tumour in children is:**
    - A. Ewing's sarcoma
    - B. Neuroblastoma
    - C. Glioma
    - D. Embryonal rhabdomyosarcoma

15. **Astrocytoma occurring in children is commonly:**
    - A. Fibrillary
    - B. Pilocytic
    - C. Anaplastic
    - D. Glioblastoma multiforme

16. **Small foci of calcification are frequently seen on X-ray of the following glioma:**
    - A. Ependymoma
    - B. Oligodendroglioma
    - C. Astrocytoma
    - D. Choroid plexus papilloma

17. **Myxopapillary ependymoma characteristically occurs at the following location:**
    - A. Lateral ventricles
    - B. Fourth ventricle
    - C. Third ventricle
    - D. Filum terminale

18. **The following brain tumour has a tendency to metastasise by haematogenous route:**
    - A. Anaplastic astrocytoma
    - B. Glioblstoma multiforme
    - C. Medulloblastoma
    - D. Ependymoma

19. **The cell of origin of meningioma is:**
    - A. Dura mater
    - B. Arachnoid cap cell layer
    - C. Pia mater
    - D. Choroid plexus

20. **Transection of axon is followed by:**
    - A. Wallerian degeneration
    - B. Axonal degeneration
    - C. Segmental degeneration
    - D. Hypertrophy of Schwann cells

21. **Angiocentric growth pattern is typical of following CNS tumour:**
    - A. Glioblastoma multiforme
    - B. Haemangioblastoma
    - C. Primary CNS lymphoma
    - D. Medulloblastoma

22. **The most common cause of dementia is:**
    - A. Parkinsonism
    - B. Alzheimer's disease
    - C. Multiple sclerosis
    - D. Perivenous encephalomyelitis

KEY

1 = B	2 = C	3 = C	4 = C
5 = B	6 = B	7 = C	8 = C
9 = C	10 = B	11 = B	12 = B
13 = B	14 = B	15 = B	16 = B
17 = D	18 = C	19 = B	20 = A
21 = C	22 = B		

29

Diagnostic Cytopathology

INTRODUCTION *(p. 922)*

In general, diagnostic cytology pertains to the interpretation of cells from the human body that either exfoliate (desquamate) spontaneously from epithelial surfaces, or are obtained from various organs/tissues by different clinical procedures. While histopathologic diagnosis is based on interpretation of changes in tissue architecture, the cytopathologic diagnosis rests upon alterations in morphology observed in single cells or groups of cells.

Role of Diagnostic Cytology *(p. 922)*

Among the numerous applications of cytodiagnostic techniques, the following are more important:

1. Diagnosis and management of cancer. e.g. a *valuable adjunct* to histopathology, *preliminary diagnosis* of cancer, in some fields, as the *primary source/method* of establishing a tissue diagnosis, detection and diagnosis of clinically silent *early cancer*, assessing *response to therapy*, in the *follow-up* of previously diagnosed/known cases of cancer.
2. Identification of benign neoplasms.
3. Intraoperative pathologic diagnosis.
4. Diagnosis of non-neoplastic/inflammatory conditions.
5. Diagnosis of specific infections.
6. Cytogenetics.
7. Assessment of hormonal status in women.
8. Identification of tissues/cells.

For cytomorphological *recognition of cancer, nuclear characteristics* are used to determine the presence or absence of malignancy. *Cytoplasmic characteristics* help in *typing the malignancy* e.g. keratinisation in squamous cell carcinoma, mucin droplets in adenocarcinoma, melanin pigment in melanomas.

Branches of Diagnostic Cytology *(p. 923)*

Two branches of diagnostic cytology are currently recognised: exfoliative and interventional.

EXFOLIATIVE CYTOLOGY. This is the older branch that essentially involves the study of cells spontaneously shed off (as a result of continuous growth of epithelial linings) from epithelial surfaces into body cavities or body fluids. In addition, cells for study may also be obtained by scraping, brushing, or washing various mucosal surfaces (abrasive cytology).

INTERVENTIONAL CYTOLOGY. This is the branch in which samples are obtained by clinical procedures or surgical intervention. It is dominated by, and is virtually synonymous with, Fine Needle Aspiration Cytology (FNAC) which is also known as Aspiration Biopsy Cytology (ABC).

Contrasting features and differences between exfoliative and interventional cytology are presented in Table 29.1.

EXFOLIATIVE CYTOLOGY *(p. 923)*

I. FEMALE GENITAL TRACT *(p. 923)*

Samples (smears) from the female genital tract have traditionally been known as 'Pap smears'. These smears may be prepared by different methods depending upon the purpose for which they are intended: i) Lateral vaginal

TABLE 29.1: Differences between Exfoliative and Interventional Cytology.

	FEATURE	EXFOLIATIVE CYTOLOGY	INTERVENTIONAL CYTOLOGY
1.	*Cell samples*	Exfoliated from epithelial surfaces	Obtained by intervention/ aspiration
2.	*Smears*	Require screening to locate suitable cells for study	Abundance of cells for study in most smears
3.	*Diagnostic basis*	Individual cell morphology	Cell patterns and morphology of groups of cells
4.	*Morphologic criteria of diagnostic significance*	Nuclear characteristics most important	Nuclear characteristics important; cytoplasmic character and background equally significant

smears (LVS) ii) Vaginal 'pool' or 'vault' smears iii) Cervical smears iv) Combined (Fast) smears v) Triple smears (cervical-vaginal-endocervical or CVE) vi) Endocervical and endometrial smears

CELLS IN NORMAL COMBINED SMEARS. Normally, combined smear contains two types of cells: epithelial and others:

Epithelial cells: There are 4 types of squamous epithelial cells in the cervical smear: *superficial, intermediate, parabasal and basal cells.* A few variants of morphological forms and other epithelial cells are: Navicular cells, lactation cells, endocervical cells, endometrial cells, trophoblastic cells.

Other cells: Besides epithelial cells, other cells in cervical smears are leucocytes and Döderlein bacilli.

APPLICATIONS OF PAP SMEAR *(p. 925)*

Cytohormonal Evaluation *(p. 925)*

Assessment of hormonal status is best carried out from lateral vaginal smears although vaginal 'pool' or fast smears may also be used. Ideally, at least 3 smears obtained on alternate days should be scrutinised and cytologic indices determined for each smear for accurate assessment.

Several indices are available for description of cytohormonal patterns. The most commonly used are as under:

i)   *Acidophilic index (AI):* The relative proportion of cells containing acidophilic (pink) and basophilic (blue) cytoplasm are determined by AI.

ii) *Pyknotic index (PI):* The percentage of cells having small, dark, shrunken nuclei (less than 6 μm in size) is determined by PI.

iii) *Maturation index (MI):* MI is the most widely used method. One hundred squamous cells are counted and grouped according to their type—parabasal, intermediate, or superficial (basal cells are virtually absent from normal vaginal smears). Their proportions are expressed as a percentage.

Abnormal Combined Smears *(p. 925)*

In order to evolve a system acceptable to clinicians and cytopathologists, National Cancer Institute Workshop in 1988 developed *The Bethesda System* for uniformity in evaluation as well as limitations of reporting in cervicovaginal cytopathology; this was subsequently modified in 1991 and further updated in 2001. Briefly, it has three basic components:

1.   Specimen adequacy: It is an important component of quality assurance and provides feedback regarding sampling technique. It implies properly labelled, adequately fixed smears having sufficient number of evenly spread, well preserved cells on microscopic evaluation.

2. **General categorisation:** It includes categorising the smear in one of the three broad categories: within normal limits, benign cellular changes, and epithelial cell abnormalities.

3. **Descriptive diagnosis:** Final aspect of the Bethesda system includes detailed description of the benign cellular changes or epithelial cell abnormalities in the smear.

Based on it, the cellular changes in cervical smears are discussed below under 2 headings: benign (non-neoplastic) cellular changes and epithelial cell abnormalities.

BENIGN CELLULAR CHANGES (NON-NEOPLASTIC) (p. 926)

i) **NON-SPECIFIC INFLAMMATORY CHANGES.** Inflammatory changes not associated with any specific infection/identifiable infectious agent (i.e. non-specific inflammation) are commonly seen in smears of the female genital tract.

■ *Acute inflammatory changes* are characterised by an increase in the number of parabasal cells (due to disruption of superficial layers of the epithelium resulting in exposure of deeper layers), cytoplasmic acidophilia and vacuolisation, leucocytic migration into cytoplasm, and perinuclear halos with nuclear pyknosis or enlargement.

■ *Chronic inflammatory changes (Reactive changes)* manifest in squamous cells as nuclear enlargement, hyperchromatism, and nucleolar prominence, with multinucleation in some instances.

ii) **SPECIFIC INFLAMMATORY CHANGES.** Specific inflammatory changes may be associated with a variety of infectious agents:

a) *Bacterial agents:* N. gonorrhoeae (the gonococcus), *Gardnerella vaginalis,* Tuberculosis.

b) *Viral agents:* Herpes simplex virus (HSV), Human papilloma virus (HPV).

c) *Fungal agents:* Moniliasis (infection by *Candida albicans*), *Torulopsis glabrata.*

d) *Parasitic agents:* Trichomonas vaginalis, Entamoeba histolytica (in trophozoite form).

Epithelial Cell Abnormalities—Neoplastic (p. 927)

Carcinoma of the uterine cervix still ranks high in the list as the most frequent cancer in third world countries and is the leading cause of morbidity and mortality. The vast majority of cervical cancers are of the squamous or epidermoid type, and the diagnosis of squamous cell carcinoma of the cervix may be considered the single most important role of exfoliative cytology.

Neoplastic epithelial changes are described below under 2 headings: squamous cell abnormalities and glandular cell abnormalities.

1. **SQUAMOUS CELL ABNORMALITIES:** The fully-developed invasive squamous cell carcinoma of the uterine cervix is preceded by a pre-invasive intraepithelial neoplastic process that is recognisable on histologic and cytologic examination.

Morphogenesis and nomenclature. The proliferating reserve cells develop certain atypical features i.e. hyperchromasia and increased nuclear size. The continuing proliferation of these atypical cells with loss of polarity, a concomitant increase in mitotic activity, and progressive involvement of more and more layers of the epithelium is known as *dysplasia* (disordered growth). When dysplasia involves the full thickness of the epithelium and the lesion morphologically resembles squamous cell carcinoma without invasion of underlying stroma, it is termed *carcinoma in situ (CIS)*. CIS further evolves through the stage of *microinvasive carcinoma* (with depth of stromal invasion not exceeding 3 mm) into full-blown *invasive squamous cell carcinoma*.

Previously depending on the degree of epithelial involvement, three grades of dysplasia were recognised: mild, moderate and severe. As the stages of dysplasia and CIS represented a continuous spectrum of lesions seen in the precancerous state, they were collectively termed 'cervical intraepithelial neoplasia' (CIN) and categorised as under:

CIN I	Mild dysplasia	Primitive (atypical) cells proliferating in lower third of epithelium.
CIN II	Moderate dysplasia	Involvement up to middle-third of epithelium.
CIN III	Severe dysplasia	Involvement of upper-third of epithelium.
	Carcinoma *in situ* (CIS)	Involvement of full thickness of epithelium.

Presently, the Bethesda system divides squamous cell abnormalities into four categories:

■ *Atypical squamous cells of undetermined significance (ASCUS)* which represents cellular changes falling short of intraepithelial lesion.

■ *Low-grade squamous intraepithelial lesion (L-SIL)* that includes CIN-I and cellular changes associated with HPV infection.

■ *High-grade squamous intraepithelial lesion (H-SIL)* includes CIN grade II and III as well as CIS.

■ Squamous cell carcinoma.

Cytomorphology. Precancerous states can be distinguished from invasive carcinoma on the basis of cytomorphological features observed in smears.

In dysplastic epithelium, stratification and maturation of cytoplasm occurs above the layers of proliferating primitive cells. While, nuclear abnormalities persist. Cells exfoliating from the surface, thus, display cytoplasmic maturation and differentiation with nuclear atypia and are known as *dyskaryotic cells*.

2. GLANDULAR CELL ABNORMALITIES. The Bethesda system categorises glandular abnormalities as under:

■ *Atypical glandular cells of undetermined significance(AGUS)* which represent nuclear atypia of endocervical and endometrial cells exceeding repartive changes.

■ *Endocervical* and *endometrial adenocarcinoma,* both of which can be detected from Pap smears.

■ Cells from *extrauterine cancers* may also be present in Pap smears, the majority originating from the ovaries. Clues to the extrauterine origin of cancer cells include: the absence of a tumour diathesis, arrangement of cancer cells in glandular and papillary configuration (accompanied by psammoma bodies in some instances), and absence of dysplastic changes in coexistent cervico-endometrial cells.

Automation in Cervical Cytology *(p. 928)*

Introduction of automated devices like PapNet for primary screening is a major technologic achievement in recent times. Automation offers routine pre-screening of hundreds of Pap smears, decreasing the workload of cytopathologists and at the same time providing quality assurance. It can be applied to conventional Pap smears or *thin-preps*.

II. RESPIRATORY TRACT *(p. 928)*

Cellular material from the respiratory tract may be obtained as a result of spontaneous expectoration (sputum) or by aspiration/brushing during broncho-scopic procedures.

III. GASTROINTESTINAL TRACT *(p. 929)*

Lesions in the oral cavity may be sampled by scraping the surface with wooden and metal tongue-depressors. For the oesophagus and stomach, samples are obtained under direct vision by brushing or lavage through fibreoptic endoscopes.

IV. URINARY TRACT *(p. 929)*

1. Urinary Sediment Cytology. Cytological evaluation of the urinary tract is most often carried out by examining the sediment of voided or catheterised specimens of urine.

2. Bladder Irrigation (Washings). Washings of the urinary bladder obtained at cystoscopy are preferred in symptomatic patients when bladder tumours are suspected.

3. Retrograde Catheterisation. In some instances, retrograde catheterisation and brushing of the ureter and renal pelvis are utilised for localisation of lesions.

4. Prostatic Massage. Prostatic secretions are obtained by prostatic massage and the sample is collected directly onto a glass slide and smeared.

V. BODY FLUIDS *(p. 929)*

The cytology of body fluids can conveniently be discussed under two headings:

A. Effusions *(p. 929)*

Effusion refers to the accumulation of fluid in any of the three body cavities (pleural, pericardial and peritoneal). An effusion in the peritoneal cavity is also known as ascites. Effusions have traditionally been classed as transudates or exudates.

Diagnostic cytology of effusions (on samples obtained by paracentesis) is mainly related to the identification of malignancy, and wherever possible, its classification.

B. Fluids of Small Volume *(p. 930)*

Cerebrospinal Fluid (CSF) *(p. 930)*

CSF examination is an important part of complete neurologic evaluation, both in non-neoplastic and neoplastic diseases of the central nervous system.

CSF is an ultrafiltrate of plasma with a total volume of about 150 ml (in the adult). Cell content is low (0-4/µl) comprising mainly lymphocytes or monocytes.

Neoplasms that are in direct contact with the CSF are most likely to shed cells which are recoverable for scrutiny. Metastatic cancers (leukaemia, lymphoma and adenocarcinoma), medulloblastomas, and ependymomas shed the greatest amount of material.

2. Seminal Fluid (Semen) *(p. 930)*

Examination of seminal fluid (semen analysis) is one of the tests for investigating infertile couples, and is also used to check the adequacy of vasectomy. Samples are obtained by masturbation or coitus interruptus after at least 4 days of sexual abstinence and assessed on the following lines:

1. Volume. Normal volume is between 2.5 and 5 ml.

2. Viscosity and pH. When ejaculated, semen is fairly viscid but liquefies in about 10 to 30 minutes. It is usually alkaline (pH about 8).

3. Motility. Normally, within 2 hours of ejaculation at least 60% of the spermatozoa are vigorously motile; in 6 to 8 hours 25 to 40% are still motile.

4. Count. Counting is done in a Neubauer chamber after suitable dilution. Normally, 60 million or more spermatozoa are present per ml.

5. Morphology. Stained smears are used to assess morphology. Normally, not more than 20% of spermatozoa are morphologically abnormal (e.g. double-head, pointed-head, or swollen).

6. Fructose. Seminal fructose estimation (normal levels 150-600 mg/dl) complements cytological analysis. Low levels of seminal fructose indicate obstruction at the level of ejaculatory ducts.

VI. BUCCAL SMEARS FOR SEX CHROMATIN BODIES *(p. 930)*

Sex-specific chromatin bodies are observed in interphase nuclei and comprise the Barr body (X chromatin) and the fluorescent or F body (Y chromatin). The number of Barr bodies observed in interphase nuclei is one less than the number of X chromosome (n–1), whereas the number of F bodies observed is equal to the number of Y chromosomes present (n). In effect, the Barr body is specific for females and the F body for males.

1. DEMONSTRATION OF THE BARR BODY (X CHROMATIN). In buccal smears, the Barr body appears as a plano-convex mass about 1 μm in diameter applied to the inner surface of the nuclear membrane. In normal females, Barr bodies are present in at least 20% of nuclei. Males have a Barr body count of less than 2%.

2. DEMONSTRATION OF THE F BODY (Y CHROMATIN). On staining buccal smears with quinacrine mustard, the intensely fluorescent F body is observed in about 60% of interphase nuclei in males and in less than 8% of nuclei in females.

3. COUNTING OF DRUM-STICK APPENDAGE. The presence and frequency of drum-stick appendages attached to nuclei of polymorphonuclear leucocytes on a peripheral blood film may also be used for determining sex. At least 500 neutrophilic leucocytes are scrutinised in a Romanowsky-stained blood film. Genetic females show drumsticks in 3-6% of neutrophils. In males, the frequency of drumsticks is less than 0.3%.

B. Fixation and Fixatives *(p. 932)*

All material for cytological examination must be properly fixed to ensure preservation of cytomorphological details. Methods of fixation vary depending upon the type of staining employed (e.g. Papanicolaou or Romanowsky staining). Material for exfoliative cytodiagnosis is usually *wet-fixed* (i.e. smears are immersed in fixative without allowing them to dry) for use with the Papanicolaou or haematoxylin and eosin stains. Sometimes, smears are *air-dried* for use with the Romanowsky stains (as used in haematologic studies). In Romanowsky staining, fixation is effected during the staining procedure.

1. ROUTINE FIXATIVES. The ideal fixative for routine use is Papanicolaou's fixative comprising a solution of equal parts of ether and 95% ethanol.

Smears prepared at the bedside as well as those prepared in the laboratory from fluid samples are immediately placed in 95% ethanol *without allowing them to dry prior to fixation.*

2. COATING FIXATIVES. Coating fixatives are applied as aerosol-sprays or with a dropper to the surface of freshly prepared smears.

3. SPECIAL PURPOSE FIXATIVES. Buffered neutral formalin, Bouin's fluid and picric acid are used for specific purposes when required.

4. PRESERVATION OF FLUID SAMPLES. Samples of fluids are best submitted to the laboratory in a fresh state for immediate processing. Where a delay is anticipated in despatch to the laboratory or in processing, the sample is collected in a suitable preservative for 'prefixation' so that cellular morphology is preserved.

D. Staining of Smears *(p. 934)*

Three staining procedures are commonly employed: Papanicolaou and haematoxylin and eosin (H&E) stains are used for *wet-fixed smears* while Romanowsky stains are used for *air-dried smears*.

1. PAPANICOLAOU STAIN. Papanicolaou staining is the best method for routine cytodiagnostic studies. Three solutions are used comprising a nuclear stain and two cytoplasmic counter-stains. Harris' haematoxylin is the nuclear stain. Orange G (OG-6) and eosin-alcohol (EA-65 or EA-50) are the two cytoplasmic counterstains which impart the orange and cyanophilic tints to cytoplasm respectively.

2. H&E STAIN. The stain is essentially the same as that used for histological sections. Harris' haematoxylin is the nuclear stain, and eosin is the cytoplasmic counter-stain.

3. ROMANOWSKY STAINS. Romanowsky stains used in haematological preparations may also be used for cytological smear preparations. Leishman's, May-Grünwald-Giemsa (MGG) and Wright's stains are most commonly used.

INTERVENTIONAL CYTOLOGY *(p. 934)*

In interventional cytology, samples are obtained by aspiration or surgical biopsy. This branch includes FNAC, imprint cytology, crush smear cytology and biopsy sediment cytology.

I. FINE NEEDLE ASPIRATION CYTOLOGY *(p. 934)*

Interventional cytology is virtually synonymous with Fine Needle Aspiration Cytology or FNAC. The technique has gained wide acceptance only over the past three decades and is increasingly being used to sample a wide variety of body tissues. Almost all organ systems are accessible to the fine needle and the versatility of the technique has enormously increased the scope of diagnostic cytology.

A. Applications of FNAC *(p. 934)*

In routine practice, FNAC is most often used for diagnosis of palpable mass lesions. Palpable lesions commonly sampled are: breast masses enlarged lymph nodes enlarged thyroid and superficial soft tissue masses. The salivary glands, palpable abdominal lesions and the testicles are also frequently sampled for FNAC. Other sites/lesions accessible to FNAC are: the prostate, pelvic organs, bone and joint spaces, lungs, retroperitoneum and orbit.

B. Advantages of FNAC *(p. 935)*

i)   FNAC is an office/OPD procedure and *no hospitalisation* is required.
ii) *No anaesthesia* is required.
iii) The procedure is *quick, safe and painless*.
iv) *Multiple attempts* (or repeating the procedure) are possible.
v)   Results are obtained *rapidly*.
vi) It is a low-cost procedure which is *cost-effective*.
vii) As the cytopathologist performs the procedure himself, he gains *first-hand knowledge* of the clinical findings.

C. General Procedure for FNAC *(p. 935)*

1. Materials *(p. 935)*

For performing FNAC, a syringe with a well-fitting needle, some microscopic glass slides and a suitable fixative are the only material required in most instances.

Chapter Twenty Nine

NEEDLES. Fine needles range from 25 to 20 gauge (0.6 mm to 0.9 mm outer diameter). The standard 21 gauge disposable needle of 38 mm length is suitable for routine transcutaneous FNAC of palpable masses; 25 or 24 gauge disposable needles of 25 mm length are used for lymph nodes and in children.

SYRINGES. Syringes of 10 to 20 ml capacity are suitable. Syringe holders (such as the Franzen handle, permit a single-hand grip during aspiration, employing disposable syringes. For needles with metal hubs (e.g. spinal puncture needles), disposable syringes should be used to ensure a proper fit between the needle hub and syringe nozzle.

GLASS SLIDES AND FIXATIVE. Four or six standard microscopic glass slides and a Coplin jar containing 95% ethyl alcohol (as a fixative) are the only other equipment required for routine FNAC. Prepared smears are either *wet-fixed* in 95% ethanol or *air-dried* (Table 29.2).

TABLE 29.2: General Properties of Wet-Fixed and Air-Dried Smears.

	FEATURE	WET-FIXED	AIR-DRIED
1.	*Staining*	Papanicolaou, H&E	Leishman, May-Grünwald-Giemsa
2.	*Cell size*	Comparable to tissue sections	Exaggerated
3.	*Nuclear detail*	Excellent	Fair
4.	*Nucleoli*	Well demonstrated	Not always discernible
5.	*Cytoplasmic details*	Poorly demonstrated	Well demonstrated
6.	*Stromal components*	Poorly demonstrated	Well demonstrated
7.	*Partially necrotic material*	Single intact cells, well defined	Cell details poorly defined

D. Radiological Imaging Aids for FNAC *(p. 938)*

Non-palpable lesions require some form of localisation by radiological aids for FNAC to be carried out. *Plain X-ray films* are usually adequate for lesions within bones and for some lesions within the chest. FNAC of the chest may also be attempted under *image amplified fluoroscopy* which allows visualisation of needle placement on the television monitor. *Computerised tomography (CT scans)* can also be used for lesions within the chest and abdomen. The most versatile radiological aid is *ultrasonography (USG)* which allows direct visualisation of needle placement in real time and is free from radiation hazards.

E. Limitations of FNAC *(p. 939)*

The main limitation of FNAC lies in the fact that only a small population of cells is sampled by the procedure. The reliability of the test, thus, depends upon the adequacy of the sample and its representative character. An inadequate sample which is not representative of the true lesion results in a 'false-negative' diagnosis. If the FNAC report is 'negative' despite a strong clinical suspicion of malignancy, the patient should be investigated further. FNAC may be repeated or a surgical biopsy performed to obtain a tissue diagnosis in such instances.

Lack of requisite clinical information (e.g. size, site and character of mass) or relevant investigative results (e.g. X-ray findings) further limit the utility of FNAC. Knowledge of the exact site from where the aspirate has been obtained is crucial to the accurate interpretation of FNAC smears and lack of this information severely compromises the ability of the cytopathologist to provide a diagnosis

II. IMPRINT CYTOLOGY *(P. 939)*

In imprint cytology, touch preparations from cut surfaces of fresh unfixed surgically excised mass lesions are examined. Imprints may also be obtained from draining sinuses or ulcerated areas.

For surgically resected specimens (e.g. lymph nodes) smears are prepared by bisecting or slicing the specimen and lightly touching/pressing a glass slide onto the freshly exposed surface without smearing it. Smears cannot be prepared from fixed specimens. Smears are wet-fixed or air-dried and stained as per routine.

The main advantage of the imprint smear is that the cell distribution reflects, and to some extent, recapitulates tissue architecture thus aiding in interpretation. The technique is used in the intraoperative diagnosis of malignancy as a complement to frozen-section, and is also valuable as an adjunct to histopathology in the typing of lymphomas.

III. CRUSH SMEAR CYTOLOGY *(p. 939)*

Crush smear preparations of tissue particles obtained by craniotomy have been used in the diagnosis of brain tumours. These smears are preferred by some workers as they allow recognition of tissue architecture to some degree, in addition to better cytological details.

IV. BIOPSY SEDIMENT CYTOLOGY *(p. 939)*

Biopsy sediment cytology entails the examination of sediment obtained by centrifugation of fixatives/fluids in which surgical biopsy specimens are despatched to the laboratory. The method may be useful in the rapid diagnosis of bone tumours as histological sections are usually obtained after many days on account of the delay necessitated by decalcification. For soft tissue specimens, the technique offers no particular advantage.

In conclusion, both exfoliative cytology and FNA cytology have now become a part of diagnostic pathology. It is imperative for the student in pathology as well as the clinician to be familiar with the advantages and limitations of cytologic diagnosis. It is acknowledged that a marked decline in incidence of cervical cancer in many western countries is attributable to highly successful preventive Pap smear screening programme. Similarly, large number of surgical diagnostic procedures are now avoided by rational use of FNAC. However, in view of unique responsibility of pathologist in patient management, reporting cytopathologist should be adequately trained in the skill and should not hesitate to ask for ancillary diagnostic techniques, or advise the use of core biopsy or open biopsy, wherever appropriate.

■ SELF ASSESSMENT

1. **For cytomorphological recognition of cancer, the following characteristics are used to determine the presence or absence of cancer** *except:*

   A. Cytoplasmic content   B. Nulcear size

   C. N:C ratio   D. Mitoses

2. **The following statements are true for Bethesda system** *except:*

   A. It is employed for cytologic reporting of Pap smears

   B. It divides dysplasias into three grades mild, moderate and severe

   C. All forms of dysplasias are graded into two grades—L-SIL and H-SIL

   D. Bethesda system is current modification of reporting over conventional system

3. **The number of Barr bodies observed in interphase nuclei are:**
   A. Equal to the number of X chromosomes
   B. One less than the number of X chromosomes
   C. Equal to the number of Y chromosomes
   D. One less than the number of Y chromosomes

4. **Drum-stick appendages seen in neutrophils in stained blood film in females are:**
   A. > 20%   B. 10-20 %
   C. 3-6%   D. < 0.3%

5. **CSF should be despatched to the laboratory for immmediate processing as under failing which it is useless for cytologic examination:**
   A. Within 1 hour   B. Within 1-4 hours
   C. Within 4-12 hours   D. Within 12-24 hours

6. **For pleural effusion, if a delay of more than 12 hours is anticipated for processing, it should be fixed in:**
   A. 95% ethanol
   B. Equal volume of 10% formalin
   C. Bouin's fluid
   D. Picric acid

7. **Haematoxylin and eosin staining is employed as cytologic stain for:**
   A. Wet-fixed smears
   B. Air-dried smears
   C. All FNAC smears only
   D. All cases of crush smear only

8. **The following features characterise wet-fixed smears over air-dried smears *except*:**
   A. Pap and H & E stain are applied for the former
   B. The nuclear details are better seen
   C. Cytoplasmic details are better seen
   D. Cell size is comparable to tissue section

9. **Ultrasound-guided FNAC is quite helpful in the following *except*:**
   A. Thyroid nodules
   B. Soft tissue masses
   C. Superficial abdominal lesions
   D. Deep intrathoracic lesions

10. **Imprint cytology is most useful in the lesions of following organ:**
    A. Bones   B. Breast
    C. Lymph nodes   D. Brain tumours

KEY

1 = A,	2 = B	3 = B	4 = C
5 = A	6 = B	7 = A	8 = C
9 = D	10 = C		

Appendix

Normal Values

WEIGHTS AND MEASUREMENTS OF NORMAL ORGANS (p. 941)

In order to understand the significance of alterations in weight and measurement of an organ in disease, it is important to be familiar with the normal values. In the foregoing chapters normal figures are given alongside the normal structure of each organ/system that precedes the discussion of pathologic states affecting it. Here, a comprehensive list of generally accepted normal weights and measurements of most of the normal organs in fully-developed, medium-sized individual and a normal healthy newborn are compiled in Table A-1.

Single value and value within brackets are indicative of the average figure for that organ. An alphabetic order has been followed.

TABLE A-1: Weights and Measurement of Normal Organs.

ORGAN	IN ADULTS	AT BIRTH (wherever applicable)
Brain:		
Weight (in males)	1400 gm	320–420 gm
Weight (in females)	1250 gm	—
Volume of cerebrospinal fluid	120–150 ml	—
Heart:		
Weight (in males)	300–350 gm	17-30 gm
Weight (in females)	250–300 gm	—
Thickness of right ventricular wall	0.3–0.5 cm	—
Thickness of left ventricular wall	1.3–1.5 cm	—
Circumference of mitral valve	10 cm	—
Circumference of aortic valve	7.5 cm	—
Circumference of pulmonary valve	8.5 cm	—
Circumference of tricuspid valve	12 cm	—
Volume of pericardial fluid	10–30 ml	—
Kidneys:		
Weight each (in males)	150 gm	20-30 gm
Weight each (in females)	135 gm	—
Liver:		
Weight (in males)	1400–1600 (1500) gm	100-160 gm
Weight (in females)	1200–1400 (1300) gm	—
Lungs:		
Weight (right lung)	375–500 (450) gm	35-55 gm
Weight (left lung)	325–450 (400) gm	—
Volume of pleural fluid	< 15 ml	—
Oesophagus:		
Length (cricoid cartilage to cardia)	25 cm	—
Distance from incisors to gastro-oesophageal junction	40 cm	—
Ovaries:		
Weight (each)	4–8 (6) gm	—

Contd...

TABLE A-1: Weights and Measurement of Normal Organs *(contd...)*

ORGAN	IN ADULTS	AT BIRTH (wherever applicable)
Pancreas:		
Total weight	60–100 (80) gm	3-6 gm
Weight of endocrine pancreas	1–1.5 gm	—
Placenta:		
Weight at term	400–600 gm	—
Prostate:		
Weight	20 gm	—
Spleen:		
Weight	125–175 (150) gm	6-14 gm
Thymus:		
Weight	5–10 gm	10-35 gm
Thyroid:		
Weight	15–40 gm	—
Uterus:		
Weight (in nonpregnant woman)	35–40 gm	—
Weight (in parous woman)	75–125 gm	—

LABORATORY VALUES OF CLINICAL SIGNIFICANCE *(p. 942)*

Currently, the concept of 'normal values' and 'normal ranges' is replaced by 'reference values' and 'reference limits' in which the variables for establishing the values for the reference population in a particular test are well defined. Reference ranges are valuable guidelines for the clinician.

The laboratory values given here are divided into three sections: clinical chemistry of blood (Table A-2), other body fluids (Table A-3), and haematologic values (Table A-4). In general, an alphabetic order has been followed.

TABLE A-2: Clinical Chemistry of Blood.

COMPONENT	FLUID	CONVENTIONAL VALUE
Alcohol, ethyl	Serum/whole blood	Negative
mild to moderate intoxication		80-200 mg/dl
marked intoxication		250-400 mg/dl
severe intoxication		>400 mg/dl
Aminotransferases (transaminases)		
aspartate (AST, SGOT)	Serum	0-35 U/L
alanine (ALT, SGPT)	Serum	0-35 U/L
Ammonia	Plasma	10-80 µg/dl
Amylase	Serum	60-180 U/L
Bicarbonate (HCO_3^-)	Whole blood	21-30 mEq/L
Bilirubin		
total	Serum	0.3-1.0 mg/dl
direct (conjugated)	Serum	0.1-0.3 mg/dl
indirect (unconjugated)	Serum	0.2-0.7 mg/dl
Calcium, ionised	Serum	4.5-5.6 mg/dl
Calcium, total	Plasma	9.0-10.5 mg/dl
CO_2 content	Whole blood	21-30 mEq/L (arterial)
Chloride (Cl^-)	Serum	98-106 mEq/L

Contd...

TABLE A-2: Clinical Chemistry of Blood *(contd...)*

COMPONENT	FLUID	CONVENTIONAL VALUE
Cholesterol	Serum	
total desirable for adults		<200 mg/dl
borderline high		200-239 mg/dl
high undesirable		>240 mg/dl
LDL-cholesterol, desirable range		<130 mg/dl
HDL-cholesterol, protective range		>60 mg/dl
triglycerides		<160 mg/dl
Copper	Serum	70-140 µg/dl
Creatine kinase (CK)	Serum	
males		25-90 U/L
females		10-70 IU/L
Creatine kinase-MB (CK-MB)	Serum	0-7 µg/L
Creatinine	Serum	0.5-1.5 mg/dl
Gases, arterial		
HCO_3^-	Whole blood	21-30 mEq/L
pH	Whole blood	7.38-7.44
pCO_2	Whole blood	35-45 mmHg
pO_2	Whole blood	80-100 mmHg
Glucose (fasting)	Plasma	
normal		70-110 mg/dl
impaired fasting glucose (IFG)		110-126 mg/dl
diabetes mellitus		>126 mg/dl
Glucose (2-hr post-prandial)	Plasma	
normal		<140 mg/dl
impaired glucose tolerance (IGT)		140-200 mg/dl
diabetes mellitus		>200 mg/dl
Lactate dehydrogenase (LDH)	Serum	100-190 U/L
pH	Blood	7.38-7.44
Phosphatases		
acid phosphatase	Serum	0-5.5 U/L
alkaline phosphatase	Serum	30-120 U/L
Phosphorus, inorganic	Serum	3-4.5 mg/dl
Potassium	Serum	3.5-5.0 mEq/L
Proteins	Serum	
total		5.5-8 g/dl
albumin		3.5-5.5 g/dl (50-60%)
globulin		2.0-3.5 g/dl (40-50%)
Renal blood flow		1200 ml/min
Sodium	Serum	136-145 mEq/L
Troponins, cardiac (cTn)		
troponin I (cTnI)	Serum	0-0.4 ng/ml
troponin T (cTnT)	Serum	0-0.1 ng/ml
Urea	Blood	20-40 mg/dl
Urea nitrogen (BUN)	Blood	10-20 mg/dl
Uric acid	Serum	
males		2.5-8.0 mg/dl
females		1.5-6.0 mg/dl

TABLE A-3: Other Body Fluids.

COMPONENT	FLUID	CONVENTIONAL VALUE
Cerebrospinal fluid (CSF)	CSF	
CSF volume		120-150 ml
CSF pressure		60-150 mm water
leucocytes		0-5 lymphocytes/µl
pH		7.31-7.34
glucose		40-70 mg/dl
proteins		20-50 mg/dl

Contd...

TABLE A-3: Other Body Fluids *(contd...)*

COMPONENT	FLUID	CONVENTIONAL VALUE
Glomerular filtration rate (GFR)	Urine	180 L/day (about 125 ml/min)
Seminal fluid	Semen	
liquefaction		Within 20 min
sperm morphology		>70% normal, mature spermatozoa
sperm motility		>60%
pH		>7.0 (average 7.7)
sperm count		60-150 million/ml
volume		1.5-5.0 ml
Urine examination	24-hr volume	600-1800 ml (variable)
specific gravity	urine (random)	1.002-1.028 (average 1.018)
protein excretion	24-hr urine	<150 mg/day
protein, qualitative	urine (random)	Negative
glucose excretion	24-hr urine	50-300 mg/day
glucose, qualitative	urine (random)	Negative
porphobilinogen	urine (random)	Negative
urobilinogen	24-hr urine	1.0-3.5 mg/day
Urobilinogen	Urine (random)	Present in 1: 20 dilution

TABLE A-4: Normal Haematologic Values.

COMPONENT	FLUID	CONVENTIONAL VALUE
Erythrocytes and Haemoglobin		
Erythrocyte count	Blood	
males		$4.5\text{-}6.5 \times 10^{12}/L$ (mean $5.5 \times 10^{12}/L$)
females		$3.8\text{-}5.8 \times 10^{12}/L$ (mean $4.8 \times 10^{12}/L$)
Erythrocyte diameter		6.7-7.7 µm (mean 7.2 µm)
Erythrocyte thickness		
peripheral		2.4 µm
central		1.0 µm
Erythrocyte indices	Blood	
(Absolute values)		
mean corpuscular haemoglobin (MCH)		27-32 pg
mean corpuscular volume (MCV)		77-93 fl
mean corpuscular haemoglobin concentration (MCHC)		30-35 g/dl
Erythrocyte life-span	Blood	120 days
Erythrocyte sedimentation rate (ESR)	Blood	
Westergren 1st hr, males		0-15 mm
females		0-20 mm
Wintrobe, 1st hr, males		0-9 mm
females		0-20 mm
Ferritin	Serum	
males		15-200 ng/ml
females		12-150 ng/ml
Haematocrit (PCV)	Blood	
males		40-54%
females		37-47%

Contd...

TABLE A-4: Normal Haematologic Values *(contd...)*

COMPONENT	FLUID	CONVENTIONAL VALUE
Haemoglobin (Hb)		
adult haemoglobin (HbA)	Whole blood	
males		13.0-18.0 g/dl
females		11.5-16.5 g/dl
plasma Hb (quantitative)		0.5-5 mg/dl
haemoglobin A$_2$ (HbA$_2$)		1.5-3.5%
haemoglobin, foetal (HbF) in adults		<1%
HbF, children under 6 months		<5%
Iron, total	Serum	80-180 µg/dl
total iron binding capacity (TIBC)	Serum	250-460 µg/dl
iron saturation	Serum	20-45% (mean 33%)
Iron intake		10-15 mg/day
Iron loss		
males		0.5-1.0 mg/day
females		1-2 mg/day
Iron, total body content		
males		50 mg/kg body weight
females		35 mg/kg body weight
Iron, storage form (ferritin and haemosiderin)		30% of body iron
Osmotic fragility	Blood	
slight haemolysis		at 0.45 to 0.39 g/dl NaCl
complete haemolysis		at 0.33 to 0.36 g/dl NaCl
mean corpuscular fragility		0.4-0.45 g/dl NaCl
Reticulocytes	Blood	
adults		0.5-2.5%
infants		2-6%
Leucocytes in Health		
Total leucocyte count (TLC)	Blood	
adults		4,000-11,000/µl
infants (full term, at birth)		10,000-25,000/µl
infants (1 year)		6,000-16,000/µl
Differential leucocyte count (DLC)	Blood film	
P (polymorphs or neutrophils)		40-75% (2,000-7,500/µl)
L (lymphocytes)		20-50% (1,500-4,000/µl)
M (monocytes)		2-10% (200-800/µl)
E (eosinophils)		1-6% (40-400/µl)
B (basophils)		< l% (10-100/µl)
Platelets and Coagulation		
Bleeding time (BT)		
Ivy's method	Prick blood	2-7 min
template method		2.5-9.5 min
Clot retraction time	Clotted blood	
qualitative		Visible in 60 min (complete in <24-hr)
quantitative		48-64% (55%)
Clotting time (CT) Lee and White method	Whole blood	4-9 min at 37°C
Partial thromboplastin time with kaolin (PTTK) or activated partial thromboplastin time (APTT)	Plasma	30-40 sec
Prothrombin time (PT) (Quick's one-stage method)	Plasma	10-14 sec
Thrombin time (TT)	Plasma	<20 sec (control ± 2 sec)
Platelet count	Blood	150,000-400,000/µl

Index

*The letter **t** after page number in the index below denotes Table.*